Dupuytren's Disease and Related Hyperproliferative Disorders

Charles Eaton
Michael Heinrich Seegenschmiedt
Ardeshir Bayat • Giulio Gabbiani
Paul M.N. Werker • Wolfgang Wach
Editors

Dupuytren's Disease and Related Hyperproliferative Disorders

Principles, Research, and Clinical Perspectives

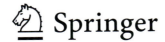

Editors

Charles Eaton, M.D.
Hand Surgeon
The Hand Center
Jupiter, FL
USA

Giulio Gabbiani, MD, PhD
Professor emeritus
Department of Pathology and Immunology
C.M.U., University of Geneva, Geneva
Switzerland

M. Heinrich Seegenschmiedt, MD, PhD
Professor and Chairman
Strahlentherapie & Radioonkologie
Strahlenzentrum Hamburg
Hamburg
Germany

Paul M.N. Werker, MD, PhD
Professor and Chair
Department of Plastic Surgery
University Medical Centre Groningen
Groningen
The Netherlands

Ardeshir Bayat, BSc (Hons), MBBS, MRCS, PhD
Principal Investigator/NIHR Clinician
Scientist
Plastic & Reconstructive Surgery Research
Manchester Interdisciplinary Biocentre
University of Manchester, Manchester
UK

Wolfgang Wach, PhD
Chairman
International Dupuytren Society
Übersee
Germany

ISBN 978-3-642-22696-0   e-ISBN 978-3-642-22697-7
DOI 10.1007/978-3-642-22697-7
Springer Heidelberg Dordrecht London New York

Library of Congress Control Number: 2011944199

© Springer-Verlag Berlin Heidelberg 2012

This work is subject to copyright. All rights are reserved, whether the whole or part of the material is concerned, specifically the rights of translation, reprinting, reuse of illustrations, recitation, broadcasting, reproduction on microfilm or in any other way, and storage in data banks. Duplication of this publication or parts thereof is permitted only under the provisions of the German Copyright Law of September 9, 1965, in its current version, and permission for use must always be obtained from Springer. Violations are liable to prosecution under the German Copyright Law.

The use of general descriptive names, registered names, trademarks, etc. in this publication does not imply, even in the absence of a specific statement, that such names are exempt from the relevant protective laws and regulations and therefore free for general use.

Product liability: The publishers cannot guarantee the accuracy of any information about dosage and application contained in this book. In every individual case the user must check such information by consulting the relevant literature.

Printed on acid-free paper

Springer is part of Springer Science+Business Media (www.springer.com)

Foreword

Why Dupuytren, Why Contracture and Why a Book?

To appreciate the surgical achievements of Baron Guillaume Dupuytren (1777–1835) we should understand that his life spanned a period of immense turmoil in France amidst riot, revolution, insurrection and war. The great pressures on the medical community from civil disturbance and cholera epidemics make Dupuytren's many contributions to anatomy and surgery all the more remarkable. In her scholarly book *Guillaume Dupuytren-A Surgeon in His Place and Time*, Hannah Barsky (1984) has eloquently described the outstanding innovations of Dupuytren and his peers as medical and surgical specialization were just beginning to emerge: Laennec's use of the stethoscope, Lisfranc's surgical procedures in both Orthopaedics and Gynaecology, Alibert father of Dermatology. L'Hotel Dieu was truly a beacon of medical and surgical inspiration, a hospital which over two or three decades has rarely seen its equal for medical and surgical advance.

As for Dupuytren, having performed the first operation for congenital dislocation of the hip and the first hemi-mandibulectomy, he would be amazed to know that the hand *Maladie* which he described would be the object of so much attention and fascination for the surgical world today. His extensive clinical observations across the whole field of surgery were both precise and perceptive including a classification of the different depths of burn injury and a medicolegal description of a round object thrust through the skin creating a linear wound, an observation later expanded upon by Karl von Langer in 1861 (translated by Gibson in 1978).

Many texts and articles have attempted to summarise the character of Dupuytren in simple and sometimes unflattering terms, but Hannah Barsky has revealed a personality so complex and a life so richly varied that only a scholarly and well researched book would do justice to the man, to the surgeon and to his competitive environment. Future journal reviewers please note!

Dupuytren certainly earned a high position in French Society being personally acquainted with cultural, intellectual and political giants: Balzac, Stendhal, Baron Alexander von Humbolt, the Rothchilds, Louis XVIII and Charles X. He travelled little but visited the great English surgeon Sir Astley Cooper, greeting him in the French manner with an embrace, much to the delight of an audience of medical students.

It was Dupuytren's description of the hand contracture and the clear description of its location in the palmar aponeurosis, no doubt supported by his prior experience as

Anatomy Prosector from the age of 17, that merits the attachment of his eponym. Dupuytren (1831) demonstrated the operation on the coachman Demarteau and in today's terms this procedure would be described as an open fasciotomy. By contrast Goyrand (1833) advised a longitudinal incision and excision of fascia and this treatment controversy persists to this day.

The original reports of Paillard and Marx have been translated and reported in scholarly articles by David Elliot (1988a, b, 1989), who has also compiled all of the nineteenth century articles on the condition (1999). It would be difficult for any future scholar to produce more accurate or clearer insights in to these early texts. Following literature sources into the twentieth century, Tord Skoog (1948), a pupil of Sir Archibald MacIndoe, in a truly remarkable doctoral thesis accomplished the extensive task of analyzing and digesting literature from many languages, an extremely time consuming task prior to photocopies and online databases.

John Hueston (1961) popularized the condition and the still common operation of limited fasciectomy. Robert McFarlane once observed of Hueston that he intuitively adapts new scientific concepts (My recollection is that the term 'jumps on the bandwagon' was appropriate) and when others gather the evidence 'they usually find that Hueston was right!'

In my view the turning point in our understanding of the disease was McFarlane's (1974) benchmark paper which showed that the Dupuytren's tissue was not random but the contracture followed anatomical structures forming well defined cords. I must pay personal tribute to Bob McFarlane and Hanno Millesi who invited me to a workshop in Vienna in 1982 in the company of anatomists (Graham Stack – first editor of the *Hand*, forerunner of the *JHS*, author of a personal text on the palmar fascia) and scientists (Michael Flint, whose experimental work described the influence of mechanical forces on fibroblast biology). Bob McFarlane in particular went out of his way to stimulate many basic scientists to look at this clinical problem. I went to that meeting as a surgeon anatomist and left with the inspiration to research the whole biological process of mechanotransduction: the cell and molecular interaction with physical forces which has led me to two chairs, countless grant applications, just enough being successful to collect some data and some further understanding.

As for the mechanism of contracture, McFarlane, McGrouther and Flint (1990) attempted to collate every article published in the English language and to merge basic science with clinical practice. There has been a proliferation of literature in the last two decades, but the cause of the contracture at a cell, matrix and molecular level remains as elusive as ever. Why is there so much focus on this non-life threatening disease? DD is a 'flying squirrel' – a model system lying between two quite different behaviours – not a true neoplasm but neither a simple repair process. Understanding this curious disease may be the key to understanding a whole class of diseases distinguished by the term 'fibrosis'.

And finally why a book? We have so many ways of recording and disseminating knowledge, and Wikipedia (moderated) is now the entry portal to new knowledge. But a book establishes the benchmark of where we stand at a point in time. It is much grander than a review paper assembling the wisdom of the key movers, thinkers and doers. It goes far beyond just evidence based knowledge and gives advice based on the experience, insights and speculations of scholars. We are yet a long way from having clear guidelines in Dupuytren's Disease as we cannot even agree how best to classify the disease.

A book is timely as after several years of little change the innovative team of Larry Hurst and Marie Badalamente (2009) have awakened interest through a carefully executed trial of collagenase which has made us reappraise questions of aetiology, classification and therapy.

Like the man himself, the pathology requires a book to give ready access to the complexity of the many views and practices. Well done Charlie Eaton, ringmaster.

Manchester, UK   D.A. McGrouther

References

Barsky HK (1984) Guillaume Dupuytren, a surgeon in his place and time. Vantage, New York

Dupuytren G (1831) De la rétraction des doigts par suite d'une affection de l'aponévrose palmaire. – Description de la maladie. – Operation chirurgicale qui convient dans ce cas. (Lecture given on 5th December 1831), Compte rendu de la clinique chirurgicale de l'Hôtel-Dieu par MM. les docteurs Alexandre Paillard et Marx. Journal Universel et Hebdomadaire de Medicine et de Chirurgie Pratiques et des Institutions Medicales 5, pp. 349–365. Reprinted in Medical Classics, 1939–1940, 4:127–141 (Partial translation by Koch S 1968 Plast Reconstr Surg 42:262–265)

Elliot D (1988a) The early history of contracture of the palmar fascia. Part 1: the origin of the disease: the curse of the MacCrimmons: the hand of benediction: Cline's contracture. J Hand Surg [Br] 13(3):246–253

Elliot D (1988b) The early history of contracture of the palmar fascia. Part 2: the revolution in Paris: Guillaume Dupuytren: Dupuytren's disease. J Hand Surg [Br] 13(4):371–378

Elliot D (1989) The early history of contracture of the palmar fascia. Part 3: the controversy in Paris and the spread of surgical treatment of the disease throughout Europe. J Hand Surg [Br] 14(1):25–31

Elliot D (1999) Pre-1900 literature on Dupuytren's disease. Hand Clin 15(1):175–181

Gibson T (1978) Karl Langer (1819–1887) and his lines. Br J Plast Surg 31(1):1–2

Goyrand G (1833) Nouvelles recherches sur la retraction premanente des doigts. Memoires de l'Academie Royale de Medicine 3:489–496

Hueston JT (1961) Limited fasciectomy for Dupuytren's contracture. Plast Reconstr Surg Transplant Bull 27:569–585

Hurst LC, Badalamente MA, Hentz VR, Hotchkiss RN, Kaplan FT, Meals RA, Smith TM, Rodzvilla J; CORD I Study Group (2009) Injectable collagenase clostridium histolyticum for Dupuytren's contracture. N Engl J Med 361(10):968–979

McFarlane RM (1974) Patterns of the diseased fascia in the fingers in Dupuytren's contracture. Displacement of the neurovascular bundle. Plast Reconstr Surg 54(1):31–44

McFarlane RM, McGrouther DA, Flint M (1990) Dupuytren's disease: biology and treatment. Churchill Livingstone, Edinburgh

Skoog T (1948) Dupuytren's contraction, with special reference to aetiology and improved surgical treatment. Acta Chir Scand 96(suppl 139):1–189

Preface

Do we really need another book on Dupuytren's Disease? Yes. Why? First, *Dupuytren's does not receive the attention and resources that it deserves*: it is a common disorder, affecting at least 30 million people worldwide, but because it is usually painless, progresses slowly and affects seniors, it is largely unknown to those not afflicted. For the lucky, it is simply a nuisance; for others, a nightmare which never ends. Second, *Dupuytren's is a juggernaut*: at present, it cannot be stopped. Surgeons have been the caregivers for Dupuytren's for almost 200 years, not because surgery is the best possible treatment, but because there is not yet an effective medical treatment. Third, *Dupuytren's is a flagship disease*. The abnormal biology of Dupuytren's – myofibroblast mediated contracture and fibrosis – is shared not only by related conditions of Ledderhose, Peyronie's and frozen shoulder, but also by other diseases, including pulmonary fibrosis, renal interstitial fibrosis, scleroderma, hepatic cirrhosis, arteriosclerosis as well as complications of injury ranging from problem scars to the origin of seizures after brain injury. Cracking the code of Dupuytren's pathobiology will potentially provide keys to the cure of these other even more life changing and life threatening diseases. Fourth, the treatment of Dupuytren's provides a *unique interdisciplinary challenge* for medicine, not constrained to a final, radical surgical solution. Many new and unique options have to be put in a sequential offering to affected patients, providing the right care at the right time including noninvasive and minimally invasive procedures; all therapeutic options are welcome in the competition to provide the best preventive care for disease progression at any stage of disease. Fifth, Dupuytren's is a new *challenge to provide sufficient genetic counseling* of the affected individual and their relatives.

The initial impetus for this book was an Internet based collaboration between affected patients, theoretical researchers and clinicians of various disciplines leading to the 2010 International Symposium on Dupuytren's Disease held on May 22 and 23 in Miami, FL. This conference was hosted by two organizations cooperating in finding a cure for Dupuytren's: Dupuytren Foundation and the International Dupuytren Society. Participants at this meeting came from 17 countries: Australia, Austria, Belgium, Canada, Croatia, England, Germany, Iceland, Italy, Japan, the Netherlands, Norway, Russia, Slovakia, Sweden, Switzerland and the United States. The symposium was not only overdue for presenting new research, but also for presenting new therapeutic options which will require careful assessment of side effects, recurrence intervals and guidelines for which therapeutic option is best applied when. Thus, this book spans from the basic research area to the latest clinical attempts in improving cures and functionality thereby minimizing patient suffering. It also addresses the related diseases, Ledderhose and Peyronie's, and is the first to include the patient's perspective.

This symposium and book were both inspired by several excellent efforts in the past: the 1966 Paris congress of the Groupe d'Étude de la Main organized by Gossett,

Tubiana and Hueston; the 1981 symposium in Torino, Italy and the 1983 symposium in Vienna, chaired by Millesi, McFarlane's 1985 London, Ontario congress; the 1991 Hannover symposium led by Berger, Delbrueck, Brenner and Hinzman; and finally 20 years later the 2010 Stony Brook meeting hosted by Hurst and Badalamente. Thus, the numerous efforts to find better treatment options for Dupuytren's has spanned lifetimes: there were some speakers who have contributed to many of these scientific meetings, especially Professor Millesi, who not only spoke at the 1966 congress, but has continued since, even presenting at the 2010 Miami symposium.

Is not this book just more of the same old topics which have been reviewed again and again in the past? No. While acknowledging the existing works of brilliant scientists and surgeons, this book comes from a different source and has a different purpose and goal. The ultimate goal of this book is to educate but also spur the readers with the main question *"What needs to be asked further, known or done* differently *to find a final cure for Dupuytren's?"*.

Evolved from the Miami symposium in 2010, the chapters have been regrouped and updated, some presenting even newer results. Some authors of the Symposium have withdrawn their initial presentations and papers as newer results are pointing in additional directions. The editors also decided to include some chapters of authors who were not able to attend the Miami symposium but were able to contribute additional and important aspects of Dupuytren's and related disorders.

The preface is a good place to express gratitude to all authors for their contributions and for their excellent collaboration with the editors and reviewers. All submitted chapters have been critically and independently reviewed by at least two expert peers. This effort would not have been possible without the continuous support and dedication from several reviewers in addition to the editors of this book. They have performed a tremendous valuable job providing their special expertise and improved the content of all chapters. We would like to acknowledge the following collaborators:

Marie A. Badalamente, New York, USA	Ilse Degreef, Leuven, Belgium
Hans C. Hennies, Cologne, Germany	Boris Hinz, Toronto, Canada
David B. O'Gorman, London, Canada	Ghazi M. Rayan, Oklahoma City, USA
Bert Reichert, Nuremberg, Germany	Paul Zidel, Phoenix, USA.

The bar is high to contribute to the legacy of former Dupuytren's books: monumental single and multiple author books have been published. Excerpts from the introductions to these books and monographs tell us about their impetus and perspectives to do so:

1879: *"The patients have in many instances been told that as in the contracted fingers are still useful in grasping, they should wait until they had become useless by increase of the contraction, and then take the chances of an operation."* Adams W: <u>Observations on the Contractions of the Fingers</u>

1948: *"After more than a century's dispute, the cause of this condition is still debated...The large number of techniques suggested nevertheless show that this important problem has not yet been definitively solved."* Skoog T: <u>Dupuytren's Contraction, with Special Reference to Aetiology and Improved Surgical Treatment, Its Occurrence in Epileptics, Note on Knuckle-Pads</u>

1963: *"Such an unsolved problem as Dupuytren's contracture should be reviewed regularly, to provide a picture of the present position and a basis for further study."* Hueston JT: <u>Dupuytren's Contracture</u>

1966: "[*The authors do not pretend to represent a complete monograph or even balanced treatment of contractures of the palmar fascia]*". Gosset J: <u>Maladie de Dupuytren</u>

1968: "*...surgical manipulation in the past has not been limited by instrumentation or by the coordination of the surgeon's hand, but by a lack of understanding.*" Milford: <u>Retaining Ligaments of the Digits of the Hands</u>

1973: "*There have been many descriptions of the palmar fascia by anatomists and in papers dealing with the surgical treatment of Dupuytren's contracture, but what seems to be lacking is an overall view of the problem...*" Stack G: <u>The Palmar Fascia</u>

1974: "*I am afraid, however, that despite this abundance of papers the reader will not be entirely satisfied or may even be slightly confused by this very same abundance.*" Hueston JT, Tubiana R: <u>Dupuytren's Disease</u>

1985: "*The swinging of the pendulum from conservative to radical surgery, from open wounds to skin grafting, from intrinsic to extrinsic theories of pathogenesis, makes it essential to keep abreast of current options.*" Hueston J, Tubiana R: <u>Dupuytren's Disease, Second Edition</u>

1990: "*The historical perspective is humbling when one appreciates what has been reported then lost, and later hailed as new information.*" McFarlane R, McGrouther D, Flint M: <u>Dupuytren's Disease: Biology and Treatment</u>

1991: "*...surgery is stressed as a form of injury and recurrence as a logical risk, rather than a complication.*" Seyfer A, Hueston J: <u>Hand Clinics: Dupuytren's Contracture</u>

1994: "*Although this disease has frequently been referred to as Dupuytren's contracture... disease is the more appropriate word...*" Berger A, Delbruk A, Brenner P, Hinzmann R: <u>Dupuytren's Disease: Pathobiochemistry and Clinical Management</u>

1999: "*Despite the munificence of knowledge attained, two issues remain unsolved relevant to Dupuytren's disease: its cause and its cure.*" Rayan G: <u>Hand Clinics: Dupuytren's Disease</u>

2000: "*Now, at the start of the 21*st *century, we still do not know the origin of this disease, and its treatment remains essentially palliative.*" Tubiana R, LeClercq C, Hurst L, Badalamente M, Mackin E: <u>Dupuytren's Disease</u>

2002: "*...Dupuytren's disease is indeed a systemic connective tissue disease.*" Brenner P, Rayan G: <u>Dupuytren's Disease</u>

2002 "*The individual characteristics that place a person at high risk are, thus, not obviously related to ongoing connective tissue production at time of surgery or to connective tissue activity in its conventionally used sense.*" Wilbrand S: <u>Dupuytren's Contracture: Features and Consequences</u>

2006 "*...several important problems concerning myofibroblast origin, function and participation in pathological processes remain to be solved.*" Chaponnier C, Desmoulière A, Gabbiani G: <u>Tissue Repair, Contraction and the Myofibroblast</u>

2009: "*These patients [with aggressive, therapy-resisting Dupuytren's] need help and we have to try to avoid getting them in such desperate situations...*" Degreef I: <u>Therapy-Resisting Dupuytren's Disease: New Perspectives in Adjuvant Treatment</u>

Collectively, these statements tell us about a problem for which there is not yet a good answer, a condition for which for many years treatments have changed back and forth but not truly advanced. Procedures to treat Dupuytren's have been developed empirically despite a lack of understanding of the fundamental biology, similar to Johann von Neumann's description of quantum mechanics: "In mathematics, you don't understand things. You get used to them".

This perspective is about to change, because we are at a tipping point: this is the first collaborative text to document clinically effective disease modifying treatments. We are fully aware that this book will not answer all questions, but will also raise new ones. Our honest hope is that this book will pave the way for all future conferences and texts on Dupuytren's to describe progressively more effective biological disease modifying interventions. It is time to change from a monistic surgical view to a multi-disciplinary perspective and translational research.

Jupiter, USA	Charles Eaton
Hamburg, Germany	Michael Heinrich Seegenschmiedt
Manchester, UK	Ardeshir Bayat
Geneva, Switzerland	Giulio Gabbiani
Groningen, Netherlands	Paul M.N. Werker
Übersee, Germany	Wolfgang Wach

Biographies of Editors

Dr. Charles Eaton is a private practice community hand surgeon in Jupiter, Florida. The majority of his practice involves the care of Dupuytren's disease. He maintains an ongoing academic presence by authoring hand surgery journal articles and textbook chapters, through his web site e-Hand.com and in committee activities of the American Society for Surgery of the Hand and the American Association of Hand Surgeons. Additional projects involve the application of web based multimedia, information technology and electronic archiving to hand surgery. Dr. Eaton established the nonprofit Dupuytren Foundation to promote and support global efforts, such as this book, to develop better treatment options for Dupuytren's disease and related conditions.

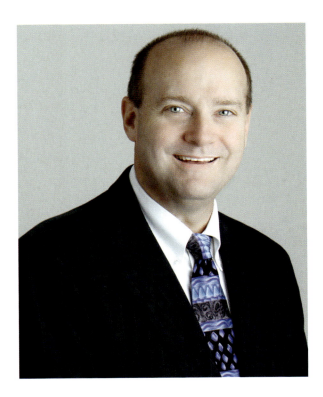

Michael Heinrich Seegenschmiedt, M.D., Ph.D., born 1955 in Erlangen (Germany), married since 1980, father of four sons and one daughter. Medical education and special training in Würzburg and Erlangen, Germany, and Philadelphia, USA. Board Certified Radiation Oncologist since 1990; member of DEGRO, ESTRO, ASTRO. Chairman Radiation Therapy and Oncology at Alfried-Krupp Krankenhaus Essen from 1996-2009. Chairman of Radiation Therapy, The X-Ray Clinic Hamburg, Germany, since 2010. Extraordinary Professor of Radiation Oncology, Westfalian University Münster, Germany. Research interests: breast cancer, palliative care, stereotactic radiotherapy/radiosurgery, non-malignant disorders responsive to radiotherapy, Quality Assurance in radiotherapy. Editor/Co-Editor of 18 books/monographs; 127 peer reviewed publications in PubMed Library.

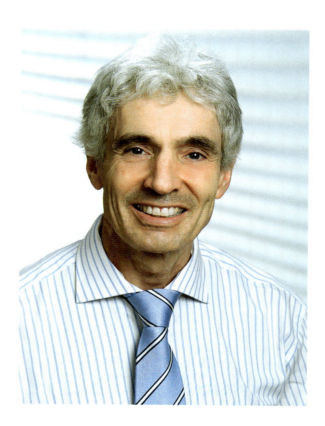

Ardeshir Bayat studied medicine and an intercalated degree in human anatomy at University College London. His surgical training was followed by a fellowship from the Royal College of Surgeons of England and MRC (UK) leading to a PhD in the molecular basis of wound repair with focus on Dupuytren's and Keloid disease at the University of Manchester, UK. His specialist training in Plastic and Reconstructive Surgery has been combined with ongoing research. He serves on editorial boards of plastic surgery and dermatology journals and has published widely. He is a National Institute of Health Research (NIHR, UK) clinician scientist and a principal investigator in plastic and reconstructive surgery. The focus of his scientific research is in tissue repair and regeneration.

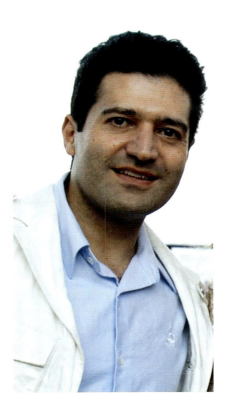

Dr. Giulio Gabbiani obtained an M.D. degree in 1961 at the University of Pavia (Italy) and a Ph.D. degree in 1965 at the University of Montreal (Canada). He is Emeritus Professor at the Department of Pathology and Immunology at the Medical Faculty, University of Geneva, Switzerland. The scientific interests of Dr. Gabbiani include soft tissue remodeling during development and pathological situations, such as wound healing and organ fibrosis. Dr. Gabbiani first described the myofibroblast, a cell type that has been shown to be responsible of connective tissue remodeling in developmental and pathological settings, such as Dupuytren's disease.

He has received several distinctions including an Honorary Doctor degree from the University of Gothenburg (Sweden) and from the University of Limoges (France).

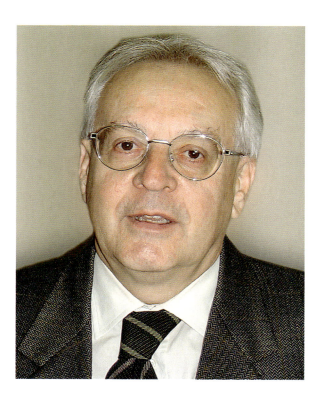

Paul Werker (1961) studied medicine in Utrecht (NL), Aberdeen (UK) and Harrow (UK). He completed a Ph.D. on free flap preservation in 1992 and trained in Utrecht (NL) to become plastic surgeon in 1996. He was fellow in reconstructive microsurgery in Louisville KY, USA, before returning to Utrecht as an assistant professor. In 1999 he became an attending plastic surgeon in Zwolle (NL), to move to Groningen (NL) in 2006, where he currently is Professor and Chair of the Department of Plastic Surgery of the University Medical Centre Groningen. He is member of national and international societies, and advisory pannels, and (co-) author of 60 peer reviewed journal papers and six book chapters. His clinical areas of interest are Dupuytren's Disease and reconstructive surgery of breast and facial palsy.

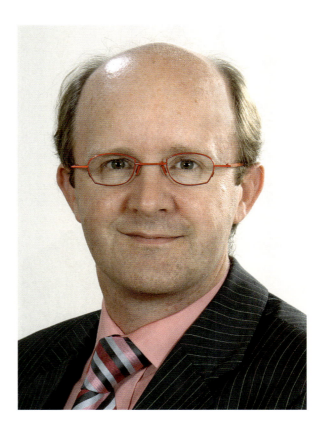

Dr. Wolfgang Wach received his Ph.D. in Solid State Physics in 1981 at the University of Munich, Germany. After 6 years of research in ion implantation he worked in microprocessor development at Siemens and as General Manager at AT&T Microelectronics. He started his own software company CAL in 1995 and the Dupuytren Society in 2003. The Dupuytren Society is an international non-profit organization with patients and physicians cooperating in informing about Dupuytren's disease and its therapeutical options, in supporting patients, and in finding a cure for Dupuytren's. He is currently one of the chairmen of the International Dupuytren Society and has been suffering from Dupuytren's and Ledderhose disease for almost 30 years.

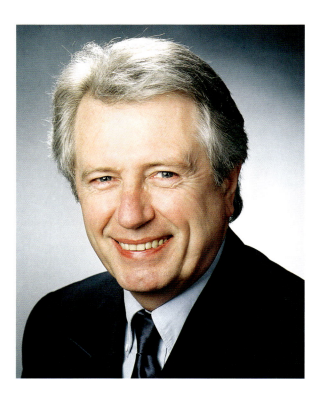

Contents

Part I Anatomy, Pathology, and Pathophysiology
Charles Eaton

1 Dupuytren's Disease: Anatomy, Pathology, and Presentation 3
Ghazi M. Rayan

**2 Palmar Fibromatosis or the Loss of Flexibility
of the Palmar Finger Tissue: A New Insight into the Disease
Process of Dupuytren Contracture** 11
Albrecht Meinel

3 Basic Thoughts on Dupuytren's Contracture 21
Hanno Millesi

**4 High Prevalence of Dupuytren's Disease
and Its Treatment in the British National Health Service:
An Ongoing Demand** 27
Karen Zaman, Sandip Hindocha, and Ardeshir Bayat

5 Treatment for Dupuytren's Disease: An Overview of Options 35
Annet L. van Rijssen and Paul M.N. Werker

6 Dupuytren's Disease and Occupation 45
Alexis Descatha

Part II The Myofibroblast
Giulio Gabbiani

**7 The Role of the Myofibroblast in Dupuytren's Disease:
Fundamental Aspects of Contraction
and Therapeutic Perspectives** 53
Boris Hinz and Giulio Gabbiani

8 Mechanisms of Myofibroblast Differentiation 61
Sem H. Phan

**9 Myofibroblasts and Interactions with Other Cells:
Contribution of the Tissue Engineering** 69
Véronique Moulin, Judith Bellemare, Daniele Bergeron,
Herve Genest, Michel Roy, and Carlos Lopez-Vallé

10 Dupuytren's Contracture Versus Burn Scar Contracture 77
Paul Zidel

Part III Genetics and Demographics
Ardeshir Bayat

11 The Genetic Basis of Dupuytren's Disease: An Introduction 87
Guido H.C.G. Dolmans and Hans C. Hennies

**12 Use of Genetic and Genomic Analyses
Tools to Study Dupuytren's Disease** 93
Barbara Shih, Stewart Watson, and Ardeshir Bayat

**13 Establishing an Animal Model of Dupuytren's Contracture
by Profiling Genes Associated with Fibrosis** 101
Latha Satish, Mark E. Baratz, Bradley Palmer, Sandra Johnson,
J. Christopher Post, Garth D. Ehrlich, and Sandeep Kathju

**14 Microarray Expression Analysis of Primary Dupuytren's
Contracture Cells** 109
Sandra Kraljevic Pavelic and Ivana Ratkaj

**15 A Clinical Genetic Study of Familial Dupuytren's Disease
in the Netherlands** 115
Guido H.C.G. Dolmans, Cisca Wijmenga,
Roel Ophoff, and Paul M.N. Werker

16 The Epidemiology of Dupuytren's Disease in Bosnia 123
Dragan Zerajic and Vilhjalmur Finsen

Part IV Collagen and Cell Biology
Charles Eaton

**17 A Primer of Collagen Biology: Synthesis, Degradation, Subtypes,
and Role in Dupuytren's Disease** 131
Susan Emeigh Hart

**18 The Expression of Collagen-Degrading Proteases Involved
in Dupuytren's Disease Fibroblast-Mediated Contraction** 143
Janine M. Wilkinson, Eleanor R. Jones, Graham P. Riley,
Adrian J. Chojnowski, and Ian M. Clark

**19 Primary Dupuytren's Disease Cell Interactions with the
Extra-cellular Environment: A Link to Disease Progression?** 151
Linda Vi, Yan Wu, Bing Siang Gan, and David B. O'Gorman

**20 Insulin-Like Growth Factor Binding Protein-6: A Potential Mediator
of Myofibroblast Differentiation in Dupuytren's Disease?** 161
Christina Raykha, Justin Crawford, Bing Siang Gan,
and David B. O'Gorman

**21 Dupuytren's Disease Shows Populations of Hematopoietic and
Mesenchymal Stem-Like Cells Involving Perinodular Fat and Skin
in Addition to Diseased Fascia: Implications for Pathogenesis
and Therapy** 167
Syed Amir Iqbal, Sandip Hindocha, Syed Farhatullah, Ralf Paus,
and Ardeshir Bayat

Contents   xxi

22 Using Laboratory Models to Develop Molecular Mechanistic Treatments for Dupuytren's Disease 175
Martin C. Robson and Wyatt G. Payne

Part V   Surgical Treatment
Paul M.N. Werker

23 Plastic Surgical Management of Scars and Soft Tissue Contractures 187
Paul M.N. Werker

24 Cline's Contracture: Dupuytren Was a Thief – A History of Surgery for Dupuytren's Contracture 195
A. Lee Osterman, Peter M. Murray, and Teresa J. Pianta

25 Cellulose Implants in Dupuytren's Surgery 207
Ilse Degreef and Luc De Smet

26 Expanded Dermofasciectomies and Full-Thickness Grafts in the Treatment of Dupuytren's Contracture: A 36-Year Experience 213
Lynn D. Ketchum

27 Minimizing Skin Necrosis and Delayed Healing After Surgical Treatment for Dupuytren's Contracture: The Mini-Chevrons Incision 221
Michael Papaloïzos

28 Skin Management in Treatment of Severe PIP Contracture by Homo- or Heterodigital Flaps 227
Bernhard Lukas and Moritz Lukas

29 The "Jacobsen Flap" for the Treatment of Stage III–IV Dupuytren's Disease at Little Finger: Our Review of 123 Cases 235
Massimiliano Tripoli, Francesco Moschella, and Michel Merle

30 A Logical Approach to Release of the Contracted Proximal Interphalangeal Joint in Dupuytren's Disease 243
Paul Smith

31 The Influence of Dupuytren's Disease on Trigger Fingers and Vice Versa 249
Bernd Kuehlein

32 No Higher Self-Reported Recurrence in Segmental Fasciectomy 255
Ilse Degreef

33 Palmar Cutaneous Branches of the Proper Digital Nerves Encountered in Dupuytren's Surgery: A Cadaveric Study 261
Robert M. Choa, Andrew F.M. McKee, and Ian S.H. McNab

Part VI Needle Release and Hand Therapy
Paul M. N. Werker

34 A Technique of Needle Aponeurotomy for Dupuytren's Contracture 267
Charles Eaton

35 Three-Year Results of First-Ever Randomized Clinical Trial on Treatment in Dupuytren's Disease: Percutaneous Needle Fasciotomy Versus Limited Fasciectomy 281
Annet L. van Rijssen, Hein ter Linden, and Paul M.N. Werker

36 Management of Dupuytren's Disease with Needle Aponeurotomy: The Experience at the Hand and Upper Limb Centre, Canada 289
Aaron Grant, David B. O'Gorman, and Bing Siang Gan

37 Percutaneous Needle Fasciotomy: A Serious Alternative? 293
Holger C. Erne, Ahmed El Gammal, and Bernhard Lukas

38 Dynamic External Fixation in the Treatment of Dupuytren's Contracture 297
George A. Lawson and Anthony A. Smith

39 Hand Therapy for Dupuytren's Contracture 305
Patricia Davis and Charles Eaton

40 Severity of Contracture and Self-Reported Disability in Patients with Dupuytren's Contracture Referred for Surgery 317
Christina Jerosch-Herold, Lee Shepstone, Adrian J. Chojnowski, and Debbie Larson

41 Night-Time Splinting After Fasciectomy or Dermofasciectomy for Dupuytren's Contracture: A Pragmatic, Multi-centre, Randomised Controlled Trial 323
Christina Jerosch-Herold, Lee Shepstone, Adrian J. Chojnowski, Debbie Larson Elisabeth Barrett, and Susan P. Vaughan

42 The Role of Static Night Splinting After Contracture Release for Dupuytren's Disease: A Preliminary Recommendation Based on Clinical Cases 333
Albrecht Meinel

Part VII Additional and New Treatment Options
M. Heinrich Seegenschmiedt

43 Injectable Collagenase (*Clostridium histolyticum*) for Dupuytren's Contracture: Results of the CORD I Study 343
Marie A. Badalamente

44 Long-Term Outcome of Radiotherapy for Early Stage Dupuytren's Disease: A Phase III Clinical Study 349
Michael Heinrich Seegenschmiedt, Ludwig Keilholz, Mark Wielpütz, Christine Schubert, and Fabian Fehlauer

45	**Outcomes of Using Bioengineered Skin Substitute (Apligraf®) for Wound Coverage in Dupuytren's Surgery**	373
	E. Anne Ouellette, Melissa Diamond, and Anna-Lena Makowski	
46	**Highly Dosed Tamoxifen in Therapy-Resisting Dupuytren's Disease**	379
	Ilse Degreef, Sabine Tejpar, and Luc De Smet	
47	**Screening of Prodrugs on Cells Grown from Dupuytren's Disease Patients**	387
	Davor Jurisic	
48	**Relaxin: An Emerging Therapy for Fibroproliferative Disorders**	393
	Chrishan S. Samuel	
49	**Cryotherapy and Other Therapeutical Options for Plantar Fibromatosis**	401
	Terry L. Spilken	
50	**Long-Term Outcome of Radiotherapy for Primary and Recurrent Ledderhose Disease**	409
	Michael Heinrich Seegenschmiedt, Mark Wielpütz, Etienne Hanslian, and Fabian Fehlauer	
51	**Medical Management of Peyronie's Disease**	429
	Ma Limin, Aaron Bernie, and Wayne J.G. Hellstrom	

Part VIII Future Perspectives

Charles Eaton

52	**The Patient's Perspective and the International Dupuytren Society**	441
	Wolfgang Wach	
53	**IDUP: Proposal for an International Research Database**	449
	Charles Eaton, Michael Heinrich Seegenschmiedt, and Wolfgang Wach	
54	**The Future of Dupuytren's Research and Treatment**	455
	Charles Eaton	
Index		471

Part I

Anatomy, Pathology, and Pathophysiology

Editor: Charles Eaton

Dupuytren's Disease: Anatomy, Pathology, and Presentation

Ghazi M. Rayan

Contents

1.1	**Anatomy**	3
1.1.1	Radial Aponeurosis	4
1.1.2	Ulnar Aponeurosis	4
1.1.3	Central Aponeurosis	4
1.1.4	Palmodigital Fascia	5
1.1.5	Digital Fascia	5
1.2	**Pathology**	5
1.2.1	Dermatopathology	5
1.2.2	Palmar Cords	5
1.2.3	Palmodigital Cords	6
1.2.4	Digital Cords	6
1.2.5	Thumb Diseased Tissue	7
1.3	**Clinical Presentation**	7
1.3.1	The Skin	7
1.3.2	The Nodule	8
1.3.3	The Cord	8
1.3.4	Disease Progression	8
1.3.5	Ectopic Dupuytren's Disease	9
1.4	**Clinical Types**	9
1.4.1	Typical Dupuytren's Disease	9
1.4.2	Non-Dupuytren's Disease	9
References		10

G.M. Rayan
Baptist Medical Centre, University of Oklahoma,
Oklahoma City, OK, USA
e-mail: ouhsgmr@aol.com

1.1 Anatomy

The palmar fascial complex (PFC) of the hand has five components (Rayan 2010), the radial, ulnar and central aponeuroses (CA), palmodigital fascia and digital fascia (Fig. 1.1).

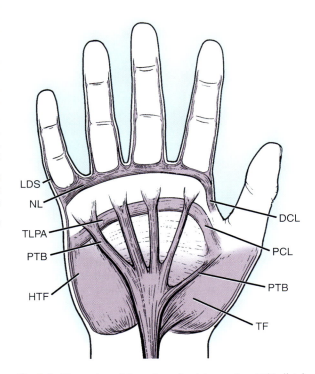

Fig. 1.1 Illustration of the palmar fascial complex. *DCL* distal commissural ligament, *HTF* hypothenar muscle fascia, *LDS* lateral digital sheet, *NL* natatory ligament, *PCL* proximal commissural ligament, *PTB* pretendinous band (small finger and thumb bands tagged), *TF* thenar fascia, *TLPA* transverse ligament of the palmar aponeurosis. (From Rayan 2010)

1.1.1 Radial Aponeurosis

Tubiana et al. (1982) described the radial aponeurosis to have four components; the thenar fascia, thumb pretendinous band, distal commissural ligament and the proximal commissural ligament. Fine operative microscope dissection (Rayan 1999a) revealed that the thenar fascia is an extension of the CA and the pretendinous band is less defined than all other bands.

1.1.2 Ulnar Aponeurosis

This consists of the hypothenar muscle fascia, pretendinous band to the small finger and abductor digiti minimi (ADM) coalescence (White 1984). The ADM tendon is enveloped by the fibers of the sagittal band (Rayan et al. 1997). Fine dissection (Rayan 1999a) revealed that the hypothenar fascia is an extension of the CA and the pretendinous band is always present and very substantial.

1.1.3 Central Aponeurosis

The CA is the core of Dupuytren's disease (DD) activity. It is a triangular fascial layer with proximal apex and distal base and its fibers are oriented into three dimensions: longitudinal, transverse, and vertical.

(a) Longitudinal fibers of the CA fan out as three pretendinous bands (PB) for the central digits and each bifurcate distally. McGrouther (1982) described three microscopic layers of insertions for the split PB. The superficial layer inserts into the dermis, the middle continues to the digit as the spiral band, and the deep layer passes almost vertically in the vicinity of the extensor tendon.

(b) Transverse Fibers of the CA encompass the natatory ligament (NL) which is distally located in the palmodigital region and the transverse ligament of the palmar aponeurosis (TLPA). The TLPA is located proximal and parallel to the NL and deep to the pretendinous bands. This ligament continues radially as the proximal commissural ligament. The TLPA gives origin to the septa of Legueu and Juvara (SLJ), protects the neurovascular (NV) structures, and provides an additional pulley to the flexor tendons.

(c) Vertical fibers of CA encompass the vertical bands of Grapow and the SLJ (Fig. 1.2).

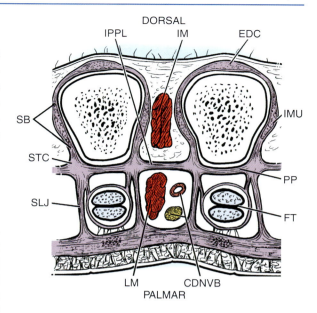

Fig. 1.2 Illustration of the interpalmar plate ligaments, septa of Legueu and Juvara, and soft tissue confluence. *CDNVB* Common digital neurovascular bundle, *EDC* extensor digitorum communis, *FT* flexor tendons, *IM* interosseous muscles, *IMU* intrinsic musculotendinous unit, *IPPL* interpalmar plate ligament, *LM* lumbrical muscle, *PP* palmar plate, *SB* sagittal band, *SLJ* septum of Legueu and Juvara, *STC* soft tissue confluence. (From Rayan 2010)

Grapow (1887) described multiple connections between the PA and palmar skin. Fine dissection shows these vertical bands to be numerous, small, strong, scattered along the PFC, and most abundant in the CA. Legueu and Juvara (1892) described the vertical septa that pass deeply from the palmar fascia forming fibro osseous compartments. Gosset (1985) observed that each of the partitions of Legueu and Juvara has proximal falciform border at a level midway between distal wrist crease and proximal digital crease. Intracompartmental arthroscopic examination (Rayan 1999a) in our laboratory revealed that each vertical septum consists of a well-developed fibrous structure that has sharp and strong proximal border and lies approximately 1 cm distal to the palmar arterial arch. A detailed anatomic study from our institute (Bilderback and Rayan 2004) identified eight septa, one radial and ulnar for each digit. The radial were longer than the ulnar septa. The septa attach to the TLPA superficially and to a soft tissue confluence deeply and distally and to the interosseous muscle fascia proximally. The soft-tissue confluence consists of the SLJ, the interpalmar plate ligaments (IPPL), palmar plate, annular pulley, and sagittal band. Three IPPLs, radial, central, and ulnar form the floor (i.e., dorsal) of the three NV web space canals.

The septa form seven compartments of two types; four flexor septal canals that contained the flexor tendons, and three web space canals that contained common digital nerves and arteries and lumbrical muscles. Grossly and histologically, the septa are thicker and consisted of organized collagen distally but not proximally.

1.1.4 Palmodigital Fascia

Gosset (1985) described several fascial structures that coalesce in the web-digital area, the most notable of these are the spiral band and NL. Each spiral band begins proximally as the middle layer of a bifurcated pretendinous band, tangential to the palm, then spirals on its axis, becoming perpendicular to the palm distally, lateral to the MP joint capsule. They course distally deep to the NV bundle and NL, and emerge distal to the NL to continue as the lateral digital sheet (LDS). The spiral band therefore is the connection between the palmar and digital fascial structures. The fibers of the NL run in a transverse plane, but the distal most fibers form a U and run longitudinally along the side of adjacent digits toward the LDS. The fibers of the NL run from side to side at the web spaces and extend radially to the first web space as the distal commissural ligament. The NL has a well-defined proximal border that becomes more pronounced when the fingers are fully abducted. The LDS therefore has deep and superficial contributions from the spiral band and NL.

1.1.5 Digital Fascia

The NV bundle in the digit is surrounded by four fascial structures; Grayson's ligament palmar, Cleland's ligaments dorsally, Gosset LDS laterally and possibly a retrovascular fascia (Thomine 1985) medially and dorsally that has not been confirmed by other studies. Some doubt the existence of the retrovascular fascia.

1.2 Pathology

Luck (1959) was the first to use the terms normal bands and diseased cords. McFarlane (1974) considered the diseased cords and nodules to be the consequence of

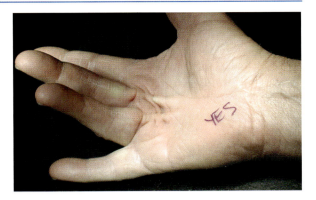

Fig. 1.3 Pretendinous bands causing metacarpophalangeal joint contracture

pathologic changes in the normal fascia. Dupuytren's nodules and cords are pathognomonic of DD. A nodule often precedes the cord, but sometimes a cord develops without a nodule. The cords typically shorten progressively leading to joint and tissue contracture. The cords are located in the palmar, palmodigital, or digital regions. Joint deformity in early stages is caused by diseased cords whereas long-standing flexion deformity can lead to capsuloligamentous tissue scarring with resultant joint contracture.

1.2.1 Dermatopathology

Microcords develop from Grapow vertical bands leading to skin thickening and tethering, which are one of the earliest manifestations of DD. *Skin pits* form from the diseased and contracted first layer of the split pretendinous band which may develop adjacent to Dupuytren's nodules and are usually located in the palm distal to the distal palmar crease.

1.2.2 Palmar Cords

The *pretendinous cord* develops from the PB and is the most frequently encountered cord in DD (Fig. 1.3).

It leads to MP joint flexion deformity as a result of the cord's attachment to the flexor tendon sheath or dermal layer of the distal palmar crease. The palmar cord sometimes extends distally and continues with digital cords. Occasionally, the pretendinous cord bifurcates distally and each branch extends to a different digit forming a commissural Y cord. The *vertical cord* (Bilderback and Rayan 2002) is less common and may be encountered as the pretendinous cord being dissected. The vertical cord is a short thick diseased tissue that departs from the pretendinous cord and extends deeply between the NV bundle and flexor tendon fibrous sheath to insert into the soft tissue confluence. This cord represents the diseased SLJ. *Extensive palmar fascial disease* is encountered in severe conditions and affects a large area of the palm leading to diffuse thickening of many components of the PFC including the TLPA.

1.2.3 Palmodigital Cords

According to McFarlane (1990) the *spiral cord* has four components of origin; pretendinous band, spiral band, lateral digital sheet, and Grayson's ligament. This cord is encountered most often in the small finger, but it may affect the ring finger. Proximally, in the palm, it is located superficial to the NV bundle. Just distal to the MP joint, in the palmodigital area, the cord then passes deep to the NV bundle. In the digit, the cord runs lateral to the NV bundle as it invades the LDS. Distally, in the digit, it becomes superficial to the NV bundle as it incorporates the Grayson's ligament. Initially, the cord spirals around the NV bundle, but as MP and PIP joint contracture becomes severe, the cord takes a straight course. The NV bundle then shifts palmar and to the midline and appears to spiral around the cord. The distorted anatomy of the NV bundle renders it at great risk of injury during surgery. The presence of a spiral nerve may be predicted by the presence of PIP joint contracture and an interdigital soft tissue mass (Ulmas et al. 1994). A spiral cord may originate proximally from the lumbrical tendon or it may attach distally to the opposite side "reverse spiral cord." (McFarlane 1985). The *natatory cord* develops from the NL and forms a transversely oriented small cord distally in the web space and may convert the U-shaped web into a V shape. The second, third, or fourth web spaces can be affected which leads to adduction contracture of the web space and limits full digital abduction. The cord extends along the dorsal lateral aspect of the adjacent digits and can be best detected by passively abducting the digits and at the same time flexing one digit and extending the other at the MP joints. This maneuver allows the natatory cord to become more prominent.

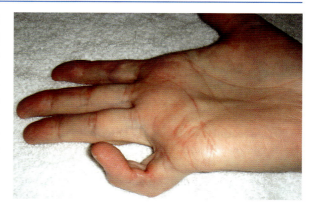

Fig. 1.4 Isolated digital cord of the small finger

1.2.4 Digital Cords

The most frequently encountered digital cords are the central, spiral, and lateral cords, which are responsible for PIP joint flexion deformity. The *central cord* is often an extension of the pretendinous cord into the digit. The origin of this cord is uncertain. It may develop from the superficial fibrofatty tissue or more likely from the second layer of the split pretendinous band. It courses in the midline and attaches into the flexor tendon sheath near the PIP joint or the periosteum of the middle phalanx on one side of the digit. The central cord usually does not displace the NV bundle. The *lateral cord* originates from the LDS and attaches to the skin or to the flexor tendon sheath near Grayson's ligament. Sometimes it causes flexion contracture of DIP joint. This cord can displace the digital NV bundle toward the midline by its volume. The *ADM cord* (Barton 1984) is also known as the isolated digital cord (Fig. 1.4).

Its relationship to the NV bundle is similar to that of the spiral band. It takes origin from the ADM tendon, but it may also arise from the nearby muscle fascia or base of the proximal phalanx. The cord courses superficial to the NV bundle and infrequently entraps and displaces it toward the midline. The cord inserts frequently on the ulnar side of the base of the middle phalanx. The cord however may attach radially or may have additional insertion in the base of the distal phalanx causing DIP joint contracture. It is unclear whether a *retrovascular cord* exists but this was suggested to be a poorly defined structure that develops from the retrovascular tissue is located deep to NV bundle near the PIP joint (McFarlane 1985). The retrovascular diseased tissue by itself does not cause PIP joint contracture, but if the tissue is not removed, full correction of PIP joint contracture may not be obtained and residual joint contracture may result.

1.2.5 Thumb Diseased Tissue

The *distal commissural cord* is the diseased distal commissural ligament, which is the radial extension of the NL whereas the *proximal commissural cord* originates from the proximal commissural ligament, which is the radial extension of the TLPA. Both of these cords cause first web space contracture. The *thumb pretendinous cord* is formed by the diseased thumb pretendinous band and causes thumb MP joint flexion deformity.

1.3 Clinical Presentation

In its early stages, DD can be difficult to diagnose even by experienced observers. Normal skin and subcutaneous alterations can mimic early skin changes that occur in DD. Certain soft tissue changes may simulate the established pretendinous cords of DD. Such nuances can bewilder skillful diagnosticians and make it difficult to ascertain the nature of these changes. The difficulty in diagnosing early DD may be a cause for disparity among epidemiologic studies regarding the prevalence of the disease. Fortunately, many cases of DD present after the confusing physical signs of early disease have elapsed and the diagnosis can be made without difficulty.

The nodule and cord are the prototypical pathologic findings in DD. In the classic scenario of typical disease the condition is ushered by skin changes followed by the formation of a nodule, possible nodule regression, cord formation, maturation and contracture and, lastly, progressive digital flexion deformity. The course and progression of an established DD however can be capricious and unpredictable.

1.3.1 The Skin

Skin alteration is the earliest manifestation of DD especially in the palm. Changes however occur in the dorsal and palmar skin. *Dorsal skin* changes are either in the form of dorsal Dupuytren's nodules (DDN) or

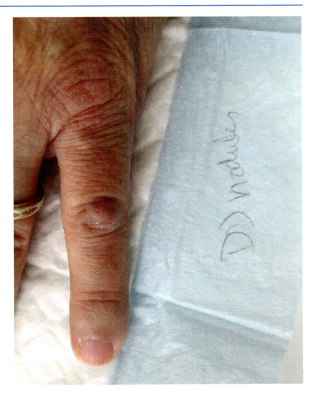

Fig. 1.5 Dorsal Dupuytren nodule over the proximal interphalangeal joint

dorsal cutaneous pads (DCP). The name Garrod's (Garrod 1904) has been associated with these changes. A case report of dorsal Dupuytren's nodule was described by Hueston (1982) to develop between the PIP and DIP joints involving the extensor mechanism with loss of DIP joint flexion. This was corrected by surgical excision of this nodular tissue. There is ambiguity about using the term knuckle pads and Garrod's nodes in the literature. We investigated the distribution and frequency of DCPs and DDNs in the normal volunteers and in DD patients (Rayan and Ali 2010). DDN are defined as subcutaneous, solid, firm, well-defined, tumor-like mass located over the dorsum of the PIP joint (Fig. 1.5).

DCPs (Fig. 1.6), sometimes referred to as Knuckle pads, are defined as painless thickening, sclerosis and loss of skin elasticity, and creases over the PIP or MCP joints.

None of the control patients had DDN while nine DD patients (18%) had DDN. Nine control patients (18%) had DCP while 11 DD patients (22%) had DCP. DCP pads were predominantly over the PIP joints and

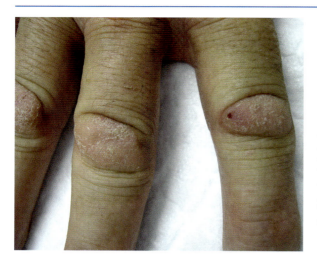

Fig. 1.6 Dorsal cutaneous pads over the proximal interphalangeal joints

had tendency for occurring in the dominant hand among males with physically demanding occupations. The index and middle fingers were most frequently affected. Patients with DDN were males, Caucasians who did not have necessarily physically demanding occupations and with lesions over the PIP joints.

Palmar skin changes begin by the formation of microcords from Grapow fibers, which connect the dermis to the palmar fascia leading to *pseudocallus* or thickening of the skin and underlying subcutaneous tissue. These vertical bands perhaps are the first anatomical structures to become afflicted by DD. As a result, the skin becomes tethered and adherent to the underlying fascial structures and loses its normal mobility. Skin thickening is often associated with surface rippling and dimpling. *Skin pits* are rarely confused or associated with other conditions. The presence of skin pits is a reliable sign for diagnosing early DD. They are caused by deep full-thickness skin retraction into the subcutaneous tissue. The diseased superficial fibers of the split pretendinous band form a dermal cord that pulls the dermal side of the skin inward.

1.3.2 The Nodule

The nodule is a firm soft tissue mass that is fixed both to the skin and deeper fascia. It seems to originate in the superficial components of the palmar or digital fascia. The nodule is usually well defined, localized, and raised above the surface, but it can be ill defined in the form of diffuse thickening of the deeper fascia. Dupuytren's nodules are encountered either in the palm or digits. *Palmar nodules* are located adjacent to the distal palmar crease often in line with the ring and small fingers and sometimes proximal to the base of the thumb and small finger. *Digital nodules* are usually located near the PIP joint and proximally at the base of the digit. Nodules are painless, but they can enlarge and become troublesome. Nodules can cause pain when associated with stenosing tenosynovitis which develops either from direct pressure by the nodule on the flexor tendons and A_1 pulley or from a vertical cord.

1.3.3 The Cord

The nodule may regress gradually giving way to the appearance of a cord. Sometimes cord maturation continues without nodule regression. Normal bands are the precursors of pathologic cords (McFarlane 1974). Early cords can be adherent to the skin and blend with the nodule making it difficult to ascertain where the nodule ends and the cord begins. The cord later becomes prominent and acquires the appearance and consistency of a tendon. Cords are located in the palm, palmodigital area or digits. Histologically, the mature cord has few cells, minimal myofibroblasts, and abundance of collagen issue.

1.3.4 Disease Progression

Palmar fascial disease or contracture may remain confined to the palm and not progress enough to cause digital flexion deformity. Palmar involvement usually precedes disease extension into the digits, but the disease can begin and remain in the digits. In order of frequency, the ring finger is the most commonly involved digit followed closely by the small, middle, and index finger and lastly the thumb. As the disease progresses, the development of palmar and digital nodules is followed by that of pretendinous and digital cords. The NV bundle anatomy can be distorted as the cord contracts especially the spiral cord. Ulmas et al. (1994) found 52% prevalence of spiral nerve intraoperatively and 42% had palpable interdigital soft tissue mass. The existence of soft tissue mass was specific (75%), but not sensitive (59%) for the presence of spiral nerve. The dis-

1 Dupuytren's Disease: Anatomy, Pathology, and Presentation

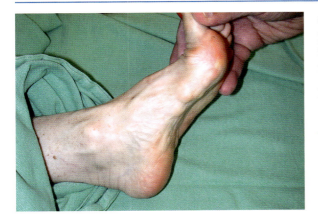

Fig. 1.7 Plantar fibromatosis or Ledderhose disease

and Meals (1981) reported a patient with DD and bilateral palmar contracture, bilateral plantar nodules, and nodular fasciitis of the popliteal space. The popliteal mass was firmly adherent to the fascia of the medial head of the gastrocnemius muscle, and fibromatosis of the popliteal tissue was confirmed histologically.

1.4 Clinical Types

There are two clinical entities responsible for palmar fascial proliferation, typical DD and non-Dupuytren's disease (NDD). These two types differ in presentation, etiology, treatment, and prognosis.

ease can be classified into early, intermediate, and late phase. Early phase entails the skin changes including loss of normal architecture and skin pit formation. Intermediate phase consists of nodule and cord formation. Late phase is the end point of joint contracture. The late phase in the typical scenario occurs in progressive contracture from the ring to the small and lastly the middle finger. This progression however is not immutable.

1.3.5 Ectopic Dupuytren's Disease

Dupuytren's disease may have a range of presentations especially in patients with strong diathesis. Patients with DD should be inquired about and assessed during evaluation for possible involvement of other areas of the body beside their hands. Ectopic disease can be either regional in the upper extremity or distant in other parts of the body. *Regional ectopic disease*: Is most often in the form of DDNs. The diseased fascia rarely extends proximal to the hand. However, reports have described DD extension to the wrist, arm, and even shoulder areas (Boyes and Jones 1967; Simons et al. 1996; Sinha 1997; Okano 1992; Bunnel 1944). *Distant ectopic disease:* This is encountered in patients with strong diathesis. These lesions affect plantar fascia, that is, Ledderhose disease and corpus cavernosum, that is,, Peyronie disease. Plantar fibromatosis (Fig. 1.7) is usually restricted to the plantar fascia, but the disease rarely presents as flexor contracture of the toes (Classen and Hurst 1992; Donato and Morrison 1996).

Most cases of plantar fibromatosis are asymptomatic, but occasionally they may cause foot discomfort. Wheeler

1.4.1 Typical Dupuytren's Disease

The patient with typical DD was described by McFarlane et al. (1990) as a Caucasian male, northern European, 57 years of age, with bilateral disease, may have more than one digit involved, and the condition is usually progressive. Patients with typical DD usually have family history, although some may not be aware of the disease existence among family members. The condition affects patients of Celtic or Scandinavian origin. This group of patients may have ectopic disease and appear to be genetically predisposed to have the disease.

1.4.2 Non-Dupuytren's Disease

In this condition the patients have no family history, are ethnically diverse (e.g., blacks can be affected), and there is no gender predilection (Rayan 1999b; Rayan and Moore 2005). The condition is confined to the hand without ectopic manifestations, unilateral, in line with a single digit without digital involvement, and nonprogressive. Environmental factors other than genetic seem to play a role in its pathogenesis such as trauma (wrist or hand fractures) and previous surgery (carpal tunnel or trigger finger releases). Frequently associated conditions include diabetes and cardiovascular disease. The condition may begin as a localized or diffuse thickening of the palmar aponeurosis forming a lesion analogous to a nodule. Longitudinal orientation of affected tissue occurs in line with the ring finger and can be reminiscent of a pretendinous cord. The condition develops 2–3 months after injury or surgery. The condition is nonprogressive or partially regressive. Surgical treatment is rarely indicated in this group of patients. The disparity among epidemiologic studies regarding DD prevalence is confusing and disconcerting. The prevalence rates differ significantly even in similar age groups and in studies from same geographical areas. The same is true for the recurrence rates after surgical treatment of DD. This disparity in literature reports of the disease prevalence, recurrence rates, and treatment outcomes is probably due to lack of distinction between these two types of palmar fascial proliferation. Future epidemiologic and outcome studies should take into consideration these two clinical entities, which should be grouped and investigated separately.

References

Barton N (1984) Dupuytren's disease arising from the abductor digiti minimi. J Hand Surg 9B:265–270

Bilderback KK, Rayan GM (2002) Dupuytren's cord involving the septa of Legueu and Juvara: a case report. J Hand Surg 27A:344–346

Bilderback KK, Rayan GM (2004) The septa of Legueu and Juvara: an anatomic study. J Hand Surg Am 29(3):494–499

Boyes J, Jones F (1967) Dupuytren's disease involving the volar aspect of the wrist. Plast Reconstr Surg 41:204–207

Bunnel S (1944) Surgery of the hand. Lippincott Company, Philadelphia, p 613

Classen D, Hurst L (1992) Plantar fibromatosis and bilateral flexion contractures: a review of the literature. Ann Plast Surg 28:475–478

Donato R, Morrison W (1996) Dupuytren's disease in feet causing flexion contracture in the toes. J Hand Surg 21B:364–366

Garrod A (1904) Concerning pads upon the finger joints and their clinical relationships. Br Med J 2:8

Gosset J (1985) Dupuytren's disease and the anatomy of the palmodigital aponeurosis. In: Hueston JT, Tubiana R (eds) Dupuytren's disease, 2nd edn. Churchill Livingstone, Edinburgh, pp 13–16

Grapow M (1887) Die Anatomie und physiologische Bedeutung der Palmaraponeurose. In: Archiv für Anatomie und Physiologie. Anatomische Abtheilung, Leipzig, pp 2–3, 143–158

Hueston J (1982) Dorsal Dupuytren's disease. J Hand Surg 7A:384–387

Legueu F, Juvara E (1892) Des aponeurosis de la paume de la main. Bull Soc Anat (Paris) 5 serie T. IV:67

Luck JV (1959) Dupuytren's contracture: a new concept of the pathogenesis correlated with surgical management. J Bone Joint Surg Am 41:635–664

McFarlane RM (1974) Patterns of the diseased fascia in the fingers of Dupuytren's contracture. Plast Reconstr Surg 54:31–44

McFarlane RM (1985) The anatomy of Dupuytren's disease. In: Hueston JT, Tubiana R (eds) Dupuytren's disease. Churchill Livingstone, Edinburgh, pp 54–71

McFarlane R (1990) The finger. In: McFarlane R, McGrouther D, Flint M (eds) Dupuytren's disease biology and treatment. Churchill Livingstone, Edinburgh, pp 155–167

McFarlane R, Botz J, Cheung H (1990) Epidemiology of surgical patients. In: McFarlane R, McGrouther D, Flint M (eds) Dupuytren's disease biology and treatment. Churchill Livingstone, Edinburgh, pp 201–238

McGrouther D (1982) The microanatomy of Dupuytren's contracture. Hand 14:215–36

Okano M (1992) Dupuytren's contracture (palmar fibromatosis) extending over the arm. Acta Derm Venereol 72(2):381–382

Rayan G (1999a) Palmar fascial complex anatomy and pathology in Dupuytren's disease. Hand Clin 15:73–86

Rayan G (1999b) Clinical presentation and types of Dupuytren's disease. Hand Clin 15:87–96

Rayan G (2010) Dupuytren's disease. In: Trumble T, Rayan G, Budoff J, Baratz M (eds) Principles of hand surgery and therapy. Elsevier, Philadelphia, pp 403–412

Rayan G, Ali M (2010) Dorsal pads versus nodules in normal population and Dupuytren's disease patients. J Hand Surg 35A:1571–1579

Rayan G, Moore J (2005) Non-Dupuytren's disease of the palmar fascia. J Hand Surg Br 30:551–556

Rayan G, Murray D, Chung K, Rohrer M (1997) The extensor retinacular system at the metacarpophalangeal joint. Anatomical and histological study. J Hand Surg 22B:585–590

Simons A, Srivastava S, Nancarrow J (1996) Dupuytren's disease affecting the wrist. J Hand Surg 21B:367–368

Sinha A (1997) Dupuytren's disease may extend beyond the wrist crease in continuity. J Bone Joint Surg 79B:211–212

Thomine JM (1985) The development and anatomy of the digital fascia. In: Hueston JT, Tubiana R (eds) Dupuytren's disease. Churchill Livingstone, Edinburgh, pp 3–12

Tubiana R, Simmons B, DeFrenne H (1982) Location of Dupuytren's disease on the radial aspect of the hand. Clin Orthop Relat Res 168:222–229

Ulmas M, Bischoff R, Gelberman R (1994) Predictors of neurovascular displacement in hands with Dupuytren's contracture. J Hand Surg 19B:644–666

Wheeler E, Meals R (1981) Dupuytren's diathesis: a broad spectrum disease. Plast Reconstr Surg 68:781–783

White S (1984) Anatomy of the palmar fascia on the ulnar border of the band. J Hand Surg 9B:50–56

Palmar Fibromatosis or the Loss of Flexibility of the Palmar Finger Tissue: A New Insight into the Disease Process of Dupuytren Contracture

2

Albrecht Meinel

Contents

2.1	**Introduction**	11
2.2	**The Skin Anchoring Fibers in the Normal and Diseased Hand**	11
2.2.1	The External View of the Soft Tissue of the Fingers	12
2.2.2	The Internal View of the Soft Tissue of the Fingers	12
2.2.3	The Loss of Mobility in Fibromatosis	16
2.3	**Discussion**	17
2.4	**Conclusion**	20
References		20

2.1 Introduction

For 400 years, the permanent finger contracture named after Dupuytren in the late nineteenth century has been understood to be a "contractio digitorum" (Plater 1614). After the European anatomist-surgeons (Elliot 1999) had ruled out the tendons as the cause 200 years ago, the flexion deformity of the fingers was attributed to a process of shrinkage in the palmar aponeurosis. Today, the substrate of the deformity is often sought in

A. Meinel
Dupuytren-Ambulanz, Kardinal-Döpfner-Platz 1 97070, Würzburg, Germany
e-mail: meinel@dupuytren-ambulanz.de

a postulated digital-palmar fibrous continuum instead of the aponeurosis. This concept has never fully divorced itself from the tendon image. Thirty years ago, I responded by introducing the notion of a contracture without contraction (Meinel 1979). With the first slice plastinates that von Hagens made available in the late 1970s (von Hagens 1979), for the first time it became possible to look into the intact soft tissue of the adult finger and comprehend clinically relevant fiber functions. Numerous findings in many years of clinical work have since confirmed the concept of an extension block in the fingers. Now I would like to apply this perspective to the disease process.

2.2 The Skin Anchoring Fibers in the Normal and Diseased Hand

Most authors today concur "that the Dupuytren's process starts somewhere within this palmar connective tissue continuum – somewhere deep to the underside of the epidermis but superficial to the transverse fibres of the palmar aponeurosis" (Flint 1990). Figure 2.1a shows the fibrofatty soft tissue in the finger of a living hand. The fibers between the skin and the divided A1 pulley run vertically and obliquely. The fat between the fibers has partially prolapsed out of the fiber formation. It is more than merely filler tissue. It acts as dividing tissue that separates the fibers and facilitates their physiologic mobility. The slice plastinate of a longitudinally sectioned flexed ring finger (Fig. 2.1b) shows how the fine, densely bundled fibers run more or less parallel between skin and tendon sheath. No longitudinally coursing fibers are detectable in the pretendinous tissue compartment. There is no connective tissue

C. Eaton et al. (eds.), *Dupuytren's Disease and Related Hyperproliferative Disorders*,
DOI 10.1007/978-3-642-22697-7_2, © Springer-Verlag Berlin Heidelberg 2012

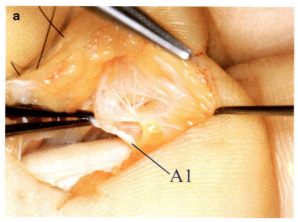

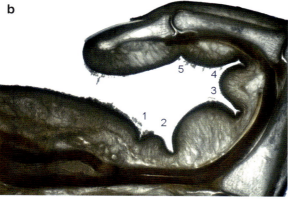

Fig. 2.1 View into the palmar soft tissue of the finger. (**a**) Palmar subcutaneous tissue; *A1*=*A1* pulley; surgical site. (**b**) Slice plastinate of a longitudinally sectioned flexed ring finger. *1+2*=palmar creases, *3*=palmar digital crease, *4+5*=proximal and distal interphalangeal joint creases

continuum, rather a densely packed fiber "discontinuum" of many individual fibers, nearly all of which function as retinacula cutis.

2.2.1 The External View of the Soft Tissue of the Fingers

Close examination of the palm reveals that there are mobile areas of tissue interspersed with stationary areas (Fig. 2.2a). The soft tissue of the fingertips is tightly anchored. The thin covering layer above the triangular center of the palm is also relatively fixed. This corresponds to the pretendinous portion of the aponeurosis. The soft tissue of the fingers between the fingertips and the area of the aponeurosis is mobile and flexible. The mobile soft tissue of the fingers overlies the fibrous tendon sheaths and extends from the distal phalanges to the metacarpophalangeal joints. The compartment of the soft tissue of the fingers is subject to considerable changes in length, to which the incompressible fibrofatty tissue responds by folding and unfolding (Fig. 2.2b). This play of the tissue is readily observable in one's own hand. The metacarpophalangeal and interphalangeal joints are ball-and-socket and hinge joints, respectively. In flexion, the distal phalanx is drawn upon the proximal phalanx. This effectively shortens the palmar length of the skeleton. When the finger is extended, the phalanx is released from its flexed position and the palmar length of the skeleton is restored. In these motions, the soft tissue of the distal phalanx is pushed into that of the proximal phalanx and pulled out of it, respectively. In the normal finger, the soft tissue structures pressed together in flexion remain separated by the cutaneous flexion creases. However, the flexion creases are not stable formations, so they are not firm borders to subcutaneous processes. The mobility of the soft tissue of the fingers appears as the smooth passive play of tissue characterized by the complete absence of any abnormal tensile stresses. Only mobile and flexible soft tissue in the fingers can ensure their free unimpaired extension.

2.2.2 The Internal View of the Soft Tissue of the Fingers

The soft tissue of the hand is supported proximally by the palmar aponeurosis and distally by the phalanges. The bones of the fingers are covered over almost their entire length by the flexor tendons and their sheaths. This fibrous skeletal structure provides the foundation for the mobile soft tissue of the fingers. The stationary fingertips lie on the portion of the distal phalanx that is not covered by tendons. In palmar fibromatosis, the mobile tissue over the tendon sheaths becomes far more important than the stationary tissue over the palmar aponeurosis. The fingertips are practically never involved.

Figure 2.3 shows the fibrous structures of the palmar soft tissue of the finger as they appear in slice plastinates

2 Palmar Fibromatosis or the Loss of Flexibility of the Palmar Finger Tissue

Fig. 2.2 Palmar soft tissue of the hand. (**a**) *Red* stationary tissue, *yellow* mobile tissue, *pcp* pars centralis palmae, *double arrow* pars digitalis palmae. (**b**) Tissue mobility over the phalanges. *1 + 2* = palmar creases, *3* = palmar digital crease, *4 + 5* = proximal and distal interphalangeal joint creases, *red* flexor tendons

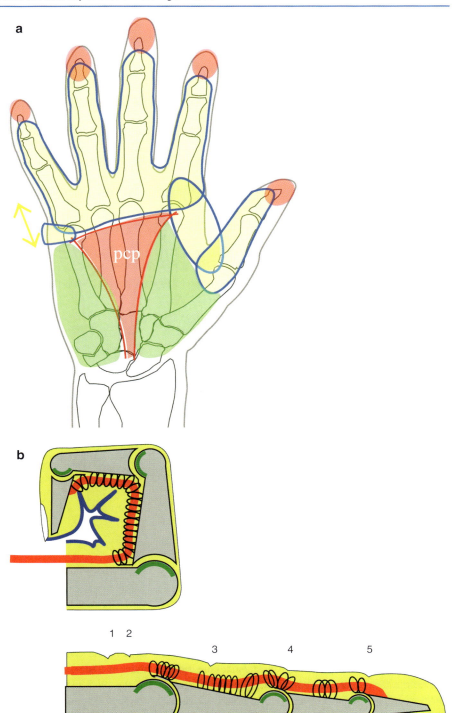

Fig. 2.3 The fibrous structure of the palmar soft tissue of the fingers. *Green* = distal margin of the palmar aponeurosis with bifurcation and pulleys. *Blue* = Cleland fibers; *black with white* cross section = palmar skin anchoring fibers. (**a**) Deep underlying structures and dorsolateral margin (Cleland fibers) with overlying nerves and arteries. (**b**) The crisscrossing peritendinous fibers covering nerves and arteries. (**c**) Cross section of the finger with Grayson fibers, cross sections of nerves and arteries and underlying Cleland fibers

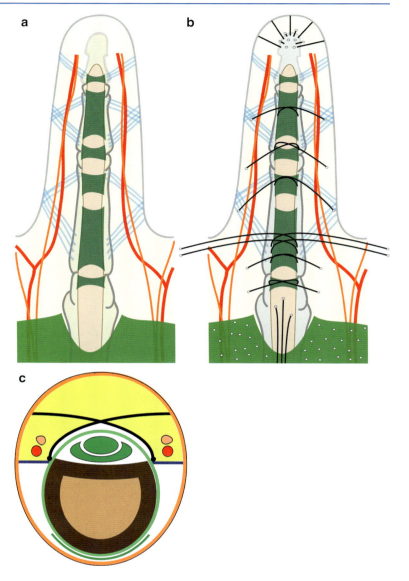

of adult hands and in many surgical findings. Figure 2.3a shows the deep layer that lies beneath the soft tissue of the fingers. This includes the osseous and fibrous finger skeleton and the lateral Cleland fibers that define the border between the palmar and dorsal soft tissue. The Cleland fibers lie immediately deep to the nerves and arteries of the finger. The neurovascular bundles enter the subcutaneous tissue as they leave the space beneath the palmar aponeurosis. Figure 2.3b presents the Grayson fibers, which cover the arteries and nerves laterally. The scissors-like or crisscrossed configuration of these fibers has long been largely ignored. These fibers overlie the lateral aspect of the tendon sheaths and course across the tendons to the skin of the contralateral side. In the extended finger, the taut fibers course obliquely to the longitudinal axis of the phalanx; as the finger is flexed, they assume a transverse direction. The fibers in the region of the natatory ligament exhibit the same crisscrossed configuration. They are merely a lot longer and bridge the adjoining interdigital space. Like the fibers in the fingers, their sole purpose is to anchor the mobile skin and soft tissue. There is no natatory ligament in the sense of a continuous transverse band (Weiss 1989).

2 Palmar Fibromatosis or the Loss of Flexibility of the Palmar Finger Tissue

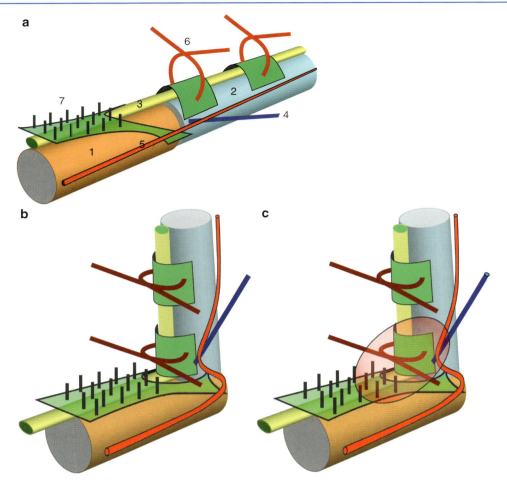

Fig. 2.4 (**a**) The joint in the extended finger - The fibers of the aponeurosis and proximal phalanx are drawn apart. 1 = Metacarpal; 2 = proximal phalanx; 3 = flexor tendon; 4 = fiber of Cleland ligament; 5 = digital artery; 6 = crisscrossing peritendinous fibers on pulley; 7 = longitudinal fascicles of the palmar aponeurosis with bifurcation (aponeurotic hiatus). Short skin anchoring fibers on the palmar aponeurosis. (**b**) The joint in the flexed finger - The fibers of the aponeurosis and proximal phalanx are pushed into each other. (**c**) The proximal phalanx is positioned within the aponeurotic hiatus. The artery is folded into loops over the Cleland fibers

Classic anatomic dissection has artificially created this "ligament." When the skin is removed, the transverse skin anchoring fibers that tethered it to deeper structures merge together to form what appears to be a continuous ligament. If there really were a transverse ligament over the proximal phalanges, then it would be impossible to flex any one finger by itself.

The two most important structural principles of the deformation of the tissue compartment are the variable length of the deep underlying structures and the crisscrossed configuration of the palmar skin anchoring fibers, which allow cross-sectional deformation (Fig. 2.3c). The tethering of the soft tissue of the fingers is thus variable in its length, width, and height. The flexor tendon sheath that is drawn out and discontinuous in the extended finger, telescopes and shortens as the finger is flexed. The aponeurotic hiatus is a particularly large anatomic gap at the junction between the tendon sheaths and the palmar aponeurosis. This gap receives the proximal phalanx (Fig. 2.4) when the finger is flexed. In this position the skin anchoring fibers are pressed tightly together above the shortened, telescoped deep underlying structures. These tissue displacements also bring the retrovascular Cleland fibers into close proximity with the fibers of the palmar aponeurosis. In purely descriptive terms, it is only the flexor tendons that actually leave the shortening tissue compartment as the fingers are flexed. All peritendinous tissue remains in situ and undergoes local deformation. The digital neurovascular structures are also unable to leave the compartment. They are folded into loops above the Cleland fibers (Fig. 2.4b). They thus assume a position in the normal flexed finger that may be observed in many Dupuytren fingers. The stationary tissue in the fingertips is tethered by radial fibers and above the aponeurotic triangle by short vertical fibers.

2.2.3 The Loss of Mobility in Fibromatosis

In fibromatosis, a disorganized hypercellular fibroblastic nodule infiltrates the fibrofatty tissue over the palmar aponeurosis and over the fibrous tendon sheaths in particular. In the normal hand, the fingers are held primarily in flexion regardless of whether the hand is working or resting. Fibromatosis therefore becomes established in the soft tissue of the fingers in its predominant compressed and shortened formation. In my opinion, this aspect has been neglected to date. This may be because the classic anatomic dissection is performed on the extended hand and we have our patients show us the extended hand during physical examination. In this setting, it is only natural to view permanently flexed fingers as contracted. However, if we assume that the disease develops in the flexed finger, then the far more plausible picture of an extension block (Fig. 2.4c) becomes apparent. This new perspective in itself renders the intuitive assumption of an abnormal contraction of the fingers untenable. This interpretation can be corroborated on every level of examination from functional anatomy to cellular biology.

The diseased hand in the stage of nodule and fold development impressively reflects the process of tissue and finger retention. In Fig. 2.5, we see a Dupuytren hand in the stage of nodule and fold development. The usual view of the open hand shows a typical nodular stage with apparent contracture of the skin and soft tissue (Fig. 2.5b). Yet when we have the patient make a fist, the resulting pattern of folds will obscure the nodules. The contour of the skin is nearly normal at the junction between the central and digital region of the palm (Fig. 2.5a). The nodule only reappears when the fingers are extended. Whereas the folded palmar soft tissue on both sides of the nodule was drawn toward the fingers in extension, the tissue adherent to the nodule was unable to unfold. Being unable to move in response to the distal traction, it creates a typical U-shaped fold. Although it resembles a skin contracture

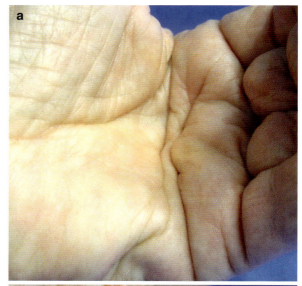

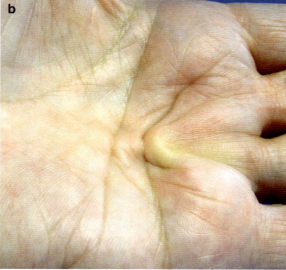

Fig. 2.5 Hand with Dupuytren nodule. (**a**) Fingers flexed; (**b**) fingers extended. Skin and tissue attached to the nodule are immobilized in the flexed position and cannot be drawn toward the fingers in extension. There is no tissue contracture!

at first glance, this pattern is in fact a sign of something totally different. The process is not one of contraction but of immobilization of tissue in the flexed position. This effectively creates an extension block. The tissue immobilized in the flexion position, as evidenced by its ischemic discoloration, is subjected to a tensile stress. This tensile stress in turn decisively influences the subsequent development of the clinical picture.

Ingrowth of new connective tissue into the fibrofatty tissue of the palm creates a pathologic conglomerate

2 Palmar Fibromatosis or the Loss of Flexibility of the Palmar Finger Tissue

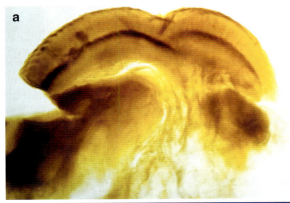

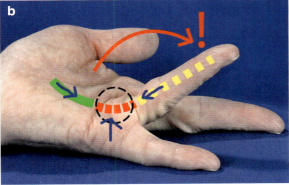

Fig. 2.6 The Dupuytren tissue. (**a**) Semitransparent section with skin and entrapped skin anchoring fibers. (**b**) The immobilized tissue blocks extension of the finger. The Dupuytren tissue and its attached structures are subjected to tensile stress

from which the fatty tissue has largely been displaced. This process transforms the physiologically discontinuous aggregate of fibers into a tissue continuum (Fig. 2.6a). Devoid of fat, the heterogeneous Dupuytren tissue of new connective tissue and entrapped skin anchoring fibers overlies the palmar aponeurosis and flexor tendon pulleys. It can extend superficially as far as the skin, which is then firmly tethered to the nodule. In the stationary tissue of the central palm, this nodule is not subjected to any significant tensile stress. There it remains in the shape of a nodule for a long time. However, the dynamics of the process develop completely differently where the nodular tissue infiltrates the mobile soft tissue of the fingers in its predominant flexion position. The individual fibers in their folded flexion configuration are bound together in a conglomerate. Extension of the fingers subjects this conglomerate to repeated tensile stresses that transform the Dupuytren tissue into a tendon-like structure in the line of the stress. All attached tissue structures – the

longitudinal fascicles of the palmar aponeurosis, vertical septa, and the Cleland fibers – are now subjected to the tensile stresses as well. They respond with functional hypertrophy (Fig. 2.6b).

In this manner the histogenesis and morphologic development of the Dupuytren tissue is decisively influenced by the specific local biomechanical conditions. Nodular tissue in the stationary compartment of the mid-palm retains its nodular shape over the long term. Dupuytren tissue occurring in the mobile soft tissue of the fingers (where it is found most often) is subject to stress adaptation. This transforms it into the typical cord-like Dupuytren tissue. The tissue in the finger axis is aligned more or less longitudinally, in the direction of the tensile stress. In the interdigital spaces, the traction produces oblique and transverse cords. Even the perplexing neurovascular dystopia can be explained as neurovascular loops trapped over hypertrophic Cleland fibers (Fig. 2.4c). The specific local tissue dynamics decisively influence the morphogenesis of the fibromatotic tissue mix and therefore the clinical picture of the disorder as well. The same applies to the ectopic foci of the disease over the interphalangeal joints, in the sole of the foot, and in the shaft of the penis.

2.3 Discussion

The concept presented here is not entirely new. Dupuytren himself noted that the disease did not involve the palmar aponeurosis but its distal prolongations (Dupuytren 1832). Dupuytren's contemporary and colleague Goyrand from Aix de Provence applied more stringent anatomic criteria and interpreted the disease as a disorder due to proliferation of new tissue (Goyrand 1833). Luck, writing over 50 years ago, saw the onset of the disorder in the occurrence of a connective tissue nodule in the subcutaneous tissue (Luck 1959) that McCallum and Hueston so aptly describe as the fibrofatty layer (MacCallum and Hueston 1962). Luck described the histogenesis of Dupuytren tissue in the three-stage model that is still in use today, in which a connective tissue nodule progresses to reactive tissue and later to residual tissue. However, Luck postulated a shortening process (which he interpreted as a process of involution) that triggers reactive hypertrophy in the attached aponeurosis. Gabbiani und Majno's description of myofibroblasts 40 years ago breathed new life into the contraction model (Gabbiani and Majno 1972).

The substrate of this process, together with the palmar aponeurosis, has been a postulated but increasingly indefinable fibrous continuum thought to connect the palm and fingers. It was Flint who introduced the term "palmar connective tissue continuum" into the discussion (Flint 1990). Intended to emphasize the role of the subcutaneous fibrofatty tissue as a functional unit, this term has unfortunately been repeatedly misinterpreted as actual anatomic fibrous continuity between the palm and fingers. Flint sees the soft tissue of the hand as a tissue mix that responds to fibromatosis with morphologic and metabolic reactions that lead to the clinical picture of Dupuytren's disease.

The infiltration of new connective tissue into the fibrofatty tissue of the fingers in particular leads to structural and functional changes. Accordingly, the clinical picture is understood as loss of mobility in the soft tissue of the fingers, which is compressed in flexion. In this view, the thickening of the palmar aponeurosis is interpreted primarily as reactive stress-induced hypertrophy, as Luck suggested. Yet, to my mind, even the thickened vertical septa of the palmar aponeurosis and the displacement and hypertrophy of the Cleland fibers may be regarded as secondary stress-induced changes. Surgical removal of tissue with reactive changes is not invariably indicated. This is especially true of cases where the cause of the tissue reaction can be eliminated. Even 50 years ago, Luck took this into account and refrained from excising the palmar aponeurosis. He only removed the active nodular tissue. Following Luck's recommendations, I began in the 1980s to leave not only the aponeurosis in situ but also the thickened vertical septa. Surgical manipulations were limited to the subcutaneous tissue of the fingers. The procedure I described initially as surgical release of the finger and later as digital fasciectomy involves manipulation within the subcutaneous tissue only. Limiting the procedure to the subcutaneous compartment further minimizes the trauma of surgery. The digital fasciectomy has proven very effective in both my own patients and those of other surgeons. Moermans went one step farther. He perfected a segmental fasciectomy that leaves not only the palmar aponeurosis but also portions of the cords in situ within the finger (Moermans 1997). This is undoubtedly a logical step to take from a pathogenetic perspective. Yet, from the standpoint of surgical technique, I personally prefer the advantages of dissection within the open, exposed soft tissue of the finger.

Figure 2.7 shows the digital fasciectomy in a ring finger with advanced extension deficits in the metacarpophalangeal and proximal interphalangeal joints.

This example is intended to demonstrate the efficacy of the digital fasciectomy and the plausibility of the new pathogenetic understanding. The aponeurotic cord tissue intraoperatively left in situ in the palm was no longer palpable within a few days postoperatively; it subsequently resolved completely. Six years postoperatively, the hand is still free of disease. One is impressed by the folds of skin (Fig. 2.7d) which has lost its mobile suspension and is now firmly attached to the Dupuytren tissue. The comparative view of the fibers on either side of the proximal phalanx is particularly important. Comparison of the two sides reveals that the thickened fibers below the ulnar neurovascular bundle (Fig. 2.7e) must be displaced hypertrophic Cleland fibers. In the unchanged tissue on the radial aspect of the same finger, the nerve and artery course across fine fibers that are clearly identifiable as Cleland fibers in their normal position (Fig. 2.7e). All these changes can be plausibly attributed to the tissue remodeling that occurs in fibromatosis and leads to loss of mobility in the tissue.

Last but not least, the percutaneous needle fasciotomy (PNF) warrants mention. The understanding of the disease process outlined above provides good arguments in favor of this surgical technique. I initially regarded percutaneous needle fasciotomy as a purely palliative measure which converts the process back to an earlier stage of the disease. However, by removing the tensile stress the fasciotomy alters the local biomechanical conditions and in so doing does indeed influence causative factors. The efficacy and sustainability of this effect can be enhanced with long-term static night splinting. I began to use percutaneous needle fasciotomy on my own patients 7 years ago. Because of the good experience with this procedure, it has become the preferred method of treatment. Its application is by no means limited solely to treating simple extension deficits in the metacarpophalangeal joints.

I will conclude with a few remarks about the significance of myofibroblasts in the finger flexion deformity process. Myofibroblasts today are generally seen as confirmation of the contraction theory, which had long been lacking a plausible morphologic correlate. The idea of a line of contraction that extends over a distance of several centimeters is difficult to reconcile with the structure and function of fibers in the

2 Palmar Fibromatosis or the Loss of Flexibility of the Palmar Finger Tissue

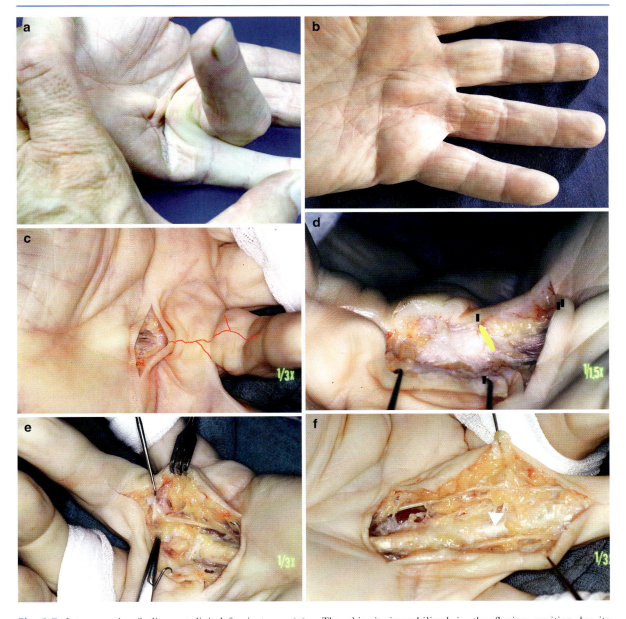

Fig. 2.7 Intraoperative findings at digital fasciectomy. (**a**) Preoperative site in the ring finger: *TPED* = 115°, Tubiana III, bloodless. (**b**) Disease-free 6 years postoperatively. (**c**) Transverse incision between the palmar creases; no dissection beneath the proximal edge of the skin incision. (**d**) The edges of the skin and cross section of the cord are marked. The skin is immobilized in the flexion position by its entrapped anchoring fibers. (**e**) The artery and nerve on the ulnar aspect are apparently displaced anteromedially over thickened Cleland fibers. (**f**) The artery and nerve on the radial aspect of the same finger course over thin Cleland fibers in their normal paratendinous position (▼)

subcutaneous tissue. On the other hand, Tomasek demonstrated in vitro that mechanical stress regulates myofibroblast differentiation (Tomasek et al. 1999). And Hinz presented a contraction model at the symposium in Miami in 2010 in which the myofibroblast is described as an isometrically contractive functional variant (Hinz 2010). Yet this is consistent with the notion of the myofibroblast as a stress-induced cell form and thus as an unspecific connective tissue reaction in palmar fibromatosis.

2.4 Conclusion

In Dupuytren's disease, new nodular tissue infiltrates the palmar subcutaneous tissue, causing it to lose its mobility that is so important for free extension of the fingers. The Dupuytren contracture is interpreted not as a result of an active contraction but of a passive retention of the fingers in their dominant flexion position – and therefore as an extension block. All histologic and clinical signs of contraction are convincingly understood as reactive isometric and not as isotonic contraction. The aponeurosis is only secondarily involved in the process of finger fixation. As a consequence, for surgical management, it is suggested to leave the aponeurosis in situ. Mechanical tensile stress is a key factor influencing histogenesis and morphogenesis of Dupuytren tissue. Efforts to mitigate this stress should be pursued, PNF being one of them. Aside from modifications of surgical technique, splinting offers a broad range of promising therapeutic options (Meinel 2012).

References

Dupuytren G (1832) Lecons orales de clinique chirurgicale Faites a L'Hôtel-Dieu de Paris. Germer Baillière, Paris, pp 2–24

Elliot DE (1999) The early history of Dupuytren's disease. Hand Clin 15(1):4

Flint MH (1990) Connective tissue biology. HUL 5 Dupuytren's disease. Churchill Livingstone, Edinburgh, pp 13–24

Gabbiani G, Majno G (1972) Dupuytren's contracture: fibroblast contraction? An ultrastructural study. Am J Pathol 66:131–146

Goyrand G (1833) Nouvelles recherches sur la rétraction permanente des doigts. Mém Acad roy Méd (Paris) 3:489–496

Hinz B (2010) Fundamental aspects of myofibroblast contraction, International symposium on Dupuytren's Disease, Miami, http://www.youtube.com/user/DupuytrenFoundation#p/u/0/fvmRS3OiWic. Accessed 20 December 2010

Luck JV (1959) Dupuytren's contracture; a new concept of the pathogenesis correlated with surgical management. J Bone Joint Surg Am 41:635–664

MacCallum P, Hueston JT (1962) The pathology of Dupuytren's contracture. Aust N Z J Surg 31:241–253

Meinel A (1979) Morbus Dupuytren: Streckhemmung statt Fingerkontraktion? Formalgenese und Pathomechanik der Palmarfibromatose. Habilitation, University of Heidelberg, Germany

Meinel A (2012) The role of night splinting after contracture release for Dupuytren disease. A preliminary recommendation based on clinical cases. In: Dupuytren's disease and related hyperproliferative disorders, pp 333–339

Moermans JP (1997) Place of segmental aponeurectomy in the treatment of Dupuytren's disease. Ph.D. thesis, University of Brussels, Belgium. http://www.ccmbel.org/These.html. Accessed 20 Dec 2010

Plater F (1614) Observationum, in hominis affectibus plerisque, corpori & animo, functionum laesione, dolore, aliave molestia & vitio incommodantibus. C. Waldkirch, Basileae, p 140

Tomasek JJ, Vaughan MB, Haaksma CJ (1999) Cellular structure and biology of Dupuytren's disease. Hand Clin 15(1):21–34

von Hagens G (1979) Impregnation of soft biological specimens with thermosetting resins and elastomers. Anat Rec 194:247–255

Weiss U (1989) Das Schwimmband. Beitrag zum anatomisch-funktionellen Verständnis des Bindegewebsgerüstes der Hand. Dissertation, University of Heidelberg, Germany

Basic Thoughts on Dupuytren's Contracture

3

Hanno Millesi

Contents

3.1	Introduction	21
3.2	**Critical Remarks**	21
3.2.1	Etiology	21
3.2.2	Pathology	22
3.2.3	Anatomy	22
3.2.4	Dynamics	22
3.2.5	Histology	22
3.2.6	Biology	22
3.3	**Functional Biomechanics of Palmar Fascia**	22
3.4	**Viscoelastic Properties of Connective Tissue**	23
3.5	**Experimental Studies of Palmar Fascia Mechanics**	24
3.5.1	Studies Comparing Viscoelastic Properties of Fiber Bundles of Flexor Tendons and Fiber Bundles of the Normal Palmar Aponeurosis	24
3.5.2	Stress–Strain Experiments with Different Stages of DD as Compared to Palmar Aponeurosis of Normal Individuals	24
3.5.3	Recovery Time in Different Stages of DD as Compared to Normal Palmar Aponeurosis	25
3.6	**Discussion**	25
3.7	**Conclusion**	26
References		26

H. Millesi
MILLESI Center, Vienna Private Clinic,
Vienna, Austria
e-mail: millesi@wpk.at

3.1 Introduction

Dupuytren's contracture has been known as such for nearly 200 years. It is a common disease in certain areas of the world. Patients suffering from the disease can have normal life expectancy. The natural course of the disease should be well known. However, our understanding of Dupuytren's has grown little in the last 100 years despite the fact that it is easy to observe and over the years has been the subject of an enormous amount of data collection, research studies, and publications. Apparently, there is something wrong with our basic concepts, which bear reexamination.

3.2 Critical Remarks

There are problems with the understanding of nearly every aspect of Dupuytren's disease (DD).

3.2.1 Etiology

Heredity is the most plausible one, but no gene causing DD has yet been defined. Racial disposition is believed, but poorly understood: is there a genetic risk for, or a genetic protection against Dupuytren's? (Slattery 2010). As far as metabolic diseases are concerned, there is a higher incidence of DD among diabetics or patients with liver diseases but the incidence is not high enough to establish a firm relationship. An enormous amount of effort has been spent to prove a relationship to certain professions or to trauma. There are arguments in favor and against but not enough to solve the problem of trauma as etiology.

C. Eaton et al. (eds.), *Dupuytren's Disease and Related Hyperproliferative Disorders*,
DOI 10.1007/978-3-642-22697-7_3, © Springer-Verlag Berlin Heidelberg 2012

3.2.2 Pathology

Pathologists classify DD as a fibromatosis: it starts with a proliferation of fibroblasts which produce collagen and ends with cords consisting of nonstructured masses of collagen. Although this classification is reasonable, the term fibromatosis does not tell the whole story. Other diseases classified as fibromatosis such as keloid, juvenile fibroma, or desmoid tumor do not have much in common with DD.

3.2.3 Anatomy

It was an important step to recognize that the disease is at the level of the palmar aponeurosis and not in the flexor tendons. Although publications on DD often describe and include an image of the palmar aponeurosis as the site of the disease, this is misleading. The disease occurs in areas where there is no defined fascia, such as the palmar side of fingers. Is this then an "ectopic" occurrence of the disease, or is our description of the palmar aponeurosis too narrow?

3.2.4 Dynamics

Does the occurrence outside of the palmar aponeurosis mean that DD is a kind of tumor of the connective tissue, and if so, why does it not occur in articular ligaments or in tendons other than the most distal segment of the palmaris longus tendon? Dupuytren and Goyrand questioned the argument of the palmar aponeurosis as site of origin of the disease in favor of the skin. Even Hueston attributed an unknown DD factor in the skin and hypodermis and hypodermis and based the dermofasciectomy on this consideration (Hueston 1985).

3.2.5 Histology

In many papers one can read: "DD was confirmed by histological examination." It is doubtful that any histologist just seeing one or two images of histological sections without knowing the macroscopic appearance and clinical data is able to establish a conclusive diagnosis.

3.2.6 Biology

The main question remains: What causes the contracture? The discovery of myofibroblasts by Gabbiani seemed to offer an easy explanation (Gabbiani and Majno 1972). Today, we know that the myofibroblasts are not specific for DD and occur in many different conditions with or without contractures (Hinz et al. 2007). The increased occurrence of type III collagen was regarded years ago as characteristic for DD but it turned out to be a common feature in wound healing in general. Many other factors described in connection with DD may have more to do with cell proliferation or collagen production than specifically with DD.

3.3 Functional Biomechanics of Palmar Fascia

The glabrous skin of the hands and feet of primates has a unique functional anatomy. It is fixed to the underlying layers in a way that skin folds are fixed, but also, ideally suited for both loose and firm grip. The subcutaneous fat tissue is compartmentalized within a firm network of collagen fibers. Pressure from the surface is transmitted to the connective tissue network around the fat lobules, which absorbs and diffuses pressure.

The baboon hand is very similar to the human. It has large fat lobules at the bases of the fingers – corresponding to the interdigital palmar monticuli of the human hand – and on the thenar and hypothenar eminence to provide an intimate "surrounding" contact with the object (Fig. 3.1).

This functional consideration helps to understand that the stiff subcutaneous connective tissue of the palmar side of the hand and fingers is a functional system which facilitates different mechanisms of grip. The palmar aponeurosis is only one part of this system (Millesi 1965). The connective tissue framework between dermis and the musculature is a functional unit which varies with location: the dorsum of the hand; the cranial skin; the palm of the hand, and the fingers. This system is called the superficial fascia in contrast to the deep fascia around and between the muscles. This anatomy affects the different distribution of early sites of DD.

3 Basic Thoughts on Dupuytren's Contracture

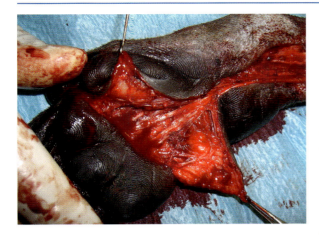

Fig. 3.1 Right palm of a baboon. The palmar connective tissue system functions to support grasping. Here, the skin of the palm is elevated toward each side. The pressure absorbing fat lobules with their connective tissue framework under the dermis at the incision lines can clearly be seen. In the center are the fibers of the palmaris longus tendon. With grasp, the palmaris longus contracts, and these fibers both flex the metacarpophalangeal joints and tighten the skin of the central palm. At the same time, the fat cushions on the radial and the ulnar side with their connective tissue framework close in around the object

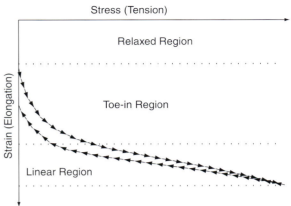

Fig. 3.2 Stress–strain test. The stress–strain test is a tool to define the viscous element in a viscoelastic system. *Stress* is the force applied; *Strain* is the length change from that force. Initially, a small force causes a significant lengthening as the wavy courses of the fiber bundles straighten (*up arrows*). Once this is complete, fiber bundle resist further elongation and the curve rises steeply. If the force is released, the fiber bundle returns due to its elasticity more or less to its original length (*down arrows*). De-elongation follows a different line as elongation. The original length is not reached but a small residual elongation remains. The residual elongation and the area between the two lines represent the viscous element of the system. An ideal elastic material without a viscous element would have no residual elongation

3.4 Viscoelastic Properties of Connective Tissue

All soft tissues and especially the connective tissues need the ability to change shape with movement and to return to their original shape when deforming forces cease. This is elasticity. *An ideal elastic material* like a steel spring deforms immediately if a deforming force acts and returns immediately to the original form if the deforming force is withdrawn: This is instantaneous elasticity. In biology such a material does not exist.

Elastic properties for connective tissues are provided by a combination of collagen fibers, elastic fibers, and ground substance. Collagen fiber bundles provide tensile strength, but have different mechanical properties depending on how much they are stretched. At rest, they are in a relaxed state with a wavy course. If longitudinal pull is applied, the undulations disappear and the fiber bundles become straight. This phase corresponds to the "toe-in" region of a stress–strain curve (Fig. 3.2). In this phase, fiber bundles lengthen with the application of a minimal force. Once the fiber bundles are completely straight, further lengthening requires movement of the ground substance between individual fibers and much more force is necessary for lengthening. This corresponds to the steeply raising "linear" region of the stress–strain curve (Fig. 3.2). If the stress is removed, elastic fibers recoil, reestablishing the length and the wavy course of the collagen fiber bundles.

An ideal elastic material will return to the original length along exactly the same line as the elongation. This is not so with living material. The return to the original state follows another line. The area between the lines is proportional to the viscous component. The original length is not immediately reestablished. There remains a residual elongation. This is also proportional to the viscous component. This combination of an elastic property with a viscous element is *viscoelasticity* (Fig. 3.2).

Another important aspect of viscoelasticity in biologic systems is *mechanical recovery time*. If a stress–strain experiment is performed and then immediately repeated, the stress–strain curve is less stiff and less force is necessary to achieve the same strain. This is due to the fact that the individual fibers remain temporarily rearranged after the first experiment. If the experiment is repeated after enough time for the fibers to fully recover, the stress–strain curve follows again the original pattern. This period of time is called the mechanical recovery time.

3.5 Experimental Studies of Palmar Fascia Mechanics

3.5.1 Studies Comparing Viscoelastic Properties of Fiber Bundles of Flexor Tendons and Fiber Bundles of the Normal Palmar Aponeurosis

In a stress–strain experiment, a significant difference between normal flexor tendons and normal palmar aponeurosis can be detected. The stress–strain curves of flexor tendons are much stiffer: much more organized to transmit force. The rise of the straight segment of the fiber bundles of normal palmar aponeurosis is significantly flatter: much less force is required for elongation. The recoiling effect is the same. This means that the fiber bundles of the palmar aponeurosis are more extensible with the same ability to return to the original length: They are more "elastic" (Fig. 3.3).

What is the functional significance of this "elasticity"? The fiber bundles *store energy*. An example is the plantar aponeurosis which forms the base line of a triangle with the middle foot and the calcaneus. Bearing weight widens the angle between the middle foot and the calcaneus. The elastic stretch of the plantar aponeurosis stores this mechanical energy, which is released later as it assists lifting the foot (Fig. 3.4).

In a similar way the energy storing effect of the palmar aponeurosis supports the hand during different gripping activities.

The energy storing effect is also important for the pressure absorbing function of the superficial fascia of the palm. The loose fiber network of this system absorbs the pressure by deformity and return to the original shape. Since the pressure is not high and distributed to a wide surface, a loose network with a few collagen fibers is sufficient.

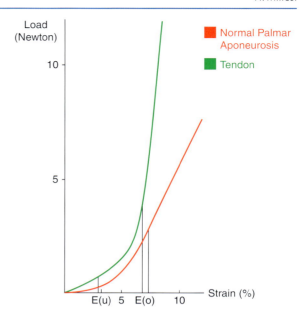

Fig. 3.3 Stress–strain test of flexor tendon and of palmar aponeurosis. Comparing the stress–strain test of fiber bundles of flexor tendon (*green*) and fiber bundles of palmar aponeurosis (*red*). The stress–strain curve of fiber bundles of flexor tendons is much stiffer, better at resisting force and transmitting stress. The curve of the fiber bundles from palmar aponeurosis is significantly less stiff. They can be elongated with much less force. They are more "elastic"

3.5.2 Stress–Strain Experiments with Different Stages of DD as Compared to Palmar Aponeurosis of Normal Individuals

We performed stress–strain tests with contracture bands and fiber bundles of palmar aponeurosis of individuals without DD. The tested tissue was elongated by 10% and the residual strain was measured. In normal palmar aponeurosis, the residual strain was well under 1 per mill. In contracture bands it was an average of 30 mm/m.

We then repeated the experiment with a lesser degree of elongation: 5% and 2.5%. The residual strain was less than with 10% elongation but the difference between contracture bands and normal palmar aponeurosis was still highly significant.

We tested also abnormally thickened fiber bundles of palmar aponeuroses without nodule formation and without contracture. We observed a significantly

3 Basic Thoughts on Dupuytren's Contracture

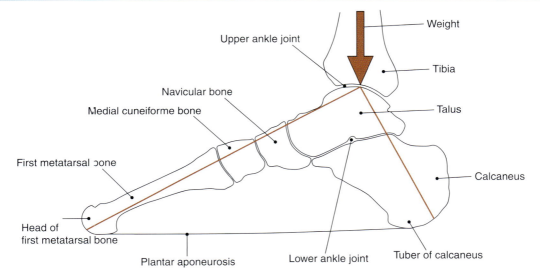

Fig. 3.4 Energy storing function of the plantar aponeurosis. The plantar aponeurosis forms the base line of a triangle with the middle foot and the calcaneus. Bearing weight widens the angle between the middle foot and the calcaneus. The elastic stretch of the plantar aponeurosis stores this mechanical energy, which later assists in lifting the foot

increased residual strain. Finally, we tested specimens from palmar aponeuroses from patients suffering from DD, which had normal appearance by macroscopic and microscopic view. After 10% elongation these specimens showed a significantly greater residual strain between 2 and 2.5 mm/m. The difference to normal palmar aponeurosis was not significant after 2.5% and 5% elongation (Table 3.1).

These results suggest that, in patients with DD, changes of the viscoelastic properties occur before other changes, such as nodules, with cell proliferation appear.

3.5.3 Recovery Time in Different Stages of DD as Compared to Normal Palmar Aponeurosis

The mechanical recovery time for normal palmar aponeurosis for persons with or without DD on average was 10 min. It was not increased in specimens with fiber thickening only. The recovery time was longer in contracture bands but it was enormously increased in tissues of active contractures. It extended up to 3 h as compared to normal values of 10 min (Table 3.2).

3.6 Discussion

I hold the view that the cellular proliferation is preceded by a stage of fibrosis with thickening of the pre-existing collagen fibers. The trigger might be the fact that fibers exposed to longitudinal stress do not relax completely after elongation and lose their wavy (undulated) course. This may be a stimulus for collagen production. In this case, the fault has to be attributed to the elastic fibers that fail to achieve complete recoilment (Millesi 1965). Longitudinal tension is certainly a factor stimulating collagen production. The thickening of the fibers changes the viscoelastic properties, causes atrophy of the loose peritendinous tissue and leads to fusion of neighboring thickening fibers to form major units. This has again an effect on the viscoelastic properties. At the same time the elastic fibers between the individual collagen fibers are changed as far as distribution and morphology are concerned. They are not anymore tiny, equally distributed fibers but show fragmentation and thickening. Frequently they are collected en masse in certain spots.

At the beginning of the disease, we see a disintegration of the sensible equilibrium that is the basis of the whole system of the energy storing devices. This consideration explains why the specially designed system

Table 3.1 Results of stress–strain test of different tissues and after different levels of elongation

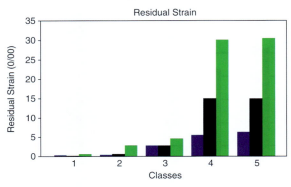

Tested tissues:
1. Palmar aponeurosis of patients without DD
2. Apparently normal segments of palmar aponeurosis of patients with DD
3. Thickened fiber bundles from Palmar aponeurosis of patients with DD before formation of cellular nodules
4. Contracture band with cell proliferation
5. Residual contracture bands

The stress–strain tests were performed using elongations of
  2.5%: black column
  5%: white column
  10%: green column

Stress–strain tests of fiber bundles of palmar aponeurosis of patients without DD showed a minimal residual elongation only at all three levels of elongations

Apparently normal palmar aponeurosis of patients with DD showed a minimal residual elongation only at 2.5% and 5% elongation. After 10% elongation however, the residual elongation of palmar aponeurosis with normal appearance of patients with DD revealed a significantly elevated residual elongation

The residual elongation was increased after elongation of all three levels in thickened fiber bundles without cell proliferation (Group 3)

It was very much increased at all three levels in groups 4 and 5

Table 3.2 Mechanical recovery

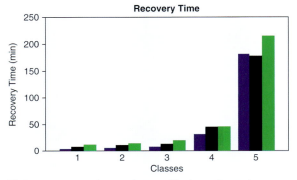

If after a stress–strain experiment with elongation and return to the original strain the experiment is immediately repeated the stress–strain curve is less stiff and less force is necessary to achieve the same strain. This is due to the fact that the individual fibers remain arranged according to the stress of the first experiment and do not need to be arranged again. If the experiment is repeated after some time and the original, less organized state has been reestablished; the stress–strain curve follows again the original pattern

The mechanical recovery time was determined for the same groups of tissue as in Table 3.1 (1–5) after elongation of 2.5% (black column), 5% (white column), and 10% (green column). The recovery time did not differ in Group 1, 2, and 3. It was somewhat elevated in group 4 (bands with cellular proliferation) but enormously elevated at all three levels in group 5 (contracture bands of the residual stage)

of the superficial fascia at the palmar side of the hand and fingers with the palmar aponeurosis as an essential part falls ill with DD and the flexor tendons – only a few mm apart and also exposed to trauma and stress – never develop a similar disease.

tissues is pressure absorption and energy storage. They have more pronounced elastic properties than other similar tissues. The pathology starts with changes of the viscoelastic properties. Wrong distribution and reduced efficiency of the elastic fibers may play a role in the initial stages of the disease. At this level hereditary factors are involved. The natural course and the treatment are not the subject of this chapter.

3.7 Conclusion

The results of these studies are the basis of the following conclusions:

  DD is a systemic disease of the superficial fascia of the palmar aspect of the hand and fingers and the plantar side of the foot and toes. A function of these

References

Gabbiani G, Majno G (1972) Dupuytren's contracture: fibroblast contraction? Am J Pathol 66:131–146

Hinz B, Phan S, Thannickal V (2007) The myofibroblast: one function, multiple origins. Am J Pathol 170(6): 1807–1816

Hueston J (1985) The role of the skin in Dupuytren's disease. Ann R Coll Surg Engl 67(6):372–375

Millesi H (1965) On the pathogenesis and therapy of Dupuytren's contracture. (A study based on more than 500 cases). Ergeb Chir Orthop 47:51–101

Slattery D (2010) Review: Dupuytren's disease in Asia and the migration theory of Dupuytren's disease. ANZ J Surg 80:495–499

High Prevalence of Dupuytren's Disease and Its Treatment in the British National Health Service: An Ongoing Demand

4

Karen Zaman, Sandip Hindocha, and Ardeshir Bayat

Contents

4.1	**Introduction**	27
4.2	**Material and Methods**	28
4.2.1	Spotlighting the High Prevalence of DD	28
4.2.2	Estimation of the Types of Surgical Procedures and Cost of DD to the Health Care System	28
4.3	**Results**	28
4.3.1	Global Identification of Epidemiology of DD	28
4.3.2	The Types of Surgical Procedures and Cost of DD to the Health Care System	29
4.4	**Discussion**	32
4.5	**Conclusion**	34
References		34

4.1 Introduction

Dupuytren's Disease (DD) is a common fibroproliferative disorder of unknown aetiology affecting 3–5% of the UK population (Gerber et al. 2011). The disease is often progressive, irreversible and commonly bilateral. DD is a late-onset disease with a mean age at onset of 55 years but can occur at younger age groups in particular in those with a strong family history of DD (Hindocha et al. 2006a). The rate of progression from palmar nodules to extreme digital contracture can vary between several months to many years. There is a general consensus that the greater the DD diathesis, the more severe the disease presentation (Hindocha et al. 2006b). DD diathesis refers to the presence of a number of factors including bilateral disease, ectopic disease presentation, early age of onset and family history, which may lead to a worse prognosis in disease outcome.

There are several therapeutic modalities available for treatment of DD. The standard treatment for DD is surgery. There are a variety of surgical approaches, which include fasciotomy (needle or open aponeurotomy) also referred to as release fasciotomy, fasciectomy (segmental, limited, radical) which can be either digital (surgery confined to the digits) or palmar (surgery confined to the palm of the hand), or dermofasciectomy. Although previous clinical studies have quoted a range of recurrence rates for these surgical interventions (Armstrong et al. 2000; Foucher and Navarro 2003), it is anticipated that a patient presenting with a strong DD diathesis has a higher recurrence rate (Hindocha et al. 2006b). As the disease is progressing, an observational approach can be taken, resulting in the disease being monitored in the outpatient department until the correct time for non-surgical (such as enzymatic injection) or surgical intervention is deemed appropriate. However, timing for surgery can be controversial, often the degree of disability and rate of progression of the disease are considered to be the determining factors (Bayat and McGrouther 2006). With no cure for the condition and high rates of disease recurrence, the cost of treating DD can be exponential. In addition, an ageing as well as a healthier, more informed population demanding functional surgical outcomes is likely to increase demand for early surgical

---

K. Zaman
Plastic & Reconstructive Surgery Research,
University Hospital of South Manchester,
Manchester, UK

S. Hindocha • A. Bayat (✉)
Plastic & Reconstructive Surgery Research,
Manchester Interdisciplinary Biocentre,
Manchester, UK
e-mail: ardeshir.bayat@manchester.ac.uk

C. Eaton et al. (eds.), *Dupuytren's Disease and Related Hyperproliferative Disorders*,
DOI 10.1007/978-3-642-22697-7_4, © Springer-Verlag Berlin Heidelberg 2012

correction and progress in this area. However, in the context of austerity and cost cutting, resource allocation and disease prioritization may also have an impact on future management of DD.

Surgical procedures can either be undertaken as an Outpatient (OP) [also referred to as Day Cases (DC)] or as an Inpatient (IP) procedure. In the UK, the main surgical specialties who perform DD surgery are Plastic Surgery and Orthopaedic Surgery. However, other clinical specialties may also undertake surgery in managing this condition. Within NHS Hospitals in the UK, variation exists in the number of these types of procedures carried out by each specialty. Coupled with this, there are differences in each specialty in the type of procedure carried out as IP versus OP. The epidemiology of DD has shown us that there are several issues which link to the health economics of DD. A previous national study in France has identified the financial constraints of DD (Maravic and Landais 2005). As a result of this, DD and its management can have an impact on healthcare economy (Maravic and Landais 2005).

There is one recent publication (Gerber et al. 2011) that relates to the cost of DD in England, UK. In this paper, it was demonstrated that fasciectomy was the most common and most costly surgical procedure carried out for management of DD in England between 2003 and 2008. They also showed that IP cases decreased as OP cases increased in number and suggested this was likely due to economic trends in the healthcare system.

In an age of economic austerity with the potential forecast of further financial burden, there have been indications that costs may not be met to treat conditions such as DD, which may become listed as conditions of low clinical priority (LCP) in the future. LCP cases are those which are not life threatening. As DD is a prevalent condition and is recurrent, the cost to the health service will be significant OP appointments, further surgery and possible IP hospital stays in some cases. However, the real cost to the patient of a 'do nothing' option is not to be negated.

The aim of this study therefore is to illustrate an estimation of the prevalence of DD, types of surgical procedures and cost of DD to the British National Health Service in England & Northern Ireland and to highlight the economic burden of this condition.

4.2 Material and Methods

4.2.1 Spotlighting the High Prevalence of DD

A thorough search of the literature on articles in relation to the epidemiology of DD included the following key words: Dupuytren's disease, contracture, history, population, prevalence, incidence and epidemiology. Numerous articles were identified as relevant to further understanding the epidemiology of DD.

4.2.2 Estimation of the Types of Surgical Procedures and Cost of DD to the Health Care System

Surgical codes for DD operations: Fasciotomy (T55), Fasciectomy (T52) and Dermofasciectomy (T56); from 2007 to 2010, procedures carried out in the NHS (England & Northern Ireland, UK) were identified and categorized into IP and OP procedures as well as being split between specialty (Plastic Surgery, Trauma & Orthopaedic and 'Other' Surgery). The national tariff was retrieved for performing each of the above (in both IP and OP). A total annual cost for treating DD was obtained.

4.3 Results

4.3.1 Global Identification of Epidemiology of DD

In relation to the use of epidemiological terms of relevance to the study, incidence was defined as the number of new cases of a disease over a defined timescale as a percentage of the population and prevalence was defined as the current number of cases of disease at a single time point. In a study by Khan et al. (2004), a British cohort demonstrated 34.4 per 100,000 men between the ages of 40 and 84 years had a gradual increase in incidence with increasing age. This is the only one study to date that has calculated the true incidence rate of DD in the British population.

Published prevalence rates have ranged from 0.2% to 56% (Finsen et al. 2002, Hindocha et al. 2009). In view of the variety of methods of data collection, it is difficult to carry out direct comparisons. However, it is clear that the prevalence of DD increases with age, a similar finding which has been reported in many previous studies. The highest prevalence rate of 56% was identified in a cohort of epileptic patients (Critchley et al. 1976). The prevalence rate for the lowest population cohort may be underestimated. The prevalence rate for the lowest population which had been calculated at 0.2% was derived using coding system data from a general practice and not data from clinical examination (Geoghegan et al. 2004). The general practice database allows a doctor to code DD under general musculoskeletal disorders as well as under DD. Not only does this affect population study data but can also have an impact on the healthcare costing system as DD can be a chronic condition requiring long-term specialist care in comparison to other short-term musculoskeletal conditions.

A consistent finding among the population studies is an increased prevalence with increasing age and that DD is more prevalent in males than females (Wilbrand et al. 1999). Not withstanding the geography of their actual study (Stadner and Pfeiffer 1987; Bayat and McGrouther 2006), they reported on the common prevalence of DD affecting Caucasians and particularly those of Northern European heritage. The other aetiological finding of significance and relevance is the familial nature of DD. The heritable nature of DD has been of great interest, with reports of the disease being present in as many as three generations (Pierce 1974) and studies suggesting forms of DD with a possible autosomal-dominant inheritance pattern (Maza and Goodman 1968; Pierce 1974). Those individuals with a positive family history of DD tend to have more severe disease and are likely to have recurrence following surgical management (Hindocha et al. 2006b). Therefore, those patients with a positive family history of DD are likely to have a greater impact on the healthcare economy.

4.3.2 The Types of Surgical Procedures and Cost of DD to the Health Care System

The three common surgical procedures currently carried out in the NHS for the management of DD are fasciectomy, fasciotomy and dermofasciectomy. Data obtained for this 3-year review across the NHS Hospitals in England and Northern Ireland revealed an average of 13,255 cases of Fasciectomy per annum compared to 571 Fasciotomies and 504 Dermofasciectomies (Table 4.1). The relevant Healthcare Resource Groups (HRG) is shown for each procedure in Table 4.1 with an average of 74% of male gender and most patients (77% on average) being operated on by trauma and orthopaedic surgery.

Fasciectomy T52 (HB51Z) in 2009/2010 attracted a tariff of £3,078 for OP procedures and £5,097 for an IP stay with an average cost of £4,087 per case, totalling an estimated yearly average expenditure of 162,515.468. Fasciotomy T55 (HB15C) in 2009/2010 attracted a tariff of £989 for both OP and IP, with an estimated yearly average spend of £1,695.146. Likewise, Dermofasciectomy T56 (HA06Z) in 2009/2010 attracted a tariff of £9,205 for both OP and IP and commanded a £13,917.960 total expenditure. Therefore, the estimated yearly average cost of DD for the last 3 years is calculated to be in the region of £59,376.291 per annum.

For the three common surgical procedures currently carried out in the NHS for the management of DD, the relevant Healthcare Resource Groups (HRG) was identified to show a split between percentage of IP carried out and those performed as OPs. The commonest age group per procedure was also highlighted. Interestingly, the mean age group for fasciotomy was significantly younger than the other two groups. The majority were performed as OP's for all three procedures (Table 4.2).

Slight variation in the average tariff for an OP appointment in 2009/2010 was noticed according to specialty with Trauma and Orthopaedics attracting £135.00 and Plastics £133.00 per new patient and follow-up attracting £74.00 and £66.00 respectively.

For all three procedures, the majority of patients were male with their surgery being performed by orthopaedic surgery–trained hand surgeons (Table 4.1). Most procedures were carried out as OP surgery with fasciotomies being the exception. This was an interesting finding as the mean age range for fasciotomy was also younger at 17–45 compared to 45–65 years for the other two procedures.

Table 4.1 Gender, frequency and speciality for the three common surgical procedures carried out in the NHS for the management of DD

Procedure	Code	M/F	Speciality	Average cases p/a
Fasciectomy	T52	78% M	80% T&O	13,255
Release fasciectomy	T55	61% M	94% T&O	571
Dermofasciectomy	T56	82% M	57% T&O	504

The relevant Healthcare Resource Groups (HRG) is shown for each procedure with a total % of gender and number of patients operated on per annum along with % undertaken by the highest specialty

Table 4.2 Mean age, percentage of inpatients and of outpatients for the three common surgical procedures currently carried out in the NHS for the management of DD

Procedure	Code	Mean age (years)	Elective (%)	Day cases (%)
Fasciectomy	T52	46–65	46	75.8
Release fasciectomy	T55	17–45	65	55.6
Dermofasciectomy	T56	45–65	50	55.4

The relevant Healthcare Resource Groups (HRG) is shown for each procedure along with the commonest age group per procedure, the % of IPs carried out and of those the % performed as OPs

Table 4.3 Yearly split of activity amongst the two main surgical specialties (Trauma & Orthopaedics; Plastic & Reconstructive Surgery) and 'other' less common surgical specialties

Fasciectomy	**T52**	**2007/2008** **13,288**		**2008/2009** **13,027**		**2009/2010** **13,449**	
		Elective split (%)	**% as DC**	**Elective split (%)**	**% as DC**	**Elective split (%)**	**% as DC**
Trauma & ortho		80	77	79	80	79	81
Plastic		19	57	18	64	19	64
Others		1	87	3	88	2	90
		100		100		100	
Release fasciectomy	**T52**	**2007/2008** **524**		**2008/2009** **523**		**2009/2010** **667**	
		Elective split (%)	**% as DC**	**Elective split (%)**	**% as DC**	**Elective split (%)**	**% as DC**
Trauma & ortho		94	51	94	58	93	58
Plastic		3	50	3	69	4	50
Others		3	39	3	29	3	44
		100		100		100	
Dermofasciectomy	**T56**	**2007/2008** **375**		**2008/2009** **546**		**2009/2010** **591**	
		Elective split (%)	**% as DC**	**Elective split (%)**	**% as DC**	**Elective split (%)**	**% as DC**
Trauma & ortho		62	61	56	74	53	71
Plastic		38	33	43	32	47	45
Others		0	0	0	0	0	0
		100		100		100	

Percentage of activity split per specialty and % of activity split undertaken as OP (DC = Day Case which is an equivalent term to OP)

The yearly split of activity amongst the three specialities along with the percentage of both IP and OP cases within each specialty showed that the majority of cases were performed by Trauma and Orthopaedic-trained hand surgeons. This figure is further broken down to demonstrate the OP percentage within the IP and OP split amongst the surgical specialties. There was an increasing trend for plastic surgery–trained hand surgeons to perform Dermofasciectomy, which showed an opposite decreasing trend in orthopaedic surgery. This variation may be accounted for by the complexity of cases necessitating an IP stay in the case-mix referred to Plastic Surgery (Table 4.3).

The percentage of IP activity by year from 2007 to 2010 and by five different age band is demonstrated for each procedure in Figs. 4.1–4.3. The percentage of IP activity is greatest for fasciectomy in the 46–65 age band for all 3 years. A similar trend is seen for dermofasciectomy. However, for fasciotomy, the greatest percentages of procedures are carried out in the 17–45 age band which remains evident for all 3 years (Figs. 4.1–4.3).

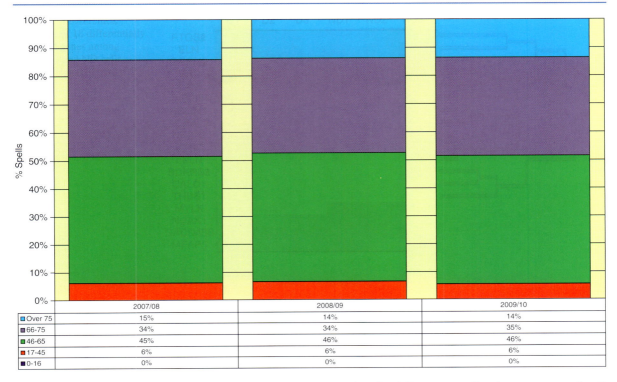

Fig. 4.1 Distribution of inpatient activity for T52: fasciectomy by year and age band. Percentage spells refers to percentage length of stay for total number of procedures

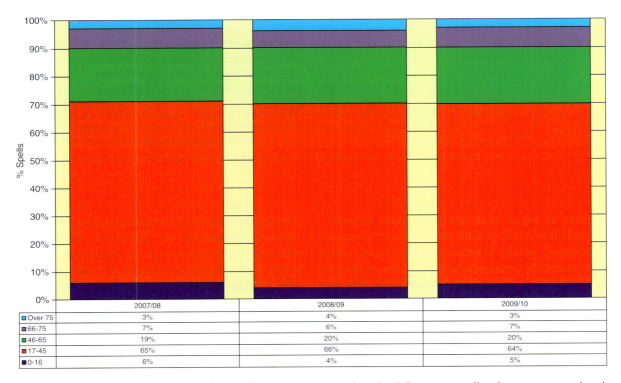

Fig. 4.2 Distribution of inpatient activity for T55: fasciotomy by year and age band. Percentage spells refers to percentage length of stay for total number of procedures

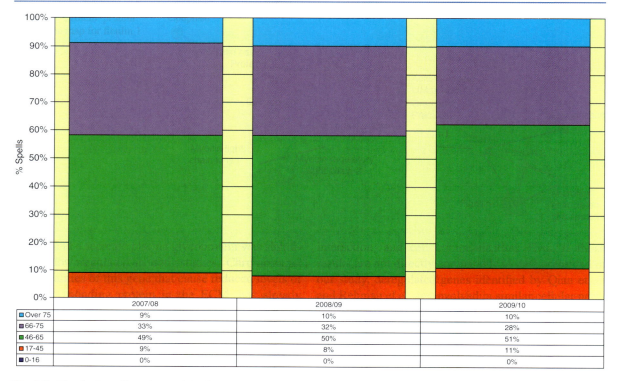

Fig. 4.3 Distribution of inpatient activity for T56: dermofasciectomy by year and age band. Percentage spells refers to percentage length of stay for total number of procedures

4.4 Discussion

This work has demonstrated the high prevalence of DD and its current surgical management in the NHS, which consists of mostly OPs of fasciectomy in male patients, within 45–65 age band carried out by Trauma and Orthopaedic hand specialists (79%). Interestingly, our findings are in agreement with those published by Gerber et al. in 2011. Additionally, this chapter has also demonstrated that the associated cost of surgical management of DD to the NHS may continue to have a significant impact on future allocation of resources.

Studies of various cohorts have identified that global prevalence of DD varies between 0.2% and 56%. One study to date only has managed to calculate the incidence of DD, estimated at 34.3 per 100,000. An estimated 25% of the population over 60 years of age or above of Northern European descent suffer from a form of DD (Burge 1999). DD is considered to be one of the most common connective tissues diseases. The Information Technology (IT) revolution of the past 20 years has empowered patients in an unprecedented way. This coupled with patient choice around specialist and desired site leaves today's patients and potentially those of the tomorrow (Luck 1959; Bayat and McGrouther 2006) better informed to find therapies and treatments in a timely fashion, as this is crucial not only for surgical intervention (Luck 1959; Bayat and McGrouther 2006) but for social and domestic factors and associated costs.

The study of population studies, incidence and prevalence rates has allowed better understanding of the geographical density. However, on the whole, the methods used for data collection were not uniform and variation between studies exists. These studies point towards patterns such as diabetes (Arkkila et al. 1997), epilepsy (Skoog 1948) and HIV (Bower et al. 1990) in the aetiology of DD.

We have highlighted the variable epidemiological nature of DD across distinct global populations and different medical subgroups. As the treatment options for DD increase and the general public become more aware of their availabilities, the treatment service provision for DD is likely to increase.

This study has shown that the cost of DD surgery can have a significant impact on the health care economy. Within hand surgery units, DD is considered to take up a large proportion of both IP and OP activity in hand surgery (Webb 2009), notwithstanding the expenses related to postoperative nursing and hand therapy follow-up of patients post-operatively. Additionally, the economic burden reviewed in this chapter does not include other nonoperative related factors such as lost wages and time off work, which in turn is greatly influenced by the type of procedure carried out; i.e. the use of fasciectomy vs. fasciotomy.

As the number of patients requiring or seeking treatment for DD increases, the types of treatment and surgical techniques will be guided at the appropriate time. Surgical treatments include fasciotomy, fasciectomy and dermofasciectomy. The fasciectomy appears to be the standard treatment option (Bayat and McGrouther 2006). Fasciotomy is a less invasive option, and its use has been rising over the last decade (Van Rijssen et al. 2006). Reasons for this could be that less severe disease, i.e. palmar disease without digital contracture, may be presenting to the hand surgery units. Alternatively, as some surgeons may find that the long-term results of this procedure for certain patients are equal to those undergoing a fasciectomy (Bryan 1998), a less invasive approach is more beneficial for the patient. In addition, fasciotomy may carry fewer surgical risks and provide a faster recovery process for the patient as it is carried out in an OP setting. As a result, there is no in-hospital stay and lower costs. The UK National Institute for Health and Clinical Excellence (NICE) has thus recommended that in those DD patients with palmar disease and mild contracture, fasciotomy (with a needle) can be used (NICE 2004). However, despite this, regular follow-up appointments and the need for further treatment are likely to be high in those patients with a high DD diathesis (Hindocha et al. 2006b). It may therefore be more cost-effective to carry out a dermofasciectomy in such patients where recurrence rates can be significantly reduced (Armstrong et al. 2000).

DD health economics may now be further guided as the use of non-surgical therapies undergoes trials and approval for use in palmar disease and mild contracture in the first instance (Bayat 2010). Non-surgical treatments in the form of collagenase injections are now available (Badalamente and Hurst 2007) and may be an alternative or a potential replacement for surgical management of DD (Hurst et al. 2009). The UK National Institute for Health and Clinical Excellence (NICE) additionally recommends radiotherapy for early DD (NICE 2010).

In order to 'soften the blow' of potential treatments costs not being covered within the UK national health service, a multidisciplinary approach to treating the disease may provide evidence for a more cost-effective approach. Although DD is treated by a multidisciplinary team, more involvement of the disciplines other than surgery may provide a more economical approach to treatment. This approach has been utilized in the treatment of chronic illnesses such as heart failure and appears to be equally beneficial to patient and health care financial structure (Wijeysundera et al. 2010).

This study was accurate as the coding for DD treatment was accurate. The conclusive statements from the authors suggesting further similar studies in countries with a high incidence of DD will enable an eco-epidemiological comparison of DD. One issue in many epidemiological studies is the methods of data collection suggesting a likely underestimation of the incidence or prevalence of DD. It will therefore be important that in the possibility of an economic analysis of DD, the prevalence or incidence data must be collected with accuracy.

With increasing financial strains on the UK healthcare system, treatment for DD is a lower clinical priority for surgical intervention in comparison to neoplastic conditions. However, the nature of this disease as a recurrent and at times aggressive condition must be considered so as to not create a false economic picture. Patients with a strong DD diathesis should have their treatment in a timely manner so as to avoid the rapid disease progression and increased risk of recurrence (Hindocha et al. 2006b).

The concept of examining 'an acceptable loss' of functionality for sufferers needs to be explored, given the condition is commonly bilateral and the failure to intervene may lead to severe disability. This in turn will have an impact of social welfare; therefore, intervention offers short- to medium- and/or medium- to long-term benefit realization to sufferers. Other non-malignant diseases such as systemic lupus erythematosus and rheumatoid arthritis have parallel economic burdens on a state-funded health system (Cooper 2000; Zhu et al. 2011). In a similar manner, DD will have a cost issue. It is imperative that timely treatments, whether surgical or non-surgical, are undertaken and that further research is carried out to better understand this debilitating condition.

4.5   Conclusion

In conclusion, this study has demonstrated the high prevalence of DD and its current surgical management in the NHS which is mostly OP fasciectomy in male patients carried out by Orthopaedic hand specialists. It is envisaged that the associated cost of surgical management of DD to the NHS may continue to have a significant impact on future allocation of resources.

Acknowledgements The data analysis was provided by Civil Eyes Research, a leading British benchmarking organisation working with clinicians and managers to use information to understand the metrics of quality and productivity within health services. Civil Eyes Research works with hospitals, GPs and the independent sector to use information to make change and share good practice. Their databases have been built up using collected information about staff, services and activity.

References

Arkkila PE, Kantola IM et al (1997) Dupuytren's disease: association with chronic diabetic complications. J Rheumatol 24:153

Armstrong JR, Hurren JS et al (2000) Dermofasciectomy in the management of Dupuytren's disease. J Bone Joint Surg Br 82:90–94

Badalamente MA, Hurst LC (2007) Efficacy and safety of injectable mixed collagenase subtypes in the treatment of Dupuytren's contracture. J Hand Surg [Am] 32(6):767–774

Bayat A (2010) Connective tissue disease: a non surgical therapy for Dupuytren disease. Nat Rev Rheumatol 6(1):7–8

Bayat A, McGrouther DA (2006) Management of Dupuytren's disease–clear advice for an elusive condition. Ann R Coll Surg Engl 88(1):3–8

Bower M, Nelson M et al (1990) Dupuytren's contractures in patients infected with HIV. BMJ 300:164–165

Bryan AS (1998) The long term results of closed palmar fasciotomy in the management of Dupuytren's contracture. J Hand Surg [Br] 13:254–256

Burge P (1999) Genetics of Dupuytren's disease. Hand Clin 15(1):63–71

Cooper NJ (2000) Economic burden of rheumatoid arthritis: a systematic review. Rheumatology 39(1):28–33

Critchley EM, Vakil SD et al (1976) Dupuytren's disease in epilepsy: result of prolonged administration of anticonvulsants. J Neurol Neurosurg Psychiatry 39:498–503

Finsen V, Dalen H et al (2002) The prevalence of Dupuytren's disease among 2 different ethnic groups in northern Norway. J Hand Surg [Am] 27A:115–117

Foucher G, Navarro R (2003) Percutaneous needle aponerectomy: complications and results. J Hand Surg [Br] 28B(5):427–431

Geoghegan JM, Forbes J et al (2004) Dupuytren's disease risk factors. J Hand Surg [Br] 29:423–426

Gerber RA, Perry R et al (2011) Dupuytren's contracture: a retrospective database analysis to assess clinical management and costs in England. BMC Musculoskelet Disord 12:73

Hindocha S, John S et al (2006a) The heritability of Dupuytren's disease: familial aggregation and its clinical significance. J Hand Surg [Am] 31:204–210

Hindocha S, Stanley JK et al (2006b) Dupuytren's diathesis revisited: evaluation of prognostic indicators for risk of disease recurrence. J Hand Surg [Am] 31(10):1626–1634

Hindocha S, McGrouther DA et al (2009) Epidemiological evaluation of Dupuytren's disease incidence and prevalence rates in relation to etiology. Hand 4:256–269

Hurst LC, Badalamente MA, Hentz VR, Hotchkiss RN, Kaplan FT, Meals RA, Smith TM, Rodzvilla J (2009) CORD I Study Group. Injectable collagenase clostridium histolyticum for Dupuytren's contracture. N Engl J Med 361(10):968–79

Khan AA, Rider OJ et al (2004) The role of manual occupation in the aetiology of Dupuytren's disease in men in England and Wales. J Hand Surg [Br] 29:12–14

Luck JV (1959) Dupuytren's contracture: a new concept of the pathogenesis correlated with surgical management. J Bone Joint Surg Am 41:635

Maravic M, Landais P (2005) Dupuytren's disease in France–1831 to 2001–from description to economic burden. J Hand Surg [Br] 30:484–487

Maza RK, Goodman RM (1968) A family with Dupuytren's contracture. Am Genet Assoc 59:155–156

NICE (National Institute for Health and Clinical Excellence) (2010) Radiation therapy for early stage Dupuytren's disease, guidance. http://guidance.nice.org.uk/IPG368. Accessed Feb 2011

NICE (National Insitute for Health and Clinical Excellence) (2004) Needle fasciotomy for Dupuytren's contracture, guidance. http://www.nice.org.uk/IPG43. Accessed Feb 2011

Pierce ER (1974) Dupuytren's contractures in three successive generations. Birth Defects Orig Artic Ser 10(5):206–207

Skoog T (1948) Dupuytren's contracture with special reference to aetiology and improved surgical treatment, its occurrence in epileptics, note on knuckle pads. Acta Chir Scand 96(39S):25–175

Stadner FUA, Pfeiffer KP (1987) Dupuytren's contracture as a concomitant disease in diabetes mellitus. Wien Med Wochenschr 137(4):89–92

Van Rijssen AL, Linden HT, Klip H, Werker PMN (2006) A comparison of the direct outcomes of percutaneous needle fasciotomy and limited fasciectomy for Dupuytren's disease: a 6 week follow up study. J Hand Surg [Am] 31:717–735

Webb JA (2009) Cost minimisation using clinic-based treatment for common hand conditions – a prospective economic analysis. Ann R Coll Surg Engl 91:135–139

Wijeysundera HC et al (2010) Cost-effectiveness of specialized multi-disciplinary heart failure clinics in Ontario, Canada. Value Health 13(8):915–921

Wilbrand S, Ekbom A et al (1999) The sex ratio and rate of reoperation for Dupuytren's contracture in men and women. J Hand Surg [Br] 24:456–459

Zhu TY, Tam LS, Li EK (2011) Cost of illness studies in systemic lupus erythematosus: a systematic review. Arthritis Care Res 63(5):751–760

Treatment for Dupuytren's Disease: An Overview of Options

5

Annet L. van Rijssen and Paul M.N. Werker

Contents

5.1	**Introduction**	35
5.2	**Diagnosis**	36
5.4	**Literature of Treatment Options**	36
5.5	**Surgical treatment**	38
5.5.1	Fasciectomy	38
5.5.2	Dermofasciectomy	39
5.5.3	Percutaneous Needle Fasciotomy or Aponeurotomy	39
5.6	**Nonsurgical Treatment**	40
5.6.1	Injections	40
5.6.2	Radiotherapy	40
5.6.3	Treatment with Splints/Splinting	41
5.7	**Conclusions**	41
References		41

This chapter has previously been published in the *Dutch Journal of Medicine* as: van Rijssen AL, Werker PM (2009) Treatment of Dupuytren's contracture; an overview of options [Article in Dutch] Ned Tijdschr Geneeskd. 153:A129. Translated and reproduced with permission.

A.L. van Rijssen (✉)
Department of Plastic Surgery, Isala Clinics,
Zwolle, The Netherlands
e-mail: annetvanrijssen@hotmail.com

P.M.N. Werker
University Medical Center Groningen,
University of Groningen, Groningen, The Netherlands
e-mail: p.m.n.werker@umcg.nl

5.1 Introduction

There are different treatment options for Dupuytren's Disease, but high level evidence of their effectiveness is limited. In this chapter, we give an overview of the different treatment options with the best available evidence (level 3 or greater).

Dupuytren's Disease (DD) is a fibromatosis of the palmer fascia of the hand and fingers, which often leads to flexion deformity of especially the ulnar fingers. Patients with digital contracture from DD may develop difficulty using their hands in daily activities. The cause of DD is not yet fully elucidated. There is some correlation between DD and smoking, excessive alcohol consumption, male gender, diabetes mellitus, epilepsy, and possibly, performing heavy manual labor (Hindocha et al. 2006a, Descatha 2012). Dupuytren's Disease is most common among Caucasians living in or originating from North-West Europe. The prevalence in a country is strongly influenced by the origin of its population and varies from 0.5 to 25% (Gudmundsson et al. 2000; Ross 1999; Thurston 2003; Wilbrand et al. 1999). Men are most often affected after the age of 50, earlier than women, but by the ninth decade, the gender ratio is nearly 1:1 (Anthony et al. 2008). There is a familial predisposition to DD, suggesting a genetic origin. The exact genetic profile of Dupuytren's Disease is not yet fully unraveled (Rehman et al. 2008; Hindocha et al. 2006b; Bayat et al. 2003), but work from a consortium of Dupuytren' study groups from the UK, Germany and initiated and coordinated in Groningen has revealed nine susceptibility loci and a role for the WNT-signaling pathway in the pathogenesis of the disease (Dolmans 2011).

C. Eaton et al. (eds.), *Dupuytren's Disease and Related Hyperproliferative Disorders*,
DOI 10.1007/978-3-642-22697-7_5, © Springer-Verlag Berlin Heidelberg 2012

5.2 Diagnosis

Dupuytren's Disease is usually easy to diagnose. The disease starts with the development of subcutaneous firm mass (nodules) and skin pitting in the palm of the hand (Fig. 5.1). Sometimes so-called knuckle pads present on the dorsum of the proximal interphalangeal joint (PIP joint). Gradually cords appear in the course of the nodules and cause the patient to be unable to fully extend the fingers (Fig. 5.2). The distal interphalangeal joint (DIP joint) is rarely directly affected, but a Boutonniere deformity may develop. Dupuytren's disease is usually located on the ulnar side of the hand and the ring finger is mostly affected (James and Tubiana 1952). Dupuytren's disease is often not only restricted to the fascia, but also the surrounding subcutaneous tissue and the skin can be affected (Meyerding et al. 1941).

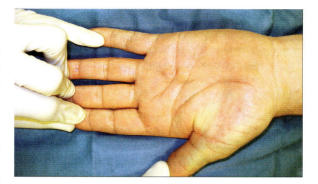

Fig. 5.1 A patient with the initial stages of Dupuytren's Disease. The fingers can still be fully extended, but in the hand palm at the level of the fourth ray, a nodule and skin pitting are visible

5.3 Prognosis

There is no cure for Dupuytren's Disease, neither can it be prevented. After treatment, the disease may recur in the previously operated field or extend to a new location. There are risk factors that influence the timing and severity of recurrence. The risk of recurrence is higher if the onset of the disease is before the age of 50; if the disease occurs in close relatives; or if ectopic lesions are present on the dorsum of the PIP joint (knuckle pads, Garrod's pads), the penis (Peyronie's Disease), or the foot (Ledderhose Disease). Bilateral disease, radial involvement and small finger involvement are other known risk factors (Abe et al. 2004). Moreover, each treatment gives its own specific risk for recurrence. All these factors together determine the prognosis; this should be taken into consideration when counseling a patient and proposing a treatment option.

5.4 Literature of Treatment Options

We have analyzed the existing literature, using Medline and the Cochrane Library without date limit. The search terms were "Dupuytren's Disease," "Morbus Dupuytren," "Dupuytren," "fasciectomy," "fasciotomy," "aponeurotomy," "radiotherapy AND Dupuytren," "splinting AND Dupuytren," and "postoperative hand therapy". For subsequent analysis, we used only the relevant articles or abstracts in English, French, or German. The relevance of an article was determined by the title or abstract. We found one relevant systematic review, ten relevant randomized clinical trials and nine case–control studies. Due to this limited number of studies, we also included the cohort studies that reported on more than 100 cases. An overview of the treatments with their advantages and disadvantages is summarized in Table 5.1. In the analysis, we followed the usual classification of levels of evidence:

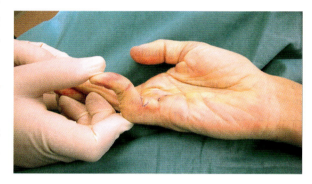

Fig. 5.2 The hand of a patient with Dupuytren's Disease. There is a contracture in the proximal interphalangeal joint of the fifth ray. The distal interphalangeal joint shows compensatory hyperextension, a Boutonniere deformity

- *Level 1*: At least one systematic review or two randomized clinical comparative studies conducted independent of each other
- *Level 2*: At least two independently conducted studies (randomized clinical trials of moderate quality of insufficient size) or other comparative studies (nonrandomized comparative cohort study or case–control study)

Table 5.1 Overview of the treatments for Dupuytren's Disease, including results and recurrence risks

Treatment	Indication	Results	Complications	Recurrence	Disadvantages	Level of evidence
Limited fasciectomy (Clibbon and Logan 2001; Foucher et al. 1992; McCash 1964; Van Rijssen et al. 2006 and 2012)	>30° contracture painful nodules (Clibbon and Logan 2001; Foucher et al. 1992; McCash 1964; Van Rijssen et al. 2006 and 2012)	79% reduction of contracture (Van Rijssen et al. 2006 and 2012)	Hematoma, skin necrosis, neurovascular damage (Clibbon and Logan 2001; McCash 1964)	41% in 5 years (Foucher et al. 1992)	Invasive treatment. Complications in 19% of patients. 6 weeks of rehabilitation (Van Rijssen et al. 2006 and 2012)	Level 2
Dermofasciectomy (Armstrong et al. 2000; Ketchum 2012)	Recurrences. Aggressive type in patients younger than 40	Comparable to limited fasciectomy.	Hematoma, loss of skin graft, infection, neurovascular damage	8.4% after 6 years (Armstrong 2000)	Most invasive treatment, further disadvantages same as with limited fasciectomy + those of skin grafting	Level 3
Percutaneous needle fasciotomy (Van Rijssen and Werker 2006; Van Rijssen et al. 2012)	Isolated cord patients >50 years postponement of limited fasciectomy (Van Rijssen et al. 2006 and 2012)	63% reduction of contracture (Van Rijssen et al. 2006 and 2012)	Nerve damage, tendon damage, skin fissures, especially in the treatment of recurrences (Van Rijssen and Werker 2006, Van Rijssen et al. 2006 and 2012)	65% in 32 months (Van Rijssen et al. 2012)	"blind technique" high risk of recurrence (Van Rijssen and Werker 2006)	Level 2
Clostridial collagenase (Badalamente and Hurst 2000 and 2007; Badalamente et al. 2002; Hurst et al. 2009; Watt et al. 2010)	Contracture associated with a palpable cord (Badalamente and Hurst 2000 and 2007; Badalamente et al. 2002; Hurst et al. 2009; Watt et al. 2010)	87% success (correction within 0–5° of full extension) (Badalamente et al. 2002; Badalamente and Hurst 2007; Hurst et al. 2009; Watt et al. 2010)	Local, temporary reaction to injection (Badalamente and Hurst 2000 and 2007; Badalamente et al. 2002; Hurst et al. 2009; Watt et al. 2010)	19% after 2 years.(Hurst et al. 2009; Watt et al. 2010)	Not selective for diseased tissue	Level 3
Radiotherapy (Adamietz et al. 2001; Betz et al. 2010; Falter et al. 1991; Keilholz et al. 1997; Seegenschmiedt et al. 2001, 2012; Weinzierl et al. 1993)	Disease in initial phase (Adamietz et al. 2001; Betz et al. 2010; Falter et al. 1991; Keilholz et al. 1997; Seegenschmiedt et al. 2012)	Delay of progression of disease (<5 years) (Adamietz et al. 2001; Betz et al. 2010; Falter et al. 1991; Keilholz et al. 1997; Seegenschmiedt et al. 2001; 2012)	Erythema and other skin conditions, long-term damage (Falter et al. 1991)	Mixed results: delay of development of contractures in stage N and Tubiana I.[2] vs. no difference between treated and nontreated patients after 7 years. (Weinzierl et al. 1993; Seegenschmiedt et al. 2012)	Only suitable in early stage	Level 3

- *Level 3*: At least one study of level 2 or a noncomparative study
- *Level 4*: Expert opinion

From our review of existing literature, 17 articles were identified with an evidence basis greater than level 4.

5.5 Surgical treatment

5.5.1 Fasciectomy

5.5.1.1 Limited Fasciectomy

In most countries, limited fasciectomy is the most frequently practiced treatment for Dupuytren's Disease. Only abnormal tissues are excised while care is taken to preserve unaffected fascia and neurovascular bundles (Fig. 5.3).

Indications: This intervention is indicated for painful nodules that do not respond to conservative measures (padded gloves) or for progressing contractures of at least 30° in one of the joints. The treatment should preferably be performed before a contracture of 60° has developed. PIP joint contracture greater than 60° is more difficult to correct, because it may be accompanied by contracture of the checkrein and collateral ligaments (Misra et al. 2007) and by lengthening of the extensor mechanism (Smith and Breed 1994).

Disadvantages: As the thickening and shortening can displace the neurovascular bundles, these could be damaged during the intervention. This complication rate is reported in 0–2% of the patients during the first surgical intervention and up to 10% of patients in recurrent cases. The total cumulative risk for complications is 19% whereby we note that apart from damage of the neurovascular bundle, most other complications are being minor such as wound healing issues (Clibbon and Logan 2001; McFarlane and McGrouther 1990). The probability of recurrence after limited fasciectomy is 41% within 5 years (Foucher et al. 1992). Recurrence rates differ enormously, from 2% to 73% (McFarlane and McGrouther 1990; Jurisic et al. 2008). Another disadvantage of limited fasciectomy is that on average, it takes 6 weeks before the patient can use the treated hand again fully. We found one randomized controlled trial on this treatment, which was compared to percutaneous needle fasciotomy (evidence level 2). The

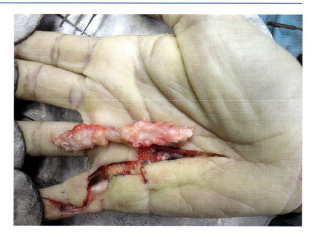

Fig. 5.3 Surgical treatment of Dupuytren's Contracture. The fibrotic tissue that caused the contracture has been removed via a zigzag Bruner incision in the finger and palm

conclusion was that 6 weeks after this operation, the extension restriction of the operated finger was reduced to an average of 79% (Van Rijssen et al. 2006). In Chapter 35 of this book, the 3-year results of this randomized controlled trial are presented and recurrence was limited to 9% following limited fasciectomy (Van Rijssen et al. 2012).

5.5.1.2 Segmental Fasciectomy

In Belgium, Moermans popularized segmental fasciectomy. In this operation, 1-cm segments of the diseased fascia are removed. The authors found decreased morbidity, quicker recovery but similar recurrence rates, when comparing their results to those reported in the literature (Moermans 1996).

5.5.1.3 Radical Fasciectomy

Radical fasciectomy, popular in the 1950s and early 1960s, fell out of favor because of a high incidence of complications (Chick and Lister 1991) and is mentioned for historical purposes. In radical fasciectomy, the fascia is widely removed but the overlying skin is preserved. Incisions may vary, but the operation usually is completed by the redistribution of elevated skin in such a way that most of the wound can be closed.

5.5.1.4 Open Palm Technique

Some advocate leaving the skin in the palm over the transverse ligament of the palmar aponeurosis open to allow for wound drainage (McCash 1964). This

5 Treatment for Dupuytren's Disease: An Overview of Options

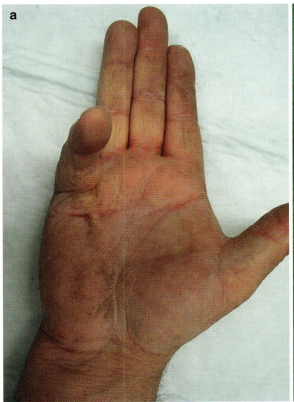 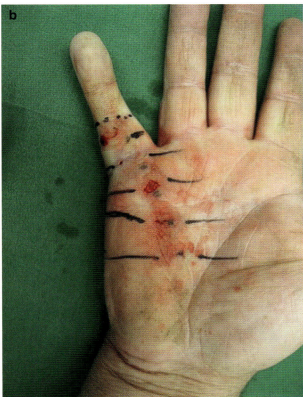

Fig. 5.4 (**a**, **b**) The hand of a patient with Dupuytren's Contracture before and after treatment with percutaneous needle fasciotomy. A palmar cord can be seen at the level of the fifth ray (**a**). The contracture is mainly in the metacarpal phalangeal joint. The contracture was cut with a needle in several places (*black lines* in **b**). Following treatment, the finger is straight (Courtesy of H. ter Linden)

technique has been found to have less complications but a slightly extended duration until complete wound healing.

5.5.2 Dermofasciectomy

Dermofasciectomy is a method where, together with the affected fascia, the overlying skin is excised. A skin graft is used to cover the skin defect. This method is indicated for patients who have either a high risk for recurrence or a recurrence with skin involvement. The rationale for the use of dermofasciectomy comes from a cohort study on 143 digits, where the skin was removed in the area between the distal palmer crease and the PIP joint. The risk of recurrence after this radical method was only 8.4% after 58 months (Armstrong et al. 1984). Similar satisfactory results with a shorter follow-up are presented elsewhere (Ketchum 2012). In addition to the disadvantages of fasciectomy, there are also the disadvantages that are associated with harvesting and application of a skin graft.

5.5.3 Percutaneous Needle Fasciotomy or Aponeurotomy

In the 1970s, a group of French rheumatologists revived and modified the original method of treatment developed by Henry Cline of London in 1777 (Cline 1777). With percutaneous needle fasciotomy (PNF), the affected cords are weakened or cut under local anesthesia with the help of an injection needle (Fig. 5.4).

5.5.3.1 Indications

This technique has recently gained wide popularity. It is a minimally invasive intervention, with a brief recovery period (see Section 6 of this book). In the only randomized trial on this treatment, the extension deficit had improved 6 weeks after the intervention with an average of 63% (van Rijssen et al. 2006). In the short term, there was no statistically significant difference between the results of the needle fasciotomy and limited fasciectomy if the contracture was less than 90° preoperatively (67–82% improvement). For more severe contractures, limited fasciectomy gave better results (van Rijssen et al. 2006; van Rijssen and Werker 2006). In experienced hands, the cumulative risk of complications is lower in needle fasciotomy than in limited fasciectomy (van Rijssen et al. 2006). The intervention is therefore seen by some as a panacea for the treatment of Dupuytren's Disease and has gained great popularity among patients on different Internet forums.

5.5.3.2 Disadvantages

Despite the advantages in the short term, this intervention also has clear disadvantages. Long-term follow-up of the comparative study showed that the recurrence rate after needle fasciotomy is much higher than after limited fasciectomy (65% after 32 months), and in some cases, fasciectomy is unavoidable in the end (van Rijssen et al. 2006; van Rijssen and Werker 2006). Three-year follow-up data of a randomized comparative study show a recurrence rate of 64% in the PNF group (Van Rijssen et al. 2012). Specifically for patients with likelihood for high recurrence rate, this treatment seems not to be the best treatment option.

5.6 Nonsurgical Treatment

5.6.1 Injections

Many nonsurgical interventions have been tried out, but so far, none have replaced surgical treatment.

5.6.1.1 Human Enzymes

From the beginning of the twentieth century, it has been tried to dissolve the thickened fascia various agents including pepsin, trypsin, hyaluronidase, and thiosinamin (Langemak 1907). As the effects of these agents were very brief, they were abandoned. Only one study in our review has been done on enzymatic

fasciotomy other than collagenase. This was a cohort study (evidence level 3) of only 10 treated hands in 9 patients injected with a mixture of lignocaine, trypsin, and hyaluronidase, with a follow-up of 6.5 years. After 2–3 years 7 patients again had a contracture with similar severity as before the treatment (McCarthy 1992).

5.6.1.2 Corticosteroids

The results of the use of local injections with corticosteroids are contradictory (Baxter et al. 1952; Ketchum and Donahue 2000). Painful nodules without contractures may become less symptomatic following local depot corticosteroid injection (Badalamente and Hurst 2000; Ketchum and Donahue 2000).

5.6.1.3 Clostridial Collagenase

In the last few years, studies have been published on the use of collagenase. (Badalamente et al. 2002; Badalamente and Hurst 2007; Hurst et al. 2009). Some of these have been conducted on the safety and efficacy of collagenase, including a double-blind randomized trial (evidence level 1). Thirty-three patients were treated with collagenase or with a placebo. In 87% of the therapy group, the treatment was successful and the contracture disappeared completely. Nineteen percent had a recurrence within 2 years. There was no effect measured in the control group. As of this writing, this treatment is FDA-approved in the United States, and in Europe, the drug is being tested in selected centers in a phase 3 trial. The treatment might be very risky in inexperienced hands because collagenase does not differentiate between normal and abnormal tissues. Clostridial collagenase acts on types 1 and 3 collagen, which are found not only in affected fibrotic cords but also tendons and retinacular fibers. Nerves have different collagen subtypes (types 2, 16, 28) (Hart 2012) and as such are resistant to Clostridial collagenase.

5.6.2 Radiotherapy

5.6.2.1 Indications

The largest experience with radiotherapy for Dupuytren's comes from Germany. Several studies have reported that local radiotherapy delays the development of contractures in patients who only have nodules or an extension deficit of less than 10° (Seegenschmiedt et al. 2001; Falter et al. 1991; Betz et al. 2010). While an older retrospective cohort study reported no difference in contracture between radiated and non-radiated hands (Weinzierl et al. 1993), a previously unpublished study of radiotherapy on Dupuytren's disease (Seegenschmiedt et al. 2012) demonstrates its efficacy by comparison with a control group.

5.6.2.2 Disadvantages

The disadvantages of this treatment are well known. Radiotherapy is potentially harmful and the side effects vary from relatively harmless erythema and dry skin to carcinogen effects in the long run (Falter et al. 1991). The risk of adverse effects is dose-dependent. Chronic toxicity events occurred in 16% (15/95) of hands treated with 30 Gy of radiation and 11% (11/103) of hands treated with 21 Gy at 3-month follow-up (Seegenschmiedt et al. 2001). Another study reports 31.7% minor long-term changes due to toxicity (Betz et al. 2010).

An added disadvantage is the induction of fibrosis, which may increase risk of later wound healing problems. Randomized clinical trials comparing radiotherapy with controls are missing and necessary to fully disclose the potential of this treatment modality, as some of the outcomes following radiotherapy might be the natural progression of early stage disease.

5.6.3 Treatment with Splints/Splinting

The benefit of preoperative use of splints to prevent contractures has proved to be of no use. Postoperative splinting is controversial and the rationale for this only comes from expert opinion, the lowest level of evidence (Rives et al. 1992; Evans et al. 2002; Jerosch-Herold et al. 2008; Larson and Jerosch-Herold 2008). At the moment, a large randomized trial on the effects of postoperative splinting is under way. An outline of the results is presented elsewhere in this book (Jerosch-Herold et al. 2012).

5.7 Conclusions

There is a wide range of treatment options for patients with Dupuytren's contracture. These options have not been compared to each other extensively. While counseling patients, one should give a realistic picture of the advantages and disadvantages of the different treatment options. The ideal treatment is one which is quick to perform, has little risk of complications, allows early recovery of function with the least possible comorbidity, and the longest possible disease-free period. A specialist who has experience in different techniques is the best to advise the patient. We believe that limited fasciectomy still is the gold-standard treatment. In a randomized trial, we proved that this method is satisfying in the short and long run for many patients, especially for those with a contracture of more than 60°. Needle fasciotomy is elegant because of the minimal invasive nature, but has a high percentage of recurrence, especially in the younger age group. Therefore, needle fasciotomy is in our view not ideal for relatively young patients with a fast progressing Dupuytren's Contracture. For this group and for the patients with a recurrence, the dermofasciectomy seems more appropriate, although comparative research should provide evidence for this. The role of radiotherapy and the injection of collagenase are not yet fully elucidated.

Acknowledgments We would like to thank Marieke Dreise very much for her help in translating our original article.

References

Abe Y, Rokkaku T, Ofuchi S, Tokunaga S, Takahashi K, Moriya H (2004) An objective method to evaluate the risk of recurrence and extension of Dupuytren's disease. J Hand Surg Br 29(5):427–430

Adamietz B, Keilholz L, Grünert J, Sauer R (2001) Radiotherapy of early stage Dupuytren disease. Long-term results after a median follow-up period of 10 years. Strahlenther Onkol 177:604–610

Anthony SG, Lozano-Calderon SA, Simmons BP, Jupiter JB (2008) Gender ratio of Dupuytren's disease in the modern U.S. population. Hand (N Y) 3(2):87–90

Armstrong JR, Hurren JS, Logan AM (2000) Dermofasciectomy in the management of Dupuytren's disease. J Bone Joint Surg Br 82:90–94

Badalamente MA, Hurst LC (2000) Enzyme injection as nonsurgical treatment of Dupuytren's disease. J Hand Surg Am 25: 629–636

Badalamente MA, Hurst LC (2007) Efficacy and safety of injectable mixed collagenase subtypes in the treatment of Dupuytren's contracture. J Hand Surg Am 32:767–774

Badalamente MA, Hurst LC, Hentz VR (2002) Collagen as a clinical target: nonoperative treatment of Dupuytren's disease. J Hand Surg Am 27:788–798

Baxter H, Schiller C, Johnson LH, Whiteside JH, Randall RE (1952) Cortisone therapy in Dupuytren's contracture. Plast Reconstr Surg 9:261–273

Bayat A, Stanley JK, Watson JS, Ferguson MW, Ollier WE (2003) Genetic susceptibility to Dupuytren's disease: transforming growth factor beta receptor (TGFbetaR) gene polymorphisms and Dupuytren's disease. Br J Plast Surg 56:328–333

Betz N, Ott OJ, Adamietz B, Sauer R, Fietkau R, Keilholz L (2010) Radiotherapy in early-stage Dupuytren's contracture. Long-term results after 13 years. Strahlenther Onkol 186(2):82–90

Chick LR, Lister GD (1991) Surgical alternatives in Dupuytren's contracture. Hand Clin 7(4):715–719, discussion 721–2

Clibbon JJ, Logan AM (2001) Palmar segmental aponeurectomy for Dupuytren's disease with metacarpophalangeal flexion contracture. J Hand Surg Br 26:360–361

Descatha A (2012) Dupuytren's Disease and Occupation. In: Dupuytren's disease and related hyperproliferative disorders, pp 45–49

Dolmans GH et al. (2011). Wnt signaling and Dupuytren's disease. N Engl J Med 365(4):307–17

Evans RB, Dell PC, Fiolkowski P (2002) A clinical report of the effect of mechanical stress on functional results after fasciectomy for Dupuytren's contracture. J Hand Ther 15:331–339

Falter E, Herndl E, Mühlbauer W (1991) Dupuytren's contracture. When operate? conservative preliminary treatment? Fortschr Med 9:223–226

Foucher G, Cornil CH, Lenoble E (1992) 'Open palm' technique in Dupuytren's disease. Postoperative complications and results after more than 5 years. Chirurgie 118:189–194

Gudmundsson KG, Arngrimsson R, Sigfusson N et al (2000) Epidemiology of Dupuytren's disease: clinical, serological, and social assessment. The Reykjavik Study. J Clin Epidemiol 53(3):291–296

Hart S (2012) A primer of collagen biology: synthesis, degradation, subtypes and role in Dupuytren's disease. In: Dupuytren's disease and related hyperproliferative disorders, pp 131–142

Hindocha S, John S, Stanley JK, Watson SJ, Bayat A (2006a) The heritability of Dupuytren's disease: familial aggregation and its clinical significance. J Hand Surg Am 31:204–210

Hindocha S, Stanley JK, Watson S, Bayat A (2006b) Dupuytren's diathesis revisited: evaluation of prognostic indicators for risk of disease recurrence. J Hand Surg Am 31(10):1626–1634

Hurst LC, Badalamente MA, Hentz VR, Hotchkiss RN, Kaplan FT, Meals RA, Smith TM, Rodzvilla J, CORD I Study Group (2009) Injectable collagenase clostridium histolyticum for Dupuytren's contracture. N Engl J Med 361(10):968–979

James J, Tubiana R (1952) Dupuytren's disease. Rev Chir Orthop Reparatrice Appar Mot 38:555–562

Jerosch-Herold C, Shepstone L, Chojnowski AJ, Larson D (2008) Splinting after contracture release for Dupuytren's contracture (SCoRD): protocol of a pragmatic, multi-centre, randomized controlled trial. BMC Musculoskelet Disord 9:62

Jerosch-Herold C, Shepstone L, Chojnowski AJ, Larson D (2012) Night-time splinting after fasciectomy or dermofasciectomy for Dupuytren's Contracture a pragmatic, multi-centre, randomized controlled trial. In: Dupuytren's disease and related hyperproliferative disorders, pp 323–332

Jurisic D, Kovic I, Lulic I, Stanec Z, Kapovic M, Uravic M (2008) Dupuytren's disease characteristics in primorsko-goranska county, croatia. Coll Antropol 32(4):1209–1213

Keilholz L, Seegenschmiedt MH, Born AD, Sauer R (1997) Radiotherapy in the early stage of Dupuytren's disease. The indications, technic and long-term results. Strahlenther Onkol 173:27–35

Ketchum L (2012) Expanded Dermofasciectomies and full-thickness grafts in the treatment of Dupuytren's contracture: a 36-year experience. In: Dupuytren's disease and related hyperproliferative disorders, pp 213–220

Ketchum LD, Donahue TK (2000) The injection of nodules of Dupuytren's disease with triamcinolone acetonide. J Hand Surg 25(6):1157–1162

Langemak GE (1907) Zur thiosinaminbehandlung der Dupuytren'schen Faschienkontraktur. Münchener Med Wochenschr 54:1380

Larson D, Jerosch-Herold C (2008) Clinical effectiveness of post-operative splinting after surgical release of Dupuytren's contracture: a systematic review. BMC Musculoskelet Disord 9:104

McCarthy DM (1992) The long-term results of enzymatic fasciotomy. J Hand Surg Br 17:356

McCash CR (1964) The open palm technique in Dupuytren's contracture. Br J Plast Surg 17:271–280

McFarlane RM, McGrouther DA (1990) Complications and their management. In: McFarlane RM, McGrouther DA, Flint M (eds) Dupuytren's disease: biology and treatment. Churchill Livingstone, Edinburgh, pp 377–382

Meyerding HW, Black JR, Broders AC (1941) The etiology and pathology of Dupuytren's contracture. Surg Gynecol Obstet 72:582–590

Misra A, Jain A, Ghazanfar R, Johnston T, Nanchahal J (2007) Predicting the outcome of surgery for the proximal interphalangeal joint in Dupuytren's disease. J Hand Surg 32(2):240–245

Moermans JP (1996) Long-term results after segmental aponeurectomy for Dupuytren's disease. J Hand Surg Br 21(6):797–800

Rehman S, Salway F, Stanley JK, Ollier WE, Day P, Bayat A (2008) Molecular phenotypic descriptors of Dupuytren's disease defined using informatics analysis of the transcriptome. J Hand Surg Am 33:359–372

Rives K, Gelberman R, Smith B, Carney K (1992) Severe contractures of the proximal interphalangeal joint in Dupuytren's disease: results of aprospective trial of operative correction and dynamic extension splinting. J Hand Surg Am 17:1153–1159

Ross DC (1999) Epidemiology of Dupuytren's disease. Hand Clin 15(1):53–62

Seegenschmiedt MH, Olschewski T, Guntrum F (2001) Optimization of radiotherapy in Dupuytren's disease. Initial results of a controlled trial. Strahlenther Onkol 177:74–81

Seegenschmiedt MH, Keilholz L, Wielpütz M, Schubert Ch., Fehlauer F (2012) Long-term outcome of radiotherapy for early stage Dupuytren's disease: a phase III clinical study. In: Dupuytren's disease and related hyperproliferative disorders, pp 349–371

Smith P, Breed C (1994) Central slip attenuation in Dupuytren's contracture: a cause of persistent flexion of the proximal interphalangeal joint. J Hand Surg 19(5):840–843

Thurston AJ (2003) Dupuytren's disease. J Bone Joint Surg Br 85(4):469–477

Van Rijssen AL, Werker PM (2006) Percutaneous needle fasciotomy in Dupuytren's disease. J Hand Surg Br 31:498–501

Van Rijssen AL, Gerbrandy FS, ter Linden H, Klip H, Werker PM (2006) A comparison of the direct outcomes of percutaneous needle fasciotomy and limited fasciectomy for Dupuytren's disease: a 6-week follow-up study. J Hand Surg Am 31:717–725

Van Rijssen AL, Ter Linden H, Werker PMN (2012) 3-year results of first-ever randomised clinical trial on treatment in Dupuytren's disease: percutaneous needle fasciotomy versus limited fasciectomy. In: Dupuytren's disease and related hyperproliferative disorders, pp 281–288

Watt AJ, Curtin CM, Hentz VR (2010) Collagenase injection as nonsurgical treatment of Dupuytren's disease: 8-year follow-up. J Hand Surg Am 35(4):534–539

Weinzierl G, Flügel M, Geldmacher J (1993) Lack of effectiveness of alternative non-surgical treatment procedures of dupuytren contracture. Chirurg 64:492–494

Wilbrand S, Ekbom A, Gerdin B (1999) The sex ratio and rate of reoperation for Dupuytren's contracture in men and women. J Hand Surg Br 24(4):456–459

Dupuytren's Disease and Occupation

6

Alexis Descatha

Contents

6.1	**Introduction**	45
6.2	**History**	45
6.3	**Association**	46
6.4	**Causation**	46
6.5	**Conclusions**	48
References		48

A. Descatha
Inserm U1018, Centre for Research
in Epidemiology and Population Health,
Population-Based Epidémiological Cohorts,
Research platform, Villejuif, France

Université de Versailles St-Quentin,
UMRS 1018, Villejuif, France

Occupational Health Unit, AP-HP,
Poincaré University Hospital, Garches, France
e-mail: alexis.descatha@rpc.aphp.fr

6.1 Introduction

For many decades, a controversy has existed regarding whether acute traumatic injury or cumulative biomechanical work exposure could contribute to the development of Dupuytren's disease (DD). Indeed, it is very surprising that DD, which was initially described as clearly work-related, is now no longer considered to be related to occupational exposure, and its traumatic etiology (isolated trauma, microtrauma) is now questioned. We review arguments for the association between work and DD.

This chapter compiles the essential results of a more detailed review paper (Descatha et al. 2011). It also discusses the causal relationship between work exposure and DD.

6.2 History

In his presentation on December 5, 1831, at the Hotel-Dieu in Paris, Baron Guillaume Dupuytren clearly identified the main lesion of the disorder as contracture of the palmar fascia, which, he asserted, could be surgically treated by incision of the palmar aponeurosis (Dupuytren 1832; Gudmundsson et al. 2003). In that lecture, Baron Dupuytren associated the disease with chronic local trauma caused by occupation: *Most people with this disease have been obliged to do work with the palm of the hand or to handle hard objects. Thus the wine merchant and the coachman whose case histories we will report were accustomed, one to broaching casks with a puncheon or to binding up staves, the other to plying his whip unceasingly on the backs of*

C. Eaton et al. (eds.), *Dupuytren's Disease and Related Hyperproliferative Disorders*,
DOI 10.1007/978-3-642-22697-7_6, © Springer-Verlag Berlin Heidelberg 2012

his jaded horses. We could also cite the example of a clerk in an office who took particular care in applying the seal to his dispatches. It is also found in masons who grasp stones with the end of their fingers, [...]. For this it is clear that the disease affects particularly those who are obliged in their work to use the palm of their hand as a pressure point (Dembe 1996). Previously, Henry Cline, Sr., a prominent London physician, recognized the disease in 1,787 as one contracted by "*laborious people*" (Dembe 1996). In 1822, Sir Astley Cooper attributed the contracture to "*excessive action of the hand, in the use of the hammer, the oar ...*" (Thurston 2003). A year after the lecture of Baron Dupuytren, Goyrand contested the role of manual work and cited the case of his hospital manager with bilateral disease who had "*never put the day of hard work*" (Thurston 2003) – thus began the debate.

In 1912, a government comity in the United Kingdom examined the possibility of the relationship between trauma and DD and found that there was no conclusive relationship (Elliot 1999).

6.3 Association

Since the middle of the twentieth century, published studies from the United Kingdom, France, Australia, and Norway described the relationship between manual work and DD with contradictory results (Herzog 1951; Hueston 1960; Early 1962; Chanut 1963; Mikkelsen 1978; Bennett 1982; Attali et al. 1987; Niezborala et al. 1995). Other authors have investigated the association between vibration and DD (Landgrot et al. 1975; Patri et al. 1982; Cocco et al. 1987; Thomas and Clarke 1992; Bovenzi 1994).

A systematic review, published in 1996 to address the apparently conflicting results regarding the possible work-related origin of this disease, examined evidence for the association between repetitive manual work or hand vibration and DD (Liss and Stock 1996). Based on ten papers included, the authors concluded that there was good evidence to support an association between vibration exposure and Dupuytren's contracture and a weaker evidence for an association with manual work: only one of the five studies satisfied the authors' criteria for methodological quality (Liss and Stock 1996).

Despite this comprehensive review, subsequent publications have not considered occupational exposure and vibration as risk factors for Dupuytren's contracture

(Burge 2004; Townley et al. 2006; Hindocha et al. 2009). Conflicting results have been published in the last 10 years: a study with a precise exposure assessment found an elevated risk in only certain job categories and did not find a significant association between vibration and exposure (Seidler et al. 2001); another large population-based study did not find increased incidence of "significant" DD based on work status (Khan et al. 2004). In contrast, other studies have supported an association between occupational work (manual work and vibration) and Dupuytren's contracture (Gudmundsson et al. 2000; Lucas et al. 2008). Table 6.1 describes all the epidemiological studies on work association with the control group and details on exposure: 10 out of 14 studies found positive association. A recent meta-analysis supported the hypothesis of an association between high levels of work exposure (meta-OR for manual work was 2.0 [1.6; 2.6] and was 2.9 [1.4; 6.1] for vibration exposure) and Dupuytren's contracture in certain cases (Descatha et al. 2011).

6.4 Causation

Association does not mean causation, and different criteria should be considered as evidence for a causal relationship. The Hill's criteria have been used and improved to study causal association in observational research (Grimes and Schulz 2002). The following summarizes a criteria-based assessment of the relationship of occupation to the presence of Dupuytren's contracture.

1. *Temporal sequence* (did exposure precede outcome?): Yes. The involved exposure is a high cumulative physical exposure during the working life based on retrospective evaluation in most studies; two longitudinal prospective studies exist (Gudmundsson et al. 2000; Godtfredsen et al. 2004).
2. *Strength of association* (how strong is the effect?): Moderate. The mean odds ratio is between 2.0 and 2.5 (Table 6.1), and the meta-OR, between 2.0 and 3.0.
3. *Consistency of association* (effect seen by others?): Yes, as stated previously (Liss and Stock 1996; Gudmundsson et al. 2000; Lucas et al. 2008).
4. *Biological gradient* (increase exposure result in more of the outcome?): Yes. Five studies found a clear dose–response relationship (Mikkelsen 1978; Cocco et al. 1987; Bovenzi 1994; Niezborala et al. 1995; Lucas et al. 2008).

Table 6.1 Studies on association in Dupuytren's disease (DD, only valid studies with control group and details on exposure have been included)

Name	Country	Type of study	Number of patients with Dupuytren's disease	Criteria for odds ratios (OR)	OR	(Confidence interval 95%)
Herzog 1951	United Kingdom	Cross-sectional	61 (including 22 steelworkers and 21 miners)	Steelworkers vs. clerical Miners vs. clerical	1.2 1.3	0.6 2.3 0.6 2.5
Early 1962	United Kingdom	Cross-sectional	151 (134 in Crewe locomotive works with manual work, 17 in office)	Manual vs. clerical	0.98	0.6 1.7
Chanut 1963	France	Cross-sectional	378 (25 in stoneworker, 130 in clerks, and 223 others)	Stonemasons vs. others	14.57	9.53 22.51
Mikkelsen 1978	Norway	Population survey	647 men with DD (including 70 in heavy manual work) and 254 women with DD (including 1 in heavy manual group)	Heavy work vs. light (men and women)	3.1	2.2 4.4
Bennett 1982	United Kingdom	Cross-sectional	17 (16 in bagging – 1 in the control group)	Bagging plant vs. nonbagging plant	5.5	0.8 36.7
Attali et al. 1987	France	Cross-sectional	78 (56 with liver disease and 22 controls)	Manual workers	2.46	1.49 4.06
Cocco et al. 1987	Italy	Case-control	180 (paired with 180 controls on sex, age, date of hospitalization)	>20 years of exposure vs. controls	3	1.3 6.7
Thomas and Clarke 1992	United Kingdom	Cross-sectional	78 (62 in the exposed group)	Vibration-exposed vs. hospital admission	2.1	1.1 3.9
Bovenzi 1994	Italy	Cross-sectional	66 (57 in workers group, 9 controls)	Quarry drillers vs. controls Masons and stonecarvers vs. controls	2.58 2.6	1.07 6.2 1.24 5.49
Niezborala et al. 1995	France	Case-control	121 (including 29 in the high-exposure group)	Case-control study (masons and lumberjack vs. others, longest job) Cross-sectional study (exposed=builders and farmers vs. others)	2.41 7.5	1.18 4.92 2.21 24.7
Gudmundsson et al. 2000	Iceland	Cohort	249 (including 38 in manual labor, 36 tradesmen)	Manual labor (seamen, farmer) vs. controls Skilled trades (masons, carpenters, blacksmith) vs. controls	1.75 1.91	1.14 2.7 1.24 2.96
Seidler et al. 2001	Germany	Case-control	317 (including 17 exposed to vibration >20 h/week and over 20 years)	>20 h/weeks over 20 years of vibration	1.3	0.6 2.7
Godtfredsen et al. 2004	Denmark	Cohort	772	Low education level (considered as a proxy for manual labor) vs. high	1.6	1.2 2.1
Lucas et al. 2008	France	Cross-sectional	212 (including 106 in high-exposure group and 47 in high-vibration group)	High cumulative work exposure vs. low	3.1	1.99 4.84

5. *Specificity of the association* (does exposure lead only to outcome?): No. Other conditions could lead to Dupuytren's disease, and high exposure of physical constraints could lead to other musculoskeletal disorders, with a probable genetic predisposition involved (McFarlane 2002; Hart and Hooper 2005; Hindocha et al. 2009).

6. *Biological plausibility* (does the association make sense?): Yes. DD is currently considered to be a fibroproliferative disorder, with dysfunction of connective tissue and fibroblast proliferation (Thurston 2003). The roles of high levels of repetitive strain and vibration exposure are plausible, especially as a result of the local hypoxia and chronic ischemia hypothesized in DD (Hart and Hooper 2005; Schubert et al. 2006). There is also a documented relationship between tissue tension and biologic activity of DD (Evans et al. 2002; Howard et al. 2003; Bisson et al. 2009), such as inflammatory changes accompanied by peripheral nervous and tissue injuries and central nervous system reorganization (Barr et al. 2004).

7. *Coherence with existing knowledge* (is the association consistent with available evidence?): Yes. There is a consistency of the association and history of Dupuytren's disease.

8. *Experimental evidence* (have randomized controlled trials been done?): Not Applicable. No randomized control trials could be ethically performed in such topic.

9. *Analogy* (is the association similar to the others?): Yes. Although odds ratios vary (Table 6.1), there is a similar magnitude of strength of association found in studies with similar high-quality design and population.

6.5 Conclusions

In conclusion, there is evidence that exposure of the hands to high cumulative physical force and/or vibration might cause or significantly aggravate Dupuytren's disease. However, only high cumulative exposure is potentially implicated, and other medical risk factors must also be considered. Long-term longitudinal studies on large samples, taking into account the effects of interactions with other risk factors, are needed to further clarify whether or not Dupuytren's disease is caused or significantly aggravated by high cumulative exposure to mechanical forces. Based on available evidence, preventative steps should be considered to reduce such exposure at the workplace, and possible aggravation or causation be considered in cases with documented high levels of occupational exposure and few other risk factors.

References

Attali P, Ink O, Pelletier G, Vernier C, Jean F, Moulton L, Etienne JP (1987) Dupuytren's contracture, alcohol consumption, and chronic liver disease. Arch Intern Med 147:1065–1067

Barr AE, Barbe MF, Clark BD (2004) Work-related musculoskeletal disorders of the hand and wrist: epidemiology, pathophysiology, and sensorimotor changes. J Orthop Sports Phys Ther 34:610–627

Bennett B (1982) Dupuytren's contracture in manual workers. Br J Ind Med 39:98–100

Bisson MA, Beckett KS, McGrouther DA, Grobbelaar AO, Mudera V (2009) Transforming growth factor-ß1 stimulation enhances Dupuytren's fibroblast contraction in response to uniaxial mechanical load within a 3-dimensional collagen Gel. J Hand Surg 34(6):1102–1110

Bovenzi M (1994) Hand-arm vibration syndrome and dose-response relation for vibration induced white finger among quarry drillers and stonecarvers. Italian Study Group on Physical Hazards in the Stone Industry. Occup Environ Med 51:603–611

Burge PD (2004) Dupuytren's disease. J Bone Joint Surg Br 86: 1088–1089

Chanut JC (1963) Dupuytren's disease. Arch Mal Prof 24: 621–625

Cocco PL, Frau P, Rapallo M, Casula D (1987) Occupational exposure to vibration and Dupuytren's disease: a case-controlled study. Med Lav 78:386–392

Dembe A (1996) Occupation and disease: How social factors affect the conception of work-related disorders. Yale University Press, Yale, New Haven and London, CT, pp p54–p56

Descatha A, Jauffret P, Chastang JF, Roquelaure Y, Leclerc A (2011) Should we consider Dupuytren's contracture as work-related? a review and meta-analysis of an old debate. BMC Musculoskel Dis 12:96

Dupuytren G (1832) Leçons orales de clinique chirurgicale, faites à l'Hôtel-Dieu. Baillère librairie, Paris, pp 2–24

Early PF (1962) Population studies in Dupuytren's contracture. J Bone Joint Surg 44B:602–612

Elliot D (1999) The early history of Dupuytren's disease. Hand Clin 15:1–19

Evans RB, Dell PC, Fiolkowski P (2002) A clinical report of the effect of mechanical stress on functional results after fasciectomy for Dupuytren's contracture. J Hand Ther 15(4): 331–339

Godtfredsen NS, Lucht H, Prescott E, Sorensen TI, Gronbaek M (2004) A prospective study linked both alcohol and tobacco to Dupuytren's disease. J Clin Epidemiol 57:358–863

Grimes DA, Schulz KF (2002) Bias and causal associations in observational research. Lancet 359:248–252

Gudmundsson KG, Arngrimsson R, Sigfusson N, Bjornsson A, Jonsson T (2000) Epidemiology of Dupuytren's disease:

clinical, serological, and social assessment. The Reykjavik study. J Clin Epidemiol 53:291–296

Gudmundsson KG, Jonsson T, Arngrimsson R (2003) Guillaume Dupuytren and finger contractures. Lancet 362:165–168

Hart MG, Hooper G (2005) Clinical associations of Dupuytren's disease. Postgrad Med J 81:425–428

Herzog EG (1951) The aetiology of Dupuytren's contracture. Lancet 257:1305–1306

Hindocha S, McGrouther DA, Bayat A (2009) Epidemiological evaluation of Dupuytren's disease incidence and prevalence rates in relation to etiology. Hand 4:256–269

Howard JC, Varallo VM, Ross DC, Roth JH, Farber KJ, Alman B, Gan BS (2003) Elevated levels of ß-catenin and fibronectin in three-dimensional collagen cultures of Dupuytren's disease cells are regulated by tension in vitro. BMC Musculoskel Dis 4(16):1–12

Hueston JT (1960) The incidence of Dupuytren's contracture. Med J Aust 47:999–1002

Khan AA, Rider OJ, Jayadev CU, Heras-Palou C, Giele H, Goldacre M (2004) The role of manual occupation in the aetiology of Dupuytren's disease in men in England and Wales. J Hand Surg Br 29:12–14

Landgrot B, Huzl F, Koudela K, Potmesil J, Sykora J (1975) The incidence of Dupuytren's contracture in workers in hazards of vibrations. Pracov Lek 27:331–335

Liss GM, Stock SR (1996) Can Dupuytren's contracture be work-related? - review of the evidence. Am J Ind Med 29:521–532

Lucas G, Brichet A, Roquelaure Y, Leclerc A, Descatha A (2008) Dupuytren's disease: personal factors and occupational exposure. Am J Ind Med 51:9–15

McFarlane RM (2002) On the origin and spread of Dupuytren's disease. J Hand Surg Am 27:385–390

Mikkelsen OA (1978) Dupuytren's disease - the influence of occupation and previous hand injuries. Hand 10:1–8

Niezborala M, Le Pors N, Teyssier-Cotte C, Tropet Y, Vichard P (1995) Arguments in favour of the occupational aetiology of Dupuytren's contracture. Arch Mal Prof 56:613–619

Patri B, Vaysseairat M, Guilmot JL, Delemotte B, Borredon JJ, Nastorg C (1982) Epidemiology and clinical evaluation of vibration white finger syndrome in lumbermen. Arch Mal Prof 43:253–259

Schubert TE, Weidler C, Borisch N, Schubert C, Hofstadter F, Straub RH (2006) Dupuytren's contracture is associated with sprouting of substance P positive nerve fibres and infiltration by mast cells. Ann Rheum Dis 65:414–415

Seidler A, Stolte R, Heiskel H, Nienhaus A, Windolf J, Elsner G (2001) Occupational, consumption-related and disease-related risk factors for Dupuytren's contracture: results of a case-control study. Arbeitsmed Sozialmed Umweltmed 36:218–228

Thomas PR, Clarke D (1992) Vibration white finger and Dupuytren's contracture: are they related? Occup Med (Lond) 42:155–158

Thurston AJ (2003) Dupuytren's disease. J Bone Joint Surg Br 85:469–477

Townley WA, Baker R, Sheppard N, Grobbelaar AO (2006) Dupuytren's contracture unfolded. BMJ 332:397–400

Part II

The Myofibroblast

Editor: Giulio Gabbiani

The Role of the Myofibroblast in Dupuytren's Disease: Fundamental Aspects of Contraction and Therapeutic Perspectives

7

Boris Hinz and Giulio Gabbiani

Contents

7.1	Introduction	53
7.2	Origin of the Myofibroblast	53
7.3	Fundamental Aspects of Myofibroblast Contraction	54
7.4	Myofibroblast Mechanics and the Stiffness of Tissue	55
7.5	Therapeutic Perspectives	56
7.6	Conclusions	58
References		58

7.1 Introduction

The identification of the myofibroblast as the prevalent cell in the Dupuytren's nodule (Gabbiani and Majno 1972) has opened the perspective that this cell is crucial for the production of contractile phenomena leading to the formation of cords and to the establishment of contracture. Myofibroblasts are characterized by the neo-expression of α-smooth muscle actin (α-SMA), the actin isoform typical of vascular smooth muscle that confers to these cells their typical contractile activity (Tomasek et al. 2002). Myofibroblasts have been shown to participate in a large number of physiological and pathological phenomena characterized by connective tissue remodeling and in many cases, as in Dupuytren's disease, by tissue deformation (Tomasek et al. 2002). Although the main biological activities of the myofibroblast, i.e., contractile force generation and collagen production (Tomasek et al. 2002), are the same in different pathological situations, they can originate from a variety of sources (Hinz et al. 2007); this suggests that the myofibroblast represents a physiological status rather than a cell type.

7.2 Origin of the Myofibroblast

It is generally accepted that myofibroblasts derive from local fibroblasts and more broadly from local mesenchymal cells, such as resident stem cells, pericytes, or smooth muscle cells (Gabbiani and Majno 1972; Humphreys et al. 2010). In most instances, this is probably the case; however, recent studies demonstrated

B. Hinz (✉)
Laboratory of Tissue Repair and Regeneration,
Matrix Dynamics Group, Faculty of Dentistry,
University of Toronto, Toronto, ON, Canada
e-mail: boris.hinz@utoronto.ca

G. Gabbiani
Department of Pathology and Immunology,
C.M.U., University of Geneva,
Geneva, Switzerland
e-mail: giulio.gabbiani@unige.ch

C. Eaton et al. (eds.), *Dupuytren's Disease and Related Hyperproliferative Disorders*,
DOI 10.1007/978-3-642-22697-7_7, © Springer-Verlag Berlin Heidelberg 2012

several hitherto unexpected origins, which open new perspectives in the interpretation of physiological and pathological mechanisms in which myofibroblasts are implicated. Epithelial–mesenchymal transition, endothelial–mesenchymal transition, and myofibroblast development from bone marrow–derived cells have been clearly demonstrated both in physiological and pathological situations, such as lung and kidney fibrosis (Li and Bertram 2010; Thiery 2002). This renders it more complex to interpret which pathways regulate tissue remodeling. The respective role of each mechanism of myofibroblast differentiation during different physiological and pathological phenomena, including Dupuytren's disease, has not yet been established (Hinz and Gabbiani 2010). Further work in these directions will be crucial to better understand: (a) organ formation during embryology, as well as (b) the pathogenesis of fibrotic lesions or of stroma reaction during epithelial carcinogenesis.

7.3 Fundamental Aspects of Myofibroblast Contraction

Myofibroblast contraction in Dupuytren's disease results in irreversible contractures of the palmar connective tissue over days, months, and even years. The basis for global tissue remodeling is the contraction of single myofibroblasts and the subsequent stabilization of the contracture by secreted collagens and other ECM molecules (Follonier Castella et al. 2010b; Tomasek et al. 2002). However, the mode of contraction at the single cell level and the mechanisms involved in this process remain largely unclear. The question of how myofibroblast contraction is controlled may partly be answered by positioning this phenotype in a continuous differentiation spectrum between fibroblastic cells and smooth muscle cells. Typical fibroblastic features of the myofibroblast are the expression collagen type I, vimentin, and non-muscle myosins (Hinz et al. 2007), whereas its characteristic smooth muscle cell features include the expression of α-SMA and the generation of high contractile force (Hinz et al. 2001). Depending on their origin and the specific in vivo or in vitro conditions, myofibroblasts may exhibit features that are closer to one or the other end of this spectrum.

The retractile nature of the connective tissue remodeling resulting in pathological scar tissue implies that myofibroblasts exert a contractile activity which is somehow

different from the classical calcium-dependent contraction of smooth muscle cells. Two principal pathways have been described to act through various stimuli and agonists in non-muscle cells and smooth muscle cells. Both pathways ultimately determine the phosphorylation state of the myosin light chain (MLC), which controls actin–myosin contraction. One pathway regulates the activity of the enzyme that phosphorylates the MLC, the MLC kinase, through changes in the concentration of cytosolic calcium interacting with calmodulin. The resulting contraction is rather rapid and transient because the phosphate is constitutively removed from the MLC by the MLC phosphatase. The second contraction-regulating pathway controls the activity of the MLC phosphatase through the small GTPase RhoA and its downstream target Rho-(associated) kinase (ROCK or ROK). Active RhoA activates ROCK which in turn inactivates MLC phosphatase (Kimura et al. 1996), resulting in continued phosphorylation of MLC and persistent actin–myosin contraction. In addition, ROCK directly phosphorylates MLC, although less effectively than MLC kinase (Amano et al. 2000).

The long-lasting and irreversible outcome of myofibroblast contraction has stimulated the idea that it is predominantly regulated by Rho/ROCK-mediated inhibition of MLC phosphatase (Parizi et al. 2000; Tomasek et al. 2006). This would be similar to what has been described for fibroblasts (Katoh et al. 2001). Other reports have suggested that myofibroblast contraction is regulated by changes in intracellular calcium concentration and MLC kinase (Follonier et al. 2008; Furuya et al. 2005; Goto et al. 1998; Levinson et al. 2004; Raizman et al. 2007), which is well described for phenotype-related smooth muscle cells (Kamm and Stull 1989). Using a two-dimensional culture system, we could recently demonstrate that calcium and Rho/ROCK regulate specific features of myofibroblast contraction which are in turn regulated separately within the same cell (Follonier Castella et al. 2010a). We simultaneously assessed: (1) intracellular calcium concentration changes using calcium-sensitive dyes, (2) subcellular stress fiber contraction by tracking ECM-coated microbeads that are linked through transmembrane integrins, and (3) overall cell contraction by recording distortions (wrinkles) in deformable silicone substrates (Fig. 7.1). We revealed that oscillations of intracellular calcium coordinate the contraction of stress fibers which are connected with beads on the cell surface, whereas Rho/ROCK controls

7 The Role of the Myofibroblast in Dupuytren's Disease: Fundamental Aspects

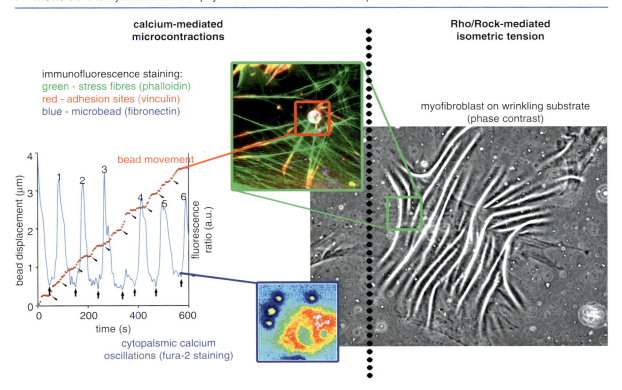

Fig. 7.1 Two modes of myofibroblast contraction. In a culture model of myofibroblasts grown on deformable (*wrinkling*) substrates, two modes of contraction function simultaneously but are controlled by different signaling pathways. Oscillating cytosolic calcium controls stress fiber microcontractions that displace matrix-coated microbeads under low mechanical resistance on the cell surface. The Rho/ROCK pathways control overall isometric cell contraction, indicated by persisting wrinkles in the elastic substrate

long-lasting isometric tension of stress fibers that are engaged with the elastic substrate (Fig. 7.1). Both mechanisms act essentially independent from each other and could be blocked separately by different effectors (Follonier Castella et al. 2010b). In cultured myofibroblasts, cytosolic calcium oscillations were shown to correlate with ~400 nm small and ~100 pN weak contractile events that occur with a regular period of ~100 s (Follonier Castella et al. 2010a). With all caution that should be taken to translate such in vitro studies to the tissue level, this would correspond to ECM shortenings of several centimeters over a period of months which is in the range of the pathological tissue contractures observed in Dupuytren's disease and fibrosis.

Based on these results, we refined the lock-step model for long-term tissue contracture proposed in earlier works (Tomasek et al. 2002): Rho/ROCK mediates strong isometric and overall cell contraction, which releases individual collagen fibrils from the tension that arises during tissue remodeling. These locally relaxed fibrils are then pulled towards the cell center by periodic calcium-dependent microcontractions until the weak subcellular contractile events are opposed by gradually increasing stress acting on the fibrils. The shorter ECM fibril configuration is subsequently stabilized by yet unexplored mechanisms and can again sustain mechanical loads. Stabilization and reorganization may include local collagen digestion, deposition of new collagen fibrils, and cross-linking with the existent ECM. To this end, myofibroblast isometric tension is no longer needed, and cells are able to re-spread. Repetitions of this cycle are expected to result in incremental and irreversible tissue contracture.

7.4 Myofibroblast Mechanics and the Stiffness of Tissue

Major clinical problems caused by the myofibroblast in Dupuytren's are progression of the disease and its reoccurrence after surgical intervention. Once myofibroblast activities have been initiated, it is clearly difficult to control and to terminate its destructive activity. Partly this is caused by the constant mechanical feedback that the cells receive from the ECM. Stiffer ECM leads to higher myofibroblast contraction and ECM secretion which again leads to further ECM stiffening. Consequently, fibrotic lesions are stiffer compared with the tissue compliance of the most non-fibrotic organs (Hinz 2010), which is obvious in Dupuytren's nodules and cords. Here, the non-compliant and shortened collagen bundles dramatically impede the movement of fingers, resisting even skeletal muscle force and resulting in functional loss of the hand.

Although this mechanical feedback mechanism has severe consequences when it becomes dysregulated, it is crucial for myofibroblast function. The overall goal of myofibroblast activity is to rapidly re-establish integrity of damaged tissue by secreting and organizing new ECM. The mechanical state of the ECM provides the reparative cells with valuable information about the progress and success of the repair process. The provisional ECM present after acute tissue injury, e.g., the fibrin clot of dermal wounds, is estimated to be very compliant with a Young's modulus of 10–1,000 Pa. The Young's modulus is defined by the force per unit area (stress) that is required to strain a given material. High stress must be applied to elongate materials with high Young's modulus. Fibroblasts cannot develop contractile features (stress fibers) and form only very small and immature adhesions with the ECM when grown on very soft (10–1,000 Pa) two-dimensional polyacrylamide gels and in three-dimensional soft collagen gels in vitro (Grinnell and Petroll 2010; Yeung et al. 2005). Stress fibers, i.e., the hallmark of the myofibroblast, are produced only on stiffer culture substrates that exhibit an elastic modulus of at least 3,000 Pa. At this stage, these so-called proto-myofibroblasts form α-SMA-negative stress fibers that terminate in mature adhesion sites (FAs) (Yeung et al. 2005). Stiffer culture substrates with a Young's modulus of ~20,000 Pa and higher are required to permit terminal myofibroblast differentiation. The differentiated myofibroblast is characterized by expression of α-SMA in stress fibers and formation of large supermature focal adhesion sites (Dugina et al. 2001; Goffin et al. 2006). Corresponding to the threshold stiffness for myofibroblast differentiation in vitro, various fibrotic tissues were shown to exhibit a Young's modulus of 25,000–50,000 Pa (Goffin et al. 2006; Li et al. 2007; Liu et al. 2010).

Since tissue stiffening seems to be both consequence and cause for myofibroblast-generated contracture, we are left with the classical chicken-and-egg question. What is initiating this vicious, mechanical loop – are fibroblasts first becoming contractile to stiffen the ECM, or is ECM stiffening preceding the fibrotic process? Studies on liver fibrosis have recently suggested that even minute increases in tissue stiffness following tissue injury and inflammation may be sufficient to trigger the mechanical cascade ultimately leading to myofibroblast formation (Georges et al. 2007; Wells 2008). It remains unknown how this initial ECM stiffening can occur even before actively remodeling fibroblasts arrive at the site of injury. One of several possibilities is initial stiffening of the collagenous ECM by cross-linking enzymes, as recently suggested for lysyl oxidase-like-2 (LOX-2) in different fibrotic conditions (Barry-Hamilton et al. 2010). It has to be noted that Dupuytren's disease is one of the few fibrotic conditions where local injection of collagen-digesting enzymes is feasible and appears to be able to halt or even resolve the progress of tissue contracture (Hurst et al. 2009). The effects of this treatment on myofibroblast persistence and re-appearance and the contribution of loss of stress have yet to be determined.

7.5 Therapeutic Perspectives

The recognition that myofibroblasts are responsible for the main phenomena resulting in fibrosis and retraction, such as mechanical force production and collagen synthesis, has indicated that these cells represent a very relevant target of therapeutic strategies for these conditions (Hinz 2009; Hinz and Gabbiani 2010). Myofibroblast differentiation depends on the coordinated action of TGF-β1 and the ED-A domain of cellular fibronectin (FN) (Serini et al. 1998). The use of TGF-β1 inhibiting drugs has been relatively unsuccessful (Howell et al. 2005; Liu et al. 2006; Meier and Nanney 2006; Varga and Pasche 2009), indicating that the control of myofibroblast activity is more complex than expected. One alternative strategy may be to prevent TGF-β1 activation in a cell type–specific manner, rather than blocking the active TGF-β1 (Jenkins 2008; Wipff and Hinz 2008). Myofibroblasts secrete TGF-β1 in a biologically latent form as part of a large complex

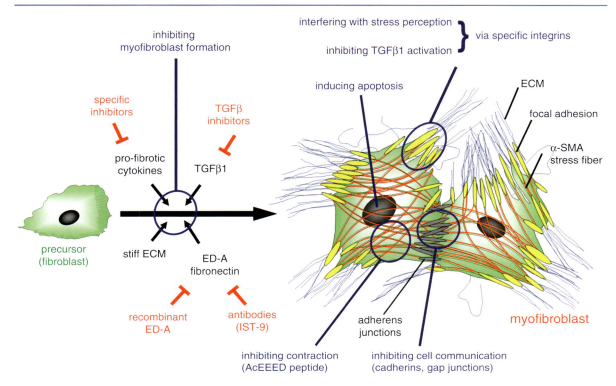

Fig. 7.2 Potential therapeutic targets in the myofibroblast. Antifibrotic therapies can potentially interfere with chemical and mechanical key elements of the pathways that control myofibroblast differentiation from different precursor cells (which is here a fibroblast). In addition, one can possibly target specific features of the differentiated myofibroblast to induce myofibroblast regression and/or apoptosis. Reproduced with permission of the Faculty of 1000 Biology Reports (Hinz and Gabbiani 2010)

that is incorporated into the ECM. One mechanism how myofibroblasts activate TGF-β1 from this reservoir is to pull the latent complex using specific integrins (Wipff et al. 2007). Inhibition of integrin αvβ6, an epithelium-specific TGF-β1 activator, protects the lung from fibrosis (Horan et al. 2008). No such treatment is available for the fibrosis in other organs promoted by myofibroblast activation of TGF-β1, and the integrins involved in this process are under investigation (Goodwin and Jenkins 2009; Margadant and Sonnenberg 2010; Nishimura 2009; Tenney and Discher 2009; Wipff and Hinz 2008). First evidence has been provided that blocking integrin αvβ5 potentially inhibits activation of latent TGF-β1 by lung myofibroblasts (Wipff et al. 2007; Zhou et al. 2010).

More generally, interference with specific ECM receptors emerges as a therapeutic approach with great potential. Recently, it has been reported that α4β7 integrin binds to ED-A FN and thus activates the kinase pathways MAPK-Erk1/2 and FAK (Kohan et al. 2010). This in turn stimulates α-SMA and collagen expression and results in increased tension production (Kohan et al. 2010). These results indicate that both the ED-A sequence and α4β7 integrin could represent targets for anti-fibrotic therapeutic strategies. Further, integrins are attractive target proteins to therapeutically intercept the myofibroblast contraction–ECM stiffening loop, either by targeting force generation, ECM adhesion, or stress perception. Inhibition of α3 integrin (Bryant et al. 2009), α11 integrin, (Carracedo et al. 2010), αvβ3 integrin (Hinz 2006), and β1 integrin (Chan et al. 2010) were all shown to inhibit myofibroblast differentiation, which may be exploited for future therapies. Figure 7.2 summarizes the possible approaches to influence myofibroblast contractile activity and hence connective tissue retraction.

Another interesting direction to decrease fibrotic changes that could be relevant for Dupuytren's disease is the induction of myofibroblast apoptosis. Several experimental attempts have been made on this direction (de Andrade and Thannickal 2009; Horowitz et al. 2007), and hopefully we shall see results based on this strategy in a near future. Interferon-γ has been shown to decrease α-SMA expression and force production in cultured myofibroblasts (Hindman et al. 2003; Pittet et al. 1994) (Tanaka et al. 2003), at least in part through its TGF-β1 inhibitory capacity. A preliminary clinical study has also indicated that interferon-γ is active in reducing the size of hypertrophic scars and Dupuytren's lesions (Pittet et al. 1994); however, these results await confirmation.

7.6 Conclusions

Although several aspects of myofibroblast biology need to be further clarified, it appears established that this cell plays a crucial role in the tissue remodeling processes characterizing fibrotic situations including Dupuytren's disease (Hinz et al. 2007). Thus, the myofibroblast appears as an ideal target for strategies aiming at reducing nodule expansion and retractile phenomena typical of this disease. As we have discussed, many approaches can be considered in order to achieve these goals; further knowledge of myofibroblast biology will certainly facilitate many of them. We have selected to work on the possibility that the α-SMA N-terminal peptide Ac-EEED reduced fibrotic changes in view of the observations that its application to cultured myofibroblasts and to experimental wound tissues reduces both granulation tissue contraction and collagen type I expression (Hinz and Gabbiani 2010; Hinz et al. 2002). It will be important to identify the putative partner of the peptide in inducing actin polymerization and stress fiber formation. The use of the peptide, once introduced safely and efficiently into myofibroblastic cells, should represent a new tool to reduce myofibroblast pathological activities and hence clinical manifestations.

Acknowledgments The work of BH is supported by grants from the Heart and Stroke Foundation Ontario (NA7086), the Collaborative Health Research Programme CHRP/NSERC (#1004005), and the Canadian Institutes of Health Research (#210820). Drs. L. Follonier Castella and L. Buscemi are acknowledged for providing expert help and images.

References

Amano M, Fukata Y, Kaibuchi K (2000) Regulation and functions of Rho-associated kinase. Exp Cell Res 261:44–51

Barry-Hamilton V, Spangler R, Marshall D, McCauley S, Rodriguez HM, Oyasu M, Mikels A, Vaysberg M,

Ghermazien H, Wai C et al (2010) Allosteric inhibition of lysyl oxidase-like-2 impedes the development of a pathologic microenvironment. Nat Med 16:1009–1017

Bryant JE, Shamhart PE, Luther DJ, Olson ER, Koshy JC, Costic DJ, Mohile MV, Dockry M, Doane KJ, Meszaros JG (2009) Cardiac myofibroblast differentiation is attenuated by alpha(3) integrin blockade: potential role in post-MI remodeling. J Mol Cell Cardiol 46:186–192

Carracedo S, Lu N, Popova SN, Jonsson R, Eckes B, Gullberg D (2010) The fibroblast integrin alpha11beta1 is induced in a mechanosensitive manner involving activin A and regulates myofibroblast differentiation. J Biol Chem 285:10434–10445

Chan MW, Chaudary F, Lee W, Copeland JW, McCulloch CA (2010) Force-induced myofibroblast differentiation through collagen receptors is dependent on mammalian diaphanous (mDia). J Biol Chem 285:9273–9281

de Andrade J, Thannickal VJ (2009) Innovative approaches to the therapy of fibrosis. Curr Opin Rheumatol 21(6):649–655

Dugina V, Fontao L, Chaponnier C, Vasiliev J, Gabbiani G (2001) Focal adhesion features during myofibroblastic differentiation are controlled by intracellular and extracellular factors. J Cell Sci 114:3285–3296

Follonier Castella L, Buscemi L, Godbout C, Meister JJ, Hinz B (2010a) A new lock-step mechanism of matrix remodelling based on subcellular contractile events. J Cell Sci 123:1751–1760

Follonier Castella L, Gabbiani G, McCulloch CA, Hinz B (2010b) Regulation of myofibroblast activities: calcium pulls some strings behind the scene. Exp Cell Res 316:2390–2401

Follonier L, Schaub S, Meister JJ, Hinz B (2008) Myofibroblast communication is controlled by intercellular mechanical coupling. J Cell Sci 121:3305–3316

Furuya K, Sokabe M, Furuya S (2005) Characteristics of subepithelial fibroblasts as a mechano-sensor in the intestine: cell-shape-dependent ATP release and P2Y1 signaling. J Cell Sci 118:3289–3304

Gabbiani G, Majno G (1972) Dupuytren's Contracture: fibroblast contraction? An ultrastructural study. Am J Pathol 66:131–146

Georges PC, Hui JJ, Gombos Z, McCormick ME, Wang AY, Uemura M, Mick R, Janmey PA, Furth EE, Wells RG (2007) Increased stiffness of the rat liver precedes matrix deposition: implications for fibrosis. Am J Physiol Gastrointest Liver Physiol 293:G1147–G1154

Goffin JM, Pittet P, Csucs G, Lussi JW, Meister JJ, Hinz B (2006) Focal adhesion size controls tension-dependent recruitment of alpha-smooth muscle actin to stress fibers. J Cell Biol 172:259–268

Goodwin A, Jenkins G (2009) Role of integrin-mediated TGFbeta activation in the pathogenesis of pulmonary fibrosis. Biochem Soc Trans 37:849–854

Goto T, Yanaga F, Ohtsuki I (1998) Studies on the endothelin-1-induced contraction of rat granulation tissue pouch mediated by myofibroblasts. Biochim Biophys Acta 1405:55–66

Grinnell F, Petroll WM (2010) Cell motility and mechanics in three-dimensional collagen matrices. Annu Rev Cell Dev Biol 26:335–361

Hindman HB, Marty-Roix R, Tang JB, Jupiter JB, Simmons BP, Spector M (2003) Regulation of expression of alpha-smooth muscle actin in cells of Dupuytren's contracture. J Bone Joint Surg Br 85:448–455

Hinz B (2006) Masters and servants of the force: the role of matrix adhesions in myofibroblast force perception and transmission. Eur J Cell Biol 85:175–181

Hinz B (2009) Tissue stiffness, latent TGF-beta1 activation, and mechanical signal transduction: implications for the pathogenesis and treatment of fibrosis. Curr Rheumatol Rep 11:120–126

Hinz B (2010) The myofibroblast: paradigm for a mechanically active cell. J Biomech 43:146–155

Hinz B, Gabbiani G (2010) Fibrosis: recent advances in myofibroblast biology and new therapeutic perspectives. F1000 Biol Rep 2:78–82

Hinz B, Celetta G, Tomasek JJ, Gabbiani G, Chaponnier C (2001) Alpha-smooth muscle actin expression upregulates fibroblast contractile activity. Mol Biol Cell 12: 2730–2741

Hinz B, Gabbiani G, Chaponnier C (2002) The NH2-terminal peptide of alpha-smooth muscle actin inhibits force generation by the myofibroblast in vitro and in vivo. J Cell Biol 157:657–663

Hinz B, Phan SH, Thannickal VJ, Galli A, Bochaton-Piallat ML, Gabbiani G (2007) The myofibroblast: one function, multiple origins. Am J Pathol 170:1807–1816

Horan GS, Wood S, Ona V, Li DJ, Lukashev ME, Weinreb PH, Simon KJ, Hahm K, Allaire NE, Rinaldi NJ et al (2008) Partial inhibition of integrin alpha(v)beta6 prevents pulmonary fibrosis without exacerbating inflammation. Am J Respir Crit Care Med 177:56–65

Horowitz JC, Rogers DS, Sharma V, Vittal R, White ES, Cui Z, Thannickal VJ (2007) Combinatorial activation of FAK and AKT by transforming growth factor-beta1 confers an anoikis-resistant phenotype to myofibroblasts. Cell Signal 19:761–771

Howell DC, Johns RH, Lasky JA, Shan B, Scotton CJ, Laurent GJ, Chambers RC (2005) Absence of proteinase-activated receptor-1 signaling affords protection from bleomycin-induced lung inflammation and fibrosis. Am J Pathol 166:1353–1365

Humphreys BD, Lin SL, Kobayashi A, Hudson TE, Nowlin BT, Bonventre JV, Valerius MT, McMahon AP, Duffield JS (2010) Fate tracing reveals the pericyte and not epithelial origin of myofibroblasts in kidney fibrosis. Am J Pathol 176:85–97

Hurst LC, Badalamente MA, Hentz VR, Hotchkiss RN, Kaplan FT, Meals RA, Smith TM, Rodzvilla J (2009) Injectable collagenase clostridium histolyticum for Dupuytren's contracture. N Engl J Med 361:968–979

Jenkins G (2008) The role of proteases in transforming growth factor-beta activation. Int J Biochem Cell Biol 40:1068–1078

Kamm KE, Stull JT (1989) Regulation of smooth muscle contractile elements by second messengers. Annu Rev Physiol 51:299–313

Katoh K, Kano Y, Amano M, Onishi H, Kaibuchi K, Fujiwara K (2001) Rho-kinase–mediated contraction of isolated stress fibers. J Cell Biol 153:569–584

Kimura K, Ito M, Amano M, Chihara K, Fukata Y, Nakafuku M, Yamamori B, Feng JH, Nakano T, Okawa K et al (1996) Regulation of myosin phosphatase by Rho and Rho-associated kinase (Rho-kinase). Science 273:245–248

Kohan M, Muro AF, White ES, Berkman N (2010) EDA-containing cellular fibronectin induces fibroblast differentiation through binding to alpha4beta7 integrin receptor and MAPK/Erk 1/2-dependent signaling. FASEB J 24:4503–4512

Levinson H, Moyer KE, Saggers GC, Ehrlich HP (2004) Calmodulin-myosin light chain kinase inhibition changes fibroblast-populated collagen lattice contraction, cell migration, focal adhesion formation, and wound contraction. Wound Repair Regen 12:505–511

Li J, Bertram JF (2010) Review: endothelial-myofibroblast transition, a new player in diabetic renal fibrosis. Nephrology (Carlton) 15:507–512

Li Z, Dranoff JA, Chan EP, Uemura M, Sevigny J, Wells RG (2007) Transforming growth factor-beta and substrate stiffness regulate portal fibroblast activation in culture. Hepatology 46:1246–1256

Liu X, Hu H, Yin JQ (2006) Therapeutic strategies against TGF-beta signaling pathway in hepatic fibrosis. Liver Int 26:8–22

Liu F, Mih JD, Shea BS, Kho AT, Sharif AS, Tager AM, Tschumperlin DJ (2010) Feedback amplification of fibrosis through matrix stiffening and COX-2 suppression. J Cell Biol 190:693–706

Margadant C, Sonnenberg A (2010) Integrin-TGF-beta crosstalk in fibrosis, cancer and wound healing. EMBO Rep 11:97–105

Meier K, Nanney LB (2006) Emerging new drugs for scar reduction. Expert Opin Emerg Drugs 11:39–47

Nishimura SL (2009) Integrin-mediated transforming growth factor-beta activation, a potential therapeutic target in fibrogenic disorders. Am J Pathol 175:1362–1370

Parizi M, Howard EW, Tomasek JJ (2000) Regulation of LPA-promoted myofibroblast contraction: role of Rho, myosin light chain kinase, and myosin light chain phosphatase. Exp Cell Res 254:210–220

Pittet B, Rubbia-Brandt L, Desmouliere A, Sappino AP, Roggero P, Guerret S, Grimaud JA, Lacher R, Montandon D, Gabbiani G (1994) Effect of gamma-interferon on the clinical and biologic evolution of hypertrophic scars and Dupuytren's disease: an open pilot study [see comments]. Plast Reconstr Surg 93:1224–1235

Raizman JE, Komljenovic J, Chang R, Deng C, Bedosky KM, Rattan SG, Cunnington RH, Freed DH, Dixon IM (2007) The participation of the Na+−Ca2+ exchanger in primary cardiac myofibroblast migration, contraction, and proliferation. J Cell Physiol 213:540–551

Serini G, Bochaton-Piallat ML, Ropraz P, Geinoz A, Borsi L, Zardi L, Gabbiani G (1998) The fibronectin domain ED-A is crucial for myofibroblastic phenotype induction by transforming growth factor-beta1. J Cell Biol 142:873–881

Tanaka K, Sano K, Yuba K, Katsumura K, Nakano T, Kobayashi M, Ikeda T, Abe M (2003) Inhibition of induction of myofibroblasts by interferon gamma in a human fibroblast cell line. Int Immunopharmacol 3:1273–1280

Tenney RM, Discher DE (2009) Stem cells, microenvironment mechanics, and growth factor activation. Curr Opin Cell Biol 21:630–635

Thiery JP (2002) Epithelial-mesenchymal transitions in tumour progression. Nat Rev Cancer 2:442–454

Tomasek JJ, Gabbiani G, Hinz B, Chaponnier C, Brown RA (2002) Myofibroblasts and mechano-regulation of connective tissue remodelling. Nat Rev Mol Cell Biol 3:349–363

Tomasek JJ, Vaughan MB, Kropp BP, Gabbiani G, Martin MD, Haaksma CJ, Hinz B (2006) Contraction of myofibroblasts in granulation tissue is dependent on Rho/Rho kinase/myosin light chain phosphatase activity. Wound Repair Regen 14:313–320

Varga J, Pasche B (2009) Transforming growth factor beta as a therapeutic target in systemic sclerosis. Nat Rev Rheumatol 5:200–206

Wells RG (2008) The role of matrix stiffness in regulating cell behavior. Hepatology 47:1394–1400

Wipff PJ, Hinz B (2008) Integrins and the activation of latent transforming growth factor beta1 - an intimate relationship. Eur J Cell Biol 87:601–615

Wipff PJ, Rifkin DB, Meister JJ, Hinz B (2007) Myofibroblast contraction activates latent TGF-beta1 from the extracellular matrix. J Cell Biol 179:1311–1323

Yeung T, Georges PC, Flanagan LA, Marg B, Ortiz M, Funaki M, Zahir N, Ming W, Weaver V, Janmey PA (2005) Effects of substrate stiffness on cell morphology, cytoskeletal structure, and adhesion. Cell Motil Cytoskeleton 60:24–34

Zhou Y, Hagood JS, Lu B, Merryman WD, Murphy-Ullrich JE (2010) Thy-1-integrin alphavbeta5 interactions inhibit lung fibroblast contraction-induced latent TGF-beta1 activation and myofibroblast differentiation. J Biol Chem 285(29): 22382–22393

Mechanisms of Myofibroblast Differentiation

8

Sem H. Phan

Contents

8.1	**Introduction**	61
8.2	**Origin of the Myofibroblast**	61
8.2.1	Fibroblastic Origin	62
8.2.2	Epithelial/Endothelial-Mesenchymal Transition	62
8.2.3	Distal Origin of the Myofibroblast	62
8.3	**Myofibroblast Differentiation**	63
8.3.1	Cell Signaling	63
8.3.2	Transcriptional Regulation	64
8.3.3	Epigenetic Regulation	65
8.4	**Conclusion**	65
References		66

8.1 Introduction

De novo genesis of the myofibroblast at sites of tissue injury, repair, and remodeling is considered to be important for wound contraction and the production of extracellular matrix that is crucial in both repair and remodeling or fibrosis (Hinz et al. 2007). Additionally, their ability to elaborate inflammatory cytokines (Phan et al. 1999) also makes them a significant player in the inflammation that accompanies injury. Their gradual disappearance as healing is successfully completed is attributed to an apoptotic process (Desmoulière et al. 1995). This is in contrast to chronic and progressive fibrosis that ensues with "unsuccessful" healing, which results in excessive matrix deposition with distortion or loss of normal parenchymal architecture and in ultimate loss of organ function. Thus, the persistence of the myofibroblast, perhaps due to lack of apoptotic stimuli and/or greater resistance to such stimuli, may be responsible for the chronicity and progressive nature of the fibrosis. Hence understanding the mechanisms for the genesis of the myofibroblast may be key in providing further insight into the pathogenesis of chronic fibrosis, and perhaps uncover novel targets for treatment of fibrotic diseases.

8.2 Origin of the Myofibroblast

Ample evidence suggests the fibroblast as the progenitor cell for the myofibroblast, although there is mixed, and in some cases controversial, evidence that it could arise also from additional sources, such as pericytes, circulating fibroblast-like cells termed "fibrocytes," and

S.H. Phan
Department of Pathology,
University of Michigan Medical School, Ann Arbor, MI, USA
e-mail: shphan@umich.edu

C. Eaton et al. (eds.), *Dupuytren's Disease and Related Hyperproliferative Disorders*,
DOI 10.1007/978-3-642-22697-7_8, © Springer-Verlag Berlin Heidelberg 2012

endothelial and epithelial cells. Thus, the possibility of a distal origin (i.e., outside of the tissue that is undergoing fibrosis) for myofibroblasts needs to be considered.

8.2.1 Fibroblastic Origin

The fibroblastic origin of myofibroblasts is assumed from their de novo genesis in injured tissue undergoing repair, wherein the preexisting cells are likely to be fibroblasts (Hinz et al. 2007). Furthermore, kinetic studies showed that in lungs, these α-SMA-expressing cells first appear at the site of early fibrosis where adventitial fibroblasts could be identified juxtaposing airways and vascular structures in lungs undergoing fibrosis (Zhang et al. 1994). Due to such proximity to vascular structures, the possibility of pericytes as an additional source of myofibroblasts is considered but deemed unlikely due to lack of α-SMA expression at these same sites in uninjured lungs. However, this is based on the assumption that pericytes normally express α-SMA, which is not detected at the comparable sites in normal lungs where de novo α-SMA expression is noted in the fibrotic lungs. Finally, isolated fibroblasts in tissue culture can be induced to differentiate to myofibroblasts in vitro upon treatment with TGFβ and other stimuli (Hinz et al. 2007). However, recent evidence also indicates that cells with certain pericyte markers along with perivascular fibroblasts are the precursors for myofibroblasts in renal fibrosis (Humphreys et al. 2010).

8.2.2 Epithelial/Endothelial-Mesenchymal Transition

Epithelial-mesenchymal transition (EMT) is a process by which differentiated epithelial cells undergo loss of epithelial markers such as E-cadherin with acquisition of mesenchymal cell markers, such as α-SMA. Hence, this process has been described as a potential source of myofibroblasts in fibrosis in the kidney and the lung for instance (Iwano et al. 2002; Willis et al. 2005; Kim et al. 2006). A similar process has been described also for endothelial cells, wherein loss of endothelial markers is accompanied by acquisition of mesenchymal cell markers (Zeisberg et al. 2007; Hashimoto et al. 2010). While EMT is well described in the development and cancer literature, in the latter case representing an essential process to enable metastasis, its occurrence and significance

in fibrosis are less clear and quite controversial with conflicting evidence, sometimes using the same animal model. For example, fibrosis using the unilateral ureteric obstruction (UUO) model of renal fibrosis, two different laboratories using sophisticated cell fate–tracking approaches arrive at opposite conclusions vis-a-vis the contribution of EMT to the myofibroblast population (Iwano et al. 2002; Humphreys et al. 2010). Another recent study also fails to show any contribution from EMT in hepatic fibrosis (Scholten et al. 2010). On the other hand, the importance of EMT in pulmonary fibrosis is suggested by evidence of co-localization of alveolar epithelial cell markers with mesenchymal cell markers, consistent with cells in the midst of transitioning from epithelial to mesenchymal phenotype (Kim et al. 2006). This is also supported in studies of animal models of pulmonary fibrosis (Willis et al. 2005). The contribution of endothelial-mesenchymal transition has also been suggested in certain models of fibrosis (Zeisberg et al. 2007; Hashimoto et al. 2010), but as with EMT, the relative contribution of this process to the overall myofibroblast population is uncertain.

8.2.3 Distal Origin of the Myofibroblast

This is of interest due to the discovery of a circulating cell with fibroblastic properties, which has been called the fibrocyte (Bucala et al. 1994). Characteristically, fibrocytes express vimentin, collagens I and III, as well as CD34 and CD45, which have been used to identify these cells in tissues. They comprise $\leq 0.5\%$ of the circulating leukocytic cell population in blood and found to be potent antigen presenting cells (Chesney et al. 1997). Based on its derivation from CD14[+] cells and expression of CD45 and CD34, they are likely derived from hematopoietic stem cells (HSCs) and not the mesenchymal stem cells (MSCs) of the bone marrow (Abe et al. 2001). Animal model studies using green fluorescence protein (GFP) bone marrow chimera mice (donor bone marrow from transgenic mice expressing GFP) provide support for their bone marrow origin. Using these mice in studies of fibrosis in skin, lung, and other organs indicate that some of the fibroblast-like cells in these distal tissues originate from the bone marrow (Hashimoto et al. 2004; Fathke et al. 2004). There is however some controversy with respect to the fate of these cells after recruitment to the site of injury and tissue remodeling. While some studies indicate

8.3.1 Cell Signaling

that myofibroblasts are mostly of local tissue origin, with minimal or no contribution from the bone marrow (Hashimoto et al. 2004; Fathke et al. 2004; Kisseleva et al. 2006; Yokota et al. 2006; Lama and Phan 2006), other studies suggest circulating fibrocytes as additional sources (Abe et al. 2001; Phillips et al. 2004; Mori et al. 2005). The basis for this discrepancy is unclear but may be related to different approaches used for tracking bone marrow–derived cells. Thus, it is uncertain at this time what the level of contribution is, if any, of precursor cells from distal sites to the de novo genesis of the myofibroblast in tissue repair and fibrosis. Nevertheless, there is evidence at least that even if these bone marrow–derived cells that migrated to the site of tissue injury do not differentiate to myofibroblasts; they can still promote fibrosis by elaborating fibrogenic mediators, such as TGFβ, to promote myofibroblast differentiation from local tissue fibroblasts (Wang et al. 2007; Dolgachev et al. 2009).

8.3 Myofibroblast Differentiation

Given the importance of the myofibroblast in tissue repair and fibrosis as noted above, understanding the mechanism of differentiation is important for providing insight into the initiation and progression of fibrotic responses, as well as to provide new targets for antifibrotic therapies. One approach is to study the mechanism that gives rise to key distinguishing phenotypic features of the differentiated myofibroblast. A key distinguishing feature of the fully differentiated myofibroblast is the expression of α-SMA, which is considered to be important for its role in wound contraction (Majno et al. 1971; Hinz et al. 2007). Additionally, myofibroblasts express vimentin and variable amounts of desmin along with other smooth muscle marker proteins such as smoothelin, caldesmon, and smooth muscle myosin heavy chain (Zhang et al. 1994; Hinz 2007). Thus, there is no single distinguishing feature between the myofibroblast and the smooth muscle cell, although OB-cadherin may show some relative specificity for the fully differentiated myofibroblast (Hinz et al. 2004). However, in vitro studies use precursor fibroblasts that do not express α-SMA, and thus its expression has been used as an indicator of differentiation. Thus, an effective approach to understand differentiation is to analyze the mechanism of regulation of α-SMA gene expression.

In addition to TGFβ, a wide variety of other soluble ligands are known to induce myofibroblast differentiation from fibroblasts (Hinz 2007). Given the prominent and key role of TGFβ in fibrosis, it has been among the most well-studied. It is known to signal via Smad proteins, although it can signal via MAP kinases as well (Derynck and Zhang 2003). Upon binding to the TGFβ types I and II receptor complex, activation of its serine/threonine kinase results in activation of Smads 2/3, which then bind Smad4 to translocate to the nucleus to affect gene expression. The critical role of Smad signaling is shown by the reduced fibrosis noted in Smad3 null mice (Bonniaud et al. 2005; Uemura et al. 2005). The MAP kinase pathway is implicated as well and thought to have modulating influences on the Smad signaling pathway (Dugina et al. 2001; Hashimoto et al. 2001; Derynck and Zhang 2003; White et al. 2006). Additional signaling pathways have also been implicated depending on the inducing stimulus. For instance, recent evidence suggests that the Wnt signaling pathway may be important in EMT (Chilosi et al. 2003; Huber et al. 2005; Kim et al. 2009), and in myofibroblast differentiation (Shafer and Towler 2009). Notch signaling has also been implicated in EMT and endothelial-mesenchymal transition with a CSL binding element identified in the α-SMA promoter (Zavadil et al. 2004; Noseda et al. 2006). Recent studies of resistin-like molecule α (RELMα or FIZZ1, found in inflammatory zone 1) indicate its important participation in pulmonary fibrosis is associated with induction of myofibroblast differentiation (Liu et al. 2004a, b). FIZZ1 is found to induce Jagged1, a ligand for Notch1, resulting in activation of this signaling pathway and activation of α-SMA gene transcription in fibroblasts (Liu et al. 2009). Inhibition of Notch signaling impairs FIZZ1 induced myofibroblast differentiation. Moreover, impaired Notch signaling in transgenic mice deficient in endogenous fucose synthesis suppresses pulmonary fibrosis with associated deficiency in myofibroblast differentiation (Liu et al. 2009). Thus, a wide variety of signaling pathways are involved in regulation of myofibroblast differentiation with downstream mediators capable of direct regulation of α-SMA gene expression. While distinct differentiation stimuli may activate specific pathways, many of these pathways do interact at some level, thus making for a complex regulatory mechanism.

8.3.2 Transcriptional Regulation

Much of the studies described above involved analysis of α-SMA as an indicator of differentiation. Moreover, the downstream gene target of the signaling pathways is often α-SMA itself. However, in addition to being a marker of differentiation, α-SMA appears to play a functional role in regulating expression of other genes characteristic of the myofibroblast and that give rise to its phenotype. For instance, it is known to be important for the upregulated collagen expression characteristic of the myofibroblast and mediates mechano-transduced gene expression (Hinz et al. 2002; Wang et al. 2005; Chaqour et al. 2006). Consequently, the focus for transcriptional regulation of myofibroblast differentiation often is directed at the α-SMA gene.

Abundant information is available on transcriptional regulation of the α-SMA gene from studies in smooth muscle cells. These early studies identified the importance of serum response factor (SRF) and the CArG elements that have been identified in the promoter. While these elements are essential for gene transcription, it appears that TGFβ-induced myofibroblast differentiation requires additional factors (Hautmann et al. 1997; Roy et al. 2001; Cogan et al. 2002). Another notable difference from smooth muscle cells is the importance in myofibroblasts of MCAT elements that bind transcription enhancer factor-1 (TEF-1) family member, RTEF-1 (Gan et al. 2007). In a search for the regulatory factors and cis-acting elements in response to TGFβ-induced α-SMA gene transcription, a proximal TGFβ control element (TCE) is identified in smooth muscle cells, which is subsequently shown to bind Krüppel-like factor (KLF) 5 as well as Sp1 and Sp3 to activate transcription, while KLF4 binding is shown to suppress promoter activity (Hautmann et al. 1997; Cogan et al. 2002). However, other studies indicate greater complexity is involved with additional factors being required in TGFβ activation of α-SMA gene expression. Thus, another region upstream of the TCE has been identified as the TGF-β hypersensitivity region (THR), which is reported to bind Sp1 and Sp3 (Cogan et al. 2002). This study also implicates Smad3 as an essential factor in myofibroblast differentiation; Smad3 is shown in another study to bind a Smad binding element (SBE) located even further upstream than the THR (Hu et al. 2003). Deficiency of Smad3 or mutation of the SBE results in significantly diminished α-SMA promoter activity.

The importance of myofibroblast differentiation in vivo is further confirmed by the observation of diminished fibrosis in the Smad3-deficient mouse (Bonniaud et al. 2005; Uemura et al. 2005; Gauldie et al. 2006). Additional factors found to be important include CCAAT enhancer–binding protein β (C/EBPβ), CSL (downstream target of Notch signaling), and c-Myb with known binding elements identified in the α-SMA promoter (Hu et al. 2004; Noseda et al. 2006; Buck et al. 2000). In the case of C/EBPβ, its long isoform known as liver activating protein (LAP) is responsible for activation of the promoter; however, its truncated isoform LIP (liver inhibitory protein) has dominant negative inhibitor activity since the activation domain is absent (Hu et al. 2004). In vitro studies of lung fibroblasts showed that IL-1β suppression of myofibroblast differentiation is dependent on the LIP isoform. However, in vivo studies using C/EBPβ-deficient mice reveal the predominant effect in pulmonary fibrosis is primarily due to the activating effects of the LAP isoform since diminished fibrosis is accompanied by significantly reduced α-SMA expression in these knockout mice (Hu et al. 2007a).

Repression by the LIP isoform of C/EBPβ suggests that an alternate and/or additional mechanism for differentiation may be induced de-repression of the α-SMA gene. By implication this would suggest that the undifferentiated state is due to active repression of this gene, perhaps by inhibitory transcription factors. In addition to LIP, several transcription factors are known to have inhibitory effects on α-SMA gene expression. As discussed previously, KLF4 is known to suppress promoter activity by competing for binding to the TCE by its activators, such as KLF5 (Hautmann et al. 1997). Additionally, it can interact with the MH2 domain of Smad3 to suppress its binding to the SBE of the α-SMA promoter with consequent diminished gene transcription (Hu et al. 2007b). PPARγ, YB-1, and Nkx2.5 represent additional candidate repressors of the α-SMA gene (Burgess et al. 2005; Zhang et al. 2005; Hu et al. 2010a). While most of these repressors are induced by appropriate stimuli, Nkx2.5 is expressed at levels sufficient to repress gene expression in the resting lung fibroblast. Upon induction of myofibroblast differentiation, this resting level is significantly reduced to allow α-SMA gene expression to occur, thus making Nkx2.5 an attractive candidate as a homeostatic repressor for maintenance of the undifferentiated state. Interestingly, its expression is enhanced by treatment of cells with FGF2, which is known to inhibit myofibroblast differentiation and with potential for treatment of hypertrophic scarring (Hu et al. 2010a). Thus derepression represents an additional mechanism in overall induction of myofibroblast differentiation that may be targeted as well in the search for novel therapies for control of chronic progressive fibrosis.

8.3.3 Epigenetic Regulation

Epigenetic regulation of gene expression is an important mechanism in development and cell differentiation and consists of modified histone–DNA interactions, DNA methylation, and more recently miRNA targeting of specific genes. There is increasing information on this mode of regulating the α-SMA gene as it relates to myofibroblast differentiation. Early evidence for its importance comes from studies using inhibitors of either histone modification or DNA methylation (Niki et al. 1999; Mann et al. 2007). Thus, the histone deacetylase (HDAC) inhibitor trichostatin A is found to inhibit differentiation, and subsequently found to be due to the important roles of HDAC4, HDAC6, and HDAC8 in this process (Glenisson et al. 2007). In the case of HDAC4, it is found to be associated with the activation of Akt in TGFβ-induced differentiation (Guo et al. 2009). Thus, while HDAC inhibition is commonly associated with activation of gene expression, its suppression of α-SMA expression implicates an indirect mechanism as suggested by effects on other genes that may have a repressive effect on α-SMA gene expression. Such an indirect mechanism is also suggested by studies of liver myofibroblasts using the DNA methylation inhibitor 5-aza-2'-deoxycytidine (Mann et al. 2007). In this case, activation of PPARγ and NFκB, known inhibitors of α-SMA gene expression, is observed upon treatment with the inhibitor. Further studies revealed the importance of the methylated DNA–binding protein MeCP2 in a complex mechanism resulting in the suppression of PPARγ expression to de-repress α-SMA expression (Mann et al. 2010). This mechanism involves upstream down-regulation of miR132, which targets MeCP2 mRNA resulting in the noted indirect effects on activation of the α-SMA gene. Direct examination of DNA methylation of the α-SMA gene itself in lung fibroblasts and alveolar epithelial type II cells (which do not normally express α-SMA) indicates methylation in three CpG islands (Hu et al. 2010b). However, the extent of methylation at the three sites is different between these two cell types, with substantial methylation in all three islands in epithelial cells while only the promoter region is highly methylated in the case of fibroblasts. Inhibition of methylation by 5-aza-2'-deoxycytidine or deficiency of DNA methyl transferases (DNMTs) activates α-SMA gene transcription in fibroblasts, while DNMT overexpression suppresses differentiation. Thus, both direct and indirect epigenetic regulation of the α-SMA gene appears to add to the complexity of the mechanisms involved in myofibroblast differentiation.

8.4 Conclusion

Chronic progressive fibrotic diseases are characterized by the persistence of myofibroblasts, which emerge de novo from precursor cells. Several precursor cell types have been described, including fibroblasts, pericytes, and epithelial and endothelial cells of local tissue origin and fibrocytes of bone marrow origin. While there is some controversy with respect to the other cellular sources, the fibroblast and hepatic stellate cell as precursor cells is undisputed. In view of the critical multifactorial importance of the myofibroblast in fibrogenesis, understanding its genesis would be critical to fully understand the fibrotic process and the basis for its persistence and progression to organ failure or severe disfigurement with functional compromise. This process is characterized by complex mechanisms involving multiple signaling pathways, downstream transcription factors, and target genes. Differentiation as viewed from the standpoint of marker gene expression is mostly focused on the α-SMA gene, which exemplifies the complexity of the process. In addition to regulation of the transcriptional level, involvement of epigenetic mechanisms, both direct and indirect, appears to be of additional significance. Further studies are needed to clarify the significant cellular sources of the myofibroblast and its genesis in vivo. For example, it is clear that the full spectrum of transcription factors that may be involved in regulating α-SMA expression in myofibroblast differentiation has not been completely identified and direct regulation at the epigenetic level remains incompletely understood. Nevertheless, the multiple targets identified thus far provide some current avenues for investigation into novel therapies.

References

Abe R, Donnelly SC, Peng T, Bucala R, Metz CN (2001) Peripheral blood fibrocytes: differentiation pathway and migration to wound sites. J Immunol 166(12):7556–7562

Bonniaud P, Margetts PJ, Ask K, Flanders K, Gauldie J, Kolb M (2005) TGF-beta and Smad3 signaling link inflammation to chronic fibrogenesis. J Immunol 175(8):5390–5395

Bucala R, Spiegel LA, Chesney J, Hogan M, Cerami A (1994) Circulating fibrocytes define a new leukocyte subpopulation that mediates tissue repair. Mol Med 1(1):71–81

Buck M, Kim DJ, Houglum K, Hassanein T, Chojkier M (2000) c-Myb modulates transcription of the alpha-smooth muscle actin gene in activated hepatic stellate cells. Am J Physiol Gastrointest Liver Physiol 278(2):G321–G328

Burgess HA, Daugherty LE, Thatcher TH, Lakatos HF, Ray DM, Redonnet M, Phipps RP, Sime PJ (2005) PPARgamma agonists inhibit TGF-beta induced pulmonary myofibroblast differentiation and collagen production: implications for therapy of lung fibrosis. Am J Physiol Lung Cell Mol Physiol 288(6):L1146–L1153

Chaqour B, Yang R, Sha Q (2006) Mechanical stretch modulates the promoter activity of the profibrotic factor CCN2 through increased actin polymerization and NF-kappaB activation. J Biol Chem 281(29):20608–20622

Chesney J, Bacher M, Bender A, Bucala R (1997) The peripheral blood fibrocyte is a potent antigen-presenting cell capable of priming naive T cells in situ. Proc Natl Acad Sci USA 94(12):6307–6312

Chilosi M, Poletti V, Zamò A, Lestani M, Montagna L, Piccoli P, Pedron S, Bertaso M, Scarpa A, Murer B, Cancellieri A, Maestro R, Semenzato G, Doglioni C (2003) Aberrant Wnt/beta-catenin pathway activation in idiopathic pulmonary fibrosis. Am J Pathol 162(5):1495–1502

Cogan JG, Subramanian SV, Polikandriotis JA, Kelm RJ Jr, Strauch AR (2002) Vascular smooth muscle alpha-actin gene transcription during myofibroblast differentiation requires Sp1/3 protein binding proximal to the MCAT enhancer. J Biol Chem 277(39):36433–36442

Derynck R, Zhang YE (2003) Smad-dependent and Smad-independent pathways in TGF-beta family signalling. Nature 425(6958):577–584

Desmoulière A, Redard M, Darby I, Gabbiani G (1995) Apoptosis mediates the decrease in cellularity during the transition between granulation tissue and scar. Am J Pathol 146:56–66

Dolgachev VA, Ullenbruch MR, Lukacs NW, Phan SH (2009) Role of stem cell factor and bone marrow-derived fibroblasts in airway remodeling. Am J Pathol 174(2):390–400

Dugina V, Fontao L, Chaponnier C, Vasiliev J, Gabbiani G (2001) Focal adhesion features during myofibroblastic differentiation are controlled by intracellular and extracellular factors. J Cell Sci 114(Pt 18):3285–3296

Fathke C, Wilson L, Hutter J, Kapoor V, Smith A, Hocking A, Isik F (2004) Contribution of bone marrow-derived cells to skin: collagen deposition and wound repair. Stem Cells 22(5):812–822

Gan Q, Yoshida T, Li J, Owens GK (2007) Smooth muscle cells and myofibroblasts use distinct transcriptional mechanisms for smooth muscle alpha-actin expression. Circ Res 101(9):883–892

Gauldie J, Kolb M, Ask K, Martin G, Bonniaud P, Warburton D (2006) Smad3 Signaling involved in pulmonary fibrosis and emphysema. Proc Am Thorac Soc 3(8):696–702

Glenisson W, Castronovo V, Waltregny D (2007) Histone deacetylase 4 is required for TGFbeta1-induced myofibroblastic differentiation. Biochim Biophys Acta 1773(10):1572–1582

Guo W, Shan B, Klingsberg RC, Qin X, Lasky JA (2009) Abrogation of TGF-beta1-induced fibroblast-myofibroblast differentiation by histone deacetylase inhibition. Am J Physiol Lung Cell Mol Physiol 297(5):L864–L870

Hashimoto S, Gon Y, Takeshita I, Matsumoto K, Maruoka S, Horie T (2001) Transforming growth Factor-beta1 induces phenotypic modulation of human lung fibroblasts to myofibroblast through a c-Jun-NH2-terminal kinase-dependent pathway. Am J Respir Crit Care Med 163(1):152–157

Hashimoto N, Jin H, Liu T, Chensue SW, Phan SH (2004) Bone marrow-derived progenitor cells in pulmonary fibrosis. J Clin Invest 113(2):243–252

Hashimoto N, Phan SH, Imaizumi K, Matsuo M, Nakashima H, Kawabe T, Shimokata K, Hasegawa Y (2010) Endothelial-mesenchymal transition in bleomycin-induced pulmonary fibrosis. Am J Respir Cell Mol Biol 43(2):161–172

Hautmann MB, Madsen CS, Owens GK (1997) A transforming growth factor beta (TGFbeta) control element drives TGFbeta-induced stimulation of smooth muscle alpha-actin gene expression in concert with two CArG elements. J Biol Chem 272(16):10948–10956

Hinz B (2007) Formation and function of the myofibroblast during tissue repair. J Invest Dermatol 127(3):526–537

Hinz B, Gabbiani G, Chaponnier C (2002) The NH2-terminal peptide of alpha-smooth muscle actin inhibits force generation by the myofibroblast in vitro and in vivo. J Cell Biol 157(4):657–663

Hinz B, Pittet P, Smith-Clerc J, Chaponnier C, Meister JJ (2004) Myofibroblast development is characterized by specific cell-cell adherens junctions. Mol Biol Cell 15(9):4310–4320

Hinz B, Phan SH, Thannickal VJ, Galli A, Bochaton-Piallat ML, Gabbiani G (2007) The myofibroblast: one function, multiple origins. Am J Pathol 170(6):1807–1816

Hu B, Wu Z, Phan SH (2003) Smad3 mediates transforming growth factor-beta-induced alpha-smooth muscle actin expression. Am J Respir Cell Mol Biol 29(3 Pt 1):397–404

Hu B, Wu Z, Jin H, Hashimoto N, Liu T, Phan SH (2004) CCAAT/enhancer-binding protein beta isoforms and the regulation of alpha-smooth muscle actin gene expression by IL-1 beta. J Immunol 173(7):4661–4668

Hu B, Ullenbruch MR, Jin H, Gharaee-Kermani M, Phan SH (2007a) An essential role for CCAAT/enhancer binding protein beta in bleomycin-induced pulmonary fibrosis. J Pathol 211(4):455–462

Hu B, Wu Z, Liu T, Ullenbruch MR, Jin H, Phan SH (2007b) Gut-enriched kruppel-like factor interaction with Smad3 inhibits myofibroblast differentiation. Am J Respir Cell Mol Biol 36(1):78–84

Hu B, Wu YM, Wu Z, Phan SH (2010a) Nkx2.5/Csx represses myofibroblast differentiation. Am J Respir Cell Mol Biol 42(2):218–226

Hu B, Gharaee-Kermani M, Wu Z, Phan SH (2010b) Epigenetic regulation of myofibroblast differentiation by DNA methylation. Am J Pathol 177(1):21–28

Huber MA, Kraut N, Beug H (2005) Molecular requirements for epithelial-mesenchymal transition during tumor progression. Curr Opin Cell Biol 17:548–558

Humphreys BD, Lin SL, Kobayashi A, Hudson TE, Nowlin BT, Bonventre JV, Valerius MT, McMahon AP, Duffield JS (2010) Fate tracing reveals the pericyte and not epithelial origin of myofibroblasts in kidney fibrosis. Am J Pathol 176(1):85–97

Iwano M, Plieth D, Danoff TM, Xue C, Okada H, Neilson EG (2002) Evidence that fibroblasts derive from epithelium during tissue fibrosis. J Clin Invest 110(3):341–350

Kim KK, Kugler MC, Wolters PJ, Robillard L, Galvez MG, Brumwell AN, Sheppard D, Chapman HA (2006) Alveolar epithelial cell mesenchymal transition develops in vivo during pulmonary fibrosis and is regulated by the extracellular matrix. Proc Natl Acad Sci USA 103(35):13180–13185

Kim KK, Wei Y, Szekeres C, Kugler MC, Wolters PJ, Hill ML, Frank JA, Brumwell AN, Wheeler SE, Kreidberg JA, Chapman HA (2009) Epithelial cell alpha3beta1 integrin links beta-catenin and Smad signaling to promote myofibroblast formation and pulmonary fibrosis. J Clin Invest 119(1):213–224

Kisseleva T, Uchinami H Feirt N, Quintana-Bustamante O, Segovia JC, Schwabe RF, Brenner DA (2006) Bone marrow-derived fibrocytes participate in pathogenesis of liver fibrosis. J Hepatol 45(3):429–438

Lama VN, Phan SH (2006) The extrapulmonary origin of fibroblasts: stem/progenitor cells and beyond. Proc Am Thorac Soc 3(4):373–376

Liu T, Dhanasekaran SM, Jin H, Hu B, Tomlins SA, Chinnaiyan AM, Phan SH (2004a) FIZZ1 stimulation of myofibroblast differentiation. Am J Pathol 164(4):1315–1326

Liu T, Jin H, Ullenbruch M, Hu B, Hashimoto N, Moore B, McKenzie A, Lukacs NW, Phan SH (2004b) Regulation of found in inflammatory zone 1 expression in bleomycin-induced lung fibrosis: role of IL-4/IL-13 and mediation via STAT-6. J Immunol 173(5):3425–3431

Liu T, Hu B, Choi YY, Chung M, Ullenbruch M, Yu H, Lowe JB, Phan SH (2009) Notch1 Signaling in FIZZ1 induction of myofibroblast differentiation. Am J Pathol 174(5):1745–1755

Majno G, Gabbiani G, Hirschel BJ, Ryan GB, Statkov PR (1971) Contraction of granulation tissue in vitro: similarity to smooth muscle. Science 173(996):548–550

Mann J, Oakley F, Akiboye F, Elsharkawy A, Thorne AW, Mann DA (2007) Regulation of myofibroblast transdifferentiation by DNA methylation and MeCP2: implications for wound healing and fibrogenesis. Cell Death Differ 14(2):275–285

Mann J, Chu DC, Maxwell A, Oakley F, Zhu NL, Tsukamoto H, Mann DA (2010) MeCP2 controls an epigenetic pathway that promotes myofibroblast transdifferentiation and fibrosis. Gastroenterology 138(2):705–714

Mori L, Bellini A, Stacey MA, Schmidt M, Mattoli S (2005) Fibrocytes contribute to the myofibroblast population in wounded skin and originate from the bone marrow. Exp Cell Res 304(1):81–90

Niki T, Rombouts K, De Bleser P, De Smet K, Rogiers V, Schuppan D, Yoshida M, Gabbiani G, Geerts A (1999) A histone deacetylase inhibitor, trichostatin A, suppresses myofibroblastic differentiation of rat hepatic stellate cells in primary culture. Hepatology 29(3):858–867

Noseda M, Fu Y, Niessen K, Wong F, Chang L, McLean G, Karsan A (2006) Smooth muscle alpha-actin is a direct target of Notch/CSL. Circ Res 98:1468–1470

Phan SH, Zhang K, Zhang HY, Gharaee-Kermani M (1999) The myofibroblast as an inflammatory cell in pulmonary fibrosis. Curr Top Pathol 93:173–182

Phillips RJ, Burdick MD, Hong K, Lutz MA, Murray LA, Xue YY, Belperio JA, Keane MP, Strieter RM (2004) Circulating fibrocytes traffic to the lungs in response to CXCL12 and mediate fibrosis. J Clin Invest 114(3):438–446

Roy SG, Nozaki Y, Phan SH (2001) Regulation of alpha-smooth muscle actin gene expression in myofibroblast differentiation from rat lung fibroblasts. Int J Biochem Cell Biol 33(7):723–734

Scholten D, Osterreicher CH, Scholten A, Iwaisako K, Gu G, Brenner DA, Kisseleva T (2010) Genetic labeling does not detect epithelial-to-mesenchymal transition of cholangiocytes in liver fibrosis in mice. Gastroenterology 139(3):987–998

Shafer SL, Towler DA (2009) Transcriptional regulation of SM22α by Wnt3a: convergence with TGFβ1/Smad signaling at a novel regulatory elemen. J Mol Cell Cardiol 46:621–635

Uemura M, Swenson ES, Gaca MD, Giordano FJ, Reiss M, Wells RG (2005) Smad2 and Smad3 play different roles in rat hepatic stellate cell function and alpha-smooth muscle actin organization. Mol Biol Cell 16(9):4214–4224

Wang J, Fan J, Laschinger C, Arora PD, Kapus A, Seth A, McCulloch CA (2005) Smooth muscle actin determines mechanical force-induced p38 activation. J Biol Chem 280(8):7273–7284

Wang JF, Jiao H, Stewart TL, Shankowsky HA, Scott PG, Tredget EE (2007) Fibrocytes from burn patients regulate the activities of fibroblasts. Wound Repair Regen 15(1):113–121

White ES, Atrasz RG, Hu B, Phan SH, Stambolic V, Mak TW, Hogaboam CM, Flaherty KR, Martinez FJ, Kontos CD, Toews GB (2006) Negative regulation of myofibroblast differentiation by PTEN (Phosphatase and Tensin Homolog Deleted on chromosome 10). Am J Respir Crit Care Med 173(1):112–121

Willis BC, Liebler JM, Luby-Phelps K, Nicholson AG, Crandall ED, du Bois RM, Borok Z (2005) Induction of epithelial-mesenchymal transition in alveolar epithelial cells by transforming growth factor-beta1: potential role in idiopathic pulmonary fibrosis. Am J Pathol 166(5):1321–1332

Yokota T, Kawakami Y, Nagai Y, Ma JX, Tsai JY, Kincade PW, Sato S (2006) Bone marrow lacks a transplantable progenitor for smooth muscle type alpha-actin-expressing cells. Stem Cells 24(1):13–22

Zavadil J, Cermak L, Soto-Nieves N, Bottinger EP (2004) Integration of TGF-beta/Smad and Jagged1/Notch signalling in epithelial-to-mesenchymal transition. EMBO J 23:1155–1165

Zeisberg EM, Tarnavski O, Zeisberg M, Dorfman AL, McMullen JR, Gustafsson E, Chandraker A, Yuan X, Pu WT, Roberts AB, Neilson EG, Sayegh MH, Izumo S, Kalluri R (2007) Endothelial-to-mesenchymal transition contributes to cardiac fibrosis. Nat Med 13(8):952–961

Zhang K, Rekhter MD, Gordon D, Phan SH (1994) Myofibroblasts and their role in lung collagen gene expression during pulmonary fibrosis. A combined immunohistochemical and in situ hybridization study. Am J Pathol 145(1):114–125

Zhang A, Liu X, Cogan JG, Fuerst MD, Polikandriotis JA, Kelm RJ Jr, Strauch AR (2005) YB-1 coordinates vascular smooth muscle alpha-actin gene activation by transforming growth factor beta1 and thrombin during differentiation of human pulmonary myofibroblasts. Mol Biol Cell 16(10):4931–4940

Myofibroblasts and Interactions with Other Cells: Contribution of the Tissue Engineering

9

Véronique Moulin, Judith Bellemare,
Daniele Bergeron, Herve Genest, Michel Roy,
and Carlos Lopez-Vallé

Contents

9.1	Bullet Points	69
9.2	Introduction	69
9.3	The Tissue Engineering Approach	70
9.4	Role of the Myofibroblasts in the Formation of the Epidermis	71
9.5	Role of the Epidermis in the Development of Fibrosis	71
9.6	Conclusion	74
References		74

9.1 Bullet Points

- Interactions exist between epidermal cells and myofibroblasts.
- By contrast to fibroblasts, myofibroblasts cannot sustain epidermal growth.
- Pathological epidermal cells stimulate mesenchymal cells to overproduce matrix.
- Tissue engineering is an interesting method to understand interactions between cells.

9.2 Introduction

Myofibroblasts are cells that are present during wound healing and in numerous fibrous pathologies (Gabbiani et al. 1971). These cells have morphological and biochemical features between those of fibroblasts and of smooth muscle (SM) cells. The hallmark of myofibroblasts is the expression of the actin isoform present in SM cells, α-SM actin, in a large quantity in opposition to fibroblasts that have been shown to express low or no α-SM actin (Gabbiani and Badonnel 1976; Moulin et al. 1996). In vivo, these cells have first been thought to contract the wound so as to decrease the wound surface (Gabbiani 2003). This finding has been supported by the presence of myofibroblasts in several contractile pathological tissues as hypertrophic scars (Kischer et al. 1982) or Dupuytren's contracture (Berndt et al. 1994). Comprehension of the modulation of α-SM actin into cells has thus become a crucial research aim to potentially decrease the pathological contraction. Besides the role that they play in contraction, myofibroblasts have been shown to secrete collagen and several

V. Moulin (✉) • J. Bellemare • D. Bergeron
Centre LOEX de l'Université Laval,
Génie tissulaire et régénération: LOEX du Centre de recherche
FRSQ du Centre hospitalier affilié universitaire de Québec,
Québec, QC, Canada and
Département de Chirurgie, Faculté de Médecine,
Université Laval, Québec, QC, Canada
e-mail: veronique.moulin@chg.ulaval.ca

H. Genest • M. Roy
Centre hospitalier affilié Universitaire de Québec,
Québec, QC, Canada

C. Lopez-Vallé
Complexe Hospitalier de la Sagamie, Chicoutimi, QC, Canada

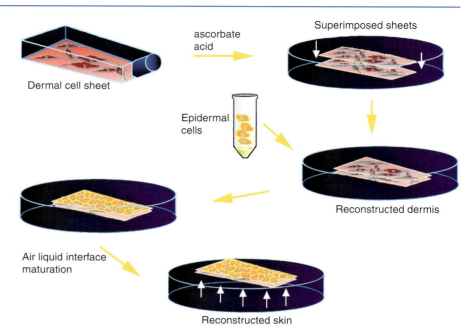

Fig. 9.1 Reconstruction of in vitro human skin using tissue engineering

other matrix proteins (Moulin et al. 1998). This points out that these cells can also play several roles during the neoformation of the tissue or during the pathological fibrosis formation, although very few studies have been performed to understand their global function in vivo.

During wound healing as well as during pathological modifications of tissues, numerous cell types are involved (Diegelmann 1997). The interactions between cells are crucial to orchestrate reorganization of the tissue (Werner et al. 2007; Moulin 1995). For example, during skin healing, inflammation, angiogenesis, tissue formation and remodeling, and reepithelialization occur in a very precise and organized fashion. Differentiation of cells into myofibroblasts has been shown to be induced by TGFß (Pierce et al. 1991; Desmoulière et al. 1993) and fibronectin ED-A isoform (Serini et al. 1998) that are secreted by numerous cells into the wound. Inversely, invasive cancer growth seems to be dependent of the myofibroblast presence (De Wever et al. 2008). However, specific interactions between myofibroblasts and other cells have not been extensively studied.

9.3 The Tissue Engineering Approach

In vitro, the culture of cells in monolayer is the most widely used method to study cells in vitro. However, cells are not in a physiological state when cultured on plastic. In contrast, cells are surrounded in vivo with an extracellular matrix that is known to have many actions on cell morphology and function (Moulin et al. 1997; Ghahary et al. 2001). Tissue engineering is a novel method arising from the field of Biomaterial. Various approaches are presently being developed in different laboratories based on the utilization of biomaterials, extracellular matrix components, and cells to produce substitutes that are morphologically similar to the studied tissue. In our laboratory, several methods are used to reproduce normal skin tissues, but also to reproduce pathological tissues such as hypertrophic scars. The most recent approach that we use is the self-assembly method that is based on the in vitro capacity of mesenchymal cells to secrete and reorganize extracellular matrix as in vivo (L'Heureux et al. 1998; Michel et al. 1999). This approach allows reconstituting an environment for the cells that is very similar to what is found in vivo: the three-dimensional environment and also the type of matrix proteins. With this technique, mesenchymal tissues with individual cells are embedded into matrix with characteristics that are similar to those that are found in in vivo tissues. It is also important to note that these cells show low cell growth and apoptosis rates (Bellemare et al. 2005), as described in vivo (Santiago et al. 2001).

Briefly, the production of the tissue-engineered skin is made in two steps (Fig. 9.1). Dermal cells are cultured with ascorbate during several weeks. The cells produce their own matrix and form sheets that can be superimposed to obtain a thicker dermis. Keratinocytes are then added on and, when epidermal cells become confluent, the skin model is then elevated to the air–liquid interface to induce maturation of epidermis.

To study healing mechanisms or fibrosis, we have developed a method to isolated fibroblasts or pathological myofibroblasts, and keratinocytes from the same small biopsies (normal skin or hypertrophic scar) (Rochon et al. 2001). Human wound myofibroblasts can be isolated from artificial wound performed using a sponge subcutaneously implanted into the patient (Germain et al. 1994). These cells can be used to reconstitute a tissue-engineered skin. The epidermis obtained has been described as very similar to real in vivo skin (Michel et al. 1999). The addition of these cells can help understand the role of each cell population in the morphogenesis of the normal or pathological tissues.

9.4 Role of the Myofibroblasts in the Formation of the Epidermis

In human skin, wound surface heals and decreases in size following two phenomena occurring at the same time: neodermal formation and reepithelialization (Laplante et al. 2001; Coulombe 2003). A contraction phenomenon can also occur but represents a small percentage of the closure in humans in comparison to other mammals. One of the first steps of wound repair is the infiltration of fibroblasts where they proliferate and differentiate into wound myofibroblasts that then play a preponderant role in neodermal formation and contraction (Schürch et al. 1992). The other event implicated in the healing process is the migration and growth of keratinocytes on neodermis followed by the formation of a complete basement membrane that ensures the structural and mechanical stability of the dermo-epidermal junction.

Two different models using tissue engineering method have been realized to analyze possible interactions existing between wound myofibroblasts and keratinocytes. The first model comes from the first tissue-engineered model of Bell (Bell et al. 1979) using collagen gel that is seeded with keratinocytes (Moulin et al. 2000). The second model is the self-assembly method described above. In both models, the use of

human fibroblasts to form dermis induces a very well-differentiated epidermis with a regular basal layer and several suprabasal layers. In contrast, when wound myofibroblasts are used, the epidermis is thin and irregular with more disorganized basal layer and differentiated cells in the suprabasal layers (Fig. 9.2). When cells are absent from the dermis or replaced by smooth muscle cells, the same disorganized histology is observed.

Formation of the basement membrane has been previously described as the result of keratinocyte–fibroblast interactions (Smola et al. 1998). We have thus studied the deposition of proteins of the basement membrane in both models. We have found that in the presence of fibroblasts, the link between dermis and epidermis is highly organized with deposition of collagen IV and laminin 5. In contrast, when wound myofibroblasts or smooth muscle cells are used, a delay in the formation of the basement membrane as well as a weak deposition of these proteins can be observed (Moulin et al. 2000).

Wound myofibroblasts play a crucial role during healing, secreting matrix, and contracting the edges of the wound. Interactions between fibroblasts and keratinocytes have been shown to be crucial to the growth and differentiation of the epidermal cells. As differentiated cells from fibroblasts, myofibroblasts should keep the capacity to support the epidermis formation. Using the tissue engineering approach, we have demonstrated that in contrast to the results obtained with fibroblasts, wound myofibroblasts cannot support keratinocyte growth and differentiation. The epidermis samples obtained in the presence of wound myofibroblasts or of smooth muscle cells and in the absence of dermal cells are similar and are very poorly differentiated. This brings postulate that factors secreted by fibroblasts to stimulate keratinocyte growth are absent in the culture of other tested mesenchymal cells.

9.5 Role of the Epidermis in the Development of Fibrosis

Mesenchymal cells are known to be crucial for the growth of epidermal cells (Barreca et al. 1992). However, it has also been observed that interactions between both cell types are also important for the mesenchymal cells. In addition to secreting autocrine proteins, keratinocytes also secrete cytokines in a paracrine

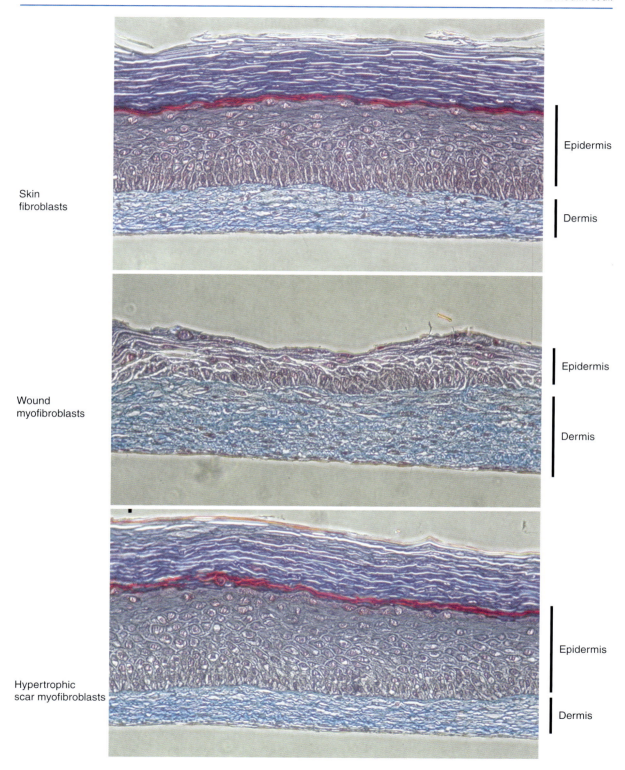

Fig. 9.2 Histology of human skin equivalent when mesenchymal cells used were skin fibroblasts (*upper*), wound myofibroblasts (*middle*), or pathological myofibroblasts (*lower*)

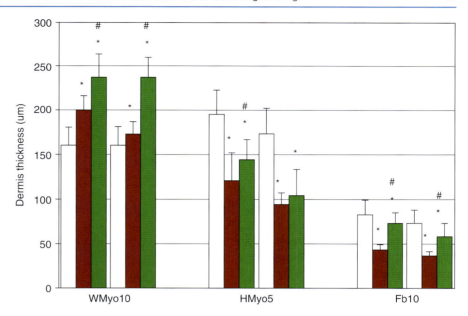

Fig. 9.3 Thickness of the dermis according to the origin of epidermal cells. Dermis was reconstructed using wound myofibroblasts (*WMyo10*), pathological scar myofibroblasts (*HMyo5*), or skin fibroblasts (*Fb10*) in the absence of keratinocytes (*white bars*), with normal skin keratinocytes (*red bars*) or hypertrophic scar keratinocytes (*green bars*). The statistical significance was determined using SNK's test to compare dermal thickness with those obtained without keratinocytes (*$p<0.05$) or with those obtained with normal skin keratinocytes (#$p<0.05$). (From Bellemare et al. 2005)

fashion, stimulating monolayer-cultured fibroblasts to proliferate (Maas-Szabowski et al. 1999; Lim et al. 2001). Depending on the authors, the role of keratinocytes on matrix component secretion is however controversial, inhibiting or stimulating collagen as well as matrix metalloproteinase (MMP) synthesis (Lacroix et al. 1995; Guo et al. 2002; Ghahary et al. 2004).

Hypertrophic scars are disfiguring pathological scars that result from an aberrant response to a cutaneous injury. They are characterized by fibroblastic hyperproliferation, overproduction of extracellular matrix, and by the persistence of myofibroblasts. Since the main characteristic of this pathology is fibrosis, authors usually postulate that the origin of hypertrophic scarring is from mesenchymal cells that are the matrix-secreting cells. However, several indications support the hypothesis that the epidermis also plays a role in fibrosis development. For example, hypertrophic scars frequently occur after reepithelialization has been delayed (Deitch et al. 1983). Furthermore, some cytokines are decreased (IL1a), while others are increased (PDGF) in pathological epidermis compared to the normal scar epidermis (Niessen et al. 2001).

Extracellular matrix formation is strongly dependent of two parameters: the number of cells that is dependant of the growth and the death rate of the cells and the matrix quantity, conditional not only to the secretion but also to the degradation of the matrix components. The majority of the studies on epidermal–dermal interactions have been performed using monolayer cell culture with a short-term culture model or conditioned medium techniques. The important role of the matrix in determining cell features has however been demonstrated. It is thus of great interest to study epidermal–dermal crosstalk in a context as close to reality as possible. We thus used the self-assembly skin model developed in our lab to study any interactions between epidermis and dermis in a context as close to the in vivo skin. This model also allows studying the results of interactions after 3 weeks of culture, the formation of fibrosis being a long-term process.

To test the hypothesis that pathological keratinocytes have a role to play during fibrosis formation, three different populations of dermal cells – hypertrophic scar myofibroblasts, wound myofibroblasts, and skin fibroblasts – were used. These three cell populations have been used to reconstitute dermis. Epidermis was reconstructed with pathological or normal keratinocytes, as described in Fig. 9.1. Histological analysis was then performed to evaluate dermal thickness, depending on the origin of the keratinocytes. For all the populations that we have tested, we noted that the addition of pathological keratinocytes induce a thicker dermis than when skin keratinocytes were used (Bellemare et al. 2005) (Fig. 9.3). This increase can be explained by an increase of collagen I secretion, a decrease of

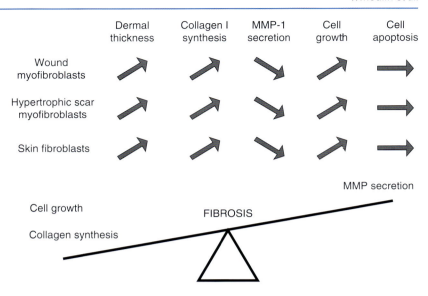

Fig. 9.4 Changes in several fibrotic parameters when epidermal cells were isolated from pathological scar instead of normal skin. Every change converges to swing the pendulum going to an increase matrix deposition and fibrosis

MMP-1 production, and an increase of cell growth without any changes in apoptosis rate (Fig. 9.4).

Thus, hypertrophic scar keratinocytes seem to induce fibrotic responses that are very close to the characteristics of hypertrophic scar pathology described in vivo. This study clearly demonstrates, for the first time, that epidermis plays a role in pathological fibrosis development in the dermis by influencing the proliferation of dermal cells and matrix accumulation.

9.6 Conclusion

Myofibroblasts are specialized cells that play a crucial role during normal healing but also during pathological deposition of the matrix and contraction of the tissues. However, these cells are not the only ones present in the tissues and can be strongly modulated by other cells that cannot secrete matrix but that can secrete mediators that can modulate myofibroblast phenotype. The role of the other cells present in tissues has thus to be studied to better understand fibrosis. Tissue engineering is an interesting method to study the interactions that can exist between cells and develop new tools to treat pathological tissues.

Acknowledgments These studies were supported by the Canadian Institute of Health Research and Foundation des Hopitaux Enfant-Jésus/Saint-Sacrement. VM was a recipient of scholarships from FRSQ.

References

Barreca A, De Luca M, Del Monte P, Bondanza S, Damonte G, Cariola G, Di Marco E, Giordano G, Cancedda R, Minuto F (1992) In vitro paracrine regulation of human keratinocyte growth by fibroblast-derived insulin-like growth factors. J Cell Physiol 151:262–268

Bell E, Ivarsson B, Merrill C (1979) Production of a tissue-like structure by contraction of collagen lattices by human fibroblasts of different proliferative potential in vitro. Proc Natl Acad Sci USA 76:1274–1278

Bellemare J, Roberge CJ, Bergeron D, Lopez-Valle CA, Roy M, Moulin VJ (2005) Epidermis promotes dermal fibrosis: role in the pathogenesis of hypertrophic scar. J Pathol 206:1–8

Berndt A, Kosmehl H, Katenkamp D, Tauchmann V (1994) Appearance of the myofibroblastic phenotype in Dupuytren's disease is associated with a fibronectin, laminin, collagen type IV and tenascin extracellular matrix. Pathobiology 62:55–58

Coulombe PA (2003) Wound epithelialization: accelerating the pace of discovery. J Invest Dermatol 121:219–230

De Wever O, Demetter P, Mareel M, Bracke M (2008) Stromal myofibroblasts are drivers of invasive cancer growth. Int J Cancer 123:2229–2238

Deitch EA, Wheelahan TM, Rose MP, Clothier J, Cotter J (1983) Hypertrophic burn scars: analysis of variables. J Trauma 23:895–8948

Desmoulière A, Geinoz A, Gabbiani F, Gabbiani G (1993) Transforming growth factor-b1 induces a-smooth muscle actin expression in granulation tissue myofibroblasts and in quiescent and growing cultured fibroblasts. J Cell Biol 122:103–111

Diegelmann RF (1997) Cellular and biochemical aspects of normal and abnormal wound healing: an overview. J Urol 157:298–302

Gabbiani G (2003) The myofibroblast in wound healing and fibrocontractive diseases. J Pathol 200:500–503

Gabbiani G, Badonnel MC (1976) Contractile events during inflammation. Agents Actions 6:277–280

Gabbiani G, Ryan GB, Majno G (1971) Presence of modified fibroblasts in granulation tissue and their possible role in wound contraction. Experientia 27:549–550

Germain L, Jean A, Auger F, Garrel DR (1994) Human wound healing fibroblasts have greater contractile properties than dermal fibroblasts. J Surg Res 57:268–273

Ghahary A, Marcoux Y, Karimi-Busheri F, Tredget EE (2001) Keratinocyte differentiation inversely regulates the expression of involucrin and transforming growth factor beta1. J Cell Biochem 83:239–248

Ghahary A, Karimi-Busheri F, Marcoux Y, Li Y, Tredget EE, Taghi Kilani R, Li L, Zheng J, Karami A, Keller BO, Weinfeld M (2004) Keratinocyte-releasable stratifin functions as a potent collagenase-stimulating factor in fibroblasts. J Invest Dermatol 122:1188–1197

Guo S, Zhang L, Wang Z, Liu J (2002) Effects of conditionned medium derived from different keratinocytes on proliferation and collagen synthesis of hypertrophic scar fibroblasts. Zhonghua Zheng Xing Wai Ke Za Zhi 18:83–85

Kischer CW, Thies AC, Chvapil M (1982) Perivascular myofibroblasts and microvascular occlusion in hypertrophic scars and keloids. Hum Pathol 13:819–824

L'Heureux N, Paquet S, Labbé R, Germain L, Auger FA (1998) A completely biological tissue-engineered human blood vessel. FASEB J 12:47–56

Lacroix C, Bovy T, Nusgens BV, Lapière CM (1995) Keratinocytes modulate the biosynthetic phenotype of dermal fibroblasts at a pretranslational level in a human skin equivalent. Arch Dermatol Res 287:659–664

Laplante A, Germain L, Auger F, Moulin V (2001) Mechanisms of wound reepithelialization: hints from a tissue-engineered reconstructed skin to long-standing questions. FASEB J 15: 2377–2389

Lim IJ, Phan T-T, Song C, Tan WTL, Longaker MT (2001) Investigation of the influence of keloid-derived keratinocytes on fibroblast growth and proliferation in vitro. Plast Reconstr Surg 107:797–808

Maas-Szabowski N, Shimotoyodome A, Fusenig NE (1999) Keratinocyte growth regulation in fibroblast cocultures via a double paracrine mechanism. J Cell Sci 112:1843–1853

Michel M, L'Heureux N, Pouliot R, Xu W, Auger FA, Germain L (1999) Characterization of a new tissue-engineered human skin equivalent with hair. In Vitro Cell Dev Biol Anim 35: 318–326

Moulin V (1995) Growth factors in skin wound healing. Eur J Cell Biol 68:1–7

Moulin V, Castilloux G, Jean A, Garrel DR, Auger FA, Germain L (1996) In vitro models to study wound healing fibroblasts. Burns 22:359–362

Moulin V, Auger FA, O'Connor-McCourt M, Germain L (1997) Fetal and postnatal sera differentially modulate human dermal fibroblast phenotypic and functional features in vitro. J Cell Physiol 171:1–10

Moulin V, Castilloux G, Auger FA, Garrel D, O'Connor-McCourt M, Germain L (1998) Modulated response to cytokines of human wound healing myofibroblasts compared to dermal fibroblasts. Exp Cell Res 238:283–293

Moulin V, Auger F, Garrel D, Germain L (2000) Role of wound healing myofibroblasts on reepithelialization of skin. Burns 26:3–12

Niessen FB, Andriessen MP, Schalkwijk J, Visser L, Timens W (2001) Keratinocyte-derived growth factors play a role in the formation of hypertrophic scars. J Pathol 194:207–216

Pierce GF, Vande Berg J, Rudolph R, Tarpley J, Mustoe TA (1991) Platelet-derived growth factor-BB and transforming growth factor beta 1 selectively modulate glycosaminoglycans, collagen, and myofibroblasts in excisional wounds. Am J Pathol 138:629–646

Rochon MH, Gauthier MJ, Auger FA, Germain L (2001) Simultaneous isolation of keratinocytes and fibroblasts from a human cutaneous biopsy for the production of autologous reconstructed skin. Can J Chem Eng 79:663–667

Santiago B, Galindo M, Rivero M, Pablos JL (2001) Decreased susceptibility to Fas-induced apoptosis of systemic sclerosis dermal fibroblasts. Arthritis Rheum 44:1667–1676

Schürch W, Seemayer TA, Gabbiani G (1992) Myofibroblast. In: Sternberg S (ed) Histology for pathologists, vol 5. Raven, NY, pp 109–114

Serini G, Bochaton-Piallat M-L, Ropraz P, Geinoz A, Borsi L, Zardi L, Gabbiani G (1998) The fibronectin domain ED-A is crucial for myofibroblastic phenotype induction by transforming growth factor-ß1. J Cell Biol 142:873–881

Smola H, Stark HJ, Thiekötter G, Mirancea N, Krieg T, Fusenig NE (1998) Dynamics of basement membrane formation by keratinocyte-fibroblast interactions in organotypic skin culture. Exp Cell Res 239:399–410

Werner S, Krieg T, Smola H (2007) Keratinocyte-fibroblast interactions in wound healing. J Invest Dermatol 127:998–1008

Dupuytren's Contracture Versus Burn Scar Contracture

10

Paul Zidel

Contents

10.1	**Introduction**	77
10.2	**Results and Questions**	78
10.3	**Discussion and More Questions**	81
10.4	**Conclusions**	81
References		82

10.1 Introduction

This is a philosophic essay of unanswered questions leaving open, thought-provoking issues.

Curiosity and inspiration should help provoke us to think anew and question the truth. One may start by considering that all we know may be wrong.

Cicatrix or scar formation and resultant contracture can be considered the body's response to an untoward event. Dupuytren's contractures and burn scar contractures share significant similarities. The purpose of this presentation is to review the intersection of burn scar and Dupuytren's contractures. The goal of this treatise is to question these two boxes from a different perspective from within and from outside as to their overlap and apply that knowledge to further better treatment of both.

P. Zidel
Department of Surgery, Maricopa Medical Center,
Phoenix, AZ, USA
e-mail: paul_zidel@dmgaz.org

Interestingly enough, there is a significant historical fact connecting burn scar contractures and Dupuytren's contractures. In 1832, Baron Guillaume Dupuytren first classified burns according to depth and divided thermal injuries into six degrees of severity (Dupuytren 1832).

There is a recent trend in Dupuytren's treatment popularized by French rheumatologists, i.e., needle aponeurotomy, (Lermusiaux and Debeyre 1979). But this is going back to similar procedures done in the 1800s by Cooper and Adams, which implies either that our evaluation of what works is lacking in astuteness or there are other factors in our treatment evolution. When we see burns and Dupuytren's, we are comparing apples and oranges but may realize the properties as defined are more similar than divergent. The scientific difference between apples and oranges is not common knowledge. Can an apple be considered both a fruit and vegetable based on what and whose definition? Using infrared transmission spectrometry, they are very similar (Sandford 1995). What function does a fruit serve for the overall organism perhaps other than propagation? In conclusion, they are more similar and tasty than divergent and provide food for thought analogous to our thesis.

Scar is the body's response to an insult, both internal, external, and/or emotional. But does the body react with the same scar cascade for all, with modifications based on what internal and/or external milieu factors? The mechanisms of injury are obviously different between burns and Dupuytren's. The burn insult is usually a single, inciting external event causing superficial to deep progression. The causation though can be quite diverse in nature such as scald, contact, fire, chemical, electric, etc. Also, the degree and duration, age of the skin and the degree of the initial inflammatory response also define the process. On the other hand, Dupuytren's disease is an insidious, internal event with an unknown, inciting event and an unpredictable, usually progressive course. The end result is the development of contracture, sometimes barely perceptible and sometimes quite severe. Is Dupuytren's by definition a scar? Will that idea help us in our understanding? But what is this scar and why does excessive scar form? What are the multifactorial components that lead from contraction to contracture? It is the identification of these atypical patients and their response to intervention which successfully alters the deteriorating cascade that is exciting. The burn scar contracture and the Dupuytren's contracture have significant commonality to warrant further combined data sharing to alter long-term effect.

Given the insightful and diverse basic research presented at this Symposium, it may be beneficial to consider a standard wound healing picture of the conceptual stages of healing and learn how and why there are deviations (Al-Qattan 2006). What is our present knowledge and what is our future focus can lead to ramifications in all fields of medicine including pulmonary fibrosis, intestinal adhesions, and many conditions characterized by fibrosis and scar (Robson 2003).

We certainly may be able to learn and lean in new directions as our outlook widens. As Dr. Charles Eaton said at this Symposium: to solve an impossible problem, question convention.

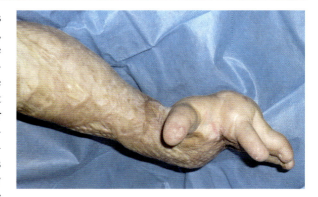

Fig. 10.1 Burn scar contracture – severe

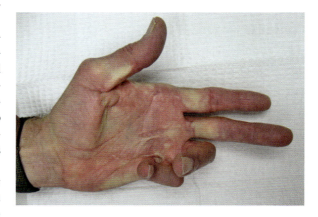

Fig. 10.2 Dupuytren's contracture

10.2 Results and Questions

It is commonly accepted that wounds progress through three main phases of healing. Initially there is the Inflammatory or Lag Phase followed by the Proliferative or Collagen Phase and then the Maturation Phase. This leads to scar and contraction as determined by the tensile strength of collagen reorganization and reorientation by cross-linking. It is the Maturation Phase that is the key to our dilemma. It is here where the burn wound strengthens and there is contraction (as opposed to wound "contracture"). The continually remodeling scar subsequently softens, relaxes, and matures. An equilibrium exists which balances cellular remodeling and extracellular degradation through collagen synthesis, degradation, and reformation (Kwan et al. 2009). What factors are in play at this time? Normally, the scar contraction softens. Abnormally, the scar can become excessively hypertrophic and/or form a contracture

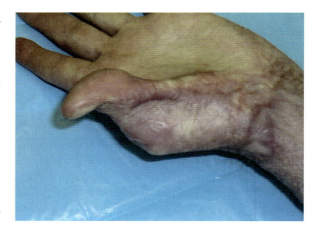

Fig. 10.3 Comparable burn scar contracture

(Figs. 10.1–10.3). Is hypertrophic scar related to contracture? (Linares 2002) In burn scar contractures, this balance is shifted and the wound becomes dysfunctional, much like in Dupuytren's contracture.

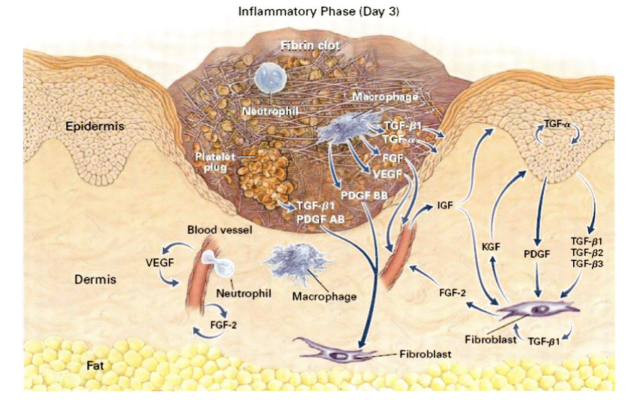

Fig. 10.4 A cutaneous wound 3 days after injury. Growth factors to be necessary for cell movement into the wound are shown. *TGF-β1*, *TGF-β2*, and *TGF-β3* denote transforming growth factor β1, β2, and β3, respectively; *TGF-α* transforming growth factor α, *FGF* fibroblast growth factor, *VEGF* vascular endothelial growth factor, *PDGF*, *PDGF AB*, and *PDGF BB* platelet-derived growth factor, platelet-derived growth factor AB, and platelet-derived growth factor BB, respectively; *IGF* insulin-like growth factor and *KGF* keratinocyte growth factor

Granulation tissue may form which some consider "healthy"; yet this healthy granulation tissue removed prior to grafting to get better wounds. What is granulation tissue and when is it healthy? (Scott et al. 2000) In general, the longer the wound is not healed or not closed, the more scar formation (Deitch et al. 1983). Closure or coverage brings about apoptosis in fibroblasts and less scar. What models best simulate wound healing? (Greenhalgh 2005)

The questions are thus. What causes the scar to mature? What causes the wound to contract and form contractures? Is it related to the initial degree of inflammatory response? What can be done to induce the abnormal contracture path not to proliferate (Kraljevic Pavelic et al. 2009) to be reoriented to the maturation road?

Many molecular and cellular forces are at work in the evolving wound scar. A classic review article by Singer and Clark (Singer and Clark 1999) demonstrates that the collagen degradation is controlled by matrix metalloproteinases which are proteolytic enzymes secreted by macrophages, epidermal and endothelial cells, and fibroblasts (Figs. 10.4 and 10.5). Myofibroblasts play a significant role in wound healing but also in fibrocontractive diseases whose hypertrophic scars contain significant numbers of these cells (Gabbiani and Majno 1972; Tomasek et al. 2002; Cordova et al. 2005). "Mechanical tension stimulates the transdifferentiation of fibroblasts into myofibroblasts in human burn scars" (Junker et al. 2008). How do the cells interact with extracellular matrix? Is there stress shielding within this environment? (Nekouzadeh et al. 2008) Is this behavior mediated by pO2 tension, vascularity, or which other factors? There are molecular and cellular causes of scarring (Scott et al. 2002). There appears to be a critical depth for a wound to develop scar (Dunkin et al. 2007). Subpopulations of fibroblasts based on

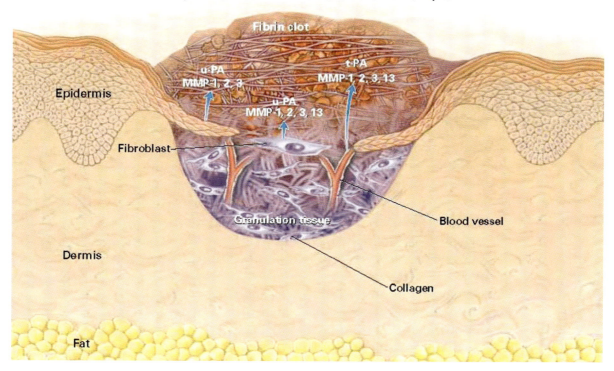

Fig. 10.5 A cutaneous wound 5 days after injury. Blood vessels are seen sprouting into the fibrin clot as epidermal cells resurface the wound. Proteinases thought to be necessary for cell movement are shown. The abbreviation *u-PA* denotes urokinase-type plasminogen activator, *MMP*-1, 2, 3, and 13 matrix metalloproteinases 1, 2, 3, and 13 (collagenase 1, gelatinase A, stromelysin 1, and collagenase 3, respectively); and *t-PA* tissue plasminogen activator

depth of injury influence scar formation (Wang et al. 2008). Modifying forces cause resistance as new collagen is synthesized along lines of stress. How could distal radius fractures affect pain syndromes and Dupuytren's flare? "Mechanical strain alters gene expression in an in vitro model of hypertrophic scarring" (Derderian et al. 2005).

The wound healing sequence is appreciably modified by external forces and internal factors. Why do mammalian embryos heal wounds with no scar and can that process be manipulated? (Ferguson and O'Kane 2004) Internal modulation of a collagen scar occurs by a long list of substances including cytokines (Polo et al. 1997), collagenase secretion, Tamoxifen (Kuhn et al. 2002), Relaxin, Calcium-channel blockers (e.g., Verapamil), Putrescine (Fibrostat), TGF-beta 1, 2 and 3, IGF-1, T-lymphocytes, other cytokines, Interferon (Pittet et al. 1994; Sahara et al. 1993), osteopontin, oxygen-free radicals, TNF IL-6,8, PDGF, bFGF, GM-CSF, proteases MMPs, corticosteroids, etc.

(Rayan et al. 1996). The list grows when including stem cells and genetic manipulation (Bayat et al. 2002; Shih et al. 2010; Branski et al. 2009). There are external, mechanical treatment options for burn scar contractures, which may apply to Dupuytren's contractures (Mustoe et al. 2002). Modalities which have been used for scar management include silicone (Perkins et al. 1983), corticosteroids, pressure garments, gel pressure sheets, splints (Larson et al. 1971), serial casting, continuous passive motion, negative pressure, hyperbarics, laser therapy (Leclère and Mordon 2010), cryosurgery, external fixation distracters, dynamic splinting, and progressive splinting. Collagenase is being used for both the treatment of burns and in Dupuytren's. One important question involves whether Dupuytren's and burn scar contractures can be stretched out and have permanent plastic deformation with no recurrence and if so, how exactly to do it in relation to time, tension, cycling, and type. Clearly much needs to be learned about the contracture process.

Given the insightful and diverse basic research presented at this Symposium, it may be beneficial to consider a different, more encompassing, internal and external, conceptual wound healing picture. There are significant overlaps of scar formation by burns and Dupuytren's to warrant further investigation with excruciatingly detailed, randomized, prospective outcome monetary studies.

10.3 Discussion and More Questions

Reading the Proceedings of the Dupuytren's Symposium based on the 1966 meeting, I was struck by the questions of Iselin and Hueston (Hueston 1974).

Etiological Questions in Dupuytren's Contracture – John T. Hueston
- Who gets it?
- What course does it run?
- What therapy influences it?
- What is its structure?
- What is its mechanism of production?
- Finally then, can it be prevented?

Mysterious Aspects of Dupuytren's Contracture – Marc Iselin (1974)
- Why does this spread like a malignant tumor?
- How does this go beyond the palmar aponeurosis?
- Why is it involved in only certain spots?
- Why is the natural history so unpredictable?

The Questions continue here comparing Dupuytren's contractures to burn scar contractures:

Does a Dupuytren's contracture serve a useful teleological purpose? Why does this happen? Can Dupuytren's contracture be considered a wound healing issue gone awry? What is the association with Peyronie's Disease and Ledderhose Disease and what can we learn from them? How is Dupuytren's disease related to diabetes etc.? Why are other areas of fascia or aponeurosis not affected? Why is Dupuytren's so variable and unpredictable? What causes some Dupuytren's contractures to progress and not others? What is a Dupuytren's flare? Is there a psychological association with Dupuytren's? Is there an animal model for Dupuytren's contractures? Why not? Why is there conflicting information regarding stretching Dupuytren's contractures? Static, progressive splinting, dynamic, digit-widget. What would allow the latter to work long term once it is removed. Are there critical details important for success, i.e., the amount of tension, pressure, timing, intermittent versus constant or progressive. Tearing with subsequent scar versus "Wolfe's Law" of stretch remodeling applied to collagen, ligaments with permanent "plastic" deformation. Tearing versus stretching.

Why do fetal wounds heal without scar? What is the genetic basis of healing? Why do burn wounds usually mature and soften while Dupuytren's fasciitis progresses. What turns one process off and the other on? Do the three main phases of healing and contracture really apply to Dupuytren's disease?

It would seem that if this phase can be "turned on" in Dupuytren's, the wounds would resolve instead of contract. How best to research the factors responsible for the maturation phase of wound healing. How do we evaluate scar for comparison? (Duncan 2006)

What causes some burns to become contractures, some hypertrophic and some hypertrophic contractures and not others? Does hypertrophic scarring perform a useful function? Why does hypertrophic scarring and contractures for both burns and Dupuytren's occur virtually only in humans? Why is there no good burn scar or Dupuytren's animal model (beyond perhaps the nude mouse)? (Polo et al. 1998; Robb et al. 1987; Morris et al. 1997).This implies the animal scar matures and resolves better than humans. Why and how and what can we learn from that?

Is there an overlap between those people who form hypertrophic burn scar contractures and those who form significant severe Dupuytren's contractures? Is there an allele for that common to both? Can a Dupuytren's nodule and cord be related to a hypertrophic burn and keloid? Do pressure garments work on burn maturation or other modalities, CPM, negative pressure, silicone, splinting, steroid impregnated silicone compression distractor? Can it work on Dupuytren's contraction given the right parameter of time, intensity, cycling, etc.?

We all want a magic bullet, a laser at? X wavelength or a topical potion penetrating the skin that will modify cross-linking or scar contracture properties if we cannot prevent the process.

10.4 Conclusions

Healing and proliferative scarring is an enigma (Robson 2003). This portion of the Symposium sought to bring a different perspective on Dupuytren's from a seemingly opposite process to stimulate questions and thought.

Will we be asking these same questions next century? Or can we change the ending of "The Blind Men and the Elephant" poem by John Godfrey Saxe (18…) where we "Rail on in utter ignorance…of what each other mean"?

References

Al-Qattan MM (2006) Factors in the pathogenesis of Dupuytren's contracture. J Hand Surg Am 31(9):1527–1534

Bayat A, Watson JS, Stanley JK, Alansari A, Shah M, Ferguson MWJ, Ollier WER (2002) Genetic susceptibility in Dupuytren's disease – TGF-beta 1 polymorphisms and Dupuytren's disease. J Bone Joint Surg Br 84(2):211–215

Branski LK, Gauglitz GG, Herndon DN, Jeschke MG (2009) A review of gene and stem cell therapy in cutaneous wound healing. Burns 35(2):171–180

Cordova A, Tripoli M, Corradino B, Napoli P, Moschella F (2005) Dupuytren's contracture: an update of biomolecular aspects and therapeutic perspectives. J Hand Surg Br 30:557–562

Deitch EA, Wheelahan TM, Rose MP, Clothier J, Cotter J (1983) Hypertrophic burn scars: analysis of variables. J Trauma 23(10):895–898

Derderian CA, Bastidas N, Lerman OZ, Bhatt KA, Lin S, Voss J, Holmes JW, Levine JP, Gurtner GC (2005) Mechanical strain alters gene expression in an in vitro model of hypertrophic scarring. Ann Plas Surg 55(1):69–75

Duncan JAL, Bond JS, Mason T, Ludlow A, Cridland P, O'Kane S, Ferguson MWJ (2006) Visual analogue scale scoring and ranking: a suitable and sensitive method for assessing scar quality? Plast Reconstr Surg 118(4):909–918

Dunkin CSJ, Pleat JM, Gillespie PH, Tyler MPH, Roberts AHN, McGrouther DA (2007) Scarring occurs at a critical depth of skin injury: precise measurement in a graduated dermal scratch in human volunteers. Plast Reconstr Surg 119(6):1722–1732

Dupuytren G (1832) Lecons orales de clinique chirurgicale faites a l'Hotel-dieu de Paris. Bailliere, Paris, 1: pp 413–516. In: Burns of the upper extremity, salisbury and pruitt, Vol. XIX. In: Major problems of clinical surgery. W.B. Saunders, Philadelphia, 1976 and in Total burn care, 2nd edition. Herndon (ed) Saunders, London, 2002

Ferguson MWJ, O'Kane S (2004) Scar-free healing: from embryonic mechanisms to adult therapeutic intervention. Philos Trans R Soc Lond B Biol Sci 359(1445):839–850

Gabbiani G, Majno G (1972) Dupuytren's contracture: fibroblast connection? an ultrastructional study. Am J Pathol 66: 131–146

Greenhalgh DG (2005) Models of wound healing. J Burn Care Rehabil 26(4):293–305

Hueston JT (1974) Aetological questions in Dupuytren's contracture. In: Hueston JT, Tubiana R (eds) Dupuytren's Disease. Grune & Stratton, New York, pp 29–36

Iselin M (1974) Mysterious aspects of Dupuytren's Contracture. In: Hueston JT, Tubiana R (eds) Dupuytren's Disease. Grune & Stratton, New York, pp 67–70

Junker JPE, Kratz C, Tollbäck A, Kratz G (2008) Mechanical tension stimulates the transdifferentiation of fibroblasts into myofibroblasts in human burn scars. Burns 34(7):942–946

Kraljevic Pavelic S, Bratulic S, Hock K, Jurisic D, Hranjec M, Karminski-Zamola G, Zinic B, Bujak M, Pavelic K (2009) Screening of potential prodrugs on cells derived from Dupuytren's disease patients. Biomed Pharmacother 63(8): 577–585

Kuhn M, Wang X, Payne W, Ko F, Robson M (2002) Tamoxifen decreases fibroblast function and down regulates TGFB2 in Dupuytren's affected palmar fascia. J Surg Res 103:146–152

Kwan P, Hori K, Ding J, Tredget E (2009) Scar and contracture: biological principles. Hand Clin 25:511–528

Larson DL, Abston S, Evans EB, Dobrokovsky M, Linares HA (1971) Techniques for decreasing scar formation and contractures in the burned patient. J Trauma 1(10):807–823

Leclère FM, Mordon SR (2010) Twenty-five years of active laser prevention of scars: what have we learned? J Cosmet Laser Ther 12(5):227–34

Lermusiaux JL, Debeyre N (1979) Le traitment medical de la maladie de Dupuytren. In: de Seze S, Ryckewaert A, Kahn MF, Kuntz D, Dryll A, Meyer O et al (eds) L'actualite rhumatologique. Expansion Scientifique, Paris, pp 3383–3443

Linares HA (2002) Pathophysiology of the burn scar. In: Herndon DN (ed.) Total burn care, 2nd edition, Chap. 44. Saunders, London, pp 544–559

Morris DE, Wu LL, Zhao L, Bolton L, Roth SI, Ladin D, Mustoe TA (1997) Acute and chronic animal models for excessive dermal scarring: Quantitative studies. Plast Reconstr Surg 100(3):674–681

Mustoe TA, Cooter RD, Gold MH, Hobbs R, Ramelet A-A, Shakespeare PG, Stella M, Téot L, Wood FM, Ziegler U (2002) International clinical recommendations on scar management for the International Advisory Panel on Scar Management. Plast Reconstr Surg 110:560

Nekouzadeh A, Pryse KM, Elson EL, Genin GM (2008) Stretch-activated force-shedding, force recovery, and cytoskeletal remodeling in contractile fibroblasts. J Biomech 41(14): 2964–2971

Perkins K, Davey RB, Wallis KA (1983) Silicone Gel: a new treatment for burn scars and contractures. Burns 9(3):201–204

Pittet B, Rubbia-Brandt L et al (1994) Effect of γ-interferon on the clinical and biologic evolution of hypertrophic scars and Dupuytren's disease: an open pilot study. Plast Recontsr Surg 93(6):1224–1235

Polo M, Ko F, Busillo B, Cruse C, Krizek T, Robson M (1997) The 1997 Moyer Award: cytokine production in burn patients with hypertrophic scars. J Burn Care Rehabil 18:477–483

Polo M, Kim Y, Kucukcelebi A, Hayward PG, Ko F, Robson MC (1998) An in vivo model of human proliferative scar. J Surg Res 74:187–195

Rayan GM, Parizi M, Tomasek JJ (1996) Pharmacologic regulation of Dupuytren's fibroblasts contraction in vitro. J Hand Surg Am 21:1065–1070

Robb EC, Waymack JP, Warden GD, Nathan P, Alexander JW (1987) A new model for studying the development of human hypertrophic burn scar formation. J Burn Care Rehabil 8(5):371–375

Robson MC (2003) Proliferative scarring. Surg Clin North Am 83:557–569

Sahara K, Kucukcelebi A, Ko F, Phillips L, Robson M (1993) Suppression of in vitro proliferative scar fibroblast contraction by interferon alpha-2â. Wound Repair Regen 1:22–27

Sandford S (1995) Apples and Oranges — a comparison. AIR 1(3)

Scott PG, Gharary A, Tredget EE (2000) Molecular and cellular aspects of fibrosis following thermal injury. Hand Clin 16(2):27

Scott PG, Ghahary A, Tredget EE (2002) Molecular and cellular basis of hypertrophic scarring. In: D. Herndon (ed). Total burn care, 2nd edition, Chapt. 43. Saunders, London, pp 536–543

Shih B, May T, Watson J, McGrouther D, Bayat A (2010) Genome-Wide High-Resolution Screening in Dupuytren's Disease Reveals Common Regions of DNA Copy Number Alterations. J Hand Surg Am 35A:1172–1183

Singer AJ, Clark RAF (1999) Cutaneous wound healing. N Engl J Med 341(10):738–746

Tomasek JU, Gabbiani G, Hinz B, Chaponnier C, Ra B (2002) Myofibroblasts and mechano-regulation of connective tissue remodeling. Nat Rev Mol Cell Biol 3:349–363

Wang J, Dodd C, Shankowsky HA, Scott PG, Tredget EE (2008) Deep dermal fibroblasts contribute to hypertrophic scarring. Lab Invest 88:1278–1290

Part III

Genetics and Demographics

Editor: Ardeshir Bayat

The Genetic Basis of Dupuytren's Disease: An Introduction

11

Guido H.C.G. Dolmans and Hans C. Hennies

Contents

11.1	**Introduction**	87
11.2	**Linkage Analysis**	88
11.3	**Association Analysis**	88
11.4	**Epidemiology of Dupuytren's Disease**	88
11.5	**Susceptibility Genes for Dupuytren's Disease**	90
References		91

Abbreviations

CNV	Copy number variant
HWE	Hardy–Weinberg equilibrium
LD	Linkage disequilibrium
LOD	Logarithm of the odds
SNP	Single-nucleotide polymorphism

11.1 Introduction

The application of Mendelian principles to heredity in man (Bateson 1906) has opened the particular field of human genetics and the experimental study of human traits. It was not before 2001, when the draft sequence of the human genome was published and thus the sequence of the nucleotides, the chemical base pairs that make up DNA (and genes), mostly determined (Lander et al. 2001; Venter et al. 2001), that we could study the human genome in its entirety rather than one gene at a time.

Genetic variation, mostly represented by single-nucleotide polymorphisms (SNPs) and copy number variants (CNVs) is frequent; any two humans are different in about 0.5% of their DNA sequence. Mutations, that is, permanent changes in the genome including point mutations affecting single nucleotides and structural changes of chromosomes, can predispose to developing disease, modify the course of disease, or cause the disease itself. Virtually any disease is the result of the combined action of genes and environment but the relative role of the genetic component may be large or small. In a simplistic way we can distinguish monogenic and multifactorial diseases.

G.H.C.G. Dolmans
Department of Plastic Surgery,
University Medical Center of Groningen,
University of Groningen, Groningen, The Netherlands

Department of Genetics, University Medical Center Groningen,
University of Groningen, Groningen, The Netherlands
e-mail: g.h.c.g.dolmans@umcg.nl

H.C. Hennies (✉)
Division of Dermatogenetics, Cologne Center for Genomics,
University of Cologne, Weyertal 115b, 50931 Cologne,
Germany

Cluster of Excellence on Cellular Stress Responses
in Aging-Associated Diseases,
University of Cologne, Cologne, Germany
e-mail: h.hennies@uni-koeln.de

C. Eaton et al. (eds.), *Dupuytren's Disease and Related Hyperproliferative Disorders*,
DOI 10.1007/978-3-642-22697-7_11, © Springer-Verlag Berlin Heidelberg 2012

Monogenic disease is the result of a single mutated gene. These diseases, such as cystic fibrosis and Huntington's disease, usually exhibit obvious inheritance patterns in families according to the laws of Mendel. These patterns can be autosomal dominant, recessive, or X-linked. Most of such single-gene diseases are rare, with a frequency as high as 1 in 500 or 1,000 individuals but usually much less. Genetic disorders may also be complex, meaning that they are associated with the effects of multiple genes (polygenic) in combination with environmental factors (multifactorial). Multifactorial diseases include, among many others, forms of diabetes, cancer, cardiovascular disease, and psoriasis.

Dupuytren's disease can be considered as a multifactorial disease as well. Although complex genetic diseases often cluster in families, they do not have a clear (Mendelian) pattern of inheritance. Multifactorial diseases have a major impact on the entire population. The identification of genes involved in Dupuytren's disease will further our understanding of the pathogenesis and also provide insight into new treatment modalities.

Two fundamental approaches are available for identifying genes involved in diseases or, more generally, in traits: linkage analysis and association analysis (Risch 2000; Terwilliger and Göring 2000).

11.2 Linkage Analysis

The first approach, linkage analysis, is family based. Linkage analysis is a method that allows us to determine regions of chromosomes that are likely to contain a risk gene, and rule out areas where there is a low chance of finding a risk gene. This technique works by investigating the segregation of genetic markers to reveal recombination events between any two chromosomal loci. Currently, mostly SNPs are used as genetic markers. The location of approximately three million SNPs is presently known in the human genome. This means that there is one genetic marker (SNP) available in every 1,000 base pairs of our DNA.

Linkage analysis involving specific genetic disease models is especially powerful for the study of rare single-gene diseases. In linkage studies, researchers are searching for a marker locus that is consistently inherited with a disease. To this end, marker alleles are experimentally determined and their segregation followed in a pedigree. When a marker is found that co-segregates with the disease, the marker locus and the disease locus are said to be linked and assumed to be located near each other on a chromosome. The statistical estimate of whether two loci are linked to each other and therefore likely inherited together is called a LOD score. A LOD score above 3 is considered significant.

11.3 Association Analysis

The second approach, association analysis, is population based. Association analysis is performed to determine whether a genetic variant (SNP) is associated with a disease. This technique is especially powerful for more common, genetically complex diseases (The Wellcome Trust Case Control Consortium 2007; Pearson and Manolio 2008). Most often a case/control study design is used. The allele frequencies of hundreds of thousands of markers (SNPs) spread over the genome are compared between cases (individuals with the disease) and controls from the same population. A significant difference in the frequency of an allele of a SNP between cases and controls indicates that the SNP is associated with the disease and may increase the risk of developing this disease. However, an associated SNP identified in an association study is usually not a disease-causing variant but located on a stretch of DNA adjacent to this variant. This concept is called linkage disequilibrium (LD): the nonrandom association of alleles at two or more loci in a population. An associated SNP therefore pinpoints a very small region of DNA with strong LD, which usually harbors only a few genes.

Because hundreds of thousands of markers have to be tested in a genome-wide association study, the possibility to detect false positive results is high. The easiest way to reduce false positive findings is a stringent significance threshold. Generally, a value $p < 5.0 \times 10^{-8}$ is accepted in studies of up to 1×10^6 markers. Another drawback in association analysis is population stratification. Population stratification is the presence of a systematic difference in allele frequencies between subpopulations, usually due to a different ancestry. Hence, cases and controls must be from the same population. In order to provide evidence that associations are not false positive, it is furthermore important to replicate results in other study cohorts preferably from different populations.

11.4 Epidemiology of Dupuytren's Disease

Dupuytren's disease is a multifactorial disease. It has a strong genetic component, as demonstrated by concordance rates in twin studies and familial clustering

(Burge 1999). The recurrence risk for persons with an affected sibling, for instance, was determined as $\lambda_s = 2.9$ in a population from England (Hindocha et al. 2006). However, a geographical imbalance has been described in the frequency of Dupuytren's disease. It seems to be more prevalent in Northern European populations, with a prevalence of 9.4% in males and 2.8% in females from Norway (Mikkelsen 1972) and a prevalence of 13.3% in an Icelandic study (Gudmundsson et al. 1999). The familial incidence has been reported as high as 44% and 74%, respectively, in populations from Sweden and Iceland (Skoog 1948; Gudmundsson et al. 2000). Cases of Dupuytren's disease were also described in several other populations all over the world. The prevalence of Dupuytren's disease in Germany has been estimated as 2.5% (Brenner et al. 2001). In a comparison of prevalence rates in studies from various countries worldwide, the mean prevalence was reported as below 5% and similar in males and females in persons up to 45 years of age. It rises to 33% in males older than 65 years and 23% in females older than 75 years (Hindocha et al. 2009). The authors also pointed out that the rather large differences described in the prevalence of Dupuytren's disease in various regions might well reflect different diagnostic criteria. These numbers also indicate that Dupuytren's disease is probably underdiagnosed in several countries (Degreef and De Smet 2010) and is, after all, an entity with worldwide occurrence.

We have recently established Dupuytren's disease study groups comprising experienced hand surgeons from Germany and the Netherlands and documented detailed clinical and epidemiological data.

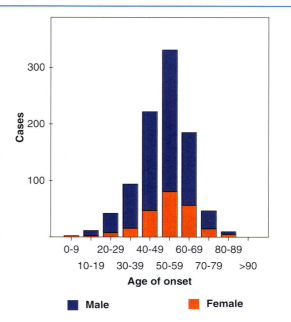

Fig. 11.1 Onset of Dupuytren's disease. Age at onset in 1,000 Dutch patients with Dupuytren's disease. The fractions of male (*blue bars*) and female (*red bars*) patients are shown separately

In 1,000 patients from the Netherlands, the age at onset clearly peaks in the sixth decade of life (Fig. 11.1). In 550 cases from Germany and Switzerland, we found a distribution between male and female patients of 4:1. The age at first surgery was 58±10 years of age in male and 61±9 years of age in female patients, ranging from 22 to 87 years (Fig. 11.2). In cases with a known family background for Dupuytren's disease (40%), the onset tends to be earlier and the course of the disease more severe: the age at first surgery was

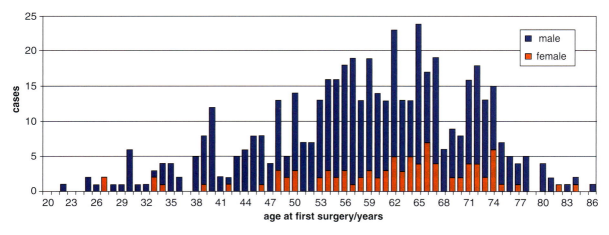

Fig. 11.2 Age at first-hand surgery. Distribution of ages at the first-hand surgery in 550 German patients with Dupuytren's disease. Male patients are represented by *blue bars*, female patients by *red bars*

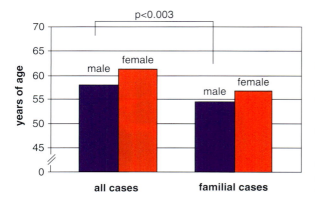

Fig. 11.3 Mean age at first surgery in familial cases compared to all cases analyzed. The mean age at first-hand surgery was clearly lower in familial cases, both in male (*blue bars*) and female (*red bars*) patients, indicating a more severe course in familial Dupuytren's disease

lower, and the number of cases with both hands affected was higher (Fig. 11.3).

In a preliminary evaluation, we did not identify significant effects of risk factors. Eleven percent of the patients also had diabetes mellitus, which might confirm a positive association of Dupuytren's disease with diabetes. We did not see, however, an association with nicotine or alcohol consumption; the ratios of smokers and continued alcohol consumers were rather the same as in the general population according to the figures from German federal institutions.

11.5 Susceptibility Genes for Dupuytren's Disease

There are few reports of extended pedigrees with a transmission of Dupuytren's disease, which demonstrate an autosomal dominant inheritance with reduced penetrance. In one pedigree from Sweden, a whole-genome linkage analysis has been conducted (Hu et al. 2005). It has localized a candidate region on chromosome 16; an underlying mutation, however, has not yet been identified. Other studies have used a case/control design for the analysis of an association with particular functional candidate genes such as those involved in the TGF-β pathways. Markers in the genes for TGF-β1, TGF-β2, or TGF-β receptors have not proven an association so far. Only a SNP in the gene for transcription factor Zf9, which may activate TGF-β1, showed an association with an odds ratio of 1.9 (Bayat et al. 2003).

In order to systematically elucidate the genetic basis for Dupuytren's disease, we have decided to use our study cohorts for genome-wide association studies in a case/control study design. As outlined above, large sample numbers are necessary for whole-genome association studies in order to gain sufficient power to obtain significant results. The 2010 International Symposium on Dupuytren's Disease has initiated the collaboration of research groups from Germany, the Netherlands, and UK, involving the institutions of the authors, departments from Oxford (UK), and several others. Until now we have incorporated more than 1,000 Dutch cases, more than 600 German cases, and more than 700 UK cases. This joint endeavor made it possible to perform a large-scale genome-wide association study including the chip-based analysis of very large numbers of SNPs, that is, up to 1×10^6 markers distributed over the human genome. Experimental procedures and data analysis are done in an automated manner. The data analysis also involves several statistical tools to remove false positive findings and test against systematic genotyping errors, genetic selection, and population stratification. These and other problems are for instance addressed by strictly taking account of the Hardy–Weinberg equilibrium (HWE), which regards the genotype distribution at a single locus in the population. Finally, our collaborations also allow for powerful replication studies, which are considered as an important part of a strong genome-wide association study. The most significant results of this cooperative study identifying several loci associated with Dupuytren's disease will soon be published elsewhere. These approaches are only first steps to characterize the genetic basis for Dupuytren's disease. However, they are an important undertaking, since only the subsequent characterization of the molecular etiology will lead to the development of more effective and possibly causal treatment opportunities for Dupuytren's disease.

Acknowledgments We are grateful to all individuals with Dupuytren's disease and control persons for participating in this study. We wish to thank Kerstin Becker, Sigrid Tinschert, Peter Nürnberg, Paul M. Werker, Roel A. Ophoff, Cisca Wijmenga, and Dominic Furniss for their contributions to the study. The project would not be possible without the immense help of the members of the Dutch and the German Dupuytren Study Groups and the UK BSSH GODD Consortium.

References

Bateson W (1906) On Mendelian heredity and its application to man. Br Med J 2:61–67

Bayat A, Watson JS, Stanley JK, Ferguson MW, Ollier WE (2003) Genetic susceptibility to dupuytren disease: association of Zf9 transcription factor gene. Plast Reconstr Surg 111:2133–2139

Brenner P, Krause-Bergmann A, Van VH (2001) Die Dupuytren-Kontraktur in Norddeutschland. Epidemiologische Erfassungsstudie anhand von 500 Fällen. Unfallchirurg 104:303–311

Burge P (1999) Genetics of Dupuytren's disease. Hand Clin 15:63–71

Degreef I, De Smet L (2010) A high prevalence of Dupuytren's disease in Flanders. Acta Orthop Belg 76:316–320

Gudmundsson KG, Arngrimsson R, Sigfusson N, Jonsson T (1999) Prevalence of joint complaints amongst individuals with Dupuytren's disease – from the Reykjavik study. Scand J Rheumatol 28:300–304

Gudmundsson KG, Arngrimsson R, Sigfusson N, Bjornsson A, Jonsson T (2000) Epidemiology of Dupuytren's disease: clinical, serological, and social assessment. The Reykjavik study. J Clin Epidemiol 53:291–296

Hindocha S, John S, Stanley JK, Watson SJ, Bayat A (2006) The heritability of Dupuytren's disease: familial aggregation and its clinical significance. J Hand Surg [Am] 31:204–210

Hindocha S, McGrouther DA, Bayat A (2009) Epidemiological evaluation of Dupuytren's disease incidence and prevalence rates in relation to etiology. Hand (N Y) 4:256–269

Hu FZ, Nystrom A, Ahmed A, Palmquist M, Dopico R, Mossberg I et al (2005) Mapping of an autosomal dominant gene for Dupuytren's contracture to chromosome 16q in a Swedish family. Clin Genet 68:424–429

Lander ES, Linton LM, Birren B, Nusbaum C, Zody MC, Baldwin J et al (2001) Initial sequencing and analysis of the human genome. Nature 409:860–921

Mikkelsen OA (1972) The prevalence of Dupuytren's disease in Norway. A study in a representative population sample of the municipality of Haugesund. Acta Chir Scand 138:695–700

Pearson TA, Manolio TA (2008) How to interpret a genome-wide association study. JAMA 299:1335–1344

Risch NJ (2000) Searching for genetic determinants in the new millennium. Nature 405:847–856

Skoog T (1948) Dupuytren's contraction. Acta Chir Scand 96:29

Terwilliger JD, Göring HH (2000) Gene mapping in the 20th and 21st centuries: statistical methods, data analysis, and experimental design. Hum Biol 72:63–132

The Wellcome Trust Case Control Consortium (2007) Genome-wide association study of 14,000 cases of seven common diseases and 3,000 shared controls. Nature 447:661–678

Venter JC, Adams MD, Myers EW, Li PW, Mural RJ, Sutton GG et al (2001) The sequence of the human genome. Science 291:1304–1351

Use of Genetic and Genomic Analyses Tools to Study Dupuytren's Disease

12

Barbara Shih, Stewart Watson, and Ardeshir Bayat

Contents

12.1	Introduction	93
12.2	Genetic Research Material and Tools	93
12.3	Observational Approaches	94
12.4	Gene-Specific Approaches	95
12.5	Genome-Wide Approaches	96
12.6	Discussion	98
References		99

B. Shih • A. Bayat (✉)
Plastic & Reconstructive Surgery Research,
Manchester Interdisciplinary Biocentre, Manchester, UK
e-mail: ardeshir.bayat@manchester.ac.uk

S. Watson
Department of Plastic & Reconstructive Surgery,
University Hospital of South Manchester, Manchester, UK

12.1 Introduction

Dupuytren's disease (DD) is a nodular fibromatosis of unknown cause, commonly affecting the hands. Several observations, including families with multiple members presenting with the disease, occurrences in homozygous twins, high prevalence in the Caucasian population, are suggestive of genetic causation in the disease etiology. To date, a large number of studies have been carried out to gain a greater understanding of the genetics of DD. Following the completion of the Human Genome Project (International Human Genome Sequencing Consortium 2004), the first phase of the HapMap project (International HapMap Consortium 2005) and the first phase of the Encyclopaedia of DNA Elements project in 2007, (Birney et al. 2007), a wide range of genetic research tools and resources have become available. These resources have facilitated a greater understanding of the genetic, physical, and transcript maps of the genomes, as well as allowed the rapid development of new genetic research tools (Feero et al. 2008). This review aims to summarize the approaches and genetics tools that have been used in DD research to date and their respective findings.

12.2 Genetic Research Material and Tools

Over the years, investigators have utilized a number of different genetics-based approaches, both gene-specific and genome wide, to decipher the genetic contribution to the disease. Earlier studies focused on gene-specific approaches, which were restricted to molecules that had

C. Eaton et al. (eds.), *Dupuytren's Disease and Related Hyperproliferative Disorders*,
DOI 10.1007/978-3-642-22697-7_12, © Springer-Verlag Berlin Heidelberg 2012

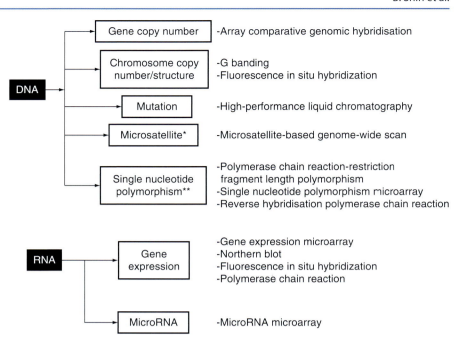

Fig. 12.1 Genetic analysis tools that have been used to study DNA and RNA abnormalities implicated in Dupuytren's disease. *Microsatellite markers have been previously used in determining family linkage. **Single nucleotide polymorphism has been used for genome-wide association studies, candidate gene studies, and HLA-typing between case–control association studies

previously been suggestive of involvement in fibrosis. However, recent studies have involved the analysis of the entire human genome, which is suggestive of being less biased as it does not focus on specific candidate genes based on previous biological data. The genetic analysis tools used in DD studies are outlined in Fig. 12.1.

The main sources of genetic research materials that can be obtained from individuals with DD include blood samples, and disease tissue (palmar and digital cord, nodule, perinodular fat, skin overlying the nodule). The genetic features of these materials can be compared to internal or external controls, which include blood from healthy individuals, fascia, skin and fat from individuals undergoing carpal tunnel decompression. Additionally, genetic research can be carried out on primary fibroblasts derived from these tissues, as it is acknowledged that myofibroblasts are involved in the pathogenesis of DD. From these genetic research materials, DNA and RNA may be extracted for analysis (Fig. 12.2).

12.3 Observational Approaches

It was Dupuytren's assistant, Goyrand, who first noted the link between DD and its familial predisposition in 1833 (Goyrand 1833). Since then, several reports have suggested the presence of familial tendency in DD. Average figures for family incidence have been reported to vary from 10% to 30%; however, studies with specific enquiries and clinical examination of relatives of DD cases have demonstrated a higher positive family history, with rates as high as 44–68% (Skoog 1948; Ling 1963). In 1963, Ling interviewed 50 DD cases and reported that 16% had a positive family history, however, after examination of the hands of 832 relatives of the 50 DD cases, Ling reported a familial incidence of 68% (Ling 1963). A later study reported a sibling recurrence-risk ratio of 2.9 in the North Western England population, suggesting that those with a sibling affected by DD are 2.9 times more likely to present with DD (Hindocha et al. 2006). Early case reports have documented monozygotic twins presenting the disease simultaneously (Couch 1938). Individuals with a strong family history of DD may develop more severe forms of the disease, and at a younger age (Hindocha et al. 2006). Thus, observations in twin studies and family studies suggest a strong element of heritability in DD.

The inheritance mode for DD is unclear. Ling (1963) suggested it to be a Mendelian autosomal dominant pattern of inheritance with strong penetrance affecting a single gene. Later studies have demonstrated that DD is an oligogenic disorder with a suggested complex gene–environment interaction (Bayat et al. 2003a). Additionally, Hu et al. reported a family with an autosomal dominant mode of inheritance with incomplete penetrance (Hu et al. 2005).

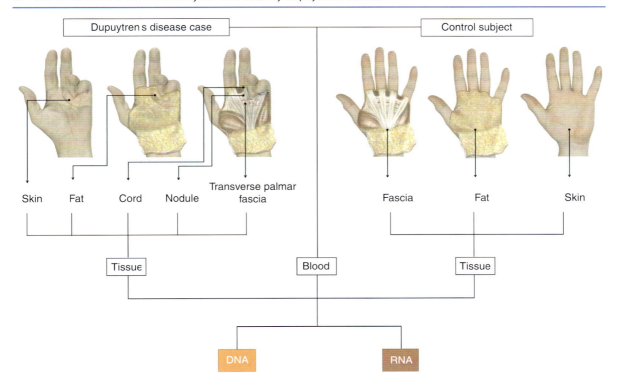

Fig. 12.2 Dupuytren's disease and control tissue phenotypes used in genetic research. The above figure describes the sources of materials that genetic studies of Dupuytren's disease employ. Disease affected tissues, including skin and fat adjacent to the disease site, nodule, and cord may be obtained from Dupuytren's disease patients who undergo surgery. Internal controls that may be used include transverse palmar fascia and blood while external control tissues include skin, fat, and fascia from individuals undergoing other surgical procedures, such as carpal tunnel decompression. In addition, blood from Dupuytren's disease patients may also be compared to blood from unaffected individuals in case–control studies

12.4 Gene-Specific Approaches

A number of previous studies selected specific genes for their investigation. These specific genes were chosen on the basis of known biological functions, previous reports of possible involvement in DD pathogenesis from genome wide studies, or association with other fibrotic diseases of relevance. These selected genes have been studied at a DNA or transcript (RNA) level. At the DNA level, transforming growth factor (TGF)-β family and its receptors, (Bayat et al. 2002a, b, 2003a) Zf9 transcription factor, (Bayat et al. 2003b) mitochondrial DNA (Bayat et al. 2005), and human leukocyte antigen (HLA) alleles (Brown et al. 2008) have been studied. Additionally, a large number of genes have been studied at the transcript level, including cytokines, growth factors, extracellular matrix (ECM) proteins, cell–cell and cell–matrix interaction proteins, metalloproteinases and their inhibitors (Gonzalez et al. 1992; Baird et al. 1993; Magro et al. 1995; Shin et al. 2004; Lee et al. 2006; Rehman et al. 2008; Zhang et al. 2008; Shih et al. 2009; Vi et al. 2009).

A possible role for TGF-β in DD has been suggested. Case–control studies have been carried out to assess an association between DD susceptibility and single nucleotide polymorphisms (SNP) in genes of the TGF-β pathway. These studies have focused on TGF-β1, TGF-β2, TGF-β receptor 1 (TGF-βRI), TGF-βRII and TGF-βRIII (Bayat et al. 2002a, b, 2003a). Although there is a lack of association between DD and almost all of these SNPs, it is possible that other uninvestigated regions of the genes may still contain DD causative polymorphisms or mutations. A polymorphism at the 3′ untranslated region of the gene for TGF-βRI has shown a statistically significant difference when it was analyzed in a recessive mode of inheritance (Bayat et al. 2003a). The authors suggested that the marginal significance value for this association may be due to the SNP being in linkage disequilibrium with a disease causative gene rather than being disease causative itself (Bayat et al. 2003a).

Increased activation or expression of TGF-β1 can be induced by Zf9 transcription factors or mitochondrial alterations (partial mitochondrial depletion or treatment with mitochondrial inhibitors) (Bayat et al. 2003b, 2005). A positive association has been determined with susceptibility to DD and the presence of a SNP at position 1140 of the Zf9 transcription factor gene (Bayat et al. 2003b). In addition, we reported an association of DD susceptibility and a heteroplasmic mutation located within the mitochondrial 16S rRNA region (Bayat et al. 2005).

The possible role of the HLA system in DD pathogenesis has been previously reviewed (McCarty et al. 2010). HLA-DRB1*15 has been positively associated with DD in a Caucasian population (Brown et al. 2008).

There is a gradation in expression of certain genes in DD tissues (cords and nodules) compared to internal/external control fascia, or DD fat to external control fat. The analysis at the transcript level is usually carried out using reverse-transcription quantitative polymerase chain reaction (RT-qPCR). Genes that have been found to be significantly up- or downregulated are demonstrated in Fig. 12.3.

12.5 Genome-Wide Approaches

In these approaches, the investigators attempt to identify regions or genes of interest by comparing the genetic materials from DD cases to internal or external controls. Most of these whole genome approaches are based on microarray technology nowadays, which allow up to a few million targets to be analyzed in one experiment.

Early cytogenetic studies, where DD cell cultures are established from tissue biopsy and chromosomes prepared for G-banding or fluorescence in situ hybridization, have shown cases with structural and numerical chromosomal abnormalities in cells grown from DD tissue samples compared to normal palmar fascia (Bowser-Riley et al. 1975; Sergovich et al. 1983; Wurster-Hill et al. 1988; Bonnici et al. 1992; Casalone et al. 1997; Dal Cin et al. 1999). These studies demonstrated a variable number of abnormalities in affected tissue, compared to normal palmar fascia. Multiple studies demonstrated trisomy 7, trisomy 8, and Y chromosome abnormalities (Sergovich et al. 1983; Wurster-Hill et al. 1988; Bonnici et al. 1992; Casalone et al. 1997). However, the transverse fascial tissue used as the control showed similar chromosomal aberrations as the DD nodular tissue. Evidence for chromosome trisomy 8 is also found in other benign tumors (Bridge et al. 1999). Various structural changes have also been reported in these studies, however, there is no consensus on whether they may or may not contribute to DD pathogenesis (Bowser-Riley et al. 1975; Sergovich et al. 1983; Wurster-Hill et al. 1988; Bonnici et al. 1992; Casalone et al. 1997).

Array-based comparative genomic hybridization (CGH) is a more recent molecular cytogenetic technique that involves hybridizing two sources of DNA, each labeled in a different color, onto the same microarray platform, allowing comparisons of copy numbers of the genome segments between two DNA sources. Two studies have been carried out to examine copy number variations (CNVs) in DD (Kaur et al. 2008; Shih et al. 2010). While Kaur et al. reported no gene copy number changes in 18 DD cases, Shih et al. found several regions of the genome showing copy number changes in four patients (Kaur et al. 2008; Shih et al. 2010). Specific gene loci with copy number changes, however, have not been validated in a larger sample comparison (Shih et al. 2010). Trisomy 7 or 8 have not been found in either of the CGH experiments, which may be due to the use of tissue; data generated using cell cultures should be interpreted with caution (Kaur et al. 2008).

Hu et al. have established a 6-cM region on chromosome 16q (between markers D16S419 and D16S3032) in a five-generation Swedish family with an autosomal dominant inheritance of DD, with a maximal two-point logarithm of odds (LOD) score of 3.18 at D16S415 (Hu et al. 2005). A genome-wide association study has also been carried out in 40 DD cases and controls, from which the authors determined an association in regions on chromosomes 6, 11, and 16 using a combination of mapping by SNP analysis and admixture linkage disequilibrium analysis (Ojwang et al. 2010). However, the stringency of the analysis that led to these conclusions has been challenged by Furniss et al. (2011). Dolmans et al. carried out a genome-wide association study in 960 DD-affected individuals and 3117 controls from the same population in the Netherlands (Dolmans et al. 2011). This led to the identification of 35 SNPs which were most strongly associated with DD and were selected and further validated in three additional, independent populations from Germany, the United Kingdom, and the Netherlands (comprising a total of 1365 affected individuals and 8445 controls) (Dolmans et al. 2011). Penultimate analysis revealed eleven SNPs from 9 different loci, which were significantly associated with DD

12 Use of Genetic and Genomic Analyses Tools to Study Dupuytren's Disease

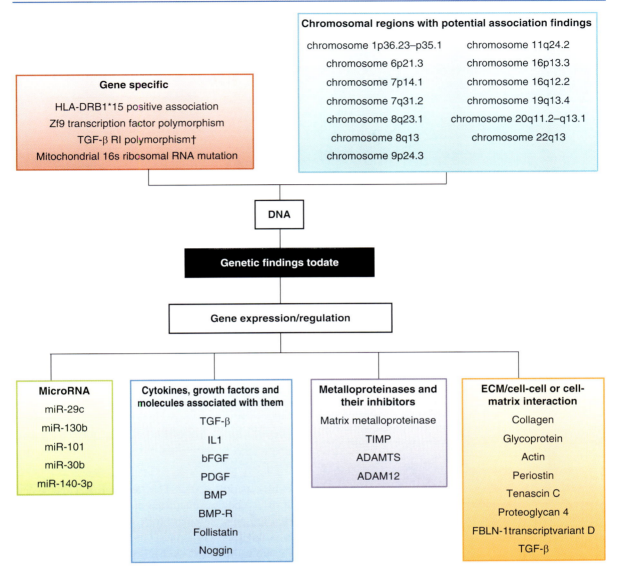

Fig. 12.3 Summary of the genetic findings in Dupuytren's disease. The above figure summarizes the major findings on the molecular genetics of DD based on previous DNA or RNA studies. *ADAM* a disintegrin and metalloproteinase domain, *ADAMTS* a disintegrin and metalloproteinase with thrombospondin motifs, *bFGF* basic fibroblast growth factor, *BMP* bone morphogenetic protein, *HLA* human leukocyte antigen, *IL* interleukin, *PDGF* platelet-derived growth factor, *SNP* single nucleotide polymorphism, *TGF* transforming growth factor, *TIMP* tissue inhibitor of metalloproteinases, Zf9 transcription factor, zinc finger transcription factor. †Significant only when the disease is assumed to be of a recessive inheritance mode

following relevant tests of replication and joint analysis (Dolmans et al. 2011). They also noted that 6 out of the 9 loci associated with DD contained genes known to be involved in the Wnt-signalling pathway, including WNT4, secreted frizzled-related protein 4 (SFRP4), WNT2, R-spondin 2 homolog (RSPO2), sulfatase 1 (SULF1) and WNT7B (Dolmans et al. 2011).

Transcriptome (the complete set of mRNA transcripts produced by the genome at a given time) profiling may not only be predictive of disease progression but also of disease phenotype. The number of target genes in the microarray platforms used for analyzing gene expression from fibroblast cultures and tissue biopsies have ranged from 1,176 genes to approximately 48,000 transcripts (Pan et al. 2003; Qian et al. 2004; Lee et al. 2006; Rehman et al. 2008; Satish et al. 2008; Vi et al. 2009). These studies indicate changes in expression of a large number of genes associated with DD formation.

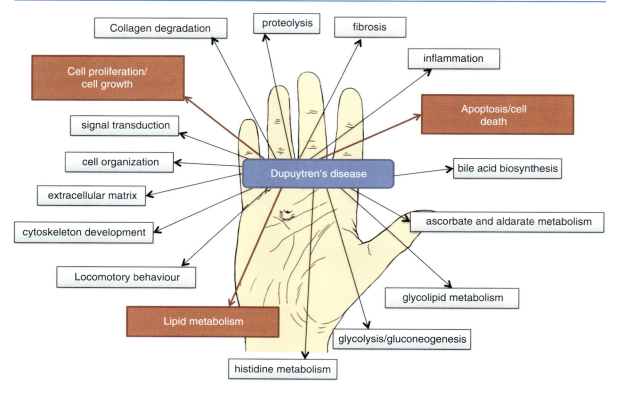

Fig. 12.4 Annotation of the genes suggested to be involved in Dupuytren's disease in three microarray studies. Genes reported with differential expression in Dupuytren's disease microarray studies are known to be associated with several molecular functions, biological processes, and cellular components. The ones that have been suggested in multiple studies include lipid metabolism, apoptosis/cell death, and cell proliferation/cell growth

Later microarray-based gene expression studies have grouped the dysregulated genes according to their molecular functions, biological process, and gene pathways that they are involved in. The biological processes reported by multiple microarray studies include cell proliferation, apoptosis, and lipid metabolism (Qian et al. 2004; Rehman et al. 2008; Satish et al. 2008) (Fig. 12.4). Gene families, including matrix metalloproteinase (MMP) and their inhibitors, collagen and ECM molecules, have been reported to be dysregulated. One microarray study has explored the possible contribution of alternative transcripts in DD; Satish et al. (2008) reported fibulin-1 transcript variant D to be differentially expressed in DD tissues. In addition to mRNA transcripts, Mosakhani et al. (2010) has found microRNAs, that regulate a disintegrin and metalloproteinase domain 12 (ADAM12), wingless-type MMTV integration site family, member 5A (WNT5A), Zic family member 1 (ZIC1), collagen, type V, alpha 2 (COL5A2), v-maf musculoaponeurotic fibrosarcoma oncogene homolog B (MAFB), periostin (POSTN), tenascin C (TNC), and TGF-β1, to be downregulated in DD. The authors suggested the possible contribution of the β-catenin pathway as WNT5A, ZIC1, and TGF-β1 are important to the β-catenin pathway (Mosakhani et al. 2010).

12.6 Discussion

Genetic studies may provide clues for molecular mechanisms involved in DD pathogenesis and may help further development of strategies for diagnosis, therapy, and prophylaxis in DD. The major genetics findings involved in DD has been summarized in Fig. 12.3. An enhanced understanding of DD may allow early diagnosis/treatment in those with susceptibility genes, and prevention of the disease in individuals who are susceptible to the disease by reducing their exposure to suspected environmental risk factors. An understanding of the genes involved may allow better diagnosis of the disease by classifying different subtypes of the disease. For instance, DD patients with higher expression of MMPs and a disintegrin and metalloproteinase with thrombospondin motifs (ADAMTSs) have been correlated to a higher recurrence rate in the 1-year clinical outcome (Johnston et al. 2008). Being able to identify patients at risk of recurrence preoperatively, may allow better postsurgical management. These patients may wish to consider procedures such as dermofasciectomy that is shown to reduce the risk of recurrence of the disease. Alternatives to surgeries, such as collagenase injection, may also be considered when risk of a further surgical procedure maybe outweighed by the high risk of disease recurrence in certain individuals.

References

Baird KS, Crossan JF et al (1993) Abnormal growth factor and cytokine expression in Dupuytren's contracture. J Clin Pathol 46(5):425–428

Bayat A, Alansar A et al (2002a) Genetic susceptibility in Dupuytren's disease: lack of association of a novel transforming growth factor beta(2) polymorphism in Dupuytren's disease. J Hand Surg [Br] 27(1):47–49

Bayat A, Watson JS et al (2002b) Genetic susceptibility in Dupuytren's disease. TGF-beta1 polymorphisms and Dupuytren's disease. J Bone Joint Surg Br 84(2):211–215

Bayat A, Stanley JK et al (2003a) Genetic susceptibility to Dupuytren's disease: transforming growth factor beta receptor (TGFbetaR) gene polymorphisms and Dupuytren's disease. Br J Plast Surg 56(4):328–333

Bayat A, Watson JS et al (2003b) Genetic susceptibility to dupuytren disease: association of Zf9 transcription factor gene. Plast Reconstr Surg 111(7):2133–2139

Bayat A, Walter J et al (2005) Identification of a novel mitochondrial mutation in Dupuytren's disease using multiplex DHPLC. Plast Reconstr Surg 115(1):134–141

Birney E, Stamatoyannopoulos JA et al (2007) Identification and analysis of functional elements in 1% of the human genome by the ENCODE pilot project. Nature 447(7146):799–816

Bonnici AV, Birjandi F et al (1992) Chromosomal abnormalities in Dupuytren's contracture and carpal tunnel syndrome. J Hand Surg [Br] 17(3):349–355

Bowser-Riley S, Bain AD et al (1975) Chromosome abnormalities in Dupuytren's disease. Lancet 2(7948):1282–1283

Bridge JA, Swarts SJ et al (1999) Trisomies 8 and 20 characterize a subgroup of benign fibrous lesions arising in both soft tissue and bone. Am J Pathol 154(3):729–733

Brown JJ, Ollier W et al (2008) Positive association of HLA-DRB1*15 with Dupuytren's disease in Caucasians. Tissue Antigens 72(2):166–170

Casalone R, Mazzola D et al (1997) Cytogenetic and interphase cytogenetic analyses reveal chromosome instability but no clonal trisomy 8 in Dupuytren contracture. Cancer Genet Cytogenet 99(1):73–76

Couch H (1938) Identical Dupuytren's contracture in identical twins. Can Med Assoc J 39(3):225–226

Dal Cin P, De Smet L et al (1999) Trisomy 7 and trisomy 8 in dividing and non-dividing tumor cells in Dupuytren's disease. Cancer Genet Cytogenet 108(2):137–140

Dolmans GH, Werker PM et al (2011) Wnt signaling and Dupuytren's disease. N Engl J Med 365(4):307–17

Feero WG, Guttmacher AE et al (2008) The genome gets personal–almost. JAMA 299(11):1351–1352

Furniss D, Dolmans GH et al (2011) Genome-wide association scan of Dupuytren's disease. J Hand Surg [Am] 36(4): 755–756

Gonzalez AM, Buscaglia M et al (1992) Basic fibroblast growth factor in Dupuytren's contracture. Am J Pathol 141(3):661–671

Goyrand G (1833) Nouvelles recherches sur la rétraction permanente des doigts. Mém Acad R Méd 3:489

Hindocha S, John S et al (2006) The heritability of Dupuytren's disease: familial aggregation and its clinical significance. J Hand Surg [Am] 31(2):204–210

Hu FZ, Nystrom A et al (2005) Mapping of an autosomal dominant gene for Dupuytren's contracture to chromosome 16q in a Swedish family. Clin Genet 68(5):424–429

International HapMap Consortium (2005) A haplotype map of the human genome. Nature 437(7063):1299–1320

International Human Genome Sequencing Consortium (2004) Finishing the euchromatic sequence of the human genome. Nature 431(7011):931–945

Johnston P, Larson D et al (2008) Metalloproteinase gene expression correlates with clinical outcome in Dupuytren's disease. J Hand Surg [Am] 33(7):1160–1167

Kaur S, Forsman M et al (2008) No gene copy number changes in Dupuytren's contracture by array comparative genomic hybridization. Cancer Genet Cytogenet 183(1):6–8

Lee LC, Zhang AY et al (2006) Expression of a novel gene, MafB, in Dupuytren's disease. J Hand Surg [Am] 31(2):211–218

Ling RS (1963) The genetic factor in Dupuytren's disease. J Bone Joint Surg Br 45:709–718

Magro G, Lanzafame S et al (1995) Co-ordinate expression of alpha 5 beta 1 integrin and fibronectin in Dupuytren's disease. Acta Histochem 97(3):229–233

McCarty S, Syed F et al (2010) Role of the HLA system in the pathogenesis of Dupuytren's disease. Hand 5(3):241–250

Mosakhani N, Guled M et al (2010) Unique microRNA profile in Dupuytren's contracture supports deregulation of beta-catenin pathway. Mod Pathol 23(11):1544–1552

Ojwang JO, Adrianto I et al (2010) Genome-wide association scan of Dupuytren's disease. J Hand Surg [Am] 35(12):2039–2045

Pan D, Watson HK et al (2003) Microarray gene analysis and expression profiles of Dupuytren's contracture. Ann Plast Surg 50(6):618–622

Pereira RS, Black CM et al (1986) Antibodies to collagen types I-VI in Dupuytren's contracture. J Hand Surg [Br] 11(1): 58–60

Qian A, Meals RA et al (2004) Comparison of gene expression profiles between Peyronie's disease and Dupuytren's contracture. Urology 64(2):399–404

Rehman S, Salway F et al (2008) Molecular phenotypic descriptors of Dupuytren's disease defined using informatics analysis of the transcriptome. J Hand Surg [Am] 33(3):359–372

Satish L, LaFramboise WA et al (2008) Identification of differentially expressed genes in fibroblasts derived from patients with Dupuytren's contracture. BMC Med Genomics 1:10

Sergovich FR, Botz JS et al (1983) Nonrandom cytogenetic abnormalities in Dupuytren's disease. N Engl J Med 308(3): 162–163

Shih B, Wijeratne D et al (2009) Identification of biomarkers in Dupuytren's disease by comparative analysis of fibroblasts versus tissue biopsies in disease-specific phenotypes. J Hand Surg [Am] 34(1):124–136

Shih BB, Tassabehji M et al (2010) Genome-wide high-resolution screening in Dupuytren's disease reveals common regions of DNA copy number alterations. J Hand Surg [Am] 35(7):1172–1183, e1177

Shin SS, Liu C et al (2004) Expression of bone morphogenetic proteins by Dupuytren's fibroblasts. J Hand Surg [Am] 29(5):809–814

Skoog T (1948) Dupuytren's contraction, with special reference to aetiology and improved surgical treatment. Its occurrence in epileptic: notes on knuckle-pads. Acta Chir Scand 96(Suppl):139

Vi L, Feng L et al (2009) Periostin differentially induces proliferation, contraction and apoptosis of primary Dupuytren's disease and adjacent palmar fascia cells. Exp Cell Res 315(20):3574–3586

Wurster-Hill DH, Brown F et al (1988) Cytogenetic studies in Dupuytren contracture. Am J Hum Genet 43(3):285–292

Zhang AY, Fong KD et al (2008) Gene expression analysis of Dupuytren's disease: the role of TGF-beta2. J Hand Surg Eur Vol 33(6):783–790

Establishing an Animal Model of Dupuytren's Contracture by Profiling Genes Associated with Fibrosis

13

Latha Satish, Mark E. Baratz, Bradley Palmer, Sandra Johnson, J. Christopher Post, Garth D. Ehrlich, and Sandeep Kathju

Contents

13.1	**Introduction**	101
13.2	**Materials and Methods**	102
13.2.1	Clinical Specimens	102
13.2.2	Primary Cell Culture	102
13.2.3	Nude Rats	102
13.2.4	Experimental Procedure	103
13.2.5	RNA Extraction	103
13.2.6	Quantitative Real-Time RT-PCR	103
13.3	**Results**	103
13.3.1	Fibroblast Morphology Was Not Affected by the Addition of Vybrant™ DiR	103
13.3.2	DD-Derived Fibroblasts Persisted Successfully in the Forepaw of Nude Rats	104
13.3.3	DD-Derived Fibroblasts in Nude Rat Forepaws Continued to Express High Levels of Type I Collagen and A-SMA	105
13.4	**Discussion**	106
13.5	**Conclusions**	107
	References	107

L. Satish (✉) • S. Johnson • J.C. Post • G.D. Ehrlich
S. Kathju
Allegheny-Singer Research Institute,
Center for Genomic Sciences, Pittsburgh, PA, USA
e-mail: lsatish@wpahs.org; sjohnson@wpahs.org;
cpost@wpahs.org; gehrlich@wpahs.org; skathju@wpahs.org

M.E. Baratz • B. Palmer
Division of Upper Extremity Surgery,
Department of Orthopaedics,
Allegheny General Hospital, Pittsburgh, PA, USA
e-mail: mebaratz@gmail.com; palmarislongus@gmail.com

13.1 Introduction

Dupuytren's disease (DD) is a fibroproliferative disorder that affects the palmar fascia of the hand and leads to digital flexion contractures. Typically, the disease is characterized by nodules in the palm of the hand that progressively develop into cords which extend proximally and distally from the distal palmar crease (McFarlane 1974; Rayan 1999). The nodule is a relatively vascular tissue containing a dense population of fibroblasts, with a high proportion being myofibroblasts (Gabbiani and Majno 1972; Vande Berg et al. 1984). Myofibroblasts are specialized fibroblasts, identified by their expression of α-smooth muscle actin (α-SMA) (Gabbiani et al. 1973). In contrast to the nodule, the cord is a collagen-rich structure that is relatively avascular, acellular, and with a reduced (but still significant) abundance of myofibroblasts. While several studies have indicated that nodular tissue is inherently more "biologically active" than cord tissue in vivo (Dave et al. 2001; Bisson et al. 2003; Rehman et al. 2008; Seyhan et al. 2006), many have also noticed that primary cells derived from either of these structures are very similar in appearance and responsiveness to transforming growth factor-beta (TGF-β) (Rehman et al. 2008; Seyhan et al. 2006). These observations correlate with more recent studies indicating that cells derived from primary nodule and cord have similar gene expression profiles (Shih et al. 2009).

The exact process of disease progression is still unknown. However, studies by several investigators have pointed out multiple potential contributory factors including: disturbance in collagen metabolism; changes in extracellular matrix protein levels, including

C. Eaton et al. (eds.), *Dupuytren's Disease and Related Hyperproliferative Disorders*,
DOI 10.1007/978-3-642-22697-7_13, © Springer-Verlag Berlin Heidelberg 2012

fibronectin (Howard et al. 2004) and periostin (Vi et al. 2009); as well as variation in the levels of growth factors (TGF-β_1 and TGF-β_2, platelet-derived growth factor [PDGF] and basic fibroblast growth factor [bFGF]) (Badalamente et al. 1996; Terek et al. 1995; Gonalez et al. 1992; Alioto et al. 1994). Other significant changes that have been implicated in contractures in Dupuytren's disease are low oxygen levels (Hueston and Murrell 1990), abnormal androgen receptors (Pagnotta et al. 2002), and high levels of the protein tyrosine phosphorylated beta-catenin (Howard et al. 2003). Perhaps the most important factor to which progression of DD has been imputed is the proliferation of fibroblasts and their transformation to a myofibroblast phenotype, as evidenced by increased levels of α-smooth muscle actin (Hindman et al. 2003). There is also substantial evidence pointing to larger changes in sets of gene expression in Dupuytren's disease at both the tissue and cellular level (Pan et al. 2003; Satish et al. 2008).

Current surgical therapy for DD is plagued by relapse, with reported contracture recurrence rates ranging from 27% to 80% (Badalamente and Hurst 2007). Other complications, which may include hematoma, seroma, necrosis, and injury to neurovascular structures, range from 3% to 26% in primary surgeries and increase significantly for secondary surgeries after recurrence (Hogemann et al. 2009). Nonsurgical treatments have generally been found to be ineffective, unsuitable for clinical use, or bothersome due to the need for repeated intervention (Hurst and Badalamente 1999). More recently, injectable collagenase clostridium histolyticum (Hurst et al. 2009) has produced some encouraging results. Alternative treatment options, including nonsurgical molecular therapies to halt the progression of DD, would be a welcome addition.

Since DD is known to naturally occur only in humans, the development of alternative therapeutic options for DD has been hindered by the lack of a well-established animal model. The current study was designed to investigate if an animal model of palmar fascia fibrosis could be established by transplanting primary cultures of human DD-derived fibroblasts into the forepaw of nude rats. Our main purpose was to investigate if the transplanted fibroblasts would persist in situ, would recapitulate gene expression patterns associated with fibrosis, and ultimately result in physiologically notable palmar fascial fibrosis and contracture. Such a model would allow for more defined and more accessible investigations into the pathophysiology and molecular mechanisms governing the progression of the disease, and serve as a baseline against which novel therapeutic strategies may be evaluated.

13.2 Materials and Methods

13.2.1 Clinical Specimens

Dupuytren's disease (DD) cord samples were surgically resected at the Division of Upper Extremity Surgery, Department of Orthopaedic Surgery, Allegheny General Hospital, Pittsburgh, PA. The study protocol confirmed to the ethical guidelines of the 1975 Declaration of Helsinki. All specimens were collected after obtaining written informed consent under Institutional Review Board approval. The specimens were collected in strict compliance by the physician performing the surgeries.

13.2.2 Primary Cell Culture

Primary cultures of fibroblasts were isolated from freshly resected DD cord as previously described (Howard et al. 2004; Satish et al. 2008; Vi et al. 2009). The cultures were maintained in α-MEM-medium supplemented with 10% fetal bovine serum (FBS, Invitrogen Corporation, Carlsbad, CA) and 1% antibiotic-antimycotic solution (Sigma-Aldrich, St Louis, MO). Cultures were maintained until a maximum of six passages, during which no changes in the cell morphology were observed. While in culture, just prior to transplantation, fibroblasts were tagged in vitro with Lipophilic Cell Tracer Vybrant™ DiR (D12731; Invitrogen, Carlsbad, CA) as per the manufacturer's instructions. DiR is a dialkylcabocyanine dye with excitation and emission maxima in the near infrared region. DiR was added directly to normal culture media to uniformly label the adherent cultured cells.

13.2.3 Nude Rats

All studies on "nude" (athymic) rats were performed in compliance with and after approval by the Institutional Animal Care and Use Committee (IACUC) of the Allegheny General Hospital. The outbred nude rats were commercially purchased from Charles River Laboratories (Willmington, MA). All animals were male, weighing between 250 and 300 g, and were housed for 2 weeks prior to the experimental procedure in an ASRI animal facility accredited by the Association for the Assessment and Accreditation of Laboratory Animal Care. Animals were housed in pathogen-free individual cages before and after the experimental procedure. All supplies including food, water, bedding, etc. were sterilized to prevent infection. Persons handling the rats wore caps, masks, sterile gowns and gloves, and shoe covers.

13.2.4 Experimental Procedure

Male athymic rats were anesthetized with an intraperitoneal injection containing a loading dose of ketamine at 50 mg/kg and xylazine at 5 mg/kg. Fibroblasts derived from DD cord explants were transplanted subcutaneously using a tuberculin syringe into the forepaws of the nude rats. The labeled cells in the rat forepaws were tracked at regular intervals by placing the animal in a light-tight chamber, and images were generated over a 10 s exposure using a cryogenically cooled charge-coupling device camera (the IVIS Lumina II, Caliper Life Sciences, Hopkinton, MA) to quantify photons emitted by the animal. The visual output represents the number of photons emitted/cm^2 as a pseudocolor image where the maximum is red and minimum is purple.

At 8 weeks posttransplantation, animals were sacrificed and rat forepaw tissues were harvested. In harvesting the specimens, the overlying rat skin was dissected away from subjacent structures, and the remaining forepaw contents were taken en bloc up to bone.

13.2.5 RNA Extraction

Tissues harvested from the rat forepaws were stored immediately in RNAlater® (Ambion, Austin, TX). Total RNA was extracted using the RNeasy Mini Kit (Qiagen Inc. USA, Valencia, CA). The quality and quantity of total RNA obtained were determined by measuring the OD 260/OD 280 ratio using an ND-1000 spectrophotometer (Nanodrop Technologies Inc., Wilmington, DE) and by capillary electrophoresis with

the Agilent 2100 BioAnalyzer (Agilent Technologies Inc., Palo Alto, CA).

13.2.6 Quantitative Real-Time RT-PCR

Real-time RT-PCR was performed using kits obtained from Applied Biosystems (Foster City, CA) that utilize FAM™Taqman®MGB probes and a Taqman® Universal PCR Master Mix. Assays were performed on two gene products, namely, human type I collagen and human α-SMA using human GAPDH as an endogenous normalizing control. Reverse transcription was performed on 125 ng of total RNA with random primers at a concentration of 100 ng/μl and with M-MLV-reverse transcriptase (Invitrogen Corporation, Carlsbad, CA). Subsequent PCR amplification and detection of template was carried out using Applied Biosystems transcript-specific assays including: type I collagen assay (ID-HS0102897_m1) and α-SMA assay (ID-HS00426835_g1) using 15 ng/μl of cDNA and 20× final concentration of Gene Expression Mix which contains both forward and reverse primers along with the gene-specific probes adjusted to final volume of 15.0 μl. The reaction set up and the thermal cycling protocol were as previously described (Satish et al. 2008). Using the comparative critical cycle (Ct) method the expression levels of the target genes were normalized to the GAPDH endogenous control (ID-HS99999905_m1) and the relative abundance was calculated. Data were analyzed using the 7900 HT SDS software version 2.1 provided by Applied Biosystems.

13.3 Results

13.3.1 Fibroblast Morphology Was Not Affected by the Addition of Vybrant™ DiR

The addition of Vybrant™ DiR, a lipophilic dye that is only weakly fluorescent in aqueous solution but is strongly fluorescent and photostable when resident in cell membranes, uniformly and effectively labeled the attached cells (Fig. 13.1c) with no light detected in unlabeled cell population (Fig. 13.1d). There was no apparent distortion of cell morphology nor any apparent cytotoxicity in labeled cells in comparison to unlabeled cells (Figs. 13.1a, b).

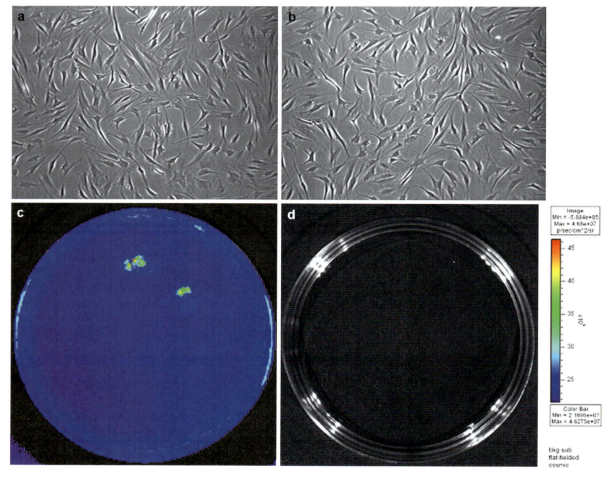

Fig. 13.1 Fibroblasts exhibited normal cellular morphology when exposed to lipophilic cell tracer Vybrant™ DiR. (**a**) and (**b**) show the phase contrast images of labeled and unlabeled DD-derived fibroblasts, which do not exhibit any significant differences in the cellular morphology. The images captured with the IVIS Lumina II camera show presence of light in the DD-derived fibroblasts labeled with Vybrant™ DiR (**c**), but there was no light detected in unlabeled DD-derived fibroblasts (**d**)

13.3.2 DD-Derived Fibroblasts Persisted Successfully in the Forepaw of Nude Rats

After determining that fibroblasts were uniformly labeled with the tracing dye, as an initial study, we injected various concentrations of DD-derived fibroblasts into the forepaws of nude rats. Our first trials showed that cell concentrations ranging from 5×10^5 to 1.5×10^6/paw did not allow us to detect significant fluorescent signal accumulation, nor could we detect significant human gene expression (data not shown). In subsequent experiments, we increased the cell number and reconstituted the cells in 0.1% low melting point agarose to increase the chances of cell survival. We utilized 5×10^6, 1.0×10^7, or 1.5×10^7 labeled fibroblasts resuspended in 0.1% low melting point agarose and transplanted by subcutaneous injection into the forepaw of nude rats. We determined that administration of both 1.0×10^7 and 1.5×10^7 cells/paw demonstrated successful persistence of cells over 8 weeks as evidenced by the continued detection of fluorescent signal emitted from the forepaw (Fig. 13.2a, b). (We observed that administration of 5×10^6 cells/paw persisted successfully for 4 weeks, but thereafter fluorescent signal was lost or minimal [data not shown].)

13 Establishing an Animal Model of Dupuytren's Contracture by Profiling Genes Associated with Fibrosis

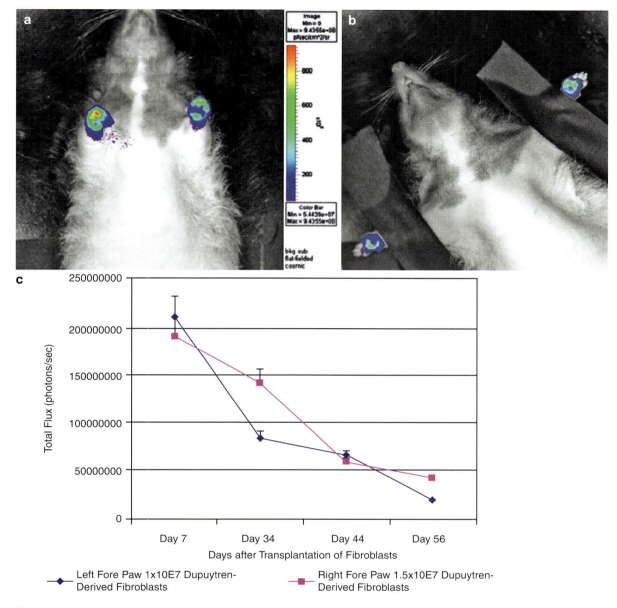

Fig. 13.2 In vivo imaging of forepaw exhibited persistent light emission in nude rat forepaws injected with labeled fibroblasts. Photons/second/pixel were determined at the forepaws of nude rats on various days after transplantation. A representative image of rats imaged on Day 7 and Day 44 is presented in (**a**) and (**b**) respectively. In (**a**) and (**b**) the left and right sides of the animal were transplanted with 1×10^7 and 1.5×10^7 labeled DD-derived fibroblasts respectively. The images are presented as a pseudocolored scale and superimposed on a black-and-white image of the animal. (**c**) Time course quantification of light accumulation in left and right forepaws of the nude rats. Images and quantification results shown here is a representation of two independent experiments

13.3.3 DD-Derived Fibroblasts in Nude Rat Forepaws Continued to Express High Levels of Type I Collagen and A-SMA

Total RNA was isolated after 8 weeks from the palmar fascia of the forepaws of nude rats receiving 1.0×10^7 and 1.5×10^7 labeled fibroblasts along with the forepaws of nude rats receiving only 0.1% low melting point agarose in balanced salt solution. RNA was also isolated from the overlying nude rat skin, and from DD-derived fibroblasts in culture, which served as a control. Our initial determinations showed that control

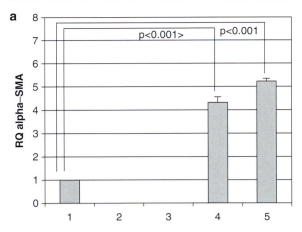
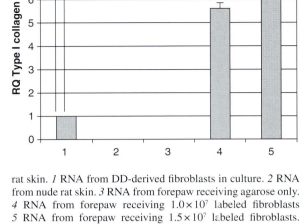

Fig. 13.3 qRT-PCR demonstrated elevated levels of α-SMA and type I collagen in the forepaws injected with DD-derived fibroblasts. Real-time RT-PCR performed on RNA isolated from transplanted palmar tissue showed increased expression levels of α-smooth muscle actin (**a**) and type I collagen (**b**) in forepaws treated with 1.0×10^7 and 1.5×10^7 labeled fibroblasts. Human probes did not detect any gene expression in the RNA isolated from forepaw of rats that received agarose only, nor from nude rat skin. *1* RNA from DD-derived fibroblasts in culture. *2* RNA from nude rat skin. *3* RNA from forepaw receiving agarose only. *4* RNA from forepaw receiving 1.0×10^7 labeled fibroblasts *5* RNA from forepaw receiving 1.5×10^7 labeled fibroblasts. Human GAPDH was used as endogenous control. Values are means ± SEM of samples obtained from two independent experiments performed in duplicate. Statistical analyses were performed using Student's *t* test. ***$p<0.001$; **$p<0.01$

and experimental RNA subjected to qRT-PCR using human probes detected greatly increased mRNA expression levels of α-SMA and type I collagen in forepaws receiving 1.0×10^7 and 1.5×10^7 labeled fibroblasts. We also showed that human α-SMA and type I collagen mRNA was not detected in either nude rat skin nor in the forepaws receiving agarose only (Fig. 13.3). This both confirms the specificity of the probes used in detecting only human genes, and also indicates that fibroblasts from affected DD tissues continue to express gene products that may contribute to the genesis of the fibrotic phenotype when injected into the palmar fascia of nude rats.

13.4 Discussion

It has been over 175 years since Dupuytren published a description of two patients with palmar fascia fibrosis, but we remain without any effective therapy to halt the progression of Dupuytren disease. This delayed progress may be due to the lack of a validated animal model, which has hindered an understanding of the pathogenesis of the disease and the development of new treatment strategies. In an attempt to develop an animal model, Larsen et al. (1960) produced Dupuytren's-like lesions in monkeys by traumatic disruption of palmar fascial fibers, but utilization of this model is limited by lack of follow-up studies (and, practically, the expense of a primate model system). Kischer et al. (1989) sought to determine if diseased DD tissue placed into subcutaneous pockets in the suprascapular area of nude mice could survive with the characteristics of Dupuytren's tissue. Their study showed that the histologic character and electron microscopic structure of the tissue were preserved, and they concluded that this may be a useful model for further experimental studies with further validation. Kuhn et al. (2001) demonstrated the maintenance of viable DD-affected palmar fascia explants for up to 60 days by using a vascularized sandwich flap model in the abdominal skin of nude rats. This study found that tissue samples obtained after perfusing the Dupuytren's tissue xenografts with TGF-β_1 demonstrated increased type I and III collagen production. Conversely, neutralizing antibody to TGF-β_2 reduced collagen production in tissue samples obtained at 30 days after administration. Furthermore, the authors also demonstrated that fibroblasts obtained from samples of explants perfused with TGF-β_2 increased DNA synthesis and protein production.

In each of the above described animal models utilizing human tissue, affected explants from DD tissues have been placed at anatomic sites distant from the observed site of disease in humans (the palmar fascia). In the present study, we transplanted DD-derived fibroblasts specifically to the nude rat forepaw, the orthologous location for the expected pathology, and demonstrated their persistence at that location fluorometrically over a period of 8 weeks. Thus, this model is the first to attempt to recapitulate an actual disease-specific cellular phenotype in an anatomically relevant site. Although we did not observe the formation of actual cords or nodules, this may be due to the fact that in some patients the progression of disease only becomes apparent after a protracted period. Alternatively, other as yet unidentified factors might also contribute to the lack of gross phenotypic changes in our model thus far.

These initial studies showed that fibroblasts derived from human DD tissues are capable of surviving in the nude rat forepaw for up to 8 weeks, albeit with apparently declining numbers. The hallmark feature of DD is the presence of myofibroblasts, which are thought to play a key role in the pathogenesis of the disease. Myofibroblasts are thought to develop from fibroblasts after specific external stimuli or from circulating mesenchymal precursor cells (Bucala et al. 1994). Myofibroblasts possess several distinguishing physiological characteristics, especially their expression of α-SMA. Myofibroblasts are responsible not only for remodeling of extracellular matrix proteins (ECM), but also both produce and respond to growth factors that can promote complex or abnormal regulation of cellular proliferation (Tomasek et al. 1986, 2002; Baird et al. 1993). Understanding the exact cellular and molecular basis of myofibroblast persistence and function may therefore represent a potential means of addressing the fibroproliferative pathology of DD. Initial results from our study show that there is increased expression in the mRNA levels of human α-SMA in tissues obtained 56 days after transplantation of DD-derived fibroblasts. This is a clear indication that transplanted fibroblasts survived and have maintained the myofibroblast phenotype. Thus, this animal model represents a first step in establishing a baseline in which agents to reverse myofibroblastic transformation may be examined.

Our ongoing studies with this model examine further differences in gene expression patterns of other ECM components, namely, type III collagen, fibronectin, and tenascin; we are also attempting to validate expression differences in mRNA at the protein level. Further refinements of the animal model are underway as well, including observation over even longer time frames, observation after repeated administration of diseased cells, and comparison of the physiology observed when DD-affected fibroblasts are compared with phenotypically normal fibroblasts derived from patients undergoing surgery for carpal tunnel syndrome.

13.5 Conclusions

- This study is the first attempt to establish a DD animal model which recapitulates a disease-specific cellular phenotype in an anatomically relevant site.
- We show that fibroblasts derived from human DD tissues are capable of surviving in the nude rat forepaw for up to 8 weeks.
- Initial results from our study show that there is increased expression in the mRNA levels of α-SMA in tissues obtained 56 days after transplantation of DD-derived fibroblasts, showing that transplanted fibroblasts have maintained the myofibroblast phenotype.

Acknowledgments The authors thank Allegheny-Singer Research Institute, The Pittsburgh Foundation, and Pennsylvania Department of Health for their financial support toward this study. We also thank the staff of Lab Animal Resource Facility of ASRI for their support toward this research protocol.

References

Alioto RJ, Rosier RN, Burton RI, Puzas JE (1994) Comparative effects of growth factors on fibroblasts of Dupuytren's tissue and normal palmar fascia. J Hand Surg [Am] 19:442–452

Badalamente MA, Hurst LC (2007) Efficacy and safety of injectable missed collagenase subtypes in the treatment of Dupuytren's contracture. J Hand Surg [Am] 32:767–774

Badalamente MA, Sampson SP, Hurst LC, Dowd A, Miyasaka K (1996) The role of transforming growth factor-beta in Dupuytren's disease. J Hand Surg [Am] 21:210–215

Baird KS, Crossan JF, Ralston SH (1993) Abnormal growth factor and cytokine expression in Dupuytren's contracture. J Clin Pathol 46:425–428

Bisson MA, McGrouther DA, Mudera V, Grobbelaar AO (2003) The different characteristics of Dupuytren's disease fibroblasts derived from either nodule or cord: expression of alpha-smooth muscle actin and the response to stimulation by TGF-beta1. J Hand Surg [Br] 28:351–356

Bucala R, Spiegel LA, Chesney J, Hogan M, Cerami A (1994) Circulating fibrocytes define a new leukocyte subpopulation that mediates tissue repair. Mol Med 1:71–81

Dave SA, Banducci DR, Graham WP 3rd, Allison GM, Ehrlich HP (2001) Differences in alpha smooth muscle actin expression between fibroblasts derived from Dupuytren's nodules or cords. Exp Mol Pathol 71:147–155

Gabbiani G, Majno G (1972) Dupuytren's contracture: fibroblast contraction? Am J Pathol 66:131–146

Gabbiani G, Majno G, Ryan GB (1973) The fibroblast as a contractile cell: the myofibroblast. In: Kulonen E, Pikkarainen J (eds) Biology of the fibroblast. Academic, New York, p 139

Gonalez AM, Buscaglia M, Fox R, Isacchi A, Sarmientos P et al (1992) Basic fibroblast growth factor in Dupuytren's contracture. Am J Pathol 141:661–671

Hindman HB, Marty-Roix R, Tang JB, Jupiter JB, Simmons BP, Spector M (2003) Regulation of expression of alpha-smooth muscle actin in cells of Dupuytren's contracture. J Bone Joint Surg Br 85:448–455

Hogemann A, Wolfhard U, Kendoff D, Board TN, Olivier LC (2009) Results of total aponeurectomy for Dupuytren's contracture in 61 patients: a retrospective clinical study. Arch Orthop Trauma Surg 129:195–201

Howard JC, Varallo VM, Ross DC, Roth JH, Faber KJ, Alman B, Gan BS (2003) Elevated levels of beta-catenin and fibronectin in three-dimensional collagen cultures of Dupuytren's disease cells are regulated by tension in vitro. BMC Musculoskelet Disord 4:16

Howard JC, Varallo VM, Ross DC, Faber KJ, Roth JH, Seney S, Gan BS (2004) Wound healing-associated proteins Hsp47 and fibronectin are elevated in Dupuytren's contracture. J Surg Res 117:232–238

Hueston JT, Murrell GA (1990) Cell-controlling factors in Dupuytren's contracture. Ann Chir Main Memb Super 9: 135–137

Hurst LC, Badalamente MA (1999) Nonooperative treatment of Dupuytren's disease. Hand Clin 15:97–107

Hurst LC, Badalamente MA, Hentz VR, Hotchkiss RN et al (2009) Injectable collagenase clostridium histolyticum for Dupuytren's contracture. N Engl J Med 361:968–979

Kischer CW, Pindur J, Madden J, Shetlar MR, Shetlar CL (1989) Characterization of implants from Dupuytren's contracture tissue in the nude (athymic) mouse (42859). Proc Soc Exp Biol Med 190:268–274

Kuhn MA, Payne WG, Kierney PC, Lu LL, Smith PD, Siegler K et al (2001) Cytokine manipulation of explanted Dupuytren's affected human palmar fascia. Int J Surg Invetig 2:443–456

Larsen R, Takagishi N, Posch J (1960) The pathogenesis of Dupuytrens' contracture. Experimental and further clinical observations. J Bone Joint Surg [Am] 42:993–1007

McFarlane RM (1974) Patterns of the diseased fascia in the fingers in Dupuytren's contracture. Plast Reconstr Surg 54:31–44

Pagnotta A, Specchia N, Greco F (2002) Androgen receptors in Dupuytren's contracture. J Orthop Res 20:163–168

Pan D, Watson HK, Swigart C, Thomson JG, Honig SC, Narayan D (2003) Microarray gene analysis and expression profiles of Dupuytren's contracture. Ann Plast Surg 50:618–622

Rayan GM (1999) Clinical presentation and types of Dupuytren's disease. Hand Clin 15:87–96

Rehman S, Salway F, Stanley JK, Ollier WE, Day P, Bayat A (2008) Molecular phenotypic descriptors of Dupuytren's disease defined using informatics analysis of the transcriptome. J Hand Surg [Am] 33:359–372

Satish L, Laframboise WA, O'Gorman DB, Johnson S, Janto B, Gan BS, Baratz ME, Hu FZ, Post JC, Ehrlich GD, Kathju S (2008) Identification of differentially expressed genes in fibroblasts derived from patients with Dupuytren's contracture. BMC Med Genomics 1:10

Seyhan H, Kopp J, Schultze-Mosgau S, Horch RE (2006) Increased metabolic activity of fibroblasts derived from cords compared with nodule fibroblasts sampling from patients with Dupuytren's contracture. Plast Reconstr Surg 117:1248–1252

Shih B, Wijeratne D, Armstrong DJ, Lindau T, Day P, Bayat A (2009) Identification of biomarkers in Dupuytren's disease by comparative analysis of fibroblasts versus tissue biopsies in disease-specific phenotypes. J Hand Surg [Am] 34:124–136

Terek RM, Jiranek WA, Goldberg MJ, Wolfe HJ, Alman BA (1995) The expression of platelet-derived growth-factor gene in Dupuytren's contracture. J Bone Joint Surg Am 77:1–9

Tomasek JJ, Schultz RJ, Episalla CW, Newmann SA (1986) The cytoskeleton and extracellular matrix of the Dupuytren's disease "myofibroblast": and immunofluorescence study of a non muscle type. J Hand Surg [Am] 11:365–371

Tomasek JJ, Gabbiani G, Hinz B, Chaponnier C, Brown RA (2002) Myofibroblasts and mechano-regulation of connective tissue remodeling. Nat Rev Mol Cell Biol 2:349–363

Vande Berg JS, Gelberman RH, Rudolph R, Johnson D, Sicurello P (1984) Dupuytren's disease: Comparative growth dynamics and morphology between cultured myofibroblasts (nodule) and fibroblasts (cord). J Orhtop Res 2:247–256

Vi L, Feng L, Zhu RD, Wu Y, Satish L, Gan BS, O'Gorman DB (2009) Periostin differentially induces proliferation, contraction and apoptosis of primary Dupuytren's disease and adjacent palmar fascia cells. Exp Cell Res 315:3574–3586

Microarray Expression Analysis of Primary Dupuytren's Contracture Cells

14

Sandra Kraljevic Pavelic and Ivana Ratkaj

Contents

14.1   **Introduction** 109

14.2   **Material and Methods** 110

14.3   **Results and Discussion** 110

14.4   **Summary** 112

References 113

14.1 Introduction

Dupuytren's contracture (DC) is a connective tissue disorder characterized as nodular palmar fibromatosis which causes permanent contraction of one or more fingers. This is an old disease described in the nineteenth century in northern Europe (Early 1962) and it has been called the "Viking disease." Scientific and clinical investigation has given a well-understood pathology while the disease etiology remains elusive (Al-Qattan 2006). Surgery remains the most widely used treatment for the disease, but this line of action

does not represent permanent solution because it does not eliminate processes that lead to disease recurrence. Indeed, up to 77% of patients are subject to recurrence and may need a new surgery (Bulstrode et al. 2005; Wong and Mudera 2006). Some of the risk factors linked to DC are trauma, diabetes, alcoholism, epilepsy, and liver disease (Al-Qattan 2006; Loos et al. 2007; Cordova et al. 2005; McFarlane 2002). Although there is a high correlation between these factors and development of disease, it is still unclear in what way are they related to the progression of disease. Myofibroblasts are essential component of DC nodules and express contractile force (Gabbiani and Majno 1972; Tomasek et al. 2002; Rayan et al. 1996). Literature data suggest that disease onset may be the result of a wound repair process that has gone wrong (Mosakhani et al. 2010). After trauma occurs, myofibroblasts migrate to the damaged area and, due to their contractile capabilities, close the wounded region. After regeneration of damaged tissue, myofibroblasts enter apoptosis in normal tissues. When the proliferating signals and contractive phenotype of myofibroblasts persist, this leads to pathological changes that might result in DC. There is a strong genetic component in the etiology of DC, like unstable protein forms of transcription factors ZF9 (Bayat et al. 2003), mutations within mitochondrial DNA leading to an abnormally high concentration of free radicals which stimulate fibroblast differentiation (Bayat et al. 2005), and polymorphism in TGF-β (Transforming Growth Factor) gene (Bayat et al. 2002), but they have not been linked with DC recurrence. It is more likely that these changes only make individuals more prone to develop the disease (Burge 1999).

K. Pavelic (✉) • I. Ratkaj
Department of Biotechnology,
University of Rijeka, Rijeka, Croatia
e-mail: sandrakp@biotech.uniri.hr; iratkaj@biotech.uniri.hr

C. Eaton et al. (eds.), *Dupuytren's Disease and Related Hyperproliferative Disorders*,
DOI 10.1007/978-3-642-22697-7_14, © Springer-Verlag Berlin Heidelberg 2012

Table 14.1 Taqman primer sets used for RT-PCR analyses

Gene Symbol	Assay ID
ABLIM1	Hs 01046520_m1
ELN	Hs 00355783_m1
FBLN1	Hs 00197774_m1
GREM2	Hs 00254699_m1
MBP	Hs 00921945_m1
MYLK	Hs 00981464_m1

14.2 Material and Methods

For the purpose of this investigation, primary cell cultures were cultured according to previously established protocols (Tse et al. 2004; Kraljevic Pavelic et al. 2009) from 20 different patients. Cells were cultured from affected tissue – the affected palmar fascia localized in palmodigital and digital area (D), as well as from patient matched healthy fascia tissue as a biopsy from macroscopically unaffected area at the edge of primary incision (ND).

Total RNA was isolated by RNeasy mini kit (Qiagen) and further used for microarray expression analysis (HG-U133A array, Affymetrix). Data was analyzed with software MAS5, GeneSpring and GENEMAPP which gave a list of 18 genes that were differentially expressed (t-test, $p \leq 0.5$, fold change ≥ 2) among D and ND cells. Selected genes were further analyzed by a TaqMan probe-based real-time PCR assay (RT-PCR) in triplicate (Table 14.1) and the results were processed with geNorm, rest-384-beta, and comparative C_T method for relative quantification.

14.3 Results and Discussion

A high-throughput technology, the transcriptomic analysis of whole-genome, has been employed to study gene expression in primary cells derived from Dupuytren's contracture tissue. Upon data analysis (Fig. 14.1) 18 genes were found to be differentially expressed. Hierarchical clustering of differentially expressed genes that was additionally performed based on a signal intensity, revealed two clusters of genes with a similar expression pattern (Fig. 14.2).

All genes identified as differentially expressed between cells grown from affected tissue D and cells grown from unaffected fasciae ND, were further studied by use of RT-PCR. RT-PCR results showed a slight variability in the expression level of studied genes among cells cultured from different DC patients (data not shown). This was partially expected due to high rates of interindividual variability among different subjects. Still, we managed to confirm the expression

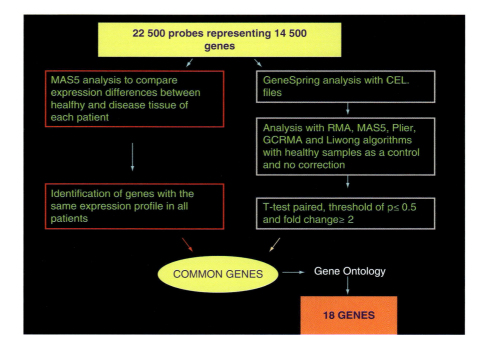

Fig. 14.1 Workflow of microarray results analysis

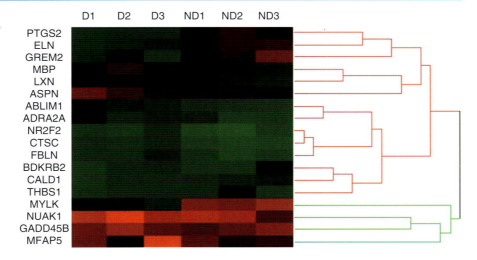

Fig. 14.2 Hierarchical clustering of 18 differentially expressed genes among primary D and ND cells based on signal intensity

Table 14.2 List of differentially expressed genes in primary DC cells that have a possible role in rise of typical palmar contraction and biological function of proteins encoded by these set of genes

Gene name and function	Expression	Fold change
ELN – Elastin (Supravascular aortic stenosis Williams–Beuren syndrome)-dominant extracellular matrix protein with regulatory functions on VSMC through activation of G-protein coupled signaling pathway	Upregulated	7
GREM2 – Gremlin 2, cystein knot superfamily, homology (Xenopus leavis)-a member of bone morphogenic protein antagonist family, it plays a role in regulating organogenesis, body patterning and tissue differentiation	Upregulated	2.1
MBP – myelin basic protein, the protein encoded by the classic MBP gene is a major constituent of the myelin sheath of oligodendrocytes and Schwann cells in the nervous system	Upregulated	2
ABLIM1 – a cytoskeletal LIM protein that binds to actin filaments, plays key roles in the regulation of developmental pathways, and functions as protein-binding interfaces	Downregulated	1.8
FBLN1 – Fibulin 1- encoded protein secretes glycoprotein that incorporates into a fibrillar extracellular matrix	Downregulated	1.5
MYLK – Myosin, light chain kinase – a muscle member of Ig gene superfamily, it is Ca and calmodulin dependent, it phosphorylates myosin regulatory light chains to facilitate myosin interactions with actin to produce contracture activity	Upregulated	1.8

Note: Results are obtained by RT-PCR analysis and presented as fold change (up- or downregulation of gene expression)

of a majority of genes (a total of 10 genes) identified as differentially expressed by microarray analysis. Among these genes, we were particularly interested in biological function of genes that might play a role in development of DC palmar contracture, namely, elastin (ELN), gremlin 2 (GREM2), myelin basic protein (MBP), a cytoskeletal LIM protein (ABLIM1), fibulin-1 (FBLN), and myosin light chain kinase (MYLK) (Table 14.2). Indeed, these genes are known to be involved in regulation of the extracellular matrix (ECM) and actin–myosin interactions.

Results obtained in our study might be partially comparable with those obtained by Satish et al. that performed gene expression studies of primary Dupuytren's contracture cells by use of microarray platforms other than Affymetrix (Satish et al. 2008). In spite of different microarray platforms used for transcriptomic studies, our results were in consistence with those obtained by Satish et al.; we similarly identified extracellular matrix and myosin regulatory genes to be differentially expressed in DC primary cells. In particular, the fibulin 1 gene which encodes both an extracellular matrix

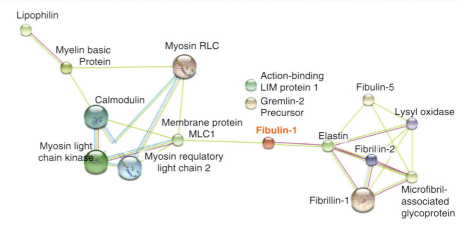

Fig. 14.3 Protein–protein interaction map for fibulin 1

protein and a secreted plasma glycoprotein was significantly downregulated in both studies. Chromosomal abnormalities of this gene that cause reduced levels of the corresponding protein in the ECM, has already been connected with a congenital disorder characterized by a union of fingers or toes and/or increase in the number of toes or fingers (Debeer et al. 2002). Moreover, biological function of fibulin-1 includes tight interactions with proteins encoded by genes MYLK1, ELN, and MBP that were identified in our study as well (Fig. 14.3). It therefore seems that fibulin-1 might be among potential candidates for development of typical DC symptoms.

Transcriptomic approach has also been applied in the research on Dupuytren's contracture tissues and unveiled specific "transcriptomic signatures" pointing to cellular events that might account for DC pathogenesis. Qian et al. (2004) profiled Dupuytren's nodules against the unaffected adjacent tendons. They identified 16 upregulated and 3 downregulated genes in the nodules. Overexpressed genes were involved in collagen degradation, generation of the contractile force, myofibroblasts differentiation, oxidative stress, regulation of apoptosis, proteolysis and inflammation, fibrosis and ossification. Further on, transcriptomic study performed by Rehman et al. (2008) compared expression profiles between Dupuytren's contracture tissues versus transversal carpal fascia of control subjects (external control), as well as Dupuytren's contracture cords and nodules from the palm versus the unaffected, patient-matched transversal palmar fascia (internal control). Results revealed deregulated genes that were involved in molecular processes such as cell growth, proliferation, differentiation, regulation of cell death, biological cell adhesion, extracellular matrix–receptor interaction, and cell communication. Even if those results are not directly comparable to data presented in our study, deregulated genes identified by Qian et al. and Rehman et al. are involved in similar cellular pathways and biological processes, that is, regulation of ECM and cytoskeletal changes that can be linked with reported DC symptoms. Observed difference in the expression status between the major deregulated genes either from the nodules and cords and cells cultured from these tissues clearly underlines the potential of transcriptomic profiling for discerning DC phenotype.

In conclusion, our preliminary research on primary cells isolated from affected palmar fascia localized in palmodigital and digital area (D), as well as from patient-matched healthy nondiseased fascia (ND) identified 18 differentially expressed genes. Among them, expression patterns of only ten genes validated by RT-PCR correlated with microarray data. These genes, in particular fibulin-1, are important ECM and cytoskeleton proteins involved in actin–myosin interactions, therefore playing an important role in development of DC symptoms.

14.4 Summary

- Dupuytren's contracture is a multifactorial and polygenic disease.
- Microarray analysis of primary DC cell cultures resulted in 18 differentially expressed genes examined and further validated by use of RT-PCR.
- Among differentially expressed genes, FBLN1, MYLK, ABLIM1, MBP, GREM2, and ELN genes might be involved in development of palamar contracture in DC.

Acknowledgments We acknowledge Croatian Ministry of Science, Education and Sport (grants: 335-0000000-3532 and 335-0982464-2393) and Professor Kresimir Pavelic, Ph.D., M.D., Head of the Department of Biotechnology, University of Rijeka, Croatia.

References

Al-Qattan MM (2006) Factors in the pathogenesis of Dupuytren's contracture. J Hand Surg [Am] 31:1527–1534

Bayat A, Watson JS, Stanley JK, Alansari A, Shah M, Ferguson MWJ, Ollier WER (2002) Genetic susceptibility in Dupuytren's disease – TGF-beta 1 polymorphisms and Dupuytren's disease. J Bone Joint Surg Br 84:211–215

Bayat A, Watson JS, Stanley JK, Ferguson MW, Ollier WE (2003) Genetic susceptibility to Dupuytren disease: association of Zf9 transcription factor gene. Plast Reconstr Surg 111:2133–2139

Bayat A, Walter J, Lambe H, Watson JS, Stanley JK, Marino M, Ferguson MWJ, Ollier WER (2005) Identification of a novel mitochondrial mutation in Dupuytren's disease using multiplex DHPLC. Plast Reconstr Surg 115:134–141

Bulstrode NW, Mudera V, McGrouther DA, Grobbelaar AO, Cambrey AD (2005) 5-fluorouracil selectively inhibits collagen synthesis. Plast Reconstr Surg 116:209–221

Burge P (1999) Genetics of Dupuytren's disease. Hand Clin 15:63–71

Cordova A, Tripoli M, Corradino B, Napoli P, Moschella F (2005) Dupuytren's contracture: an update of biomolecular aspects and therapeutic perspectives. J Hand Surg [Br] 30:557–562

Debeer P, Schoenmakers EFPM, Twal WO, Argraves WS, De Smet L Fryns J-P, Van de Ven WJM (2002) The fibulin-1 gene (FBLN1) is disrupted in a t(12;22) associated with a complex type of synpolydactyly. J Med Genet 39:98–104

Early PF (1962) Population studies in Dupuytren's contracture. J Bone Joint Surg [Br] 44:602–613

Gabbiani G, Majno G (1972) Dupuytren's contracture: fibroblast contraction? An ultrastructural study. Am J Pathol 66: 131–146

Kraljevic Pavelic S, Bratulic HK, Jurisic D, Hranjec M, Karminski-Zamola G, Zinic B, Bujak M, Pavelic K (2009) Screening of potential prodrugs on cells derived from Dupuytren's disease patients. Biomed Pharmacother 63:577–585

Loos B, Puschkin V, Horch RE (2007) 50 years experience with Dupuytrens contracture in the Erlangen University Hospital-A retrospective analysis of 2919 operated hands from 1956 to 2006. BMC Musculoskelet Disord 8:60–69

McFarlane RM (2002) On the origin and spread of Dupuytren's disease. J Hand Surg [Am] 27:385–390

Mosakhani N, Guled M, Lahti L, Borze I, Forsman M, Pääkkönen V, Ryhänen J, Knuutila S (2010) Unique microRNA profile in Dupuytren's contracture supports deregulation of β-catenin pathway. Mod Pathol 23:1544–1552

Qian A, Meals RA, Rajfer J, Gonzalez-Cadavid NF (2004) Comparison of gene expression profiles between Peyronie's disease and Dupuytren's contracture. Urology 64:399–404

Rayan GM, Parizi M, Tomasek JJ (1996) Pharmacologic regulation of Dupuytren's fibroblasts contraction in vitro. J Hand Surg [Am] 21:1065–1070

Rehman S, Salway F, Stanley JK, Ollier WE, Day P, Bayat A (2008) Molecular phenotypic descriptors of Dupuytren's disease defined using informatics analysis of the transcriptome. J Hand Surg [Am] 33:359–372

Satish L, LaFramboise WA, O'Gorman DB, Johnson S, Janto B, Gan BS, Baratz ME, Hu FZ, Post JC, Ehrlich GD, Kathju S (2008) Identification of differentially expressed genes in fibroblasts derived from patients with Dupuytren's Contracture. BMC Med Genomics 1:10

Tomasek JU, Gabbiani G, Hinz B, Chaponnier C, Brown RA (2002) Myofibroblasts and mechano – regulation of connective tissue remodeling. Nat Rev Mol Cell Biol 3: 349–363

Tse R, Howard J, Wu Y, Gan BS (2004) Enhanced Dupuytren's disease fibroblast populated collagen lattice contraction is independent of endogenous active TGF-beta2. BMC Musculoskelet Disord 5:41

Wong M, Mudera V (2006) Feedback inhibition of high TGF-beta 1 concentrations on myofibroblast induction and contraction by Dupuytren's fibroblasts. J Hand Surg [Br] 31:473–483

A Clinical Genetic Study of Familial Dupuytren's Disease in the Netherlands

15

Guido H.C.G. Dolmans, Cisca Wijmenga,
Roel Ophoff, and Paul M.N. Werker

Contents

15.1	Introduction	115
15.2	Material and Methods	116
15.3	Results	117
15.3.1	Demographics and Mode of Inheritance	117
15.3.2	Description of Selected Pedigrees	117
15.4	Discussion	121
15.5	Conclusions	122
References		122

G.H.C.G. Dolmans (✉) • P.M.N. Werker
Department of Plastic Surgery,
University Medical Centre Groningen,
Groningen, The Netherlands
e-mail: g.h.c.g.dolmans@umcg.nl;
p.m.n.werker@umcg.nl

C. Wijmenga
Department of Medical Genetics,
University Medical Centre Groningen,
Groningen, The Netherlands

R. Ophoff
Department of Medical Genetics,
Rudolf Magnus Institute of Neuroscience,
University Medical Centre Utrecht, Utrecht, The Netherlands

15.1 Introduction

Dupuytren's disease is a benign, progressive fibrosing disorder of the palmar fascias of the hand and fingers, which leads to the formation of nodules and cords, and may lead to disabling extension deficits of the finger joints. Treatment consists of division or surgical excision of pathologic cords, but there is a high recurrence rate after surgery in patients with the Dupuytren's disease diathesis (Hueston 1963).

Dupuytren's disease has been recognized for several centuries and was first described as a medical condition by Plater of Basle in 1614 (Elliot 1988). Its pathogenesis remains largely unknown. The reported prevalence of Dupuytren's disease varies from 3% to 42% (Ross 1999), with the highest incidence in Caucasians, while it is rarely seen in Africans (Sladicka et al. 1996). Men are seven times more often affected than women, but in later life the incidence in women increases to the same as men (Ross 1999). Some suggest that the disease symptoms are milder in women and therefore may remain unnoticed for a longer period (Burge 1999).

The clustering of Dupuytren's disease in families suggests a genetic influence on the onset of the disease. Several studies on the genetic origin of Dupuytren's disease have been performed (Badalamente et al. 1996; Bayat et al. 2002a, b, 2003a, b, 2005; Burge 1999; Hindocha et al. 2006; Hu et al. 2005; Lee et al. 2006; Qian et al. 2004), but its mode of inheritance is still not clear. Multiple reports describe Dupuytren's disease as an autosomal dominant disease with varying penetrance (Ling 1963; Matthews 1979; Maza and Goodman 1968). An allele with a reduced penetrance means that some disease gene carriers do not develop the disease

C. Eaton et al. (eds.), *Dupuytren's Disease and Related Hyperproliferative Disorders*,
DOI 10.1007/978-3-642-22697-7_15, © Springer-Verlag Berlin Heidelberg 2012

Table 15.1 Review of the English language literature

Author	Year	Journal	No. of families	Affected/total no. family members	Mode of inheritance
Ling et al.	1963	J Bone Joint Surg Br	34	151/832	Autosomal dominant
Maza et al.	1968	J Hered	1	4/16	Autosomal dominant
Matthews et al.	1979	Br J Plast Surg	1	13/42	Autosomal dominant[a]
Hu et al.	2005	Clin Genet	1	18/50	Autosomal dominant

[a]Matthews et al. reported a family with predominantly affected females (males:females = 4:9)

phenotype. Table 15.1 presents an overview of the family studies performed in Dupuytren's disease.

The most recent one was published by Hu et al. who presented a single Swedish family with a clear autosomal dominant mode of inheritance (Hu et al. 2005). But there are many sporadic (nonfamilial) cases of the disease that are not compatible with a Mendelian inheritance pattern (Burge 1999). In a review in 1999, Burge et al. suggested that recessive inheritance still remains a viable hypothesis for Dupuytren's disease (Burge 1999). In two candidate-gene association studies by Bayat et al., the genes for TGFβR and Zf9 were only significantly associated with Dupuytren's disease when using a recessive model (Bayat et al. 2003a, b). Another possible hypothesis is that Dupuytren's disease is a complex trait in which several genes and risk factors are involved, each conferring a certain (limited) risk to developing the disease. It is known that factors such as smoking, use of alcohol, antiepilepsy drugs, and medical conditions including liver disease and diabetes, are associated with a higher prevalence of the disease (Legge 1985; Ross 1999), complicating the picture even further. Since Dupuytren's disease is considered to be one of the most common hereditary connective tissue disorder in Caucasians (Hindocha et al. 2006), finding genes for this disease is of utmost importance to understanding the disease pathogenesis and for developing diagnostic and prognostic protocols.

We investigated the clinical characteristic of families with Dupuytren's disease and examined the mode of inheritance. Here, we describe 11 pedigrees with familial Dupuytren's disease from the Netherlands. The results of this work will significantly aid in designing proper genetic studies to identify the underlying gene(s).

15.2 Material and Methods

We identified Dupuytren patients visiting the outpatient clinics, who had two or more first-degree relatives with the disease. They were asked to participate in this study and family members were contacted via the proband. All participants signed an informed consent and this study was approved by the Medical Ethics Committees.

All the subjects (including probands, affected and unaffected family members) of five families were personally examined by trained clinical researchers or plastic surgeons with substantial clinical experience in treating Dupuytren's disease. The diagnosis was based on the presence of characteristic Dupuytren nodules and/or cords in the palm of the hand and/or digits, with or without contractures of the digits. All probands and affected family members were asked to complete a questionnaire on the age of onset, presence of suggested risk factors (diabetes, alcohol consumption, liver disease, antiepileptic medication), occupation, hobbies, and the presence of recurrent disease. In most cases the hands of the affected individuals were also photographed. Information about deceased family members was gathered via the proband and other family members.

In the six remaining families, the diagnosis of Dupuytren's disease was based on information provided only by the proband; the family members were not clinically examined.

Data were entered into a database (Excel 2003; Microsoft, US). To investigate the genetic transmission of Dupuytren's disease in these families, pedigree charts were reconstructed from the data obtained from all 11 families using pedigree-drawing software (Cyrillic; Cyrillic software, UK). The mean age of onset of Dupuytren's disease in patients with a positive family history in a study by Hindocha et al. was 49 years (Hindocha et al. 2006). Therefore, unaffected family members under the age of 49 were included in the pedigrees, but were not considered in the analysis of the inheritance pattern, because of the age-dependent penetrance of Dupuytren's disease. Healthy family members suspected of being a carrier of the disease gene were used in the analysis of the transmission pattern. These unaffected carriers have at least one affected first-degree family member and one affected child. All the families who participated in this study between January and December 2007 are described in this paper.

The pedigrees encompassed 475 family members, with 66 subjects diagnosed with Dupuytren's disease. Of the affected family members, 44 (67%) were male and 22 (33%) were female. Five of the pedigrees spanned three generations and six pedigrees spanned four generations.

15.3 Results

15.3.1 Demographics and Mode of Inheritance

We describe the mode of inheritance of 11 pedigrees with Dupuytren's disease (Table 15.2) and the detailed clinical characteristics of five of these families (Table 15.3). All family members were Caucasians and originated from the northern part of the Netherlands.

In the selected pedigrees, two individuals were thought to be unaffected carriers because they had transmitted the disease to the next generation. This suggested an incomplete penetrance in at least 3% (2/68) of the Dupuytren carriers, assuming a dominant model of inheritance. All types of transmission were observed (male to male, male to female, female to female, female to male). Paternal transmission was observed in 45% of cases and maternal transmission in 55%. Fifty-two percent of the offspring of the affected individuals have Dupuytren's disease. The inheritance pattern of Dupuytren's disease in these pedigrees was compatible with an autosomal dominant mode of inheritance with slightly reduced penetrance (95%). Penetrance is the proportion of individuals carrying a disease gene that also expresses this disease.

15.3.2 Description of Selected Pedigrees

15.3.2.1 Family 1

This family spanned four generations and consisted of 76 family members, with nine affected. Of the affected family members, five were male and four were female. The family members in the fourth generation were all younger than 40 years. Family member II:11 and his children III:30 and III:32 displayed an early onset of the disease (before age 40).

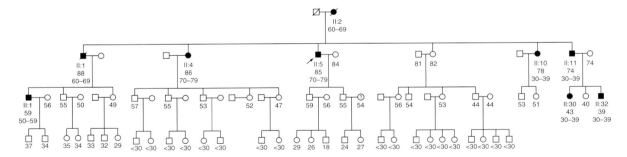

Fig. 15.1 Family 1

Table 15.2 Characteristics of 11 Dupuytren families

Family	Generation	No. of affected members	Unaffected carriers	Affected, M:F	Ethnicity	Total no. of family members	Family members, M:F	Paternal transmission	Maternal transmission	% offspring of affected parents who also have DD[a]	Compatible with autosomal dominant transmission
1	4	9	0	5:4	Caucasian	76	38:38	2	6	40% (8/20)	+
2	3	3	0	2:1	Caucasian	33	16:17	3	0	60% (3/5)	+
3	3	8	0	6:2	Caucasian	54	28:26	1	6	54% (7/13)	+
4	3	7	1	5:1	Caucasian	48	21:27	5	0	38% (5/13)	+
5	4	5	0	3:2	Caucasian	19	8:11	2[b]	4[b]	50% (4/8)	+
6	3	5	1	3:2	Caucasian	56	27:29	2	3	44% (4/9)	+
7	3	5	0	3:2	Caucasian	25	14:11	3	3	60% (3/5)	+
8	4	6	0	5:1	Caucasian	44	27:17	?	?	75% (6/8)	+
9	4	5	0	3:2	Caucasian	52	28:24	4	0	29% (4/14)	+
10	4	9	0	4:5	Caucasian	45	25:20	0	8	80% (8/10)	+
11	4	4	0	4:0	Caucasian	23	9:14	3	0	43% (3/7)	+
Total	39	66	2	44:22		475	241:234	25 (45%)	30 (55%)	52%	+

DD Dupuytren's disease

[a]Unaffected individuals under the age of 49 were not considered in the analyses, unaffected carriers were used

[b]Transmission of Dupuytren disease from the second to third generation could be paternal, maternal, or both

Table 15.3 Clinical characteristics of affected individuals in five Dupuytren families

Family	Individual	Sex	Age of onset	Recurrent disease	Manual laborer	Other disease locations	Comorbidity	Smoking
1	I:2	f	60–69	–	+	–		
1	II:1	m	60–69	–	–	–	–	–
1	II:4	f	70–79	–	–	–	–	–
1	II:5	m	70–79	–	–	–	–	–
1	II:10	f	30–39	–	+	–	–	–
1	II:11	m	30–39	+	+	–	–	–
1	III:1	m	50–59	–	+	–	–	–
1	III:30	f	30–39	–	+	–	–	+
1	III:32	m	30–39	–	+	–	–	–
2	II:4	f	50–59	+	+	–	–	+
2	II:5	m	50–59	+	–	–	–	–
2	II:7	m	40–49	–	–	–	–	+
3	II:3	m	60–69	+	+	kn	–	–
3	II:4	m	60–69	–	–	–	–	–
3	II:6	m	40–49	+	–	–	–	–
3	II:11	f	60–69	–	+	–	–	–
3	II:15	m	50–59	+	–	kn	–	–
3	II:17	m	50–59	–	+	–	Epilepsy	Stopped 1974
3	III:9	m	30–39	–	–	–	–	–
4	II:5[a]	m	?	?	?	?	?	?
4	III:1	m	40–49	+	+	–	Diabetes	–
4	III:3	m	40–49	–	+	–	–	+
4	III:5	m	40–49	+	–	led	–	Stopped 1998
4	III:21	f	50–59	–	–	–	–	+
4	III:24	m	40–49	+	–	–	–	Stopped 2000
5	II:1	m	50–59	+	+	–	–	–
5	II:2	f	60–69	–	+	–	–	–
5	III:1	m	40–49	+	–	kn/led	–	–
5	III:3	m	30–39	+	+	kn/led/pe	–	–

kn knuckle pads, *led* Ledderhose's disease, *pe* Peyronie's disease
[a]The clinical characteristics of individual II:5 in family 4 are unknown

15.3.2.2 Family 2

This family spanned three generations, with 33 family members, of whom three were affected. In the first generation the grandparents, who were unrelated, did not develop the disease, however the grandfather (I:1) died at the early age of 39 years. Except for individual III:1 (50 years), the entire third generation was younger than 49 years old.

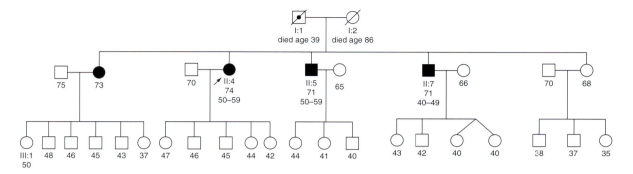

Fig. 15.2 Family 2

15.3.2.3 Family 3

In this three-generation family, 8 out of 54 family members were affected. In the second generation, 6 out of 12 individuals were affected. Individual III:9 (42 years), who developed the disease before the age of 40, was the only affected family member in the third generation. His father, II:6, was the only affected person in the second generation who demonstrated Dupuytren's disease before the age of 50.

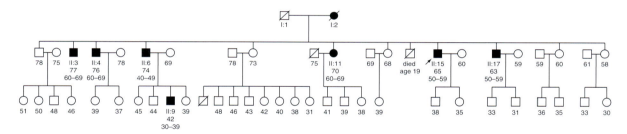

Fig. 15.3 Family 3

15.3.2.4 Family 4

This three-generation family had 48 members, of whom six were affected. It is not known whether the grandparents were affected. Individual II:1 was presumed to be an unaffected carrier. The fourth generation is not shown, since they are all younger than 40 years and so far unaffected.

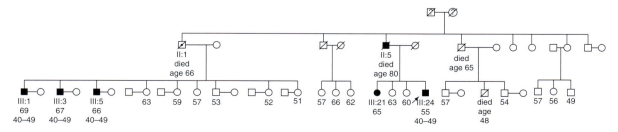

Fig. 15.4 Family 4

15.3.2.5 Family 5

In this small family, both parents in the second generation (II:1 and II:2) were affected by Dupuytren's disease, with the father having an age of onset between 50 and 59 years and the mother between 60 and 69 years. Individuals III:1 and III:3 showed the first signs of the disease before the age of 44. They have both been treated three times with a selective fasciectomy. III:1 and III:3 not only display the disease in both hands including Garrod's pads, but also in their feet (Ledderhose's disease), while individual III:3 also has a benign progressive fibrosing disorder affecting the penis (Peyronie's disease). All pedigrees were compatible with an autosomal dominant mode of inheritance.

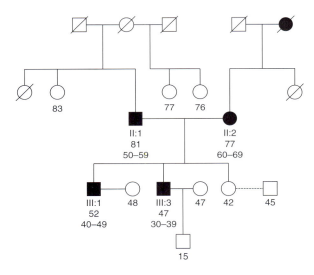

Fig. 15.5 Family 5

15.4 Discussion

We describe the mode of inheritance and the clinical characteristics of families with Dupuytren's disease in order to further elucidate the genetics of this familial disorder. Probands and their relatives of five families were interviewed and examined. Information on six additional families was collected via six other probands.

The sex distribution of affected individuals male:female was 2:1 (67%:33%). As noted by Ross, women develop Dupuytren's disease approximately a decade later and the sex distribution will consequently be nearly equal by the ninth decade of life (Ross 1999). This explains the relatively small difference in the sex distribution found in this study.

Paternal and maternal transmission was observed in 45% and 55% of cases, respectively. Fifty-two percent of the offspring of affected individuals was also affected at age 49 years or older. These data, in combination with the appearance of the pedigrees, is compatible with an autosomal dominant mode of inheritance for a late-onset disease in these families.

From the families described, it is apparent that the decade of onset of the disease seen in the parents also predicts the age of onset for their offspring. For instance, in family 1, individual II:11 developed Dupuytren's disease in the fourth decade (30–39 years) just as his offspring (III:30 and III:32). In family 3, III:9 was the only affected person in the third generation so far. His father (II:6) was the only individual affected under the age of 50 in the second generation of this family.

In family 2, the grandfather (I:1) might have been a carrier of the disease. He died aged 39 and had probably not developed Dupuytren's disease at that stage.

In family 5 individuals III:1 and III:3 not only displayed an earlier onset than their parents, but also a far more aggressive form and at different locations. The coexistence of Dupuytren's disease with Ledderhose's disease and Peyronie's disease has been noted frequently. Since both their parents are affected, individuals III:1 and III:3 could be homozygous for the mutation of this apparently dominant disease. Ling et al. also observed a more severe clinical manifestation of the disease in individuals with both parents affected (Ling 1963).

Table 15.3 shows the clinical characteristics of the affected individuals in the five families, but there are no apparent patterns. Two factors complicate the resolving of the genetic mechanism of Dupuytren's disease: the late age of onset and its fairly high incidence in the general population. Our data suggest that the most likely mode of inheritance in these families with Dupuytren's disease is autosomal dominant with a reduced penetrance, which confirms previously published data.

Since only Dupuytren patients with two or more affected first-degree relatives were asked to participate in this study, there will have been an ascertainment bias. Sporadic cases of the disease were excluded in this design, hence alternative modes of inheritance cannot be ruled out. To prevent this bias, all Dupuytren patients presenting at the outpatient clinics should have been included. Furthermore, to improve the power of this study more families need to be included and all family members should be examined by an experienced clinician.

The large pedigrees with multiple affected patients with Dupuytren's disease will be instrumental in the genetic mapping and identification of genetic factors involved in Dupuytren's disease by using classical linkage approaches. Genes identified in this way may also help to resolve the disease etiology of the sporadic form of Dupuytren's disease. This knowledge will ultimately lead to improved diagnosis and possibly to alternative treatments.

15.5 Conclusions

- Our data suggest an autosomal dominant mode of inheritance with a reduced penetrance for familial Dupuytren's disease.
- Knowing the mode of inheritance will be instrumental in genetic mapping and identification of genetic factors involved in Dupuytren's disease.

Acknowledgment We thank Jackie Senior for critically reading the chapter.

References

Badalamente MA, Sampson SP, Hurst LC, Dowd A, Miyasaka K (1996) The role of transforming growth factor beta in Dupuytren's disease. J Hand Surg [Am] 21(2):210–215

Bayat A, Alansar A, Hajeer AH, Shah M, Watson JS, Stanley JK, Ferguson MW, Ollier WE (2002a) Genetic susceptibility in Dupuytren's disease: lack of association of a novel transforming growth factor beta(2) polymorphism in Dupuytren's disease. J Hand Surg [Br] 27(1):47–49

Bayat A, Watson JS, Stanley JK, Alansari A, Shah M, Ferguson MW, Ollier WE (2002b) Genetic susceptibility in Dupuytren's disease TGF-beta1 polymorphisms and Dupuytren's disease. J Bone Joint Surg Br 84(2):211–215

Bayat A, Stanley JK, Watson JS, Ferguson MW, Ollier WE (2003a) Genetic susceptibility to Dupuytren's disease: transforming growth factor beta receptor (TGFbetaR) gene polymorphisms and Dupuytren's disease. Br J Plast Surg 56(4):328–333

Bayat A, Watson JS, Stanley JK, Ferguson MW, Ollier WE (2003b) Genetic susceptibility to dupuytren disease: association of Zf9 transcription factor gene. Plast Reconstr Surg 111(7):2133–2139

Bayat A, Walter J, Lambe H, Watson JS, Stanley JK, Marino M, Ferguson MW, Ollier WE (2005) Identification of a novel mitochondrial mutation in Dupuytren's disease using multiplex DHPLC. Plast Reconstr Surg 115(1):134–141

Burge P (1999) Genetics of Dupuytren's disease. Hand Clin 15(1):63–71

Elliot D (1988) The early history of contracture of the palmar fascia. Part 1: the origin of the disease: the curse of the MacCrimmons: the hand of benediction: cline's contracture. J Hand Surg [Br] 13(3):246–253

Hindocha S, John S, Stanley JK, Watson SJ, Bayat A (2006) The heritability of Dupuytren's disease: familial aggregation and its clinical significance. J Hand Surg [Am] 31(2):204–210

Hu FZ, Nystrom A, Ahmed A, Palmquist M, Dopico R, Mossberg I, Gladitz J, Rayner M, Post JC, Ehrlich GD, Preston RA (2005) Mapping of an autosomal dominant gene for Dupuytren's contracture to chromosome 16q in a Swedish family. Clin Genet 68(5):424–429

Hueston JT (1963) Recurrent Dupuytren's contracture. Plast Reconstr Surg 31:66–69

Lee LC, Zhang AY, Chong AK, Pham H, Longaker MT, Chang J (2006) Expression of a novel gene, MafB, in Dupuytren's disease. J Hand Surg [Am] 31(2):211–218

Legge JW (1985) Dupuytren disease. Surg Annu 17:355–368

Ling RS (1963) The genetic factor in Dupuytren's disease. J Bone Joint Surg 45:709–718

Matthews P (1979) Familial Dupuytren's contracture with predominantly female expression. Br J Plast Surg 32(2):120–123

Maza RK, Goodman RM (1968) A family with Dupuytren's contracture. J Hered 59(2):155–156

Qian A, Meals RA, Rajfer J, Gonzalez-Cadavid NF (2004) Comparison of gene expression profiles between Peyronie's disease and Dupuytren's contracture. Urology 64(2):399–404

Ross DC (1999) Epidemiology of Dupuytren's disease. Hand Clin 15(1):53–62, vi

Sladicka MS, Benfanti P, Raab M, Becton J (1996) Dupuytren's contracture in the black population: a case report and review of the literature. J Hand Surg [Am] 21(5):898–899

The Epidemiology of Dupuytren's Disease in Bosnia

16

Dragan Zerajic and Vilhjalmur Finsen

Contents

16.1 Introduction 123

16.2 Methods 123

16.3 Results 124

16.4 Discussion 126

16.5 Conclusions 127

References 127

16.1 Introduction

The etiology of Dupuytren's disease is still unclear. There are indications that diabetes mellitus (Ravid et al. 1977; Lawson et al. 1983; Noble et al. 1984; Attali et al. 1987; Stradner et al. 1987; Quintana Guitian 1988; Jennings et al. 1989; Arkkila et al. 1997), alcohol consumption (Bradlow and Mowat 1986; Attali et al. 1987; Burge et al. 1997), and smoking (Attali et al. 1987; An et al. 1988; Burge et al. 1997; Gudmundsson et al. 2000) are risk factors. It is generally agreed that the prevalence is much higher among Europeans than among other ethnic groups (Maes 1979; Zarowski and Mann 1979; Mennen and Gräbe 1979; Chow et al. 1984; Muguti and Appelt 1993; Ross 1999) and that the prevalence in Europe is higher in northern compared to Mediterranean countries (Ross 1999). A fairly high prevalence has, however, been reported in Spain (Quintana Guitian 1988). We have not found other studies from southern Europe.

The purpose of the present study was to determine the prevalence of Dupuytren's disease in the southern European country of Bosnia and Herzegovina and to evaluate the prevalence of some of the suggested risk factors.

16.2 Methods

An effort was made to survey all the three ethnic groups living in the old Bosnia and Herzegovina. The data for the study were collected in 2001 by the first author in the mainly Serb populated towns of Banja Luka (population 143,079) and Trebinje (30,979); the mainly Moslem populated towns of Tuzla (83,770), Zenica (96,027), and

D. Zerajic
Faculty of Medicine, Norwegian University
of Science and Technology, Trondheim, Norway

V. Finsen (✉)
Faculty of Medicine, Norwegian University
of Science and Technology, Trondheim, Norway

Department of Orthopaedic Surgery,
St. Olav's University Hospital, Trondheim, Norway
e-mail: vilh.finsen@ntnu.no

C. Eaton et al. (eds.), *Dupuytren's Disease and Related Hyperproliferative Disorders*,
DOI 10.1007/978-3-642-22697-7_16, © Springer-Verlag Berlin Heidelberg 2012

Table 16.1 The number of individuals found with Dupuytren's disease (DD+) in the general population and the age-specific prevalence (DD%)

Age	Men			Women		
	Total	DD+	DD%	Total	DD+	DD%
50–54	152	26	17	178	20	11
55–59	121	33	27	135	16	12
60–64	98	32	33	91	12	13
65–69	61	21	34	71	10	14
70–74	98	47	48	56	13	23
75–79	40	30	75	32	13	41
80+	40	24	60	34	10	29
All	610	213	31	597	94	16

Konjic (13,729); and the Croat and Moslem populated city of Mostar (126,643). In rural areas, the survey was undertaken in the mainly Serb populated community of Nevesinje (4,068); mainly Croat, Neum (1,651), Grude (3,598), and Stolac (5,530); and the mainly Moslem Tesanj (5,621) and Jablanica (4,457).

In the main part of the study, members of the public were approached at random on the street and in other public places by the second author and asked to take part in the study. He was a medical student who had received instruction on how to recognize Dupuytren's disease. The only criterion for approaching someone was that they looked as if they might be over the age of 50 years. Almost everyone approached seemed happy to take part in the study. It was extremely uncommon for anyone to refuse. Those who consented were asked their year of birth and their ethnic background, whether they had had surgery for Dupuytren's disease, and whether they smoked tobacco or consumed alcohol or suffered from diabetes mellitus ("Do you have sugar?"). They were not asked if the diabetes was insulin dependent (IDDM) or diet-regulated (NIDDM). The respondents hands were then examined for signs of Dupuytren's disease which was graded into three stages: Stage 1 when there were only palpable nodules and skin tethering in the palm and no flexion contracture of the digit, stage 2 when there was less than 90° total contracture of the metacarpophalangeal and interphalangeal joints, and stage 3 when there was more than 90° contracture of the digit. The degree of contracture was estimated visually.

The age-specific prevalence among men and women was calculated and also the prevalence for various subgroups.

In a separate part of the study, we also examined the hands of 237 patients at a diabetes clinic. These were inpatients and consecutive patients at the outpatient clinic. Data from these patients were kept separate from those of the main study.

Statistical significance was tested with the Mantel–Haenszel summary chi-square test, and the Mantel–Haenszel weighted odds ratios (OR) and Cornfield 95% confidence limits were calculated (Statcalc, Epiinfo 2000, Centers for Disease Control and Prevention, Atlanta, Georgia, USA). P values lower than 0.05 were taken to indicate statistically significant differences.

16.3 Results

A total of 1,287 individuals were interviewed in the main part of the study. Of these, 80 (5 with Dupuytren's disease) were excluded because they proved to be under the age of 50 years. Dupuytren's disease was found in the hands of 210 men and 94 women among the 1,207 individuals over the age of 50. A stage 2 disease was found in 72 men and 16 women, and a stage 3 disease in 7 men and 1 woman. The prevalence was highly age-dependent, ranging from 17% for men between 50 and 54 years to 60% in the oldest men (Table 16.1). The prevalence among women was lower (Table 16.1).

Dupuytren's disease was detected in a total of 775 finger rays (Table 16.2). Of these, 608 were without contracture of the digit (stage 1). A total of 16 (2.6%) men and 7 (1.2%) women stated that they had been operated for Dupuytren's disease. In 3 of the men and 2 of the women, no typical Dupuytren's disease–associated changes could be detected and it seems possible that they had in fact been operated for other conditions. Changes were equally distributed in the right and left hands in women, while they were found more than three times as often in the right hands as in the left hands of men. The ring and little finger rays were most often affected, and the thumb and index finger rays least often.

The prevalence of Dupuytren's disease was significantly lower among Muslim men than among Serbian and Croatian men (Table 16.3: $p=0.018$; OR 1.61;

16 The Epidemiology of Dupuytren's Disease in Bosnia

Table 16.2 The number of digital rays affected by Dupuytren's disease

Stage:	Right hand				Left hand			
	1	2	3	All	1	2	3	All
Men								
Thumb	5	0	0	5	2	0	0	2
Index	6	0	0	6	2	0	0	2
Long	45	8	0	53	9	4	0	13
Ring	146	41	3	190	57	8	1	66
Little	90	56	5	151	27	7	1	35
All	292	105	8	405	97	19	2	118
Women								
Thumb	0	0	0	0	0	0	0	0
Index	0	0	0	0	0	0	0	0
Long	5	2	0	7	15	1	0	16
Ring	59	7	0	66	69	8	0	77
Little	41	6	1	48	30	8	0	38
All	105	15	1	121	114	17	0	131

Stage 1: only palmar changes; Stage 2: less than 90° contracture of digit; Stage 3: more than 90° contracture of digit

Table 16.3 The prevalence of Dupuytren's disease (DD%) among Serbian, Croat, and Muslim men

Age	Serbian			Croat			Muslim		
	Total	DD+	DD%	Total	DD+	DD%	Total	DD+	DD%
50–59	66	16	24	84	25	30	123	18	15
60–69	49	18	37	58	18	31	52	17	33
70–79	54	30	56	50	31	62	34	16	47
80+	16	10	63	14	9	64	10	5	50
All	185	74	35	206	83	33	219	56	25

Table 16.4 The prevalence of Dupuytren's disease (DD%) among self-reported diabetics and nondiabetics and the prevalence of self-reported diabetes mellitus

	Diabetics			Nondiabetics			
	Total	DD+	DD%	Total	DD+	DD%	Diabetes %
Men							
50–59	65	24	37	208	35	17	24
60–69	53	24	45	106	29	27	33
70–79	44	32	73	94	42	45	32
80+	9	7	78	31	17	55	23
Women							
50–59	48	14	29	265	22	8	15
60–69	40	8	20	122	14	11	25
70–79	22	10	45	66	16	24	25
80+	11	4	36	23	6	26	32

95% confidence interval 1.08–2.41). This was not the case for women ($p=0.6$; OR 1.17; 95% confidence interval 0.71–1.92).

There was no significant difference in the prevalence of Dupuytren's disease between smokers and nonsmokers, between those admitting to drinking alcohol and teetotalers, or between those living in urban areas and those living in rural areas. The prevalence was, however, far higher among those who stated that they suffered from diabetes mellitus (Table 16.4. Men: $p=0.00000033$; OR 2.75; 95% confidence interval 1.83–4.11; women: $p=0.000034$; OR 2.79; 95% confidence interval 1.70–4.81).

The separate examination of 125 male and 112 female patients at a diabetes clinic show that 92 men and 64 women had Dupuytren's disease (Table 16.5).

Table 16.5 The number of individuals found with Dupuytren's disease (DD+) at a diabetes clinic and the age-specific prevalence

Age	Men			Women		
	Total	DD+	DD%	Total	DD+	DD%
50–59	30	19	63	25	14	56
60–69	48	36	75	36	22	61
70–79	43	34	79	41	24	58
80+	4	3	75	10	4	40
All	125	92	69	112	64	57

16.4 Discussion

In 1991, the population of the old Bosnia and Herzegovina was 44% Muslim, 31% Greek Orthodox Serb, and 17% Roman Catholic Croat. The inhabitants are, however, all descendants of the South Slavs who migrated into the Balkans in the sixth and seventh centuries A.D. Little attention was paid to ethnic labels until the war of 1992–1995, particularly in the cities where intermarriage had blurred the lines between the groups and religious devoutness was uncommon. After the "ethnic cleansing" of the war that took place in the 1990s, the country has been divided into Bosnia, inhabited mainly by Croats and Muslims, and the Serbian Republic with a mainly Serbian population. Rural and urban areas in both parts of Bosnia and Herzegovina were visited in order to obtain a representative sample of the population during the collection of data for this study.

There are considerable differences between studies of the prevalence of Dupuytren's disease in various geographic areas. The highest prevalence has been found in Scandinavia and the British Isles (Lund 1941; Mikkelsen 1972; Bergenudd et al. 1993; Lennox et al. 1993; Gudmundsson et al. 2000; Finsen et al. 2002). Contrary to previous opinion, we found a high prevalence of Dupuytren's contracture in Bosnia and Herzegovina. It was even higher than the reported prevalence in northern Europe. Most cases had only palmar changes, and even for those with moderate contracture of the fingers, it may not seem worthwhile to seek medical advice in this relatively poor country, which has a health-care system that is in crisis after the war. It seems possible that factors such as these may explain why the prevalence has been perceived to be low up to now.

The manner of sampling the population in this study is not ideal. Hardly anyone refused to participate in the study, but groups such as the incarcerated and the bedridden are obviously not included. It seems unlikely that this has influenced the findings materially, and we were unable to devise a better sampling method in a country in which detailed demographic data to a great extent are lacking. Even so, it seems probable that our study comes closer to revealing the true prevalence than the occasional anecdotal reports of orthopedic and plastic surgeons that have been the basis of the present view. It is sometimes difficult to distinguish Dupuytren's disease from other pathology in the hand, but this is true also for the other population-based epidemiological studies that have been reported.

A predilection for the right hand has also been reported by others (Mikkelsen 1972). Furthermore, Mikkelsen and coworkers (1999) and Gudmundsson et al. (2001a) have found an increased death rate among individuals with Dupuytren's disease, and this, together with the high prevalence of diabetes mellitus, may explain the lower prevalence of Dupuytren's disease among the oldest individuals in our study.

Ethnic differences in the prevalence of Dupuytren's disease have been documented (Maes 1979; Zarowski and Mann 1979; Mennen and Gräbe 1979; Chow et al. 1984; Muguti and Appelt 1993; Ross 1999). However, as there are no true ethnic differences between the populations of Bosnia and Herzegovina, only religious and social differences, it is surprising to find lower prevalence among Bosnian Muslim than Bosnian Serb and Croat men. It is possible that this is a spurious finding, particularly as no such difference was found among women, but it may also be due to some, as yet undetermined, difference in social factors.

Some studies have shown a correlation between smoking habits and Dupuytren's disease (Attali et al. 1987; An et al. 1988; Burge et al. 1997; Gudmundsson et al. 2000). This association was not found by Bergenudd et al. (1993), nor was it in the present study. Many studies report a relationship between alcohol consumption and Dupuytren's disease (Bradlow and Mowat 1986; Attali et al. 1987; Burge et al. 1997). In the present investigation, in keeping with some other reports (Mikkelsen 1972; Houghton et al. 1983; Quintana Guitian 1988; Gudmundsson et al. 2001b), no significant correlation could be found.

Diabetes mellitus has been related to Dupuytren's disease in numerous reports (Ravid et al. 1977; Lawson et al. 1983; Noble et al. 1984; Attali et al. 1987; Jennings et al. 1989; Arkkila et al. 1997), and they were found to be associated in the present study. In the main material, the diagnoses of diabetes mellitus are self-reported and therefore open to question. The diagnoses of diabetes are not in doubt in the separate data from a diabetic clinic, and the prevalence of Dupuytren's disease among these patients was even higher than among the self-reported diabetics. The prevalence of diabetes mellitus seems extremely high in the population we have studied, but we do not know of figures for self-reported diabetes in other populations.

16.5 Conclusions

Contrary to previous opinion, we find that Dupuytren's disease is common in Bosnia. The prevalence is highly age-dependent and is strongly associated with diabetes mellitus. Other suggested risk factors such as smoking and alcohol consumption appear to be less important in this population.

This chapter was previously published in similar form in BMC Musculoskel Disord 2004, 5:10.

References

An HS, Southworth SR, Jackson WT, Russ B (1988) Cigarette smoking and Dupuytren's contracture of the hand. J Hand Surg [Am] 13:872–874

Arkkila PET, Kantola IM, Viikari JSA (1997) Dupuytren's disease: association with chronic diabetic complications. J Rheumatol 24:153–9

Attali P, Ink O, Pelletier G, Vernier C, Jean F, Moulton L, Etienne J-P (1987) Dupuytren's contracture, alcohol consumption, and chronic liver disease. Arch Intern Med 147:1065–1067

Bergenudd H, Lindgärde F, Nilsson BE (1993) Prevalence of Dupuytren's contracture and its correlation with degenerative changes of the hands and feet and with criteria of general health. J Hand Surg [Br] 18:254–257

Bradlow A, Mowat AG (1986) Dupuytren's contracture and alcohol. Ann Rheum Dis 45:304–307

Burge P, Hoy G, Regan P, Milne R (1997) Smoking, alcohol and the risk factor of Dupuytren's contracture. J Bone Joint Surg Br 79:206–210

Chow SP, Luk KDK, Kung TM (1984) Dupuytren's contracture in Chinese. J R Coll Surg Edinb 29:49–51

Finsen V, Dalen H, Nesheim J (2002) The prevalence of Dupuytren's disease among 2 different ethnic groups in northern Norway. J Hand Surg [Am] 27:115–117

Gudmundsson KG, Arngrimsson R, Sigfusson N, Bjornsson A, Jonsson T (2000) Epidemiology of Dupuytren's disease. Clinical, serological, and social assessment. The Reykjavik study. J Clin Epidemiol 53:291–196

Gudmundsson KG, Arngrimsson R, Sigfusson N, Jonsson T (2001a) Increased total mortality and cancer mortality in men with Dupuytren's disease: a 15-year follow-up study. J Clin Epidemiol 54:1–6

Gudmundsson KG, Arngrimsson R, Jonsson T (2001b) Dupuytren's disease, alcohol consumption and alcoholism. Scand J Prim Health Care 19:186–190

Houghton S, Holdstock G, Cockerell R, Wright R (1983) Dupuytren's contracture, chronic liver disease and IgA immune complexes. Liver 3:220–224

Jennings AM, Milner PC, Ward JD (1989) Hand abnormalities are associated with the complications of diabetes in type 2 diabetes. Diabet Med 6:43–47

Lawson PM, Maneschi F, Kohner EM (1983) The relationship of hand abnormalities to diabetes and diabetic retinopathy. Diabetes Care 6:140–143

Lennox IAC, Murali SR, Porter R (1993) A study of repeatability of the diagnosis of Dupuytren's contracture and its prevalence in the Grampian region. J Hand Surg [Br] 18:258–261

Lund M (1941) Dupuytren's contracture and epilepsy. Acta Psychiar Neurol 16:465–492

Maes J (1979) Dupuytren's contracture in an oriental patient (letter). Plast Reconstr Surg 64:251

Mennen U, Gräbe PR (1979) Dupuytren's contracture in a Negro: a case report. J Hand Surg [Am] 4:451–453

Mikkelsen OA (1972) The prevalence of Dupuytren's disease in Norway. Acta Chir Scand 138:695–700

Mikkelsen OA, Høyeraal HM, Sandvik L (1999) Increased mortality in Dupuytren's disease. J Hand Surg [Br] 24:515–518

Muguti GI, Appelt B (1993) Dupuytren's contracture in black Zimbabweans. Cent Afr J Med 39:129–132

Noble J, Heathcote JG, Cohen H (1984) Diabetes mellitus in the aetiology of Dupuytren's disease. J Bone Joint Surg Br 66:322–325

Quintana Guitian A (1988) Various epidemiologic aspects of Dupuytren's disease. Ann Chir Main 7:256–262

Ravid M, Dinai Y, Sohar E (1977) Dupuytren's disease in diabetes mellitus. Acta Diabetol Lat 14:170–174

Ross DC (1999) Epidemiology of Dupuytren's disease. Hand Clin 15:53–62

Stradner F, Ulreich A, Pfeiffer KP (1987) Dupuytren's palmar contraction as an attendant disease of diabetes mellitus. Wien Med Wochenschr 137:89–92

Zarowski RE, Mann RJ (1979) Dupuytren's contracture in a black patient. Plast Reconstr Surg 63:122–124

Part IV
Collagen and Cell Biology

Editor: Charles Eaton

A Primer of Collagen Biology: Synthesis, Degradation, Subtypes, and Role in Dupuytren's Disease

17

Susan Emeigh Hart

Contents

17.1	**Introduction**	131
17.2	**Collagens: Structurally and Functionally Diverse Proteins with Common Features**	132
17.3	**Collagen Remodeling: Process and Controls**	133
17.3.1	Collagen Deposition	134
17.3.2	Collagen Degradation	135
17.4	**Roles of Collagen in Dupuytren's Disease**	137
17.4.1	Structural Role of Collagen (Imbalance in Collagen Remodeling)	137
17.4.2	Functional Role of Collagen (Mechanotransduction and Fibroblast Responses to Force)	138
17.5	**Conclusions**	140
References		140

17.1 Introduction

Historically, investigations into the pathogenesis of Dupuytren's disease have focused on the roles of genetic and epigenetic factors (such as growth factors, trauma, concurrent medications and/or disease states) and their influence on the cellular components of the subcutaneous tissues (fibroblasts and myofibroblasts) (reviewed in Cordova et al. 2005; Al-Qattan 2006; Rayan 2007) The collagen matrix (the primary constituent of the cords found in late stage Dupuytren's contracture) has been considered merely a biomarker of the cellular processes, with little importance as a therapeutic target (except as an inert structure whose disruption or removal will result in symptomatic relief to the patient).

However, more recent investigations into the genomics and proteomics of cells and tissues isolated from surgically excised Dupuytren's tissue have revealed significant overlap with the patterns of gene and protein expression in normal wound healing. These findings suggest that the abnormalities in Dupuytren's disease may represent an aberrant or exaggerated wound healing response in affected patients, a process which is largely mediated through the interaction of the fibroblast with the extracellular matrix, specifically via attachments to collagen fibers. The genomic and proteomic changes detected at the cellular level, coupled with structural differences in collagen components of Dupuytren's tissue compared to those in normal palmar fascia, indicate an additional contribution to the pathogenesis of this disease from an upset in the normal balance of extracellular matrix remodeling.

Thus, the collagen matrix continues to represent a key therapeutic target in Dupuytren's disease, both as

S.E. Hart
Intrexon Corporation, Germantown, MD, USA
e-mail: SHart@intrexon.com

C. Eaton et al. (eds.), *Dupuytren's Disease and Related Hyperproliferative Disorders*,
DOI 10.1007/978-3-642-22697-7_17, © Springer-Verlag Berlin Heidelberg 2012

Table 17.1 Functional/structural classification and tissue distribution of collagen subtypes

Classification	Types	Tissue distribution	General functions
Fibril forming	I, II, III, V, XI, XXIV, XXVII	Skin, bone, tendon, blood vessels, cornea (I, III)	Primary structural components of extracellular matrix (ECM)
		Reticular fibers (III)	
		Associated with Type I (V) or Type II (XI)	
		Cartilage, intervertebral disk, vitreous (II)	
		Developing/embryonic tissues (XXIV, XXVII)	
Network	IV, VIII, X	Widespread, all basement membranes (IV)	Adhesion
		Descement's membrane, endothelial cells (VIII)	Occlusion
		Hypertrophic cartilage (X)	Source of matricryptins (IV, VIII)[b]
Anchoring fibrils	VII	Dermal–epidermal junctions (skin, oral mucosa, genitourinary tract)	Anchoring
FACIT	IX, XII, XIV, XIX, XX, XXI, XXII	Widespread, esp. corneal epithelium (XX)	Integration, stabilization, and structural regulation of ECM
		Associated w. Type I (XII, XIV) or Type II (IX)	Signal transduction
		Skeletal muscle (XIX)	
		Cornea and vitreous (IX)	
		Blood vessel wall (XXI)	
Transmembrane (MACIT)	XIII, XVII, XXIII, XXV	Hemidesmosomes (XVII)	Cell–cell/cell–matrix adhesion
		Neuromuscular junction (XIII)	Regulation of embryonic development
Beaded filament (microfibrillar)	VI , XXVIII	Widespread in connective tissues, especially adipose and synovial membranes (VI)	Integration
		Peripheral nerves (XXVIII)	Myelination (XXVIII)
		Associated with Type VI in blood vessels (VI)	
Endostatin producing (multiplexins[a])	XV, XVI, XVIII	Associated with basement membranes (widespread), but especially blood vessels, skeletal muscle (XV), and eye (XVIII)	Antiangiogenic
			Source of matricryptins[b]
Unknown	XXVI	Testis and ovary (during development), elastic fibers	Unknown

Information from the following sources: van der rest and Garrone (1991); Prockop and Kivirikko (1995); Kuo et al. (1997); Zeichen et al. (1999); Ortega and Werb (2002); Gelse et al. (2003); Ricard-Blum and Ruggerio (2005); Khoshnoodi et al. (2006); Veit et al. (2006); Shoulders and Raines (2009)
FACIT *F*ibril *A*ssociated *C*ollagens with *I*nterrupted *T*riple Helices, MACIT *M*embrane *A*ssociated *C*ollagens with *I*nterrupted *T*riple Helices
[a]Multiplexin indicates collagen with multiple triple-helix domains and interruptions
[b]Matricryptin indicates C-terminal fragment with growth factor or other pharmacologic effect derived by proteolytic cleavage from the parent collagen molecule

a structural and as a functional component. An understanding of its structure, biology, regulation, and potential roles in Dupuytren's disease are important to development of novel approaches in modulating the disease via this target.

17.2 Collagens: Structurally and Functionally Diverse Proteins with Common Features

Collagens are an extremely structurally and functionally diverse group of proteins that are defined as such based on the following common features:

- Somewhere within the molecule, one or more triple-helical motifs consisting of three polypeptide chains (McAlinden et al. 2003; Khoshnoodi et al. 2006)
- The presence of multiple Gly-X-Y repeats (with X and Y usually being proline or hydroxyproline), which permit the formation of the helical structures (van der Rest and Garrone 1991; Ricard-Blum and Ruggerio 2005)
- A high content (up to 50% of the proline residues) of hydroxyproline, required for stabilization of the triple helix (Gelse et al. 2003; Shoulders and Raines 2009)

To date, 28 different types of collagen (the products of 34 distinct genes) have been identified; these have been

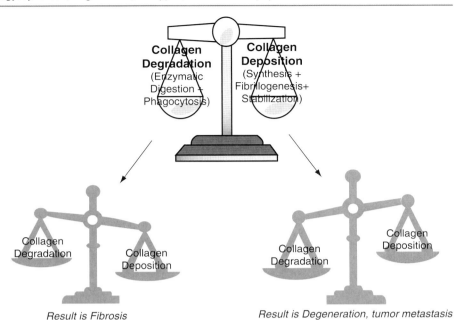

Fig. 17.1 Remodeling of the extracellular matrix. Remodeling of the extracellular matrix requires both removal and deposition of collagen. The processes are normally balanced so that there is no net increase or decrease in the amount of matrix present. The balance is altered in pathologic conditions. Increased deposition or decreased degradation results in fibrosis; the opposite scenario results in tissue degeneration and facilitation of tumor metastasis (Mansell and Bailey 2004)

classified, based on their structural and/or functional similarity, into eight different classes (reviewed in van der Rest and Garrone 1991; Prockop and Kivirikko 1995; Gelse et al. 2003; Ricard-Blum and Ruggerio 2005; Khoshnoodi et al. 2006). An overview of collagen classification and tissue distribution is presented in Table 17.1.

The fibrillar collagens are the most abundant class of collagens and are the best characterized; all of them consist almost exclusively of triple-helical collagen composed of Gly-X-Y repeats which is deposited in the extracellular space in the form of overlapping fibrils. Type I is the primary structural component of the extracellular matrix in most tissues. In fibrils, it is usually found as a complex protein in combination with Type V collagen, which serves as a nucleus for fibril formation. Type III collagen fibrils are also referred to as reticulin; this collagen type is found in healing wounds, embryonic connective tissues, and as a primary structural component in tissues such as skin, lung, and blood vessels where greater elasticity is needed (reviewed in Prockop and Kivirikko 1995; Ricard-Blum and Ruggerio 2005; Kadler et al. 2008; Shoulders and Raines 2009). An increase in the content of Type III relative to Type I collagen compared to the normal palmar fascia is considered a hallmark feature of Dupuytren's disease tissue, regardless of the stage of the disease (Hanyu et al. 1984; Melling et al. 1999, 2000).

Other collagens can be found within Dupuytren's tissue or associated with adjacent structures, although they have not been implicated in the pathogenesis of this condition. These include Type IV (a primary component of epidermal and vascular basement membranes as well as perineural structures), Type VI (an important component of synovial membranes and blood vessel basement membranes), and Type VII (plays a role in anchoring the epidermis to the dermis).

17.3 Collagen Remodeling: Process and Controls

The components of the extracellular matrix are in a constant state of flux, with the changes in the composition and quantity of the matrix collagen dictated by environmental stimuli and stage of development. In order for new collagen to be deposited, the existing collagen must be removed; these two processes occur simultaneously in a balanced fashion in normal tissues so that there is no net change in either the quantity or composition of the extracellular matrix present (Fig. 17.1). Disruption of the dynamic balance between these two processes can occur in response to physiologic need but also occurs in a number of pathologic conditions, including Dupuytren's disease (Mansell and Bailey 2004; Stetler-Stevenson 1996).

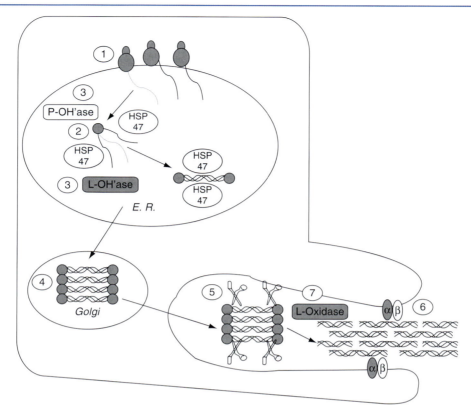

Fig. 17.2 Key control points in collagen synthesis. The rate of collagen deposition is determined by the sum of the following processes: (*1*) the rate of COL gene expression and translocation of collagen monomers into the endoplasmic reticulum (ER), (*2*) aggregation of monomers into trimers via their C propeptides, which initiates triple-helix formation. Heat shock protein 47 (Hsp47) is required to prevent "tangling" of the monomers and to slow helix formation to allow for (*3*) hydroxylation of proline and lysine residues by prolyl-hydroxylase (P-OH'ase) and lysyl hydroxylase (L-OH'ase) and formation of intramolecular cross-links by these hydroxy amino acids, stabilizing the triple helix, (*4*) translocation into the Golgi apparatus and aggregation into fibril "stacks" (speed of translocation depends on speed and effectiveness of triple-helix formation), (*5*) deposition of stacks into the extracellular space via the formation of "fibripositors" and cleavage of the N- and C-terminal propeptides by N- and C-terminal propeptidases (represented by scissors), (*6*) overlapping aggregation of collagen tripeptides into fibrils, enhanced by the presence of β_1 integrins ($\alpha\beta$) on the cell surface, and (*7*) stabilization of the collagen fibrils by intermolecular cross-links through the action of lysyl oxidase (L-oxidase) (Figure adapted from material in Kadler et al. 1996; Persikov and Brodsky 2002; Canty and Kadler 2005; Khoshnoodi et al. 2006; Kadler et al. 2008)

Of the two processes involved in collagen remodeling, the process of collagen deposition is more complex and thus can be regulated at multiple levels. In contrast, collagen degradation is primarily regulated by controlling the quantity and activity of collagen digesting enzymes.

17.3.1 Collagen Deposition

The transformation of labile newly synthesized collagen polypeptides into the stable collagen fibrils present within the extracellular matrix is a slow and complex process. The rate and effectiveness of collagen deposition (the net result of synthesis and fibrillogenesis) is thus governed at many levels (as depicted in Fig. 17.2). These are described specifically as they relate to the fibrillar collagens in the following sections.

As with all proteins, the rate of collagen deposition can be regulated by up- or downregulation of the *COL* genes responsible for the synthesis of the collagen α chains. These are synthesized directly into the endoplasmic reticulum to undergo the posttranslational modifications needed for both the formation and stabilization of triple-helical procollagen. Assembly of collagen trimers from the monomeric α chains occurs due to the interaction of the C-NC domains located near the C termini of these molecules (Khoshnoodi et al. 2006).

Once trimerization is complete, triple-helix formation commences in a C to N direction; formation and stabilization of the helix requires conversion of proline residues located in the −Y position of the Gly-X-Y collagen motif to hydroxyproline through the action of prolyl-4-hydroxylase and its essential cofactor, ascorbic acid (vitamin C). Further stabilization of the triple helix results from the action of lysyl hydroxylase which generates hydroxylysine from lysine residues within the collagen molecule; the hydroxylysine residues provide sites for the addition of glucose and galactose molecules to the procollagen molecules and are also critical to extracellular cross-linking of collagen fibrils. These modifications serve to increase the thermal stability of the collagen molecules (Prockop and Kivirikko 1995; Persikov and Brodsky 2002; Canty and Kadler 2005).

Additional stabilization of the forming procollagen triple helices results from their association with the molecular chaperone heat shock protein 47 (Hsp47). This protein becomes associated with the newly synthesized collagen α chains, facilitating trimerization; it also is critical to the correct formation of the procollagen triple helix by preventing premature and incorrect "folding" of the procollagen monomers as well as preventing their thermal denaturation until the necessary posttranslational modifications of proline and lysine are complete and triple-helix formation can take place. Additionally, Hsp47 assists with the translocation of the completed procollagen trimers into the Golgi apparatus for transportation to the extracellular space (Prockop and Kivirikko 1995; Canty and Kadler 2005).

Within the Golgi apparatus, the procollagen trimers are aligned into stacks and are transported to the cell membrane of the fibroblasts in specialized elongated vacuoles; these fuse with the plasma membrane surface to form specialized structures known as "fibripositors" in which the lumen of the vacuole is contiguous with the extracellular space but is still somewhat protected from the extracellular environment (Canty et al. 2004). The process known as "fibrillogenesis" is initiated; this requires cleavage of the C- and N-terminal propeptides by the appropriate peptidases, assembly of the cleaved collagen triple helices into fibrils, and stabilization of the forming fibrils by cross-linking the individual triple-helical collagen monomers through their hydroxylysine residues by the activity of extracellular lysyl oxidase. The confinement of these processes within the fibripositor not only protects the labile collagen monomers from degradation until stable fibrils can be formed but also directs the placement

of the forming collagen fibrils where they are needed, along the lines of force (Gelse et al. 2003; Canty and Kadler 2005; Canty et al. 2006).

Once the propeptides are cleaved, collagen monomers can self-assemble into fibrils at neutral pH, but the speed and effectiveness of fibrillogenesis as well as the thermal and enzymatic stability of the resulting fibrils are enhanced when this process is assisted (Prockop and Kivirikko 1995). Cell surface β_1 integrins (primarily α_2 and α_5) can bind to collagen fibrils and assist in fibrillogenesis by keeping the monomers in close proximity with each other (facilitating cross-linking) as well as with Type V collagen fibrils (which serve as a nucleus for the formation of mature Type I collagen fibrils) and cell surface bound fibronectin (which assists in fibril assembly and protects newly formed fibrils from degradation) (Wenstrup et al. 2004; Kadler et al. 2008). Fibrillogenesis is also potentiated by the action of the matricellular protein periostin, which also plays a role in determining the ultimate diameter and orientation of newly laid collagen fibrils (Norris et al. 2007).

Additional stabilization of the collagen fibrils occurs once fibrillogenesis is complete. Covalent modification of the maturing fibrils (lysyl oxidase mediated cross-linking, along with enzymatic and nonenzymatic glycation), association with matrix proteins and small leucine-rich proteoglycans (such as periostin, decorin, and the FACIT collagens), increased fibril length and/or diameter, and increased mechanical tension all serve to increase the resistance of the collagen fibrils to enzymatic and thermal degradation (Canty and Kadler 2005; Minond et al. 2006; Norris et al. 2007; Hamilton 2008; Perumal et al. 2008; Flynn et al. 2010; Kalamajski and Oldberg 2010).

17.3.2 Collagen Degradation

17.3.2.1 Collagenases

The collagen triple helix, once stabilized by intra- and intermolecular cross-linking, is remarkably resistant to degradation, as the labile peptide bonds are buried within the interior of the collagen molecule. For an enzyme to effectively initiate degradation of an intact triple-helical collagen molecule, it must possess the ability to identify and bind to "weaker" sites on the molecule, locally unwind the triple helix, and successfully cleave one or more strands of the triple helix. A collagenase is defined as an enzyme which can effectively perform all three of these activities (Lauer-Fields et al. 2002).

Table 17.2 Mammalian collagenases and their substrates

Enzyme designation	Common name(s)	Substrate(s)	Function(s)
MMP-1	Collagenase 1	Fibrillar collagens (Type III preferred)	Extracellular cleavage (physiologic and pathologic)
	Interstitial collagenase	Collagens VI, VII, X, IX	Wound healing
	Fibroblast collagenase	Gelatin	
	Synovial collagenase		
MMP-2	Gelatinase A	Gelatin (preferred)	Pericellular collagenolysis (phagocytosis)
		Fibrillar collagens	Inflammation
		Collagens IV, V, VII, X, XI	Activates proMMPs (8, 9, 13)
MMP-3	Stromelysin 1	Gelatin (preferred)	Activates most proMMPs
		Collagens III, IV, V, VII, IX, X, XI	
MMP-7	Matrilysin 1	Gelatin (preferred)	Activates many proMMPs
		Collagens I and V	
MMP-8	Collagenase 2	Fibrillar collagens (Type I preferred)	Inflammation
	Neutrophil collagenase		Wound healing
MMP-9	Gelatinase B	Gelatin	Inflammation
		Collagen I(?)	Pathologic remodeling
		Collagens IV, V, VII, X, XI	
MMP-10	Stromelysin 2	Gelatin (preferred)	Activates many proMMPs
		Collagens I, III, IV, V, IX, X	Wound healing
MMP-12	Metalloelastase	Gelatin	Basement membrane remodeling
		Collagens I, IV	
MMP-13	Collagenase 3	Gelatin	Cartilage and bone remodeling
		Fibrillar collagens (Type II preferred)	Wound healing
		Collagens VI, IX, X, XIV	
MMP-14	MT1-MMP[a]	Fibrillar collagens	Activates proMMPs (2, 8, 13)
		Gelatin	Pericellular collagenolysis (phagocytosis)
			Fibroblast migration
MMP-15	MT2-MMP[a]	Gelatins	Activates proMMP-2
		Collagen III	
MMP-16	MT3-MMP[a]	Fibrillar collagens	Activates proMMP-2

Information from the following sources: Everts et al. (1996); Stetler-Stevenson (1996); Sternlicht and Werb (2001); Lauer-Fields et al. (2002); Visse and Nagase (2003); Gutiérrez-Fernández et al. (2007); Barbolina and Stack (2008); Sabeh et al. (2009); Minond et al. (2006); Nagase et al. (2006); Pasternak and Aspenberg (2009)
[a]MT-MMP indicates membrane-associated (transmembrane) MMP. These are not secreted but remain associated with the cell membrane and are activated intracellularly by furin-mediated cleavage

Mammalian collagenases fall into two enzyme classes: the zinc-dependent metalloproteinases (represented by a subset of the 23 known mammalian matrix metalloproteinases, or MMPs) and the cysteine proteases (represented by cathepsins K and L). Of the two classes, the MMPs are the primary enzymes responsible for both physiologic and pathologic remodeling of extracellular matrix collagen (Lauer-Fields et al. 2002; Pasternak and Aspenberg 2009); cathepsins primarily function as lysosomal proteases but do play a role in extracellular collagenolysis in bone and cartilage remodeling (Turk et al. 2001; Daley et al. 2007). The MMPs that can act as collagenases and/or have been shown to have a role in collagen remodeling are listed in Table 17.2.

Cleavage of fibrillar collagens by MMPs occurs in the same fashion, regardless of the enzyme involved, as all of them recognize a single site on the collagen molecule (Gly_{775}-Ile/Leu_{776} on the alpha chain). Cleavage at this site results in the generation of two fragments of approximately one-fourth and three-fourths the length of the original fibril (Lauer-Fields et al. 2002; Nagase et al. 2006). The resultant cleavage fragments are known as gelatin and are rapidly cleared from the site of their formation, either by additional proteolysis (in addition to the gelatinolytic MMPs, a number of nonspecific proteases can digest gelatin), by denaturation (gelatin is thermically unstable at physiologic temperatures), and by phagocytosis, a process that is mediated in part by the β_1 integrin-mediated interaction of collagen fibrils with the fibroblast cell surface (Evanson et al. 1968; Fesus et al. 1981; Everts et al. 1996; Arora et al. 2000; Leikina et al. 2002; Stultz 2002).

17.3.2.2 Control of Collagen Degradation

Control of collagen degradation depends on tight regulation of the activity of the MMPs as well as temporal and spatial limitation of these enzymes. There are four levels at which these enzymes are regulated:

Transcription

Only a few of the MMPs (notably MMP-2 and MMP-14) are constitutively expressed, and then only at low levels and in a few tissues. As a general rule, up- and downregulation of the genes responsible for MMP synthesis is required for these enzymes; additional regulation occurs via stabilization of the transcripts (Sternlicht and Werb 2001; Ra and Parks 2007).

Activation of Inactive Enzyme

With the exception of the matrix metalloproteinases (MT-MMPs) which are activated intracellularly, most MMPs are synthesized and secreted as inactive zymogens as the result of a direct internal interaction between a cysteine on the polypeptide and the zinc bound to the catalytic site of the molecule. Disruption of this interaction (resulting in the generation of catalytically active enzyme) requires proteolytic cleavage of the proMMP. While this most commonly results from interaction with another MMP, nonspecific proteases (such as plasmin) can activate the membrane-bound MMPs; additionally, chemical disruption of the cysteine-Zn^{+2} interaction by strong oxidizing conditions, metal ions, or disulfides can also lead to MMP activation and autocatalysis of the prodomain (Somerville et al. 2003; Visse and Nagase 2003; Ra and Parks 2007).

Compartmentalization

Inactive forms of MMPs 8, 9, and 12 are retained within the secretory granules of inflammatory cells such as neutrophils and macrophages until released upon stimulation of the cell (Sternlicht and Werb 2001). MMPs that are freely secreted into the extracellular space are generally held close to the surface of the secreting fibroblast via interactions with cell surface proteins such as integrins or membrane-bound MMPs; these interactions are critical to the activity and substrate specificity of each MMP (Ra and Parks 2007).

Inactivation of Active Enzymes

Temporal and spatial regulation of MMP activity results primarily from their inhibition due to interaction with one of the four small glycoproteins known as *t*issue *i*nhibitors of *m*etalloproteinases (TIMPs). Like MMPs, these are not constitutive proteins but are regulated in response to physiologic need (the exception is TIMP-3, which is present in an inactive complex with the carbohydrate moieties of the interstitial matrix and is released in active form during matrix degradation), with the relative balance between the levels of MMP and TIMP determining the net activity of matrix degradation. All MMPs are subject to inactivation by all of the TIMPs, with a few exceptions; TIMP-1 is not effective at inactivating the MT-MMPs, and TIMP-2 actually enhances the activation of proMMP-2 by MMP-14 (MT1-MMP) by facilitating the interaction between these two proteins (Baker et al. 2002; Visse and Nagase 2003). Any MMP that escapes local inactivation by TIMPS and/or enters the systemic circulation is rapidly inactivated by interaction with the nonspecific protease inhibitor α_2-macroglobulin which is ubiquitously present in the serum and interstitial fluid, and to a lesser extent by the cell-surface-associated protein *re*versin-inducing *c*ysteine-rich protein (RECK), which is widely distributed in many tissues (Cawston and Mercer 1986; Baker et al. 2002).

17.4 Roles of Collagen in Dupuytren's Disease

17.4.1 Structural Role of Collagen (Imbalance in Collagen Remodeling)

The hallmark feature of Dupuytren's contracture is the localized deposition of excess and abnormal collagen within the palmar fascia, which suggests that the normal balance of collagen remodeling has been locally perturbed in these patients. A number of studies evaluating genomic and proteomic differences in the diseased palmar fascia (cords, nodules, and/or fibroblasts) from Dupuytren's patients compared to either unaffected fascial components or palmar fascia from unaffected individuals clearly indicate the presence of a shift in this balance in favor of net collagen deposition. These studies are summarized in Table 17.3.

In addition, a number of structural and biochemical abnormalities have been identified in the collagen comprising the Dupuytren's cords that indicate an increase in the stability of the matrix to enzymatic and/or thermal degradation, which would further tip the balance by decreasing collagen degradation even when collagen degrading enzymes are present in abundance. Increased thermal and enzymatic stability of collagen fibrils resulting from increased cross-linking of collagen due to increased hydroxylysine and/or hydroxyproline and the presence of abnormal collagen cross-links (Brickley-Parsons et al. 1981; Notbohm et al. 1995) or resulting from increased or altered collagen glycation (Brickley-Parsons et al. 1981; Hanyu et al. 1984; Melling et al. 1999) has been described in Dupuytren's disease tissue. The collagen fibrils are also larger in diameter in Dupuytren's disease tissue and are more closely packed in larger fascicles with thicker fascicular sheaths (Mansell and Bailey 2004), which prevents ready access to the labile portions of the individual collagen monomers by collagenases (Perumal et al. 2008). These structural changes in Dupuytren's collagen also result in increased stiffness (decreased elasticity) in the fibrils relative to normal tissue, which renders them more effective in their role as signal transducers to fibroblasts (detailed in the following section) (Melling et al. 2000; Shoulders and Raines 2009).

17.4.2 Functional Role of Collagen (Mechanotransduction and Fibroblast Responses to Force)

More recent studies investigating the pathophysiology of Dupuytren's disease have revealed the significant degree of overlap in its morphology and biology with several phases of wound healing. Features common to the two processes include the transition of fibroblasts to myofibroblasts, generation of tension by myofibroblasts, increased deposition of Type III collagen and fibronectin, the key role of TGF-β, and upregulation of collagen remodeling resulting in shortening of the existing collagen fibrils, which causes contraction (Brickley-Parsons et al. 1981; Tomasek et al. 2002; Rayan 2007). The key difference between these two

processes is that the tissue responses in Dupuytren's disease are more exaggerated and/or prolonged than those seen in normal healing wounds. Thus, Dupuytren's disease may be regarded as a manifestation of aberrant wound healing responses.

Fibroblasts are in constant contact with their external environment and monitor the degree of static and dynamic force present through cell surface β_1 integrins (α_2, α_5 and/or α_{11}) and the Type I collagen fibrils present in the extracellular matrix. Any increase in the degree of tension present in the matrix is transmitted to the intracellular cytoskeleton; this transmission of force results in alteration of gene expression which occurs either indirectly via the release and nuclear translocation of preformed transcription factors, or directly, resulting from mechanical deformation of the nuclear DNA due to its physical association with the cytoskeletal elements that cross the nuclear membrane (Fig. 17.3) (Chiquet et al. 2003, 2007; Wang et al. 2007, 2009). The alteration of mechanical force on resting fibroblasts is the primary stimulus for the initiation of wound healing and also for physiologic remodeling to ensure that the quantity and quality of the extracellular matrix is adequate to the load.

It has been shown that the morphologic changes common to both wound healing and the early stages of Dupuytren's disease can be induced in cultured fibroblasts (normal or derived from Dupuytren's disease tissue) or granulation tissue explants by subjecting them to mechanical tension; these include proliferation, transition to myofibroblasts, secretion of TGF-β and other cytokines, generation of contractile force in myofibroblasts, increased fibroblast motility, and increased thickness and stiffness of collagen fibrils (Alman et al. 1996, Hinz et al. 2001; Tomasek et al. 2002; Balestrini and Billiar 2009; Roeder et al. 2009). In addition, many of the same genomic and proteomic differences in the diseased palmar fascia (cords, nodules, and/or fibroblasts) from Dupuytren's patients compared to either unaffected fascial components or palmar fascia from unaffected individuals can be induced in cultured fibroblasts by subjecting them to mechanical force or have been identified as being differentially expressed in tissues under stress (Table 17.3). Conversely, decreased mechanical tension on myofibroblasts results in their disappearance via apoptosis, seen in the resolution phase of wound healing and also in the late stages of Dupuytren's disease (Fluck et al. 1998; Grinnell et al. 1999; Gabbiani 2003).

Table 17.3 Gene and/or protein alterations in Dupuytrens's fibroblasts related to collagen remodeling or fibroblast responses to tension

Gene or protein	Function	Effect on collagen remodeling	Direction of change in: Dupuytren's disease tissue	Fibroblasts under tension
ADAMTS-2	N-terminal propeptidase	↑ Collagen deposition	↑↑	↑
ADAMTS-3	N-terminal propeptidase	↑ Collagen deposition	↑↑	↑
ADAMTS-14	N-terminal propeptidase	↑ Collagen deposition	↑↑	↑
COL1A1	Collagen I alpha1 chain	↑ Collagen deposition	↑↑	↑↑
COL1A2	Collagen I alpha2 chain	↑ Collagen deposition	↑↑	↑↑
COL3A1	Collagen III alpha1 chain	↑ Collagen deposition	↑	↑
COL5A1	Collagen V alpha1 chain	↑ Collagen deposition	↑	
COL5A2	Collagen V alpha2 chain	↑ Collagen deposition	↑	
Integrin β_1	Signal transduction from collagen; facilitates fibrillogenesis	↑ Collagen deposition	↑	↑
Fibronectin	Facilitates fibrillogenesis	↑ Collagen deposition	↑	↑
Hsp47	Intracellular collagen stabilization and triple-helix formation	↑ Collagen deposition	↑	↑
Lysyl oxidase-2	Extracellular collagen cross-linking (enhances fibrillogenesis and fibril stability/stiffness)	↑ Collagen deposition ↓ Collagen degradation	↑↑	↑
MMP-1	Collagenase	↑ Collagen degradation	↑	↓↓
MMP-2	Gelatinase; pericellular collagenase	↑ Collagen degradation ("local" remodeling)	↑↑	↑
MMP-3	Activates proMMPs	↑ Collagen degradation	↓↓	↑
MMP-7	Activates proMMPs	↑ Collagen degradation	↑	
MMP-8	Collagenase	↑ Collagen degradation	↓	
MMP-13	Collagenase	↑ Collagen degradation	↑	↑
MMP-14	Collagenase (membrane-associated); activates proMMPs	↑ Collagen degradation ("local" remodeling)	↑ (nodule) ↓ (cord)	
Periostin	Enhances fibrillogenesis; stabilizes extracellular collagen fibrils	↑ Collagen deposition ↑ collagen degradation	↑↑	↑
TIMP-1	Inhibits MMPs (except 14)	↑ Collagen degradation	↑↑↑	
TIMP-2	Allows activation of MMP-2 by MMP-14; inactivates MMPs	↑ Collagen degradation (via MMP-2); ↓ collagen degradation	↓	↑,↓, or no change
TIMP-3	Inhibits all MMPs	↓ Collagen degradation	↓	
TIMP-4	Inhibits all MMPs	↓ Collagen degradation	↑↑↑	

Information from the following sources: Lambert et al. (1992, 2001); Wilde et al. (2003); Qian et al. (2004); Lee et al. (2006); Webb et al. (2006); Johnston et al. (2007); Merryman et al. (2007); Hamilton (2008); Rehman et al. (2008); Kaneko et al. (2009); Vi et al. (2009); Ziegler et al. (2010)
Unless specified, gene or protein changes are in the same direction in both nodules and cords from Dupuytren's disease patients

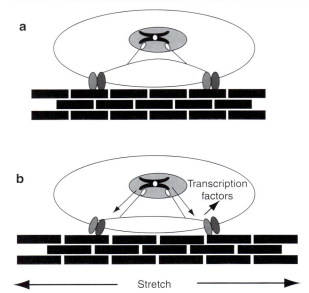

Fig. 17.3 Fibroblast and matrix responses to mechanical forces. Fibroblast responses to mechanical forces are mediated through β_1 integrin interaction with collagen fibrils in the extracellular matrix and the actin cytoskeleton. (**a**) No signaling occurs in the absence of tension on the collagen matrix or the actin cytoskeleton; note normal orientation of the integrin molecules (depicted as perpendicular to the collagen fibrils) that link the collagen matrix to the actin cytoskeleton. (**b**) Increased tension on the collagen matrix is transmitted to the actin cytoskeleton due to altered orientation of the cell surface integrins, resulting in the release of transcription factors and rapid changes in gene/protein expression. Effects may also be mediated due to direct cytoskeletal coupling of the cell membrane to the chromosomal DNA through the nuclear membrane; deformation of DNA by transferred tension results in direct alteration of gene transcription. NOTE: a decrease in the elasticity of either the collagen matrix or the actin cytoskeleton increases the intensity of the signal (Figure adapted from material in Chiquet et al. 2003, 2007; Wang et al. 2007, 2009)

17.5 Conclusions

Collagen has been described as "an unstable molecule that can form stable tissues." This property results from the careful shepherding of the unstable precursor through a highly complex process as well as close regulation over the processes that initiate its degradation, so that the quantity and quality of this essential structural component is balanced to the physical requirements of each tissue. Either as the primary structural component of the Dupuytren's cord or as the primary functional mediator of the pathophysiologic processes that underlie this disease, it remains an important target for therapeutic intervention, and a basic understanding of its biology is critical to therapeutic success.

References

Alman BA, Greel DA, Ruby LK, Goldberg MJ, Wolfe HJ (1996) Regulation of proliferation and platelet-derived growth factor expression in palmar fibromatosis (Dupuytren contracture) by mechanical strain. J Orthop Res 14:722–728

Al-Qattan MM (2006) Factors in the pathogenesis of Dupuytren's contracture. J Hand Surg 31A:1527–1534

Arora PD, Manolson MF, Downey GP, Sodek J, McCulloch CAG (2000) A novel model system for characterization of phagosomal maturation, acidification, and intracellular collagen degradation in fibroblasts. J Biol Chem 275:35432–35441

Baker AH, Edwards DR, Murphy G (2002) Metalloproteinase inhibitors: biological actions and therapeutic opportunities. J Cell Sci 115:3719–3727

Balestrini JL, Billiar KL (2009) Magnitude and duration of stretch modulate fibroblast remodeling. J Biomech Eng 131:051005-1–051005-8

Barbolina MV, Stack MS (2008) Membrane type 1-matrix metalloproteinase: substrate diversity in pericellular proteolysis. Semin Cell Dev Biol 19:24–33

Brickley-Parsons D, Glimcher MJ, Smith RJ, Albin R, Adams JP (1981) Biochemical changes in the collagen of the palmar fascia in patients with Dupuytren's disease. J Bone Joint Surg Am 63:787–797

Canty EG, Kadler KE (2005) Procollagen trafficking, processing and fibrillogenesis. J Cell Sci 118:1341–1353

Canty EG, Lu Y, Meadows RS, Shaw MK, Holmes DF, Kadler KE (2004) Coalignment of plasma membrane channels and protrusions (fibripositors) specifies the parallelism of tendon. J Cell Biol 165:553–563

Canty EG, Starborg T, Lu Y, Humphries SM, Holmes DF, Meadows RS, Huffman A, O'Toole ET, Kadler KE (2006) Actin filaments are required for fibripositor-mediated collagen fibril alignment in tendon. J Biol Chem 281:38592–38598

Cawston TE, Mercer E (1986) Preferential binding of collagenase to $\alpha 2$-macroglobulin in the presence of the tissue inhibitor of metalloproteinases. FEBS Lett 209:9–12

Chiquet M, Renedo AS, Huber F, Flück M (2003) How do fibroblasts translate mechanical signals into changes in extracellular matrix production? Matrix Biol 22:73–80

Chiquet M, Tunç-Civelek V, Sarasa-Renedo A (2007) Gene regulation by mechanotransduction in fibroblasts. Appl Physiol Nutr Metab 32:967–973

Cordova A, Tripoli M, Corradino B, Napoli P, Moschella F (2005) Dupuytren's contracture: an update of biomolecular aspects and therapeutic perspectives. J Hand Surg 30B:557–562

Daley WP, Peters SB, Larsen M (2007) Extracellular matrix dynamics in development and regenerative medicine. J Cell Sci 121:255–264

Evanson J, Jeffrey JJ, Krane SM (1968) Studies on collagenase from rheumatoid synovium in tissue culture. J Clin Invest 47:2639–2651

Everts V, van der Zee E, Creemers L, Beertsen W (1996) Phagocytosis and intracellular digestion of collagen, its role in turnover and remodeling. Histochem J 28:229–245

Fesus L, Jeleliska MM, Kope M (1981) Degradation by thrombin of denatured collagen and of collagenase digestion products. Thromb Res 22:367–373

Fluck J, Querfeld C, Cremer A, Niland S, Krieg T, Sollberg S (1998) Normal human primary fibroblasts undergo apoptosis in three-dimensional contractile collagen gels. J Invest Dermatol 110:153–157

Flynn BP, Bhole AP, Saeidi N, Liles M, DiMarzio CA et al (2010) Mechanical strain stabilizes reconstituted collagen fibrils against enzymatic degradation by mammalian collagenase matrix metalloproteinase 8 (MMP-8). PLoS One 5:e12337. doi:10.1371/journal.pone.0012337

Gabbiani G (2003) The myofibroblast in wound healing and fibrocontractive diseases. J Pathol 200:500–503

Gelse K, Pöschl E, Aigner T (2003) Collagens – structure, function, and biosynthesis. Adv Drug Deliv Rev 55:1531–1546

Grinnell F, Zhu M, Carlson MA, Abrams JM (1999) Release of mechanical tension triggers apoptosis of human fibroblasts in a model of regressing granulation tissue. Exp Cell Res 248:608–619

Gutiérrez-Fernández A, Inada M, Balbín M, Fueyo A, Pitiot AS, Astudillo A, Hirose K, Hirata M, Shapiro SD, Noël A, Werb Z, Krane SM, López-Otín C, Puente XS (2007) Increased inflammation delays wound healing in mice deficient in collagenase-2 (MMP-8). FASEB J 21:2580–2591

Hamilton DW (2008) Functional role of periostin in development and wound repair: implications for connective tissue disease. J Cell Commun Signal 2:9–17

Hanyu T, Tajima T, Tagaki T, Sasaki S, Fujimoto D, Isemora M, Yosizawa Z (1984) Biochemical studies on the collagen of the palmar aponeurosis affected with Dupuytren's disease. Tohoku J Exp Med 142:437–443

Hinz B, Mastrangelo D, Iselin CE, Chaponnier C, Gabbiani G (2001) Mechanical tension controls granulation tissue contractile activity and myofibroblast differentiation. Am J Pathol 159:1009–1020

Johnston P, Chojnowski AJ, Davidson RK, Riley GP, Donell ST, Clark IM (2007) A complete expression profile of matrix-degrading metalloproteinases in Dupuytren's disease. J Hand Surg 32A:343–351

Kadler KE, Holmes DF, Trotter JA, Chapman JA (1996). Collagen fibril formation. Biochem J. 316(Pt 1):1–11

Kadler KE, Hill A, Canty-Laird EG (2008). Collagen fibrillogenesis: fibronectin, integrins, and minor collagens as organizers and nucleators. Curr Opin Cell Biol 20(5):495–501

Kalamajski S, Oldberg Å (2010) The role of small leucine-rich proteoglycans in collagen fibrillogenesis. Matrix Biol 29: 248–253

Kaneko D, Sasazaki Y, Kikuchi T, Ono T, Nemoto K, Matsumoto H, Toyama Y (2009) Temporal effects of cyclic stretching on distribution and gene expression of integrin and cytoskeleton by ligament fibroblasts in vitro. Connect Tissue Res 50: 263–269

Khoshnoodi J, Cartailler J-P, Alvares K, Veis A, Hudson BG (2006) Molecular recognition in the assembly of collagens: terminal noncollagenous domains are key recognition modules in the formation of triple helical protomers. J Biol Chem 281:38117–38121

Kuo H-J, Maslen CL, Keene DR, Glanville RW (1997) Type VI collagen anchors endothelial basement membranes by interacting with Type IV collagen. J Biol Chem 272:26522–26529

Lambert CA, Soudant EP, Nusgens BV, Lapière CM (1992) Pretranslational regulation of extracellular matrix macromolecules and collagenase expression in fibroblasts by mechanical forces. Lab Invest 66:444–451

Lambert CA, Colige AC, Lapière CM, Nusgens BV (2001) Coordinated regulation of procollagens I and III and their post-translational enzymes by dissipation of mechanical tension in human dermal fibroblasts. Eur J Cell Biol 80:479–485

Lauer-Fields JL, Juska D, Fields GB (2002) Matrix metalloproteinases and collagen catabolism. Biopolymers (Pept Sci) 66:19–32

Lee LC, Zhang AY, Chong AK, Pham H, Longaker MT, Chang J (2006) Expression of a novel gene, MafB, in Dupuytren's disease. J Hand Surg 31A:211–218

Leikina E, Mertts MV, Kuznetsova N, Leikin S (2002) Type I collagen is thermally unstable at body temperature. Proc Natl Acad Sci 99:1314–1318

Mansell JP, Bailey AJ (2004) Collagen metabolism disorders. Encyclopedia Endo Dis 1:530–537

McAlinden A, Smith TA, Sandell LJ, Ficheux D, Parry DAD, Hulmes DJS (2003) Alpha-helical coiled-coil oligomerization domains are almost ubiquitous in the collagen superfamily. J Biol Chem 278:42200–42207

Melling M, Reihsner R, Pfeiler W, Schnallinger M, Karimian-Teherani D, Behnam M, Mostler S, Menzel EJ (1999) Comparison of palmar aponeuroses from individuals with diabetes mellitus and Dupuytren's contracture. Anat Rec 255:401–406

Melling M, Karimian-Teherani D, Mostler S, Behnam M, Sobal G, Menzel EJ (2000) Changes of biochemical and biomechanical properties in Dupuytren disease. Arch Pathol Lab Med 124:1275–1281

Merryman WD, Lukoff HD, Long RA, Engelmayr GC Jr, Hopkins RA, Sacks MS (2007) Synergistic effects of cyclic tension and transforming growth factor-beta1 on the aortic valve myofibroblast. Cardiovasc Pathol 16:268–276

Minond D, Lauer-Fields JL, Cudic M, Overall CM, Pei D, Brew K, Visse R, Nagase H, Fields GB (2006) The roles of substrate thermal stability and P_2 and $P_1{'}$ subsite identity on matrix metalloproteinase triple-helical peptidase activity and collagen specificity. J Biol Chem 281:38302–38313

Nagase H, Visse R, Murphy G (2006) Structure and function of matrix metalloproteinases and TIMPs. Cardiovasc Res 69:562–573

Norris RA, Damon B, Mironov V, Kasyanov V, Ramamurthi A, Moreno-Rodriguez R, Trusk T, Potts JD, Goodwin RL, Davis J, Hoffman S, Wen X, Sugi Y, Kern CB, Mjaatvedt CH, Turner DK, Oka T, Conway ST, Molkentin JD, Forgacs G, Markwald RR (2007) Periostin regulates collagen fibrillogenesis and the biomechanical properties of connective tissues. J Cell Biochem 101:695–711

Notbohm H, Bigi A, Roveri N, Hoch J, Acil Y, Koch HJ (1995) Ultrastructural and biochemical modifications of collagen from tissue of morbus Dupuytren patients. J Biochem 118: 405–410

Ortega N, Werb Z (2002) New functional roles for non-collagenous domains of basement membrane collagens. J Cell Sci 115:4201–4214

Pasternak B, Aspenberg P (2009) Metalloproteinases and their inhibitors – diagnostic and therapeutic opportunities in orthopedics. Acta Orthop 80:693–703

Persikov AV, Brodsky B (2002) Unstable molecules form stable tissues. Proc Natl Acad Sci 99:1101–1103

Perumal S, Antipova O, Orgel JPRO (2008) Collagen fibril architecture, domain organization, and triple-helical conformation govern its proteolysis. Proc Natl Acad Sci 105:2824–2829

Prockop DJ, Kivirikko KI (1995) Collagens: molecular biology, diseases, and potentials for therapy. Annu Rev Biochem 64:403–434

Qian A, Meals RA, Rajfer J, Gonzalez-Cavidad NF (2004) Comparison of gene expression profiles between Peyronie's disease and Dupuytren's contracture. Urology 64:399–404

Ra H-J, Parks WC (2007) Control of matrix metalloproteinase catalytic activity. Matrix Biol 26:587–596

Rayan GM (2007) Dupuytren disease: anatomy, pathology, presentation, and treatment. J Bone Joint Surg Am 89:189–198

Rehman S, Salway F, Stanley JK, Ollier WER, Day P, Bayat A (2008) Molecular phenotypic descriptors of Dupuytren's disease defined using informatics analysis of the transcriptome. J Hand Surg 33A:359–372

Ricard-Blum S, Ruggerio F (2005) The collagen superfamily: from the extracellular matrix to the cell membrane. Pathol Biol 53:430–442

Roeder BA, Kokini K, Voytik-Harbin SL (2009) Fibril microstructure affects strain transmission within collagen extracellular matrices. J Biomech Eng 131:031004-1–031004-11

Sabeh F, Li X-Y, Saunders TL, Rowe RG, Weiss SJ (2009) Secreted versus membrane-anchored collagenases: relative roles in fibroblast-dependent collageanolysis and invasion. J Biol Chem 284:23001–23011

Shoulders MD, Raines RT (2009) Collagen structure and stability. Annu Rev Biochem 78:929–958

Somerville RPT, Oblander SA, Apte SS (2003) Matrix metalloproteinases: old dogs with new tricks. Genome Biol 4:216

Sternlicht MD, Werb Z (2001) How matrix metalloproteinases regulate cell behavior. Annu Rev Cell Dev Biol 17:463–516

Stetler-Stevenson WG (1996) Dynamics of matrix turnover during pathologic remodeling of the extracellular matrix. Am J Pathol 148:1345–1350

Stultz CM (2002) Localized unfolding of collagen explains collagenase cleavage near imino-poor sites. J Mol Biol 319:997–1003

Tomasek JJ, Gabbiani G, Hinz B, Chaponnier C, Brown RA (2002) Myofibroblasts and mechanoregulation of connective tissue remodeling. Nat Rev Mol Cell Biol 3:349–363

Turk V, Turk B, Turk D (2001) Lysosomal cysteine proteases: facts and opportunities. EMBO J 20:4629–4633

Van der Rest M, Garrone R (1991) Collagen family of proteins. FASEB J 5:2814–2823

Veit G, Kobbe B, Keene DR, Paulsson M, Koch M, Wagener R (2006) Collagen XXVIII, a novel von Willebrand factor A domain containing protein with many imperfections in the collagenous domain. J Biol Chem 281:3494–3504

Vi L, Fenga L, Zhu RB, Wu Y, Satish L, Gan BS, O'Gorman DB (2009) Periostin differentially induces proliferation, contraction and apoptosis of primary Dupuytren's disease and adjacent palmar fascia cells. Exp Cell Res 315:3574–3586

Visse R and Nagase H (2003). Matrix metalloproteinases and tissue inhibitors of metalloproteinases: structure, function, and biochemistry. Circ. Res 92(8): 827–839.

Wang JH, Thampatty BP, Lin JS, Im HJ (2007) Mechanoregulation of gene expression in fibroblasts. Gene 391:1–15

Wang N, Tytell JD, Ingber DE (2009) Mechanotransduction at a distance: mechanically coupling the extracellular matrix with the nucleus. Nat Rev Mol Cell Biol 10:75–82

Webb K, Hitchcock RW, Smeal RM, Li W, Gray SD, Tresco PA (2006) Cyclic strain increases fibroblast proliferation, matrix accumulation, and elastic modulus of fibroblast-seeded polyurethane constructs. J Biomech 39:1136–1144

Wenstrup RJ, Florer JB, Brunskill EW, Bell SM, Chervoneva I, Birk DE (2004) Type V collagen controls the initiation of collagen fibril assembly. J Biol Chem 279:53331–53337

Wilde J, Yokozeki M, Terai K, Kudo A, Moriyama K (2003) The divergent expression of periostin mRNA in the periodontal ligament during experimental tooth movement. Cell Tissue Res 312:345–351

Zeichen J, van Griensven M, Albers I, Lobenhoffer P, Bosch U (1999) Immunohistochemical localization of collagen VI in arthrofibrosis. Arch Orthop Trauma Surg 119:315–318

Ziegler N, Alonso A, Steinberg T, Woodnutt D, Kohl A, Müssig E, Schulz S, Tomakidi P (2010) Mechano-transduction in periodontal ligament cells identifies activated states of MAP-kinases p42/44 and p38-stress kinase as a mechanism for MMP-13 expression. BMC Cell Biol 11:10

The Expression of Collagen-Degrading Proteases Involved in Dupuytren's Disease Fibroblast-Mediated Contraction

18

Janine M. Wilkinson, Eleanor R. Jones, Graham P. Riley, Adrian J. Chojnowski, and Ian M. Clark

Contents

18.1	**Introduction**	143
18.2	**Materials and Methods**	144
18.2.1	Cell Culture	144
18.2.2	Fibroblast-Populated Collagen Lattice (FPCL)	145
18.2.3	RNA Extraction	145
18.2.4	Synthesis of Complementary DNA	145
18.2.5	Quantitative Real-Time PCR	145
18.2.6	Hydroxyproline Assay	145
18.2.7	Statistical Analysis	146
18.3	**Results**	146
18.3.1	Contraction of FPCL	146
18.3.2	Protease Gene Expression	146
18.4	**Discussion**	147
18.5	**Conclusions**	148
References		148

J.M. Wilkinson (✉) • E.R. Jones • G.P. Riley • I.M. Clark
School of Biological Sciences,
University of East Anglia, Norwich, UK
e-mail: jmw237@cam.ac.uk

A.J. Chojnowski
Institute of Orthopaedics,
Norfolk and Norwich University Hospital, Norwich, UK

Abbreviations

ADAMTS	A disintegrin and metalloproteinase domain with thrombospondin motifs
(ADR)-FPCL	Attached delayed release fibroblast-populated collagen lattice
DD	Dupuytren's disease
ECM	Extracellular matrix
MMP	Matrix metalloproteinase
TLDA	Taqman® low density array
TIMP	Tissue inhibitor of metalloproteinases

18.1 Introduction

Dupuytren's disease (DD) is a disabling fibrotic condition affecting the palmar fascia of the hand. It was described by Baron Dupuytren in 1831. Typically, DD presents itself over three phases (Luck 1959), the first of which, the proliferative phase, shows the development of nodular tissue on the palm of the hand. These nodules contain proliferative myofibroblasts which are thought to mediate the eventual contraction of the palmar fascia leading to the irreversible contracture of the digits (most commonly the ring and little fingers). The involutional secondary phase is characterised by the alignment of the myofibroblasts along the line of stress followed by the third stage represented by the deposition of an acellular collagen-rich cord.

C. Eaton et al. (eds.), *Dupuytren's Disease and Related Hyperproliferative Disorders*,
DOI 10.1007/978-3-642-22697-7_18, © Springer-Verlag Berlin Heidelberg 2012

Incidence of DD is age, gender and genetically dependent. Men are more likely to have the disease than women, and incidence increases with age (Early 1962). The disease is often familial, but the mode of inheritance is currently unknown (Rayan 2007). Individuals with a history of alcoholism, smoking and high blood cholesterol are also at a higher risk of developing DD (Burge et al. 1997).

The most common treatment for DD is surgery, specifically fasciectomy (Rayan 2007) with recurrence of disease common. A number of pharmaceutical treatments have been proposed, but efficacy remains unproven (Rayan et al. 1996; Ketchum and Donahue 2000; Pittet et al. 1994).

The MMPs are a family of zinc endopeptidases, capable of degrading the extracellular matrix (ECM). A number of these proteases have been shown specifically to degrade the collagen triple helix, for example MMP-1, MMP-8 and MMP-13, the classical collagenases, but also MMP-2 and MMP-14 (Brinckerhoff and Matrisian 2002). A related family of metalloproteinases, the ADAMTSs (a disintegrin and metalloproteinase domain with thrombospondin motifs), also includes enzymes which are procollagen N-propeptidases, contributing to collagen biosynthesis (Porter et al. 2005). Four TIMPs regulate the activity of these enzyme families. There is broad specificity for the TIMPs in inhibition of the MMPs, though TIMP-1 is a poor inhibitor of MMP-14. TIMP-3 is the only effective inhibitor of ADAMTSs, though its action against ADAMTS-2, ADAMTS-3 and ADAMTS-14 is unproven. The homeostatic turnover of the ECM is a balance between synthesis and proteolytic breakdown with this latter a balance between proteases and their inhibitors. Any deviation away from this balance resulting in the reduced activities of the MMPs could contribute to the development of fibrotic disorders such as Dupuytren's disease. The level of circulating TIMP-1 has previously been shown to be higher in DD than controls (Ulrich et al. 2003).

We recently identified changes in the expression of specific metalloproteinases in Dupuytren's disease and correlated these with post-operative outcomes (Johnston et al. 2007). Thus, the expression of three key collagenases, *MMP1*, *MMP13* and *MMP14*, is significantly raised in DD nodule, as is the expression of a collagen biosynthetic enzyme *ADAMTS14*. *TIMP1* expression is significantly elevated in DD nodule compared to normal palmar fascia. From that study, we speculated that contraction and fibrosis in DD may result from: (1)

increased collagen biosynthesis with processing mediated by increased ADAMTS-14, (2) an elevated level of TIMP-1 blocking MMP-1 and MMP-13-mediated collagenolysis (with these enzymes elevated in an attempt to resolve the fibrosis) and (3) contraction enabled by MMP-14-mediated pericellular collagenolysis which may escape inhibition by TIMP-1 (Johnston et al. 2007). We have also followed DD patients whose tissues were used for gene profiling and assessed their disease and hand function for 2 years. Interestingly, we discovered that the expression level of some of these key proteinases (e.g. *MMP13* and *MMP14*) positively correlates with poor progression post-fasciectomy (Johnston et al. 2008). In order to investigate this further, we turned to an in vitro model of collagen contraction.

Fibroblast-populated collagen lattices (FPCLs) have been used in a variety of formats to study collagen matrix contraction in vitro (Rayan and Tomasek 1994; Daniels et al. 2003; Grinnell 2008; Dallon 2008; Tomasek et al. 1992). The attached delayed release (ADR)-FPCL allows the collagen gel to develop tension over a specific time, followed by release from the well and subsequent contraction (Tomasek et al. 1992). Contraction of the gels using this method is thought to be a response to the tension generated by the cells, rather than simply cell migration and matrix remodelling in a free-floating gel (Parizi et al. 2000). The ADR FPCL model is therefore a surrogate for the contraction seen in Dupuytren's disease. It is known that broad-spectrum inhibitors of metalloproteases can inhibit contraction in this model (Daniels et al. 2003), though this is somewhat opposed to the Dupuytren-like toxicity that some similar inhibitors showed in the cancer clinic (Hutchinson et al. 1998).

In this study, we used the (ADR)-FPCL technique to measure the expression of proteases and inhibitors involved in collagen metabolism, as well as collagen degradation itself in contracting lattices. Understanding the contribution of specific proteases to contraction and collagen remodelling may shed light on the molecular mechanisms underlying Dupuytren's disease.

18.2 Materials and Methods

18.2.1 Cell Culture

Primary fibroblasts derived from the palmar fascia of Dupuytren's disease patients undergoing fasciectomy or from patients without Dupuytren's disease undergoing carpal tunnel release (as previously described (Johnston et al. 2007)) were cultured in Dulbecco's modified Eagle's medium (DMEM) with Glutamax supplemented with 10% (vol/vol) foetal calf serum (FCS), 100 IU/mL penicillin and 100 μg/mL streptomycin at 37°C with 5% CO_2 in air. Fibroblasts were used up to and including passage 5.

18.2.2 Fibroblast-Populated Collagen Lattice (FPCL)

Collagen contraction was assessed using (ADR)-FPCL gels ($n=4$). Rat tail type 1 collagen (First Link, UK) was combined with 10× serum-free DMEM, neutralised with NaOH (10M) and combined at a ratio of 1:1 with cell suspension (serum-free DMEM). Final concentration of collagen and cells were 0.925 mg/mL and 2×10^5 cells/mL respectively. Cell suspension at 0.5 mL gel/well was allowed to set at 37°C for 1 h. Serum-free media (0.5 mL/well) were added, and collagen lattices were allowed to develop tension over 24, 48 and 72 h prior to their release or harvest. One hour before the release of gel, the serum-free medium was replaced with complete medium containing 10% FCS. All media were harvested and stored at −80°C for downstream analysis.

Cells were harvested directly in Trizol reagent after 24, 48 and 72 h of tension and also at 3 and 24 h post release. Contraction was monitored using a flatbed scanner (HP Scanjet 3800) and quantified using the image-processing program Image J (http://rsbweb.nih.gov/ij/). Images were taken at release and across the subsequent 24 h.

18.2.3 RNA Extraction

Gels (and the equivalent cells from monolayer culture) were harvested directly into Trizol (Invitrogen, UK). After complete suspension, chloroform was added (200 μL/mL Trizol), vortexed and centrifuged at 12,000 g for 15 min at 4°C. The clear aqueous layer was placed into a separate tube, and a total of 0.5 × volume of 100% ethanol was added and mixed. Samples were then placed into spin columns (RNeasy Mini Kit, Qiagen, UK) and RNA extraction performed according to the manufacturer's instructions. RNA samples were quantified using a NanoDrop spectrophotometer (NanoDrop technologies, Wilmington, DE) and stored at −80°C.

18.2.4 Synthesis of Complementary DNA

RNA (250 ng) was converted to cDNA using Superscript II reverse transcriptase (Invitrogen) in a final volume of 20 μL. Samples were stored at −20°C.

18.2.5 Quantitative Real-Time PCR

The relative quantification of gene expression was carried out on the ABI Prism 7,700 sequence detection system (Applied Biosystems) following the manufacturer's protocol. A total of 1 ng of cDNA was used for the detection of the 18S rRNA housekeeping gene. The sample was added to the PCR reaction mixture containing 50% 2× master mix, 100 nmol/L of forward and reverse primer and 200 nmol/L probe in a final volume of 25 μL. The PCR protocol involved 2 min at 50°C, 10 min at 95°C, then 40 cycles each consisting of 15 s at 95°C and 1 min at 60°C. The expression of MMPs, ADAMTSs and TIMPs, along with the β-actin housekeeping gene, was measured using Taqman® low density arrays (TLDA) (Applied Biosystems). For the amplification reactions, 100 ng/μL of cDNA was combined with master mix to a final volume of 100 μL and applied to each port of the TLDA. In order to compare expression of all genes, expression was normalised to β-actin using a transformation proportional to normalised copy number ($2_T^{-\Delta C}$), where ΔC_T is C_T of the gene of interest − C_T of β-actin (C_T is threshold cycle, the number of PCR cycles at which the signal from the PCR reaction becomes detectable above the background noise). FPCLs using nodular cells from a Dupuytren patient were used at $n=3$ to generate the TLDA data. Monolayer data originates from cells grown in culture ($n=1$).

18.2.6 Hydroxyproline Assay

In parallel to the FPCLs, hydroxyproline (OH-Pro) assays were performed on the lattice-conditioned media using a microtitre modification of the method described by Bergman and Loxley (1963) at each time point to quantify collagen release.

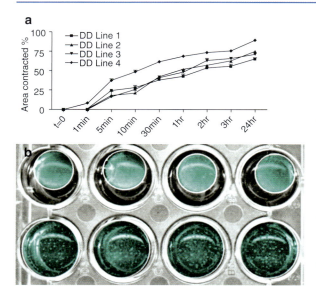

Fig. 18.1 (a) Contraction profile of four FPCLs with differing patient cell lines demonstrating ability of DD fibroblasts to contract a type 1 collagen lattice ($n=4$). (b) An example of FPCLs after 10 min release (*top row*) and immediately before release (*lower row*)

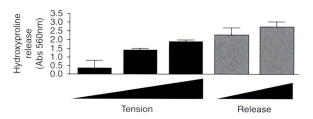

Fig. 18.2 Hydroxyproline (OH-Pro) assay result showing increasing OH-Pro released into the media as tension is increased over 72 h and released for 3 and 24 h following 48 h tension

18.2.7 Statistical Analysis

Statistical analysis utilised the Student's *t*-test. Data was analysed and presented using GraphPad Prism 4 (GraphPad Software, La Jolla, CA).

18.3 Results

18.3.1 Contraction of FPCL

Figure 18.1a shows that contraction of FPCL gels by nodule-derived Dupuytren's fibroblasts was consistently observed. Up to 90% contraction was measured over the time course of 24 h, with similar kinetics across the four lines tested. No significant difference was seen when gels were populated with Dupuytren's disease fibroblasts and those derived from normal palmar fascia (data not shown). Contraction of the gels after 10 min was already clear (Fig. 18.1b).

Hydroxyproline loss into the FPCL-conditioned medium can be measured as early as the 24-h time point (Fig. 18.2). Collagen breakdown then continues throughout the tension phase of the model. Interestingly, release of the FPCL results in even greater release of OH-Pro into the medium (compare 48 h tension to 48 h tension + 3 h release, or 72 h tension to 48 h tension + 24 h release).

18.3.2 Protease Gene Expression

Initial Taqman® low density array shows the pattern of metalloproteinase gene expression in cells cultured in monolayer at passage 5 (Fig. 18.3). It is interesting to

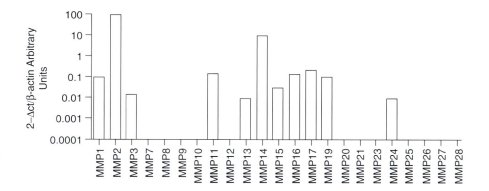

Fig. 18.3 Complete gene profile of DD fibroblasts grown in monolayer culture (passage 5), normalised to β-actin

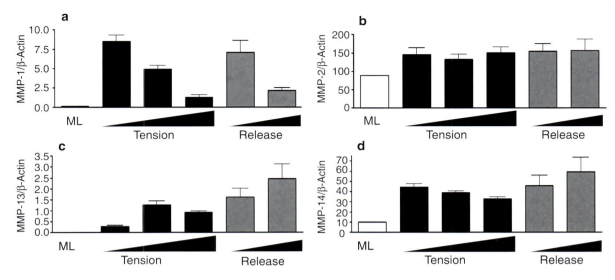

Fig. 18.4 Summary of data, normalised to β-actin. All data normalised to β-actin ($2_T^{-\Delta C}$) and shown in monolayer culture (*bar 1*), increasing tension over 24, 48 and 72 h in the FPCL (*bars 2, 3 and 4*) and at tension for 48 h followed by release over 3 and 24 h (*bars 5 and 6*). (**a**) MMP1 expression. (**b**) MMP2 expression. (**c**) MMP13 expression. (**d**) MMP14 expression

note that for several genes (MMP1, MMP2, MMP11, MMP14, ADAMTS1, ADAMTS2, TIMP1, TIMP2, TIMP3), there is a broad correlation between expression in the cultured cells and that previously reported in the DD tissue (Johnston et al. 2007). We examined expression of a subset of these genes across the FPCL model (Fig. 18.4a–d). The expression of all MMPs measured increased in the collagen gel (at $t=24$ h) compared to monolayer culture (cell pellet). The expression of MMP1 (Fig. 18.4a) and MMP14 (Fig. 18.4d), then decreased as tension developed over 72 h and increased upon release. MMP13 (Fig. 18.4c) expression increased with tension, with a further increase upon release. MMP2 (Fig. 18.4b) expression was constant across the model. MMP8 expression was not detectable. MMP3 was the most obviously tension responsive gene, with ~13-fold reduction in expression between 24 and 72 h of tension and ~96-fold induction in expression after 24 h release. MMP14 expression showed only minimal response to tension and release, with MMP2 expression showing no response to these conditions. Interestingly, ADAMTS3 and 14 showed increased expression in the collagen gel compared to monolayer culture. Furthermore, ADAMTS14 showed a similar pattern of expression to MMP1 across the FPCL model (data not shown).

18.4 Discussion

Dupuytren's disease is characterised by the progressive fibrosis and contraction of the palma fascia causing the fingers to be drawn irreversibly towards the palm of the hand. This cell-mediated contraction of the ECM has been previously studied in vitro using FPCL assays. In the format we describe, the ability of the DD fibroblasts to contract the collagen lattice is not significantly greater than that of fibroblasts derived from normal palmar fascia, though this has been described by others (Bisson et al. 2004). The format of the FPCL assay shows considerable variability across laboratories, and the concentration of collagen, derivation, culture or storage of cells may also impact upon the assay. It should also be noted that alpha-smooth muscle actin expression, measured by immunocytochemistry, is similar in cells derived from both DD and normal tissue (data not shown), and this may be an outcome of the explant outgrowth system used to derive cells.

It is interesting to note that for several genes (MMP1, MMP2, MMP11, MMP14, ADAMTS1, ADAMTS2, TIMP1, TIMP2, TIMP3), there is broad correlation between expression levels in monolayer culture and in DD tissue itself. This would suggest that these genes are regulated either by autocrine factors or in an epigenetic fashion. Measuring the level of expression across increasing cell passage may be informative.

Our previous work in DD tissue suggested (1) increased collagen biosynthesis with processing mediated by increased ADAMTS-14, (2) an elevated level of TIMP-1 blocking MMP-1 and MMP-13-mediated collagenolysis (with these enzymes elevated in an attempt to resolve the fibrosis) and (3) contraction enabled by MMP-14-mediated pericellular collagenolysis which may escape inhibition by TIMP-1.

A clear paradox here is that despite the presence of high TIMP1 expression, collagen degradation still takes place, and it is not known if the latter is required for contraction itself. MMP-14 is known to degrade collagen and to be insensitive to inhibition by TIMP-1 (Baker et al. 2002), so this is a possible explanation. Alternatively, collagen degradation is taking place in an environment in which the proteases are protected from TIMP-1 inhibition in some way (e.g. at the cell surface). Thirdly, it may be that other routes of collagen degradation are taking place (e.g. via cathepsin K or intracellularly) (Hou et al. 2001). Release of the FPCL from tension results in a further increase of hydroxyproline release, and this may simply be a mechanical process (of contraction leading to an increase in collagen degradation products in the conditioned medium) or alternatively an active process (via activation of proteolytic activity).

The expression of all the MMP genes measured increased upon culture in a three-dimensional collagen matrix, perhaps reflecting the influence of cell shape/cytoskeleton and/or integrin signalling on protease expression. For MMP1, MMP3, TIMP1 and to some extent MMP14, this decreased with time and increasing tension, then increased upon release. MMP3 was particularly responsive, and MMP-3 is a known activator of procollagenases like proMMP1 (Treadwell et al. 1986). Against this background, collagen degradation increased across the model, which is more akin to the expression of MMP13.

The gene expression of the procollagen N-propeptidase ADAMTSs was also included in this study. ADAMTS3 and 14 were both upregulated by culture in the three-dimensional collagen gel (see above) and also during tension and release in Dupuytren's fibroblasts, suggesting that some collagen biosynthesis may also be increased.

If collagen degradation is required in order to achieve contraction in the FPCL assay, then this would explain the inhibition of contraction reported with broad-spectrum metalloprotease inhibitors like Ilomastat in this assay (Daniels et al. 2003). However, in order to understand the function of specific proteases, we now plan to use siRNA to knockdown expression separately of each collagenase and measure the impact on contraction. This will identify specific proteases which may be drug targets in developing pharmaceutical interventions in Dupuytren's disease.

18.5 Conclusions

- Fibroblasts derived from Dupuytren's disease and normal palmar fascia were found to have similar contractile activity in the fixed fibroblast-populated collagen lattice model format used in this study.
- Collagen degradation increased across both tension and release phases of the contraction model despite the high expression of TIMPs, particularly TIMP1.
- The expression of many MMP and ADAMTS genes was increased in three-dimensional culture in collagen gels compared to monolayer.
- The expression of a subset of MMP genes was modulated by the development of tension in the collagen gel.
- This model can be used to delineate the role of individual metalloproteinases and inhibitors in cell-mediated contraction.

Acknowledgements Thanks go to the Furlong Research Charitable Foundation and the Gwendoline Fish Trust for supporting this research.

References

Baker AH, Edwards DR, Murphy G (2002) Metalloproteinase inhibitors: biological actions and therapeutic opportunities. J Cell Sci 115(19):3719–3727

Bergman I, Loxley R (1963) Two improved and simplified methods for the spectrophotometric determination of hydroxyproline. Anal Chem 35(12):1961–1965

Bisson MA, Mudera V, Mcgrouther DA, Grobbelaar AO, Hinz B (2004) The contractile properties and responses to tensional loading of Dupuytren's disease-derived fibroblasts are altered: a cause of the contracture? Plast Reconstr Surg 113(2):611–621

Brinckerhoff CE, Matrisian LM (2002) Matrix metalloproteinases: a tail of a frog that became a prince. Nat Rev Mol Cell Biol 3:207–214

Burge P, Hoy G, Regan P, Milne R (1997) Smoking, alcohol and the risk of Dupuytren's contracture. J Bone Joint Surg Br 79:206–210

Dallon JC (2008) A review of fibroblast-populated collagen lattices. Wound Repair Regen 16(4):472–479

Daniels JT, Cambrey AD, Occleston NL, Garrett Q, Tarnuzzer RW, Schultz GS, Khaw PT (2003) Matrix metalloproteinase inhibition modulates fibroblast-mediated matrix contraction and collagen production in vitro. Invest Ophthalmol Vis Sci 44(3):1104–1110

Early PF (1962) Population studies in Dupuytren's contracture. J Bone Joint Surg Br 44:602–613

Grinnell F (2008) Fibroblast mechanics in three-dimensional collagen matrices. J Bodyw Mov Ther 12(3):191–193

Hou WS, Li Z, Gordon RE, Chan K, Klein MJ, Levy R, Keysser M, Keyszer G, Brömme D (2001) Cathepsin K is a critical protease in synovial fibroblast-mediated collagen degradation. Am J Pathol 159(6):2167–2177

Hutchinson JW, Tierney GM, Parsons SL, Davis TRC (1998) Dupuytren's disease and frozen shoulder induced by treatment with a matrix metalloproteinase inhibitor. J Bone Joint Surg Br 80(5):907–908

Johnston P, Chojnowski AJ, Davidson RK, Riley GP, Donell ST, Clark IM (2007) A complete expression profile of matrix-degrading metalloproteinases in Dupuytren's disease. J Hand Surg Am 32(3):343–351

Johnston P, Larson D, Clark IM, Chojnowski AJ (2008) Metalloproteinase gene expression correlates with clinical outcome in Dupuytren's disease. J Hand Surg Am 33(7): 1160–1167

Ketchum LD, Donahue TK (2000) The injection of nodules of Dupuytren's disease with triamcinolone acetonide. J Hand Surg Am 25:1157–1162

Luck JV (1959) Dupuytren's contracture; a new concept of the pathogenesis correlated with surgical management. J Bone Joint Surg Am 41:635–664

Parizi M, Howard EW, Tomasek JJ (2000) Regulation of LPA-promoted myofibroblast contraction:role of Rho, myosin, light chain kinase and light chain phosphatase. Exp Cell Res 254:210–220

Pittet B, Rubbia-Brandt L, Desmouliere A (1994) Effect of gamma-interferon on the clinical and biological evolution of hypertrophic scares and Dupuytren's disease. Plast Reconstr Surg 93:1224–1235

Porter S, Clark IM, Kevorkian L, Edwards DR (2005) The ADAMTS metalloproteinases. Biochem J 386:15–27

Rayan GM (2007) Dupuytren disease: anatomy, pathology, presentation, and treatment. J Bone Joint Surg Am 89(1):189–198

Rayan GM, Tomasek JJ (1994) Generation of contractile forces by cultured Dupuytren's disease and normal palmar fibroblasts. Tissue Cell 26:747–756

Rayan GM, Parizi M, Tomasek JJ (1996) Pharmacologic regulation of Dupuytren's fibroblast contraction in vitro. J Hand Surg Am 21:1065–1070

Tomasek JJ, Haaksma CJ, Eddy RJ, Vaughan MB (1992) Fibroblast contraction occurs on release of tension in attached collagen lattices: dependency on an organised actin cytoskeleton and serum. Anat Rec 232:359–368

Treadwell BV, Neidel J, Pavia M, Towle CA, Trice ME, Mankin HJ (1986) Purification and characterization of collagenase activator protein synthesized by articular cartilage. Arch Biochem Biophys 251:715–723

Ulrich D, Hrynyschyn K, Pallua N (2003) Matrix metalloproteinases and tissue inhibitors of metalloproteinase in sera and tissue of patients with Dupuytren's disease. Plast Reconstr Surg 112:1279–1286

Primary Dupuytren's Disease Cell Interactions with the Extra-cellular Environment: A Link to Disease Progression?

19

Linda Vi, Yan Wu, Bing Siang Gan, and David B. O'Gorman

Contents

19.1 The Pathogenesis of Dupuytren's Disease 151

19.2 Methods 152
19.2.1 Adapted Nested Collagen Migration Assay 152
19.2.2 Collagen Substrate Conditioning Assay 152
19.2.3 Immunoblotting 152
19.2.4 Immunofluorescence Microscopy 153

19.3 Results 153
19.3.1 Adapted Nested Collagen Migration Assay 153
19.3.2 Collagen Substrate Conditioning Assay 155

19.4 Discussion 156

19.5 Conclusions 158

References 158

L. Vi (✉) • Y. Wu
Cell and Molecular Biology Laboratory,
Hand and Upper Limb Centre,
St. Joseph's Health Care, Lawson Health Research Institute,
University of Western Ontario, London, ON, Canada
e-mail: linda.vi@mail.utoronto.ca; wuy0815@yahoo.com

B.S. Gan • D.B.O'Gorman
Departments of Surgery,
Physiology and Pharmacology, Medical Biophysics,
Cell and Molecular Biology Laboratory,
Hand and Upper Limb Centre,
St. Joseph's Health Care, Lawson Health Research Institute,
University of Western Ontario, London, ON, Canada
e-mail: bsgan@rogers.com; dogorman@uwo.ca

19.1 The Pathogenesis of Dupuytren's Disease

The most widely accepted theory on the pathogenesis of Dupuytren's disease (DD) is that resident fibroblasts within the fascia of the palm are stimulated by as yet unidentified factor(s) to proliferate and differentiate into a nodule of myofibroblasts. This nodule develops into a contractile disease cord within the adjacent palmar fascia over a variable period of time and through a process that is poorly understood. The contractile forces that produce finger contracture are generated by these myofibroblasts. This theory is largely based on the temporal correlation between the appearance of a densely cellular nodule containing randomly orientated spindle-shaped fibroblasts with increased α-smooth muscle expression and the orientation of these cells along lines of tension at the onset of contracture (Luck 1959; Hurst et al. 1986; Iwasaki et al. 1984; Rayan et al. 1996; Rayan and Tomasek 1994; Tomasek and Rayan 1995; Tomasek et al. 1986).

It has long been surmised that components of the extra-cellular matrix (ECM) are important factors in the pathogenesis of DD (Citron and Hearnden 2003; Hueston 1992; Gupta et al. 1998; Evans et al. 2002). Replacement of the dermis by full-thickness skin grafts, which could hypothetically replace some of the disease-associated ECM, has been used to slow secondary disease recurrence in some studies (Bunyan and Mathur 2000; Rajesh et al. 2000). Members of the transforming growth factor (TGF)β family associate with the ECM and are established components of myofibroblast formation in DD (Badalamente et al. 1996; Berndt et al. 1995). As mechanical stress of the ECM

C. Eaton et al. (eds.), *Dupuytren's Disease and Related Hyperproliferative Disorders*,
DOI 10.1007/978-3-642-22697-7_19, © Springer-Verlag Berlin Heidelberg 2012

has been shown to activate latent TGFβ1 (Wipff and Hinz 2009; Hinz 2009; Wipff et al. 2007), a combination of stress and ECM modification by TGFβ deposition are plausible contributors to myofibroblast development and persistence in DD. Primary DD cells display enhanced sensitivity to TGFβ1 relative to control fibroblasts (Bisson et al. 2003), and this sensitivity can be modulated by altering their extra-cellular environment (Vi et al. 2009c). DD cells grown in collagen under tension (stressed fibroblast-populated collagen lattice, sFPCL) secrete a variety of ECM proteins including fibronectin and its splice variants (ED-B), and mechanical release triggers additional changes in the levels of β-catenin, fibronectin and ED-B within these cultures relative to patient-matched control cells (Howard et al. 2003, 2004). More recently, periostin, an ECM protein consistently upregulated in DD cord, has been shown to differentially regulate the proliferation, apoptosis and myofibroblast differentiation of primary cells derived from DD cord tissue and patient-matched, phenotypically unaffected palmar fascia when incorporated into the cell culture substrate (Vi et al. 2009a). Overall, these data implicate the ECM in playing an active role in DD progression.

The mechanism(s) by which a modified ECM might facilitate disease progression from a nodule to a collagenous disease cord are not understood. In this study, we have compared two hypothetical models of cord development (Vi et al. 2009b). The first, the "cell migration hypothesis," suggests that DD cells secrete factors into their ECM that facilitate their migration throughout the surrounding palmar fascia. Alternatively, the "ECM-mediated disease" model (Vi et al. 2009b) hypothesizes that DD cells secrete factors into their ECM that promote adjacent, quiescent fibroblasts resident in the palmar fascia to take on a "disease cell" phenotype.

19.2 Methods

19.2.1 Adapted Nested Collagen Migration Assay

Primary DD and PF cells (passage 2–6) were isolated and cast into fibroblast-populated collagen lattices (FPCLs), as described previously (Vi et al. 2009a). Cells were cultured for 3 days in α-minimal Eagle's media (MEM) supplemented with 2% fetal bovine serum (FBS) at 37°C with 5% CO_2. FPCLs were then manually released from the wells and allowed to contract overnight. The contracted FPCLs are predicted to contain a large proportion of myofibroblasts in a collagenous ECM and, in this respect, to resemble a nodule. These were embedded into cell-free collagen containing a disintegrin and metalloprotease (ADAM)12, periostin, transforming growth factor (TGF)β1 or vehicle in 35-mm plates. Where indicated, cells were also treated with 0.02 mg/mL mitomycin C to block any contribution from cell proliferation. Once polymerized, α-MEM/2% FBS media was added to the plates and migration was observed at the junction between the contracted cell-containing FPCL and the cell-free outer collagen. The collagen cultures were fixed and stained with 4′,6-diamidino-2-phenylindole (DAPI) to identify nuclei. Samples were washed two times with phosphate buffered saline (PBS), and images were captured using a black and white digital camera attached to an upright Zeiss SteREO Lumar V12 (Carl Zeiss Canada Ltd., Toronto, ON) at 60 times magnification.

19.2.2 Collagen Substrate Conditioning Assay

The standard transwell culture system was modified by the addition of type-I collagen (500 μL) in the tray well, allowing us to lightly embed the transwell into this substrate. Parallel cultures of low passage DD and PF cells (1×10^4) were plated directly onto a transwell membrane with 0.4-μm pores, sufficient to allow direct cellular interaction with the collagen substrate but too small to allow the cells to invade this substrate. After 7 days culture on this substrate in low serum media (α MEM/2% FBS), the transwell was withdrawn, leaving the conditioned collagen behind in the tray well. PF cells (1×10^4) were then cultured in low serum media on the conditioned collagen for an additional 7 days prior to processing for immunoblotting or immunofluorescence studies.

19.2.3 Immunoblotting

Cells lysates were prepared in modified radioimmunoprecipitation assay (RIPA) buffer (RIPA buffer, 1 mM Na_3VO_4, 1 mM NaF and 1 mM phenylmethanesulfonylfluoride (PMSF)). Standard bicinchoninic acid (BCA) analysis was used to determine protein concentration of samples. Samples were subjected to sodium dodecyl sulphate polyacrylamide gel electrophrosis (SDS-PAGE) using 8% resolving gels. Proteins in the gel were transferred to polyvinylidene difluoride (PVDF) membranes, and membranes were blocked with 5% non-fat skim milk in 5 mL of TBS-0.05% Tween 20, a polysorbate detergent. Membranes were probed overnight at 4°C with primary antibodies to the following molecules: β-catenin (BD Biosciences, San Jose, CA) and β-actin (Labvision, Fremont CA). The membranes were then incubated with secondary antibody conjugated to the primary antibody in 5% non-fat skim milk for 60 min at room temperature. Membranes were washed in TBS-0.05% Tween and was exposed to chemiluminescence HRP substrate (1:1, hydrogen peroxide and luminol; Millipore/Chemicon, Billerica, MA) for 5 min before detection with Chemi-Genius gel dock system (Syngene, Frederick, MD).

19.2.4 Immunofluorescence Microscopy

Collagen cultures were fixed with 4% paraformaldehyde in PBS for 30 min, washed twice with PBS and permeablized with PBS-0.1% Triton X-100 for 15 min. Fixed cultures were blocked with 5% non-fat skim milk for 60 min in PBS-0.1% Triton X-100 and washed twice with PBS. Cells were stained for DNA (DAPI) actin stress fibres (Alexa 488 phalloidin, Molecular Probes, Eugene OR) and β-catenin (TRITC-conjugated anti-β-catenin, BD Biosciences, Mississauga ON). Samples were mounted on glass slides, affixed using ProLong Gold (Invitrogen Canada Inc., Burlington, ON) mounting solution, and allowed to dry overnight in the dark. All images were captured using a black and white CoolSnap digital camera attached to an IX81 Olympus inverted microscope (Olympus America Inc., Central Valley, PA).

19.3 Results

19.3.1 Adapted Nested Collagen Migration Assay

To assess the effects of DD-ECM molecules on cell migration, a modified nested collagen migration model was used to assess cell migration out of a contracted FPCL. Initial experiments confirmed the absence of cell migration for 18–20 h after the contracted FPCLs were embedded into cell-free collagen. After this initial lag phase, cell migration became visible at the junction between the FPCL and surrounding collagen. Three-dimensional migration assays were prepared, fixed at 72 h and stained with DAPI to identify individual cell nuclei. Images of each sample were captured by immunoflourescence

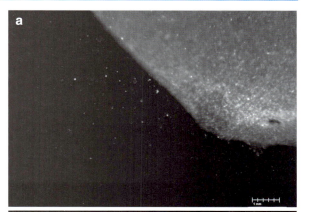

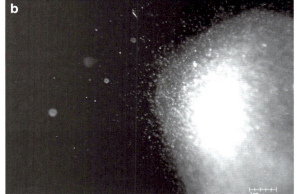

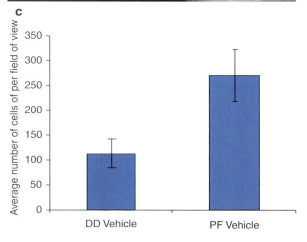

Fig. 19.1 Typical stereomicroscopy images (60×) of DD (**a**) and PF (**b**) cells migrating into the surrounding cell-free collagen treated with phosphate buffered saline and 2% fetal bovine serum, vehicle for the majority of additives used in this study. Cells are stained with DAPI to identify nuclei. (**c**) Triplicate cell counts of patient-matched DD and PF cells migrating out of the FPCLs were performed for this and all subsequent migration analyses

stereomicroscopy (Fig. 19.1). Representative cell counts from three randomly selected fields around the edge of the FPCLs showed that a greater number of PF cells migrate from the FPCLs than did the DD cells. In addition,

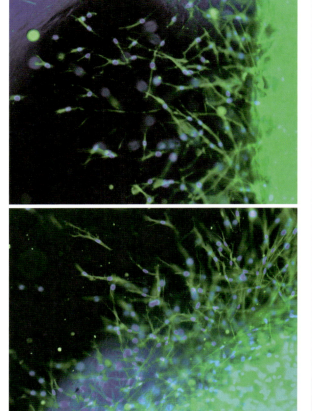

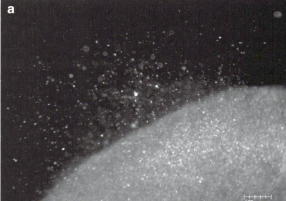

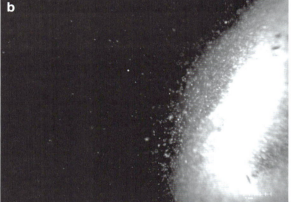

Fig. 19.2 Typical immunofluorescence microscopy images (100×) of DD (**a**) and PF (**b**) cells migrating into the surrounding cell-free collagen treated with phosphate buffered saline and 2% fetal bovine serum, vehicle for the majority of additives used in this study. Cells are stained with DAPI to identify nuclei and phalloidin to identify actin stress fibres

a subset of samples were dried and imaged by differential interference contrast (DIC) and immunofluorescence microscopy to gain higher resolution images of the migrating cells (Fig. 19.2).

The genes encoding TGFβ1, ADAM12 and periostin (*TGFB1*, *ADAM12* and *POSTN*, respectively) have all been previously identified as upregulated transcripts in DD (Rehman et al. 2008; Qian et al. 2004; Shih et al. 2009). TGFβ1, ADAM12, and periostin were therefore added to the surrounding collagen to mimic this aspect of a DD-ECM. Recombinant TGFβ1 displayed highly variable effects on DD cell migration between experiments that were not evident in PF cells tested in parallel. While TGFβ1 did not alter the three-dimensional migration of DD cells, it inhibited PF cell migration (Fig. 19.3). ADAM12 reduced both DD and

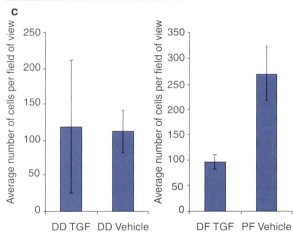

Fig. 19.3 Stereomicroscopy images (60×) of DD (**a**) and PF (**b**) cells migrating into the surrounding cell-free collagen containing 12.5 ng/mL TGFβ1. Cells are stained with DAPI to identify nuclei. (**c**) Cell count analyses of patient-matched DD (*left*) and PF (*right*) cells migrating out of the FPCLs into collagen containing TGFβ1 or vehicle

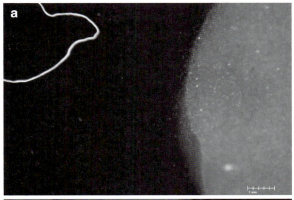
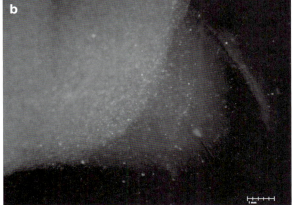
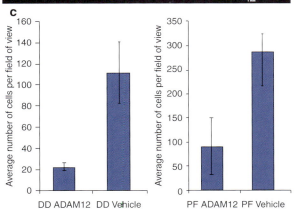
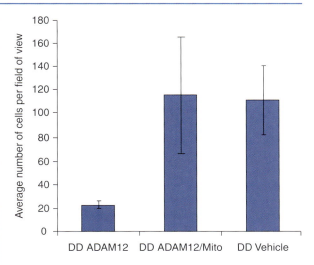

Fig. 19.5 Cell count analyses of DD pretreated with vehicle (*left*) or mitomycin C (*centre*) migrating into the surrounding cell-free collagen containing 10pM ADAM12 compared to DD cells migrating into collagen containing vehicle (*right*)

Fig. 19.4 Stereomicroscopy images (60×) of DD (**a**) and PF (**b**) cells migrating into the surrounding cell-free collagen containing 10pM ADAM12. Cells are stained with DAPI to identify nuclei. (**c**) Cell counts analyses of patient-matched DD (*left*) and PF (*right*) cells migrating out of the FPCLs into collagen containing ADAM12 or vehicle

PF cell migration relative to the vehicle controls (Fig. 19.4); however, these effects were negated by treatment with 0.02 mg/mL mitomycin C (Fig. 19.5). Periostin treatment had no discernable effects on three-dimensional migration in DD or PF cells (Fig. 19.6), although an inhibitory effect was evident in the presence of mitomycin C treatment (Fig. 19.7).

19.3.2 Collagen Substrate Conditioning Assay

To assess the ability of DD cells to modify their environment with factors that could induce a "disease cell" phenotype, DD or PF cells were cultured into a transwell embedded in a collagen substrate. After 7 days of conditioning the collagen, the transwell was removed and PF cells were cultured on the conditioned collagen in the tray well for an additional 7 days. The cells were isolated using collagenase and processed for immunoblotting analysis with a β-catenin antibody. As shown in Fig. 19.8, a DD cell-conditioned collagen substrate consistently induced β-catenin accumulation in PF cells. In contrast, PF cells growing on a PF cell-conditioned collagen substrate did not display β-catenin accumulation. To confirm the location and accumulation of β-catenin, immunofluorescence microscopy was performed on the PF cells after 7 days exposure to conditioned collagen substrates. As shown in Fig. 19.9, PF cells exposed to a DD cell-conditioned collagen substrate displayed β-catenin accumulation in the perinuclear region in the majority, but not all, cells, as well

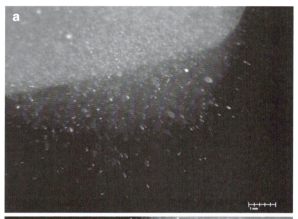
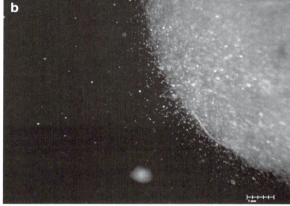
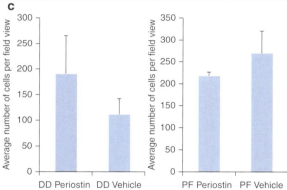

Fig. 19.6 Stereomicroscopy images (60×) of DD (**a**) and PF (**b**) cells migrating into the surrounding cell-free collagen containing 2 μg/mL periostin. Cells are stained with DAPI to identify nuclei. (**c**) Cell counts analyses of patient-matched DD (*left*) and PF (*right*) cells migrating out of the FPCLs into collagen containing periostin or vehicle

as some β-catenin localization to the cell membrane. In contrast, little or no β-catenin immunoreactivity was evident in PF cells grown on a PF cell-conditioned collagen substrate.

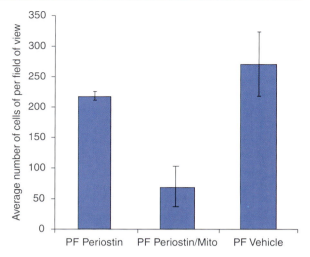

Fig. 19.7 Cell count analyses of DD pretreated with vehicle (*left*) or mitomycin C (*centre*) migrating into the surrounding cell-free collagen containing periostin compared to DD cells migrating into collagen containing vehicle (*right*)

19.4 Discussion

The three-dimensional migration data indicated that, overall, DD cells are less motile than PF cells. These findings are consistent with previous studies of migration in one and two dimensions, which have suggest that myofibroblasts may have reduced motility relative to fibroblasts (Tomasek et al. 2002; Thampatty and Wang 2007). Using microgrooved surface migration assays that monitor cell migration in one dimension, TGFβ1-treated myofibroblasts were found to be 30% less motile than untreated fibroblasts in a previous study (Thampatty and Wang 2007). DD cells cultured in FPCLs differentiate into myofibroblast, and the increased contractility and α-smooth muscle actin protein expression associated with this differentiation may decrease their migratory abilities. Inhibition of α-smooth muscle actin has also been previously shown to decrease cell adhesion (Hinz et al. 2003) and increase myofibroblast motility (Tomasek et al. 2002). This reduction in migration may also be associated with the development of supermature focal adhesions which exert much greater stress than typical focal adhesions (Goffin et al. 2006). PF cells cultured in FPCLs consistently display reduced contractility and decreased α-smooth muscle actin protein expression, potentially indicative of a "proto-myofibroblast" phenotype, and may retain a more migratory phenotype relative to the DD cells.

Fig. 19.8 Primary PF cells grown on collagen substrates conditioned for 7 days by PF or DD cells, lysed and assessed by SDS-PAGE. From left, molecular weight markers, lysates from cells grown on PF cell-conditioned collagen (*centre lane*) or DD cell-conditioned collagen (*right lane*). β-catenin immunoreactivity is evident as a primary band at 94 kDa. Smaller immunoreactive species are unidentified but may indicate β-catenin degradation products. β-actin imunoreactivity was also assessed to confirm equal loading of cell lysates in each lane

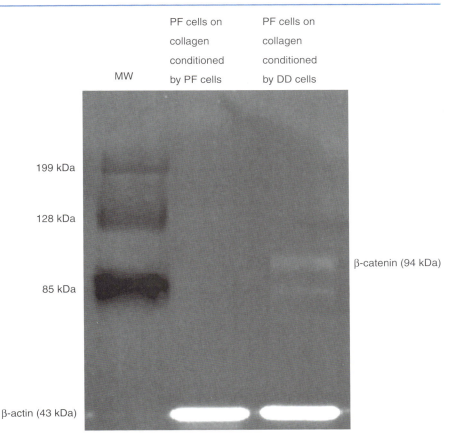

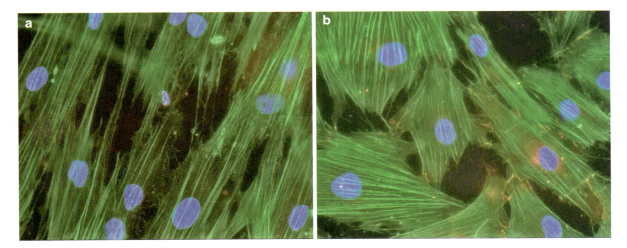

Fig. 19.9 Primary PF cells grown on collagen substrates conditioned for 7 days by PF cells (**a**) or DD cells (**b**), fixed and assessed by immunofluorescence microscopy for β-catenin accumulation (TRITC-conjugated anti-β-catenin, shown in *orange*), actin stress fibres (Alexa 488 phallodin, shown in *green*) and nuclei (DAPI, shown in *blue*)

ADAM12 consistently inhibited migration of DD and PF cells. Interestingly, when mitomycin C was utilized to inhibit cell proliferation, DD cells treated with ADAM12 showed a recovery in migration to levels similar to the vehicle-treated DD cells. This suggests that the mechanism by which ADAM12 alters DD cell migration is post-transcriptional. DD and PF cell migration were relatively unaffected by periostin treatment. Since periostin has been previously shown to induce PF cell proliferation (Vi et al. 2009a), PF cells were treated with both periostin and mitomycin C and migration was reassessed to distinguish the effects of proliferation from migration. Treated PF cells displayed decreased migration when compared to cells treated with periostin alone and vehicle-treated PF cultures. This observation implies that periostin may actually inhibit PF cell migration, while inducing PF cell proliferation, thereby inflating the apparent degree of periostin-induced PF cell migration. As periostin has also been shown to induce PF cell apoptosis (Vi et al. 2009a), further detailed analysis of these effects will be necessary before these interactions are understood in context.

The finding that DD cells, but not PF cells, can condition a collagen substrate with factors that induce β-catenin accumulation in PF cells is intriguing. TGFβ1 can induce β-catenin accumulation in fibroblasts (Cheon et al. 2006; Amini Nik et al. 2007; Caraci et al. 2008), and TGFβ1 levels are increased in DD cells (Badalamente et al. 1996; Berndt et al. 1995), making this cytokine a likely candidate for inducing this effect. Primary DD cells display enhanced sensitivity to TGFβ1 relative to control fibroblasts (Bisson et al. 2003), and β-catenin accumulation by TGFβ1 can be modulated by altering the extra-cellular environment (Vi et al. 2009c). In contrast, while ADAM12 induces β-catenin accumulation in DD cells, it does not alter the levels in PF cells, and periostin does not induce β-catenin accumulation in either cell type (our unpublished observations). Future studies will focus on determining if DD cells can secrete factors that induce disease-associated changes in gene expression in PF cells, including *TGFBI*, *POSTN* and *ADAM12* mRNA expression, as well as enhanced sensitivity to TGFβ1.

The hypotheses compared in this analysis are not mutually exclusive, i.e. it is possible that DD cells may migrate into the surrounding fascia *and* secrete factors that induce disease cell behaviours in adjacent palmar fascia fibroblasts simultaneously. Nor are these hypotheses comprehensive in terms of encompassing all of the potential interactions between DD cells, PF cells,

other cell types and the ECM. Nonetheless, these hypotheses predict interesting consequences for *in vitro* models of DD derived from surgically resected tissues. For example, the cell migration hypothesis predicts that the migratory cells are the progenitors of the disease cells that make up a DD cord. In contrast, an ECM-mediated disease hypothesis predicts that the cells that secrete ECM-associated factors to promote disease cell differentiation are not direct predecessors of cord cells but instead that cord cells arise through a series of "initiation" events. Like the quiescent fibroblasts from which they are derived, DD cells may therefore be more heterogeneous than the original nodule population (Vi et al. 2009b). The data presented here support the latter model and implicate the ECM as a mediator of disease progression. Future studies will be required to determine if therapies targeted to particular ECM molecules, rather than the cells that secrete them, have potential as alternative treatment modalities for DD.

19.5 Conclusions

- Primary Dupuytren's disease (DD) cells are less motile than adjacent, patient-matched cells derived from the palmar fascia (PF cells).
- TGFβ1, periostin or ADAM12 do not induce the motility of DD or PF cells in three-dimensional collagen cultures.
- DD cells, but not PF cells, secrete as yet unidentified factors into their collagen culture substrate that can induce PF cells to express high levels of β-catenin, a characteristic of DD cells *in vivo*.
- DD cells may be able to induce quiescent neighbouring cells in the palmar fascia to take on a disease cell-like phenotype.

Acknowledgments   We would like to acknowledge Ms Karen Nygard at the Biotron of the University of Western Ontario for her expert assistance with stereomicroscopy. We also acknowledge the Canadian Institutes of Health Research and The Lawson Health Research Institute Internal Research Fund for financial support.

References

Amini Nik S, Ebrahim RP, Van Dam K, Cassiman JJ, Tejpar S (2007) TGF-beta modulates beta-Catenin stability and signaling in mesenchymal proliferations. Exp Cell Res 313(13):2887–2895

Badalamente MA, Sampson SP, Hurst LC, Dowd A, Miyasaka K (1996) The role of transforming growth factor beta in Dupuytren's disease. J Hand Surg Am 21(2):210–215

Berndt A, Kosmehl H, Mandel U, Gabler U, Luo X, Celeda D, Zardi L, Katenkamp D (1995) TGF beta and bFGF synthesis and localization in Dupuytren's disease (nodular palmar fibromatosis) relative to cellular activity, myofibroblast phenotype and oncofetal variants of fibronectin. Histochem J 27(12):1014–1020

Bisson MA, McGrouther DA, Mudera V, Grobbelaar AO (2003) The different characteristics of Dupuytren's disease fibroblasts derived from either nodule or cord: expression of alpha-smooth muscle actin and the response to stimulation by TGF-beta1. J Hand Surg Br 28(4):351–356

Bunyan AR, Mathur BS (2000) Medium thickness plantar skin graft for the management of digital and palmar flexion contractures. Burns 26(6):575–580

Caraci F, Gili E, Calafiore M, Failla M, La Rosa C, Crimi N, Sortino MA, Nicoletti F, Copani A, Vancheri C (2008) TGF-beta1 targets the GSK-3beta/beta-catenin pathway via ERK activation in the transition of human lung fibroblasts into myofibroblasts. Pharmacol Res 57(4):274–282

Cheon SS, Wei Q, Gurung A, Youn A, Bright T, Poon R, Whetstone H, Guha A, Alman BA (2006) Beta-catenin regulates wound size and mediates the effect of TGF-beta in cutaneous healing. FASEB J 20(6):692–701

Citron N, Hearnden A (2003) Skin tension in the aetiology of Dupuytren's disease; a prospective trial. J Hand Surg Br 28(6):528–530

Evans RB, Dell PC, Fiolkowski P (2002) A clinical report of the effect of mechanical stress on functional results after fasciectomy for Dupuytren's contracture. J Hand Ther 15(4):331–339

Goffin JM, Pittet P, Csucs G, Lussi JW, Meister JJ, Hinz B (2006) Focal adhesion size controls tension-dependent recruitment of alpha-smooth muscle actin to stress fibers. J Cell Biol 172(2):259–268

Gupta R, Allen F, Tan V, Bozentka DJ, Bora FW, Osterman AL (1998) The effect of shear stress on fibroblasts derived from Dupuytren's tissue and normal palmar fascia. J Hand Surg Am 23(5):945–950

Hinz B (2009) Tissue stiffness, latent TGF-beta1 activation, and mechanical signal transduction: implications for the pathogenesis and treatment of fibrosis. Curr Rheumatol Rep 11(2):120–126

Hinz B, Dugina V, Ballestrem C, Wehrle-Haller B, Chaponnier C (2003) Alpha-smooth muscle actin is crucial for focal adhesion maturation in myofibroblasts. Mol Biol Cell 14(6):2508–2519

Howard JC, Varallo VM, Ross DC, Roth JH, Faber KJ, Alman B, Gan BS (2003) Elevated levels of beta-catenin and fibronectin in three-dimensional collagen cultures of Dupuytren's disease cells are regulated by tension in vitro. BMC Musculoskelet Disord 4:16

Howard JC, Varallo VM, Ross DC, Faber KJ, Roth JH, Seney S, Gan BS (2004) Wound healing-associated proteins Hsp47 and fibronectin are elevated in Dupuytren's contracture. J Surg Res 117(2):232–238

Hueston JT (1992) Regression of Dupuytren's contracture. J Hand Surg Br 17(4):453–457

Hurst LC, Badalamente MA, Makowski J (1986) The pathobiology of Dupuytren's contracture: effects of prostaglandins on myofibroblasts. J Hand Surg Am 11(1):18–23

Iwasaki H, Muller H, Stutte HJ, Brennscheidt U (1984) Palmar fibromatosis (Dupuytren's contracture). Ultrastructural and enzyme histochemical studies of 43 cases. Virchows Arch A Pathol Anat Histopathol 405(1):41–53

Luck JV (1959) Dupuytren's contracture; a new concept of the pathogenesis correlated with surgical management. J Bone Joint Surg Am 41(4):635–664

Qian A, Meals RA, Rajfer J, Gonzalez-Cadavid NF (2004) Comparison of gene expression profiles between Peyronie's disease and Dupuytren's contracture. Urology 64(2):399–404

Rajesh KR, Rex C, Mehdi H, Martin C, Fahmy NR (2000) Severe Dupuytren's contracture of the proximal interphalangeal joint: treatment by two-stage technique. J Hand Surg Br 25(5):442–444

Rayan GM, Tomasek JJ (1994) Generation of contractile force by cultured Dupuytren's disease and normal palmar fibroblasts. Tissue Cell 26(5):747–756

Rayan GM, Parizi M, Tomasek JJ (1996) Pharmacologic regulation of Dupuytren's fibroblast contraction in vitro. J Hand Surg Am 21(6):1065–1070

Rehman S, Salway F, Stanley JK, Ollier WE, Day P, Bayat A (2008) Molecular phenotypic descriptors of Dupuytren's disease defined using informatics analysis of the transcriptome. J Hand Surg Am 33(3):359–372

Shih B, Wijeratne D, Armstrong DJ, Lindau T, Day P, Bayat A (2009) Identification of biomarkers in Dupuytren's disease by comparative analysis of fibroblasts versus tissue biopsies in disease-specific phenotypes. J Hand Surg Am 34(1):124–136

Thampatty BP, Wang JH (2007) A new approach to study fibroblast migration. Cell Motil Cytoskeleton 64(1):1–5

Tomasek J, Rayan GM (1995) Correlation of alpha-smooth muscle actin expression and contraction in Dupuytren's disease fibroblasts. J Hand Surg Am 20(3):450–455

Tomasek JJ, Schultz RJ, Episalla CW, Newman SA (1986) The cytoskeleton and extracellular matrix of the Dupuytren's disease "myofibroblast": an immunofluorescence study of a nonmuscle cell type. J Hand Surg Am 11(3):365–371

Tomasek JJ, Gabbiani G, Hinz B, Chaponnier C, Brown RA (2002) Myofibroblasts and mechano-regulation of connective tissue remodelling. Nat Rev Mol Cell Biol 3(5):349–363

Vi L, Feng L, Zhu RD, Wu Y, Satish L, Gan BS, O'Gorman DB (2009a) Periostin differentially induces proliferation, contraction and apoptosis of primary Dupuytren's disease and adjacent palmar fascia cells. Exp Cell Res 315(20): 3574–3586

Vi L, Gan BS, O'Gorman DB (2009b) The potential roles of cell migration and extra-cellular matrix interactions in Dupuytren's disease progression and recurrence. Med Hypotheses 74(3):510–512

Vi L, Njarlangattil A, Wu Y, Gan BS, O'Gorman DB (2009c) Type-1 collagen differentially alters beta-catenin accumulation in primary Dupuytren's Disease cord and adjacent palmar fascia cells. BMC Musculoskelet Disord 10(1):72

Wipff PJ, Hinz B (2009) Myofibroblasts work best under stress. J Bodyw Mov Ther 13(2):121–127

Wipff PJ, Rifkin DB, Meister JJ, Hinz B (2007) Myofibroblast contraction activates latent TGF-beta1 from the extracellular matrix. J Cell Biol 179(6):1311–1323

Insulin-Like Growth Factor Binding Protein-6: A Potential Mediator of Myofibroblast Differentiation in Dupuytren's Disease?

20

Christina Raykha, Justin Crawford, Bing Siang Gan, and David B. O'Gorman

Contents

20.1 Introduction 161

20.2 Methods 162
20.2.1 Downregulation of IGFBP-6 Transcription and Secretion 162
20.2.2 IGFBP-6 in Contraction 162

20.3 Results 163

20.4 Discussion 163

20.5 Conclusions 165

References 165

C. Raykha • J. Crawford
Cell and Molecular Biology Laboratory,
Hand and Upper Limb Centre, St. Joseph's Health Care,
Lawson Health Research Institute,
University of Western Ontario, London, ON, Canada
e-mail: craykha@hotmail.com; jcrawfo9@uwo.ca

B.S. Gan • D.B. O'Gorman (✉)
Departments of Surgery, Physiology and Pharmacology,
Medical Biophysics, Cell and Molecular Biology Laboratory,
Hand and Upper Limb Centre, St. Joseph's Health Care,
Lawson Health Research Institute,
University of Western Ontario, London, ON, Canada
e-mail: bsgan@rogers.com; dogorman@uwo.ca

20.1 Introduction

Insulin-like growth factor binding protein (IGFBP)-6 is one of five other binding proteins in the insulin-like growth factor (IGF) family. The main function of these IGFBPs is to regulate the availability of the insulin-like growth factors, IGF-I and -II to their receptors (Baxter 2000; Firth and Baxter 2002). The type I IGF receptor (IGFIR) is a signaling receptor through which numerous effects can be initiated, relating to proliferation, differentiation, cell death as well as many other cellular processes (Firth and Baxter 2002). IGFBP-6 is unique in that it can bind IGF-II with 20–100 times more affinity than IGF-1, and as such, it is generally accepted as a relatively specific inhibitor of IGF-II actions (Bach 2005).

Gene expression analyses have identified *IGFBP6*, encoding IGFBP-6, as downregulated in both Dupuytren's Disease (DD), a benign fibromatosis, and in desmoid tumour, an aggressive fibromatosis, a potentially related fibrosis (Rehman et al. 2008; Denys et al. 2004). As the main function of this protein is to regulate levels of IGF-II available for interaction with its receptor, the effects of IGF-II in fibrotic disease are of particular interest.

A putative role for IGF-II was addressed in work by Grotendorst et al. (Grotendorst et al. 2004), which demonstrated combinatorial signaling between transforming growth factor (TGF)-β and IGF-II to induce contraction of murine fibroblasts. Furthermore, in a separate study, IGF-II was shown to increase collagen and fibronectin production in fibroblasts derived from pulmonary fibrosis (Hsu and Feghali-Bostwick 2008). A role for IGF signaling in myofibroblast differentiation has yet to be elucidated in DD.

C. Eaton et al. (eds.), *Dupuytren's Disease and Related Hyperproliferative Disorders*,
DOI 10.1007/978-3-642-22697-7_20, © Springer-Verlag Berlin Heidelberg 2012

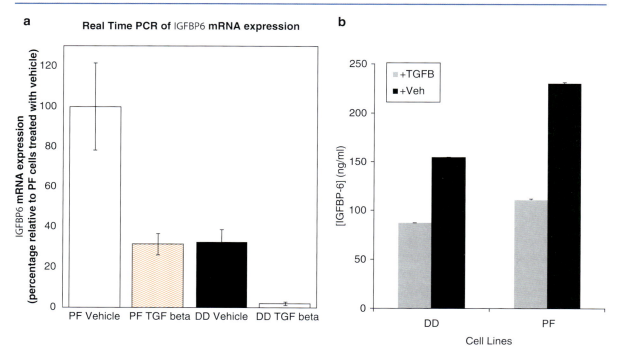

Fig. 20.1 *IGFBP6* gene expression (**a**) and protein secretion (**b**) in DD and patient matched control samples. Real-time PCR was carried out on DD and PF cells treated for 3 days with TGF-β or with vehicle on a type I collagen layer. *IGFBP6* expression was analyzed using β-2-microglobulin as an endogenous control for 45 cycles on an ABI PRISM 7700 using the comparative Ct method. With TGF-β treatment, *IGFBP6* mRNA expression is decreased. A multiplex assay (**b**) to analyze IGFBP-6 protein levels was completed on conditioned α-minimal essential media from cells treated with or without TGF-β. Compared to vehicle (0.1% bovine serum albumin in PBS and 4 mM HCl) treated samples (*black bars*), TGF-β represses IGFBP-6 protein levels in DD and PF samples

As IGF-II availability is regulated by IGFBPs, particularly IGFBP-6, we hypothesize that changes in the levels or availability of IGF-II may be contributing to the DD process through combinatorial signaling between TGF-β and IGF-II, resulting in increased myofibroblast differentiation and subsequent collagen deposition into the extracellular matrix.

20.2 Methods

20.2.1 Downregulation of IGFBP-6 Transcription and Secretion

Real time polymerase chain reaction (PCR) was conducted using TaqMan® IGFBP-6 primers to confirm Affymetrix microarray results. Fibroblasts derived from DD cord tissue (DD) as well as fibroblasts derived from phenotypically normal adjacent palmar fascia from DD patients (PF) were treated with TGF-β for 3 days on a collagen monolayer after which cells were collected and RNA was isolated using the RNeasy mini kit. IGFBP-6 mRNA levels were measured in comparison to the experimentally determined endogenous control, β-2-microglobulin. Protein levels of IGFBP-6 were analysed by multiplex assay on conditioned media from DD and PF cells. Fibroblasts were grown on a Type I collagen layer for 3 days, after which TGF-β treatment was added to the media (α-minimal essential media).

20.2.2 IGFBP-6 in Contraction

DD and PF cells were cultured in Type I collagen with IGFBP-6 +/− TGF-β, and with IGF-II (100 ng/ml) and incubated for 72 h to achieve a stressed matrix in a stressed fibroblast populated collagen lattice (sFPCL). Two different amounts of IGFBP-6 were added, 200–400 ng/ml, with or without TGF-β (12.5ng/ml). Manual release of the collagen lattices allowed for subsequent measurement of the change in surface area of the lattice using ImageJ software. Contraction was therefore measured over a period of 24 h.

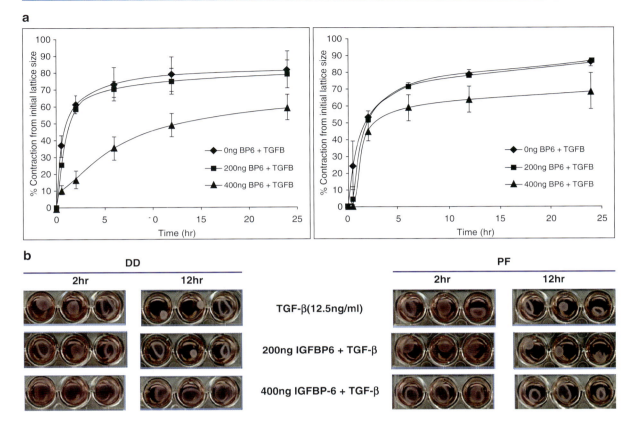

Fig. 20.2 Stressed fibroblast populated collagen lattice from DD and PF cells treated with varying amounts of IGFBP-6 and TGF-β. DD (*left*) and PF cells (*right*) were cultured in collagen for 72 h with IGFBP-6 (200 ng/ml ■ and 400 ng/ml ▲) and/or TGF-β (12.5 ng/ml ♦) to achieve a stressed matrix. Lattice was manually released and contraction rate was measured over 24 h using changes in surface area with ImageJ software. Reduction in lattice area was then plotted against time to assess differences in contraction rate with standard error (**a**). 400 ng/ml of IGFBP-6 with TGF-β inhibits contraction compared to 200 ng/ml IGFBP-6+TGF-β and the TGF-β positive control. Lattices are pictured below (**b**)

20.3 Results

Microarray analyses were confirmed with RT-PCR. DD cells were found to have lower *IGFBP6* mRNA levels when compared to PF. TGF-β treatment of these cells further repressed *IGFBP6* transcription (Fig. 20.1a).

IGFBP-6 secretion as measured by multiplex assay was also shown to be decreased in DD cells compared to the patient-matched PF control cells, and this effect was further repressed by TGF-β treatment of the cells (Fig. 20.1b).

In the dose response sFPCL with various IGFBP-6 concentrations in combination to TGF-β treatment of both DD and PF cells, we see that 400 ng/ml IGFBP-6+TGF-β results in decreased contraction and thus repressed myofibroblast differentiation (Fig. 20.2).

Conversely, IGF-II induces contraction of the sFPCLs in both DD and PF-derived fibroblasts (Fig. 20.3).

20.4 Discussion

IGFBP-6 is known to be a negative regulator of IGF-II, a growth factor that signals through the IGFIR to cause various effects on cellular processes, including differentiation. *IGFBP6* transcription is downregulated in DD compared to the patient-matched PF control by Affymetrix microarray analysis, which was confirmed by Real-time PCR on DD and PF cells (Fig. 20.1a). Interestingly, TGF-β treatment of these cells resulted in further repression of *IGFBP6* mRNA. This suggests that TGF-β signaling is repressing

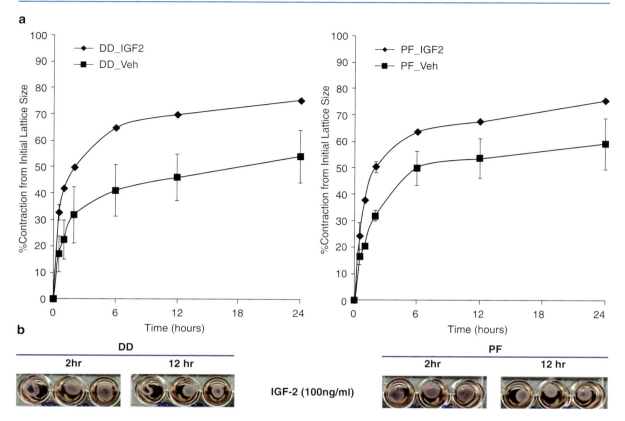

Fig. 20.3 Stressed fibroblast populated collagen lattice for DD (*left*) and PF cells (*right*) cells treated with IGF-II ♦ or vehicle ■. Cells were cultured in Type I collagen for 72 h with 100 ng/ml IGF-II or vehicle (PBS) to achieve a stressed environment. Lattices were then released and contraction was measured over 24 h from measurement of surface area using ImageJ software (**a**). IGF-II induces contraction in both cells types, compared to vehicle treated cells (**a**). Lattices are pictured below (**b**), from which surface area was measured

IGFBP6 transcription, presumably through the activation of cytoplasmic and nuclear factors.

In a study on aggressive fibromatosis, *IGFBP6* transcription was also shown to be downregulated as the result of β-catenin transactivation of the T cell factor/Lymphoid Enhancing Factor (Tcf/LEF) transcription activation complex (Denys et al. 2004). This study reports increased β-catenin levels in disease versus control cells, a trend also seen in DD (Bowley et al. 2007; Amini Nik et al. 2007). We have previously shown that TGF-β increases β-catenin levels in DD cells (Vi et al. 2009), leading to a hypothesis that TGF-β induced β-catenin accumulation in the cytoplasm, allows for its subsequent nuclear translocation and thus increased binding of β-catenin transactivation of Tcf/LEF transcription factor complex at either of the TCF1 or TCF2 sites within the *IGFBP6* promoter region. Studies in our laboratory are underway using chromatin immunoprecipitation to determine whether β-catenin binding to the Tcf/LEF complex is resulting in decreased *IGFBP6* transcription.

To confirm that IGFBP-6 protein levels were mirroring *IGFBP6* mRNA levels, we performed a multiplex assay. IGFBP-6 protein levels were increased in patient-matched PF control cell conditioned media compared to DD cell media (Fig. 20.1b). In parallel to the mRNA levels, TGF-β treatment of both cell types resulted in lower IGFBP-6 protein secretion into the media, likely due to further repression of the *IGFBP6* gene transcript.

Investigations of the effects of decreased IGFBP-6 levels are currently being assessed in our laboratory. With exogenous addition of 400 ng/ml IGFBP-6 to sFP-CLs containing DD and PF cells, TGF-β-induced contraction was inhibited (Fig. 20.2). This supports the work by Grotendorst et al. (Grotendorst et al. 2004) where IGF-II was found to have a role in contraction and myofibroblast differentiation. In this case, as IGF-II is inducing contraction (Fig. 20.3), exogenous addition of 400 ng/ml IGFBP-6 would be predicted to bind endogenous IGF-II in DD and PF cells allowing for repression of contraction, which is confirmed in Fig. 20.3a.

Currently, other effects of IGF-II on collagen production and proliferation are under evaluation. As IGF-II is expected to increase both of these phenotypes, exogenous addition of IGFBP-6 to disease and patient-matched control cells would be expected to inhibit collagen deposition and fibroblast proliferation, thereby acting as a "fibrosis suppressor". It is likely that IGFBP-6 down-regulation results in excess IGF-II bioavailability which, in combination with TGF-β, contributes to myofibroblast development and disease progression. Thus, targeting the intracellular signaling molecules induced by TGF-β that repress *IGFBP6* gene transcription, thereby allowing the recovery of normal physiological levels of IGFBP-6 in the palmar fascia and inhibition of IGF-II signaling, may be of particular interest for the future development of non-surgical interventions in DD.

20.5 Conclusions

- Transcription of the gene encoding IGFBP-6, *IGFBP6*, is consistently decreased in DD
- TGF β1, which is consistently up-regulated in DD, decreases *IGFBP6* transcription
- Replacement of the depleted IGFBP-6 in primary cultures of DD cells inhibits the ability of TGF β to induce contraction of these cells
- Blocking the repression of *IGFBP6* transcription may assist in preventing contractures and have potential for the development of novel molecular therapies for DD

References

Amini Nik S, Ebrahim RP, Van Dam K, Cassiman JJ, Tejpar S (2007) TGF-beta modulates beta-Catenin stability and signaling in mesenchymal proliferations. Exp Cell Res 313(13): 2887–2895

Bach LA (2005) IGFBP-6 five years on; not so 'forgotten'? Growth Horm IGF Res 15(3):185–192

Baxter RC (2000) Insulin-like growth factor (IGF)-binding proteins: interactions with IGFs and intrinsic bioactivities. Am J Physiol Endocrinol Metab 278(6):E967–E976

Bowley E, O'Gorman DB, Gan BS (2007) Beta-catenin signaling in fibroproliferative disease. J Surg Res 138(1):141–150

Denys H, Jadidizadeh A, Amini Nik S, Van Dam K, Aerts S, Alman BA, Cassiman JJ, Tejpar S (2004) Identification of IGFBP-6 as a significantly downregulated gene by beta-catenin in desmoid tumors. Oncogene 23(3):654–664

Firth SM, Baxter RC (2002) Cellular actions of the insulin-like growth factor binding proteins. Endocr Rev 23(6):824–854

Grotendorst GR, Rahmanie H, Duncan MR (2004) Combinatorial signaling pathways determine fibroblast proliferation and myofibroblast differentiation. FASEB J 18(3):469–479

Hsu E, Feghali-Bostwick CA (2008) Insulin-like growth factor-II is increased in systemic sclerosis-associated pulmonary fibrosis and contributes to the fibrotic process via Jun N-terminal kinase- and phosphatidylinositol-3 kinase-dependent pathways. Am J Pathol 172(6):1580–1590

Rehman S, Salway F, Stanley JK, Ollier WE, Day P, Bayat A (2008) Molecular phenotypic descriptors of Dupuytren's disease defined using informatics analysis of the transcriptome. J Hand Surg Am 33(3):359–372

Vi L, Njarlangattil A, Wu Y, Gan BS, O'Gorman DB (2009) Type-1 Collagen differentially alters beta-catenin accumulation in primary Dupuytren's Disease cord and adjacent palmar fascia cells. BMC Musculoskelet Disord 10:72

Dupuytren's Disease Shows Populations of Hematopoietic and Mesenchymal Stem-Like Cells Involving Perinodular Fat and Skin in Addition to Diseased Fascia: Implications for Pathogenesis and Therapy

21

Syed Amir Iqbal, Sandip Hindocha, Syed Farhatullah, Ralf Paus, and Ardeshir Bayat

Contents

21.1	**Introduction**	167
21.2	**Materials and Methods**	168
21.3	**Results**	169
21.4	**Discussion**	171
21.5	**Conclusion**	172
References		173

21.1 Introduction

Dupuytren's Disease (DD) is a common, benign fibro-proliferative disease of unknown origin that primarily affects the palmar fascia (Brickley-Parsons et al. 1981). DD is a progressive, irreversible, and highly recurrent condition which is often treated surgically (Bayat 2010). Myofibroblasts are considered to be the causative cellular elements involved in the formation of DD; however their origin remains unknown to date (McCann et al. 1993; Berndt et al. 1994).

DD typically involves the palmar fascia, but in progressive cases can extend into the digital fascia and subcutaneous tissues. The two principal tissue components commonly described in the fascia to be pathognomonic of the disease are the nodule and the cord (Shih et al. 2009b; Verjee et al. 2010). Myofibroblasts are found in both the nodule and the cord (Dave et al. 2001; Bisson et al. 2003). Other tissue components adjacent to the diseased fascia including the perinodular fat and the skin overlying the nodule have also been implicated in the pathogenesis of DD (Rabinowitz et al. 1983; Shih et al. 2009a). Previous studies have investigated palmar fat cells (Shih et al. 2009a, b), although the exact role of adipocytes and fat stromal cells in relation to DD pathology remains unclear. Therefore, the exact nature of the skin overlying the diseased palmar fascia plus the surrounding fat is of scientific and clinical relevance.

Mesenchymal Stem Cells (MSCs) are obvious candidates as a potential source for DD myofibroblasts but

---

S.A. Iqbal • S. Hindocha • S. Farhatullah • A. Bayat (✉)
Plastic & Reconstructive Surgery Research,
Manchester Interdisciplinary Biocentre, Manchester, UK
e-mail: ardeshir.bayat@manchester.ac.uk

R. Paus
Epithelial Sciences Research Group,
School of Translational Medicine,
University of Manchester, Manchester, UK

Syed Amir Iqbal and Sandip Hindocha have contributed equally to this work.

C. Eaton et al. (eds.), *Dupuytren's Disease and Related Hyperproliferative Disorders*,
DOI 10.1007/978-3-642-22697-7_21, © Springer-Verlag Berlin Heidelberg 2012

have not as yet been investigated (McCann et al. 1993; Berndt et al. 1994; Verjee et al. 2010). In addition, certain hematopoietic stem cells (HSCs) markers may also provide clues as to the pathogenesis and, more importantly, the explanation for disease recurrence. MSCs are multipotent cells found in the bone marrow, skin, and adipose tissue (Young et al. 2001; Zuk et al. 2001; Delorme and Charbord 2007). MSCs are thought to be able to differentiate into cells contributing to palmar fascia and fat as well as to the adjacent dermis (Azzarone et al. 1983), yet MSCs could develop into aberrant cells that may contribute to DD pathogenesis. Therefore, the identification and profiling of stem cells in DD tissue may help unravel disease origin and provide further clues in disease pathology. We have previously characterized the population of stem cells in a separate cohort of DD patients using single color Fluorescence Activated Cell Sorting (FACS) (Hindocha et al. 2011).

HSCs and MSCs are identified on the basis of their morphology and phenotype. HSCs are suspension cells while MSCs show plastic adherence when cultured in vitro. The phenotype of HSCs and MSCs is determined by the expression of cell surface markers known as cluster of differentiation (CD). HSCs are identified by their expression of CD34 while MSCs are CD34 negative. Single or multiple CD markers could be identified using FACS as described above (Fritsch et al. 1995; Delorme and Charbord 2007). Therefore, the aim of this study was not only to identify and profile stem cells in DD nodule, cord, perinodular fat, and skin and to compare normal control tissue using multicolor FACS analysis, but also to determine the progenitor cell potential of DD-derived cells compared to bone marrow (BM)-derived MSCs through in vitro differentiation assays.

21.2 Materials and Methods

Patients diagnosed with DD ($n = 13$) scheduled for elective surgery and control subjects diagnosed with carpal tunnel syndrome (CTS) undergoing open surgical release ($n = 6$) were enrolled in the study. All DD patients were Caucasians of Northern European extraction, with digital contractures involving metacarpophalangeal and proximal interphalangeal joints. Full ethical approval and consent were obtained to conduct the study.

All patients with DD had a fasciectomy with no adverse perioperative complications. DD tissue was harvested and the various tissue components including the nodule, cord, perinodular fat and skin overlying the disease were carefully dissected. The tissue was then placed into Dulbecco's modified Eagle's Medium (Invitrogen, Paisley, UK).

DD tissue components were treated with Dispase II (Roche Diagnostics, UK) and Collagenase A treatment (Roche Diagnostics, UK) as previously described (Iqbal et al. 2010). After enzymatic digestion, 2×10^5 freshly isolated cells were passed through a 70 µm cell strainer (BD Biosciences, USA) in order to avoid tissue pieces. For multicolor FACS analysis, mouse primary antibodies for CD13, CD29, CD34, CD44, and CD90 conjugated to various fluorophores were diluted (1:20) together in phosphate buffered saline (PBS). Cells were incubated in 100 µl of primary antibodies cocktail on ice for 30 min. Cells were washed once with Hank's balanced salt solution (HBSS) and passed through 50 µm filter (BD Bioscience, USA), before being analyzed on FACSAria flow cytometer (BD Biosciences, USA) that was equipped with four lasers. The cell viability was assessed through Sytox blue (Invitrogen, UK) staining and the data was analyzed on BD FACSDiva software (version 5.03).

In order to determine if the cells from DD samples were uncommitted MSCs capable of differentiating into adipogenic, osteogenic, and chondrogenic lineages, we compared their differentiation potential with bone marrow (BM)-derived MSCs. We grew cells in lineage-specific StemPro adipogenic, chondrogenic, and osteogenic differentiation media (Invitrogen, UK). Cells were washed once in PBS and resuspended at a concentration of 1.6×10^7 cells per ml in complete media (10% fetal bovine serum/Dulbecco's modified Eagle's medium supplemented with penicillin/streptomycin, L-glutamine, and nonessential amino acids). For chondrogenic pathway, 5 µl of the cell suspension was spotted in the middle of the 24-well plate wells in triplicates and incubated at 37°C/5% CO_2 for 2 h. 1×10^4 cells/cm^2 were added for adipogenic pathway and 5×10^3 cells/cm^2 were added for osteogenic pathway in 24-well plates and incubated at 37°C/5% CO_2 for 2 h, all in triplicates. After 2 h, the complete media was removed and replaced with 1,000 µl respective StemPro differentiation media. The media was changed every week for 4 weeks by removing 500 µl media and replacing it with the same volume. Detection of differentiation was performed by staining calcium deposited by osteocytes (using Alzarin Red S), lipid secreted by adipocytes (using Oil Red O), and chondrocytes were detected by staining collagen II with Alcian blue (all dyes from Sigma-aldrich, UK) as described earlier (Pittenger et al. 1999). The images

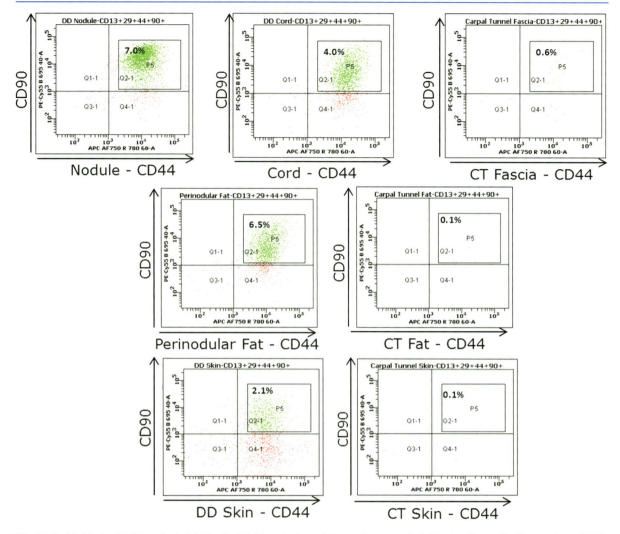

Fig. 21.1 Multicolor FACS analysis. Multicolor FACS analysis demonstrates the presence of progenitor cells in DD in comparison to control tissue obtained from patients undergoing carpal tunnel release. DD nodule and DD perinodular fat showed the highest number of cells positive for CD13$^+$29$^+$44$^+$90$^+$. Cells were isolated from DD tissue biopsies as well as from CT tissue by enzymatic digestion. In order to determine the presence of multiple markers on individual cells antibodies against CD13, CD29, CD44, and CD90 conjugated with fluorophores that could be identified simultaneously were used. Sytox blue (live cells) CD13$^+$29$^+$ cells were gated and plotted here in CD90 versus CD44 plots. Percentages shown in the graph are the mean from four patients each for DD and CT tissue samples. *CT* Carpal tunnel; *DD* Dupuytren's disease

were taken using Olympus inverted microscope (IX71) equipped with a 5 M pixel color camera.

For FACS analysis, the total number of positive cells for CD13, CD29, CD44, and CD90 were obtained and the mean is shown (Fig. 21.1). Since the total number of patients is considered to be small, the standard deviation (SD) values were omitted. On the other hand CD34$^+$ cells determined in all patients and their values are presented as mean±SD. Results are shown for each tissue component.

21.3 Results

Using the results from FACS analysis, we identified multiple subpopulations of stem-like cells within the various anatomical sites of DD compared to control tissue. Moreover, we confirmed that the cells derived from DD were able to differentiate into MSC lineage cells.

The perinodular fat and the nodule contained the highest expression of cells positive simultaneously for

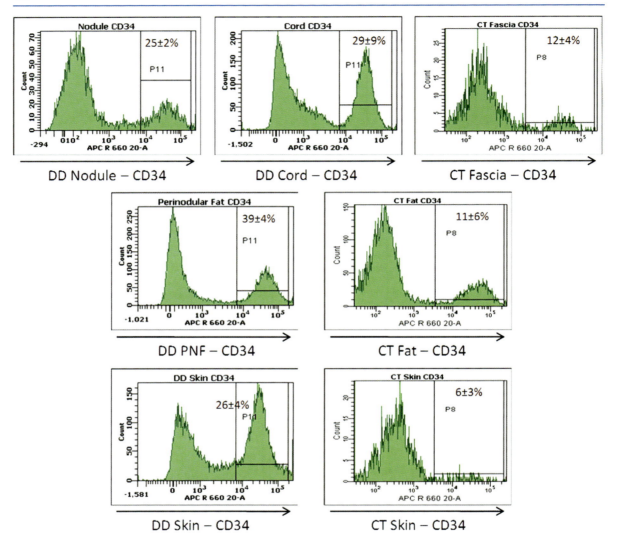

Fig. 21.2 CD34 expression on cells derived from DD and CT tissues. All DD samples showed higher expression of CD34 marker compared to CT control tissue samples. In particular, the perinodular fat was enriched in CD34+ cells. These cells were derived from DD and CT tissues after enzymatic digestion (please see explanation in the text). Minimum of 10,000 cells were counted for analysis on BD FACSAria cytometer. Live cells were selected as Sytox blue⁻ cells. Data shown as mean ± SD from 10 patients each for DD and CT tissue samples. *CT* Carpal tunnel; DD Dupuytren's disease

CD13, CD29, CD44, and CD90 in comparison to carpal tunnel control tissue (Fig. 21.1). CD90 appeared to show a lower prevalent trend of positive cells in comparison to CD13, 29, and 44 positive cells across all anatomical sites (data not shown). Therefore, there was an elevated expression of CD13 and CD29 in the perinodular fat in addition to the diseased palmar fascia (Fig. 21.1). There was a consistently elevated number of CD29 positive cells found in all DD tissue components. The cord, nodule, perinodular fat, and skin all displayed elevated numbers of CD29 positive cells compared to carpal tunnel control tissue (Fig. 21.1).

We found that CD13+29+44+90+ cells, thought to be the progenitor MSCs, were expressed more frequently in the nodule and perinodular fat compared to their CT control tissue counterparts (Fig. 21.1). Nonetheless, cord tissue showed lower expression of the above markers.

In order to identify and confirm the presence of the hematopoietic progenitor cells in DD and CT tissues,

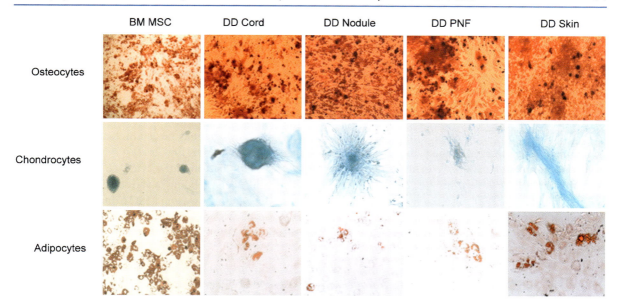

Fig. 21.3 In vitro differentiation assay. In vitro differentiation assay demonstrates the MSC progenitor potential of DD-derived cells compared to bone marrow cells. The differentiation assay was performed on cells in their 1–3 passage (please see procedure described in the text). After 4 weeks of growing in differentiation media, the cells were fixed in 10% neutral buffered formalin and stained by using Alizarin Red S for identification of osteocytes, Alcian Blue for chondrocytes, and Oil Red O for adipocytes. All DD tissue biopsies-derived cells differentiated into three lineages. All images were taken at 10× magnification. *BM MSC* bone marrow-derived mesenchymal stem cells, *DD* Dupuytren's disease, *PNF* perinodular fat

we looked for the presence of the quintessential HSC marker CD34 in all tissue samples (Fig. 21.2). The expression of CD34 in DD skin cells (16 ± 3) was greater in comparison to control carpal tunnel skin (6 ± 4%) and this trend was similar in diseased fascia, where cord (13 ± 6%) and nodule (15 ± 9%) cells expressed CD34 in almost equal numbers compared to carpal tunnel fascia (4 ± 1) (Fig. 21.2).

To further confirm the progenitor potential of MSCs, the cells derived from DD and from BM were grown in culture for up to three passages. The cells from passage 1 to 3 were used to initiate MSC trilineage differentiation assays. We found that all tissue samples obtained from DD differentiated into all three lineages of MSCs, that is, osteocytes, chondrocytes, and adipocytes (Fig. 21.3).

Only perinodular fat cells did not differentiate appreciably into chondrocytes. We found no difference in morphology or frequency of lineage forming colonies between BM MSCs and DD cells. The only difference between the two cells types was the late onset of initiation of differentiation of DD cells compared to BM MSCs. This was confirmed by monitoring cells under an inverted microscope every third day during the differentiation assay. Therefore, we concluded that the cells derived from DD also mimic MSCs and possess a potential to differentiate into cell types that identify MSCs.

21.4 Discussion

This unique study has profiled stem cell populations in not just one but multiple anatomical sites from DD using multicolor FACS and differentiation assays. We have demonstrated which progenitor cells predominate in the various anatomical sites thought to be involved in the disease process, namely, cord, nodule, perinodular fat, and the skin. This study gives a thorough description of HSCs and MSCs in different DD sites and gives evidence that the disease houses a niche for the progenitor cells which may be involved in DD development and/or recurrence.

CD13 is normally expressed on inflammatory cells, but recently it has been shown to be expressed in half of the 149 neoplastic tissue specimens stained with the anti-CD13 antibodies (Di Matteo et al. 2011). Thus, the presence of CD13 in DD cells, especially in perinodular fat gives strength to the hypothesis that DD displays a quasi-neoplastic behavior. CD13 has also been found to be a staging marker in non-small cell lung carcinoma (Ju et al. 2009). In addition to this, the relationship between fat cells and poorer prognosis in dermatofibrous tumors (Perez et al. 2009; Wang et al. 2009) is of relevance to DD as CD13 is expressed in PNF-derived cells (Fig. 21.1). Similarly, CD29 has been found to be involved in the pathogenesis of neoplasia (Seeberger et al. 2006; Yu et al. 2006), although expression of CD29 alone is not sufficient to classify a cell as an MSC. CD90, also known as thy-1, is a hematopoietic marker that is also found on fibroblasts and MSCs (Rege and Hagood 2006; Campioni et al. 2009) (Fig. 21.1). Therefore, simultaneous expression of both CD29 and CD90 is likely to exclude misidentifying fibroblasts as MSCs.

DD is known to have an altered ratio of collagen types and there is an increased deposition of extracellular matrix (ECM) components (Bailey et al. 1977; Brickley-Parsons et al. 1981). CD44 may therefore be a useful marker, as it is a cell adhesion receptor that encourages cell migration within the ECM. Some isoforms of CD44 have been associated with malignancy (Lesley et al. 1993; Naor et al. 1997). The expression of CD44 has been previously associated with tumor invasiveness and increased cell adhesion (Wielenga et al. 1993). The high expression of this marker in DD cord, nodule, and perinodular fat, in comparison to carpal tunnel controls, may suggest that these cells located within the DD cord may have locally infiltrating properties (Fig. 21.1).

All the markers discussed above cannot be used alone to identify MSCs, since all of them are found to be expressed individually not only in MSCs, but in fibroblasts as well (Halfon et al. 2011). In order to uniquely identify MSCs, we utilized multicolor FACS and found that $CD13^+29^+44^+90^+$ cells were prevalent in DD nodule, cord and perinodular fat compared to CT equivalents (Fig. 21.1). This increase in MSCs in DD, compared to CT, supports our hypothesis that these cells are the active progenitors of fibroblasts (Dennis and Charbord 2002) that proliferate in DD fascia.

CD34 is a common hematopoietic marker previously shown to be present in all tissues in the body (Erdag et al. 2008). Despite its broad distribution, CD34 is also currently used as a biomarker in fibrotic skin disorders like dermatofibrosarcoma protruberans,

(DFSP) (Aiba et al. 1992) and has been shown to be useful in identifying those patients at risk of recurrent DFSP (Abenoza and Lillimoe 1993). The increased expression of CD34 in DD skin compared to CT skin may therefore be a useful marker for identifying hematopoietic progenitor cells that are potentially involved in the pathogenesis of DD and thus predict those patients who may be at a higher risk of developing recurrent disease (Fig. 21.2).

This study has provided evidence for the presence of stem-like cells residing in various DD tissue components. In addition, by using MSC trilineage differentiation, we have shown that cells derived from DD are capable of differentiating into osteocytes, chondrocytes, and adipocytes (Fig. 21.3). These findings may have implications in the current indications for specific type and timing of surgical treatments for DD. The standard surgical treatment for DD is excision of the diseased fascia alone (fasciectomy) (Verjee et al. 2009). The introduction of dermofasciectomy, which involves excision of the skin overlying the nodule and subcutaneous tissue, in addition to the diseased fascia, has shown to significantly reduce the rate of recurrence (Tonkin et al. 1984). Dermofasciectomy is often reserved for the recurrent and severely affected cases. Individuals suffering from DD diathesis have been shown to have a higher rate of recurrence following routine fasciectomy and may therefore be candidates for dermofasciectomy as a primary procedure (Ketchum 1991; Abe et al. 2004). Our findings that skin adjacent to the nodule and fat contains progenitors of fibroblasts may indicate a potential role for consideration of the early use of dermofasciectomy in selected cases as primary procedure at an earlier stage of DD, although this preliminary proposal would require further detailed confirmatory clinical and scientific studies.

21.5 Conclusion

This study has identified the presence of specific stem-like cell markers in DD. FACS analysis identified $CD13^+29^+44^+90^+$ cells in all DD biopsies with DD nodule and DD PNF showing the highest expression. Highest number of $CD34^+$ cells was identified in DD samples compared to control tissue. All DD samples differentiated into three characteristic mesenchymal stem cell lineages, that is, osteocytes, chondrocytes, and adipocytes in vitro, except for PNF, which did not differentiate appreciably into chondrocytes. These findings raise the possibility that MSC may serve as an additional source of the abnormal myofibroblasts that induce finger contracture in DD. A possible clinical implication of this study may be to advocate the use of adipodermofasciectomy as a potential primary therapy, although this proposal would require further additional clinical and scientific research.

References

Abe Y, Rokkaku T et al (2004) Surgery for Dupuytren's disease in Japanese patients and a new preoperative classification. J Hand Surg Br 29(3):235–239

Abenoza P, Lillimoe T (1993) CD34 and factor XIIIa in the differential diagnosis of dermatofibroma and dermatofibrosarcoma protuberans. Am J Dermatopathol 15:429–434

Aiba S, Tabata N et al (1992) Dermatofibrosarcoma protuberans is a unique fibrohistiocytic tumour expressing CD34. Br J Dermatol 127(2):79–84

Azzarone B, Failly-Crepin C et al (1983) Abnormal behavior of cultured fibroblasts from nodule and nonaffected aponeurosis of Dupuytren's disease. J Cell Physiol 117(3):353–361

Bailey AJ, Sims TJ et al (1977) Collagen of Dupuytren's disease. Clin Sci Mol Med 53(5):499–502

Bayat A (2010) Connective tissue diseases: a nonsurgical therapy for Dupuytren disease. Nat Rev Rheumatol 6(1):7–8

Berndt A, Kosmehl H et al (1994) Appearance of the myofibroblastic phenotype in Dupuytren's disease is associated with a fibronectin, laminin, collagen type IV and tenascin extracellular matrix. Pathobiology 62(2):55–58

Bisson MA, McGrouther DA et al (2003) The different characteristics of Dupuytren's disease fibroblasts derived from either nodule or cord: expression of alpha-smooth muscle actin and the response to stimulation by TGF-beta1. J Hand Surg Br 28(4):351–356

Brickley-Parsons D, Glimcher MJ et al (1981) Biochemical changes in the collagen of the palmar fascia in patients with Dupuytren's disease. J Bone Joint Surg Am 63(5):787–797

Campioni D, Rizzo R et al (2009) A decreased positivity for CD90 on human mesenchymal stromal cells (MSCs) is associated with a loss of immunosuppressive activity by MSCs. Cytometry B Clin Cytom 76(3):225–230

Dave SA, Banducci DR et al (2001) Differences in alpha smooth muscle actin expression between fibroblasts derived from Dupuytren's nodules or cords. Exp Mol Pathol 71(2):147–155

Delorme B, Charbord P (2007) Culture and characterization of human bone marrow mesenchymal stem cells. Methods Mol Med 140:67–81

Dennis JE, Charbord P (2002) Origin and differentiation of human and murine stroma. Stem Cells 20(3):205–214

Di Matteo P, Arrigoni GL et al (2011) Enhanced expression of CD13 in vessels of inflammatory and neoplastic tissues. J Histochem Cytochem 59(1):47–59

Erdag G, Qureshi HS et al (2008) CD34-Positive dendritic cells disappear from scars but are increased in pericicatricial tissue. J Cutan Pathol 35(8):752–756

Fritsch G, Stimpfl M et al (1995) Characterization of hematopoietic stem cells. Ann N Y Acad Sci 770:42–52

Halfon S, Abramov N et al (2011) Markers distinguishing mesenchymal stem cells from fibroblasts are downregulated with passaging. Stem Cells Dev 20(1):53–66

Hindocha S, Iqbal SA et al (2011) Characterization of stem cells in Dupuytren's disease. Br J Surg 98(2):308–315

Iqbal SA, Syed F et al (2010) Differential distribution of haematopoietic and nonhaematopoietic progenitor cells in intralesional and extralesional keloid: do keloid scars provide a niche for nonhaematopoietic mesenchymal stem cells? Br J Dermatol 162(6):1377–1383

Ju S, Qiu H et al (2009) CD13+CD4+CD25hi regulatory T cells exhibit higher suppressive function and increase with tumor stage in non-small cell lung cancer patients. Cell Cycle 8(16):2578–2585

Ketchum LD (1991) The use of the full thickness skin graft in Dupuytren's contracture. Hand Clin 7(4):731–741, discussion 743

Lesley J, Hyman R et al (1993) CD44 and its interaction with extracellular matrix. Adv Immunol 54:271–335

McCann BG, Logan A et al (1993) The presence of myofibroblasts in the dermis of patients with Dupuytren's contracture. A possible source for recurrence. J Hand Surg Br 18(5): 656–661

Naor D, Sionov RV et al (1997) CD44: structure, function, and association with the malignant process. Adv Cancer Res 71:241–319

Perez I, Varona A et al (2009) Increased APN/CD13 and acid aminopeptidase activities in head and neck squamous cell carcinoma. Head Neck 31(10):1335–1340

Pittenger MF, Mackay AM et al (1999) Multilineage potential of adult human mesenchymal stem cells. Science 284(5411): 143–147

Rabinowitz JL, Ostermann L et al (1983) Lipid composition and de novo lipid biosynthesis of human palmar fat in Dupuytren's disease. Lipids 18(5):371–374

Rege TA, Hagood JS (2006) Thy-1 as a regulator of cell-cell and cell-matrix interactions in axon regeneration, apoptosis, adhesion, migration, cancer, and fibrosis. FASEB J 20(8):1045–1054

Seeberger KL, Dufour JM et al (2006) Expansion of mesenchymal stem cells from human pancreatic ductal epithelium. Lab Invest 86(2):141–153

Shih B, Brown JJ et al (2009a) Differential gene expression analysis of subcutaneous fat, fascia, and skin overlying a Dupuytren's disease nodule in comparison to control tissue. Hand (N Y) 4(3):294–301

Shih B, Wijeratne D et al (2009b) Identification of biomarkers in Dupuytren's disease by comparative analysis of fibroblasts versus tissue biopsies in disease-specific phenotypes. J Hand Surg Am 34(1):124–136

Tonkin MA, Burke FD et al (1984) Dupuytren's contracture: a comparative study of fasciectomy and dermofasciectomy in one hundred patients. J Hand Surg Br 9(2):156–162

Verjee LS, Midwood K et al (2009) Myofibroblast distribution in Dupuytren's cords: correlation with digital contracture. J Hand Surg Am 34(10):1785–1794

Verjee LS, Midwood K et al (2010) Post-transcriptional regulation of alpha-smooth muscle actin determines the contractile phenotype of Dupuytren's nodular cells. J Cell Physiol 224(3):681–690

Wang X, Wang Y et al (2009) NGR-modified micelles enhance their interaction with CD13-overexpressing tumor and endothelial cells. J Control Release 139(1):56–62

Wielenga VJ, Heider KH et al (1993) Expression of CD44 variant proteins in human colorectal cancer is related to tumor progression. Cancer Res 53(20):4754–4756

Young HE, Steele TA et al (2001) Human reserve pluripotent mesenchymal stem cells are present in the connective tissues of skeletal muscle and dermis derived from fetal, adult, and geriatric donors. Anat Rec 264:51–62

Yu Y, Fuhr J et al (2006) Mesenchymal stem cells and adipogenesis in hemangioma involution. Stem Cells 24(6):1605–1612

Zuk PA, Zhu M et al (2001) Multilineage cells from human adipose tissue: implications for cell-based therapies. Tissue Eng 7:211–228

Using Laboratory Models to Develop Molecular Mechanistic Treatments for Dupuytren's Disease

22

Martin C. Robson and Wyatt G. Payne

Contents

22.1	**Introduction**	175
22.2	**Methodology of the Laboratory Models**	176
22.2.1	In Vitro Model	176
22.2.2	In Vivo Model	177
22.3	**Results Obtained from Use of the Laboratory Models**	178
22.3.1	In Vitro Model	178
22.3.2	In Vivo Model	179
22.4	**Discussion**	180
22.4.1	Role of TGF-B	180
22.4.2	Pharmacologic Manipulation of TGF-B Activity	180
22.5	**Conclusions**	181
References		181

M.C. Robson (✉)
Division of Plastic Surgery,
University of South Florida, Tampa, FL, USA
e-mail: robsonmd1@gmail.com

W.G. Payne
Division of Plastic Surgery,
University of South Florida, Tampa, FL, USA

Institute for Tissue Regeneration, Repair, and Rehabilitation,
Bay Pines Veterans Administration Healthcare Center,
Bay Pines, FL, USA

22.1 Introduction

It has been over 175 years since Dupuytren's initial description of a progressive fibrosis affecting human hands and digits (Verheyden 1983; Dupuytren 1834). The flexion deformities localized to the palmodigital aponeurosis associated with Dupuytren's Disease have been compared with other progressive human fibrotic conditions. It has been postulated that many of the same factors that contribute to the development of other progressive human fibrotic conditions such as hypertrophic scar, keloid, rhinophyma, and periprosthetic breast capsules also play a role in the development of Dupuytren's Disease (Kuhn et al. 2000, 2001, 2002; Payne et al. 2002; Pu et al. 2000; Robson 2003). These data suggest that these apparently diverse human physiologic disorders are pathophysiologically related (Kuhn et al. 2002). It is a known fact that a small percentage of Dupuytren's patients will simultaneously have other fibrosing conditions (Gonzalez-Martinez et al. 1995).

Both the cellular processes and the humoral messengers or mediators of the wound repair scheme have been discussed in relation to many of these fibrotic disorders (Robson 2003). An array of cytokines and growth factors orchestrate the sequence of normal wound repair. There are now significant data demonstrating that cytokines also play critical roles in abnormal wound repair and the formation of various human proliferative-type scars (Kuhn et al. 2001, 2002; Robson 2003). Evidence points to transforming growth factor beta (TGF-B) as the key cytokine that initiates and terminates normal tissue repair, and with sustained production participates in the development of pathologic progressive tissue fibrosis (O'Kane and Ferguson 1997). Data in animals suggest

C. Eaton et al. (eds.), *Dupuytren's Disease and Related Hyperproliferative Disorders*,
DOI 10.1007/978-3-642-22697-7_22, © Springer-Verlag Berlin Heidelberg 2012

that persistent overexpression or dysregulated activation of the cytokine TGF-B may lead to excessive scarring (Border and Rouslahti 1992; Border and Noble 1994), and other fibrotic conditions such as lung fibrosis, cirrhosis, glomerulonephritis, and scleroderma (Border and Noble 1994; O'Kane and Ferguson 1997; Robson 2003; Shah et al. 1995).

Of the isoforms of TGF-B, TGF-B1 and TGF-B2 have been associated with fibrotic conditions, whereas TGF-B3 tends to decrease fibrosis and scarring (Cox 1995; O'Kane and Ferguson 1997; Shah et al. 1995; Wang et al. 1999). Peripheral blood mononuclear cells from patients with proliferative scars have been shown to have higher levels of TGF-B2 than matched patients who did not develop proliferative scars (Polo et al. 1997). This work suggested that the fibroblast was an end organ that was responding to messages of a different intensity than those sent for normal mature wound repair (Robson et al. 2001). Fibroblasts from overexuberant fibrotic conditions, such as keloids, Dupuytren's Disease, rhinophyma, and periprosthetic breast capsules, show either overexpression of TGF-B2 or increased reactivity to TGF-B1, TGF-B2, or both (Kuhn et al. 2000, 2001; Lee et al. 1999; Younai et al. 1994, 1996; Wang et al. 1999).

It has repeatedly been demonstrated that TGF-B2 plays an important role in the fibrogenic nature of Dupuytren's Disease (Kloen et al. 1995; Viljanto et al. 1971). Fibroblasts are abundant within the affected palmar fascia and TGF-B has been demonstrated to be a stimulus for both collagen and noncollagen production by these cells (Badalamente and Hurst 1999; Hurst and Badalamente 1999; Lee et al. 1999).

One of the major problems in studying Dupuytren's Disease and other fibrotic disorders such as keloids is that they are known to be naturally occurring conditions only in humans and, until recently, there was no reproducible animal model. This has restricted the investigation of Dupuytren's Disease to in vitro techniques. In recent years, two laboratory models have been demonstrated to allow molecular and mechanistic studies to be performed on tissue harvested from human cases of Dupuytren's Disease and to fully evaluate the role of various TGF-B isoforms in the pathophysiology of this fibrotic condition. These models also allow new therapies to be proposed for treatment of Dupuytren's Disease. This review will discuss the methodology of these models and the data that have been obtained from them.

22.2 Methodology of the Laboratory Models

22.2.1 In Vitro Model

22.2.1.1 Fibroblast-Populated Collagen Lattice

The fibroblast-populated collagen lattice (FPCL) has been demonstrated to be the ideal in vitro model for the study of Dupuytren's Disease and other proliferative scarring and fibrosing conditions. There are differences in the normal wound healing process of fibroplasias with an overabundant deposition of collagen seen with excessive scarring in all organ systems (Murray and Pinnell 1992). These differences include increased collagen synthesis and deposition and decreased collagenolysis despite increased levels of collagenase (Robson 2003). A persistent imbalance in synthesis and breakdown of collagen favoring a net increase in fibroplasias results (Ketchum et al. 1974).

The process of contraction also is different in excessive scarring and fibrosis compared with "normal" healing. Although contraction is a normal process of wound repair, there appears to be an abnormal continuation of contraction in proliferative scarring (Robson et al. 1992; Robson 2003). It is possible that the excess of collagen encountered in overabundant scar impairs the activity of activated fibroblasts or myofibroblasts, rendering them unable to control a proper fibrillar arrangement toward normal repair (Linares 1988). Another possibility for the enhanced contraction is the excess production of isoforms of TGF-B, which have been shown to increase the contraction of FPCLs (Robson et al. 2001; Smith et al. 1999).

Since the fibroblast has been implicated in fibrosing disorders, the FPCL has proved useful for understanding these conditions. The methodology for the FPCL has been reported and is divided into four steps: preparation of fibroblast cultures, preparation of collagen lattices, assay for gel contraction, and immunoassay of the supernatant for TGF-B2 (Kuhn et al. 2002; Payne et al. 2006).

22.2.1.2 Preparation of Fibroblast Cultures

Primary cultures of fibroblasts can be obtained from Dupuytren's affected palmar fascia. Control fibroblasts can be obtained from the palmar fascia of carpal tunnel syndrome patients. From the primary cultures, cells from passages 3 to 5 are used for experiments. Following incubation and rinsing, the cells are subcultured until 80% confluence is obtained (Kuhn et al. 2002; Payne et al. 2006). After addition of trypsin-ethylenediaminetetraacetic acid, incubation, and addition of a trypsin inhibitor, the cultures are centrifuged, rinsed and resuspended three times (Kuhn et al. 2002; Payne et al. 2006). The cells are then counted and trypan blue is used to determine cell viability. The cell density is then adjusted to 5×10^5 cells/mL (Kuhn et al. 2002; Payne et al. 2006).

22.2.1.3 Preparation of Collagen Lattices

The collagen lattices can be prepared from Type I rat tail collagen as recommended by the manufacturer (Upstate Biotechnology, Lake Placid, NY). Undiluted collagen is placed in 35 mm culture dishes and 1 mL evenly spread. The dishes are then placed in an ammonia vapor chamber to solidify. Four rinses of distilled water are used to remove excess ammonia, and then the collagen gel lattices are incubated for 24 h at 4°C (Kuhn et al. 2002; Payne et al. 2006). An 18 gauge needle is used to detach the collagen lattices from the surface of the culture dishes so that they are loose and suspended in saline. Enough lattices are prepared to allow triplicate measurement from each specimen. Two milliliters of the 5×10^5 cells/mL suspension are placed on the surface of the prefabricated collagen gel lattices. If it is desirable to test potential treatment, such as an agent to abrogate or neutralize TGF-B, it can be added to the seeded lattices at this point (Kuhn et al. 2002; Payne et al. 2006).

22.2.1.4 Assay for Gel Contraction

The FPCLs are incubated at 37°C in a humidified atmosphere of 5% carbon dioxide. The amount of gel contraction can be measured every 24 h for 5 days. Acetate overlays are used to trace the area of the gels. Gels are performed in triplicate and measurements are calculated using digital planimetry and Sigma Scan software (Jandel Scientific, Corte Madera, CA). Each collagen gel area measurement is then converted to reflect the percentage of area remaining over time and subsequently the percentage of gel contraction (Kuhn et al. 2002; Payne et al. 2006).

22.2.1.5 Immunoassay for TGF-B2

The supernatant obtained from the culture medium following completion of the FPCL contraction is retained and used for a Quantikine human TGF-B2 immunoassay (R&D Systems, Minneapolis, MN).

22.2.2 In Vivo Model

22.2.2.1 Choice of the Nude Rat Model

In a condition which only occurs in humans, in vivo models of the pathologic disorder are difficult to design. Dupuytren's lesions have been produced in monkeys by traumatic disruption of palmar fascial fibers, but the capacity for study purposes has been limited (Larsen et al. 1960). Dupuytren's affected palmar aponeurosis explants have been maintained in an athymic mouse from which characteristics of histologic and electron microscopic structural changes following extended specimen explantation were determined (Kischer et al. 1989). The problem with the athymic mouse model is that only very small tissue specimens can be implanted, making repeated biopsy observations difficult.

The athymic "nude" rat model described by Polo and colleagues solves that problem and has proved extremely useful for the study of human proliferative fibrotic disorders (Polo et al. 1998). Outbred, congenitally "nude" (athymic) rats can be used to explant human tissue. These animals can be purchased commercially (Harlan Sprague Dawley, Inc., Indianapolis, IN). The animals are housed in pathogen-free barrier facilities, in cages with sealed air-filters, animal isolators, laminar flow units, and laminar flow rooms (Kuhn et al. 2001). All supplies including food, water, bedding, etc., must be sterilized to prevent infection in these immunologically compromised animals. Persons handling the rats need to wear caps, masks, sterile gowns, gloves, and shoe covers. All surgical operations on the "nude" rats are carried out under a unidirectional airflow biological hood.

In reported experiments, affected palmar fascia specimens from patients with Dupuytren's Disease are explanted into the "nude" rats in a two-stage procedure (Polo et al. 1998). The first stage is creation of a sandwich flap. The abdominal skin of the rat is incised along three sides, creating a flap based on the superficial inferior epigastric vascular pedicle. The prepared human Dupuytren's specimen is sutured to the inner surface of the flap. The flap is then returned to its bed, in the normal anatomic position. This surgical procedure results in a sandwich flap, which receives the entirety of its blood supply from the

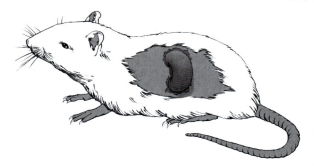

Fig. 22.1 Explanted tissue in tubed flap. A "nude" rat with a tubed abdominal island flap containing explanted human tissue from a patient with Dupuytren's Disease. The human tissue remains viable, isolated, and intact and can be manipulated and studied longitudinally over time

superficial inferior epigastric vessels (Kuhn et al. 2001; Polo et al. 1998).

22.2.2.2 The Sandwich-Island Flap

The final step in the preparation of the flap is initiated 3 weeks later. The femoral vessels, which arise 3–4 mm distal to the origin of the superficial inferior epigastric vessels are surgically isolated and divided, thus maximizing blood flow into the sandwich flap through the superficial inferior epigastric vessels. The sandwich flap can then be raised while isolated on its neurovascular bundle and tubed, converting it to a sandwich-island flap (Fig. 22.1). The flap, on its isolated pedicle, is then moved through a subcutaneous tunnel to the ipsilateral flank where it can be externalized and sutured in place on the dorsum of the rat (Kuhn et al. 2001). The abdominal donor site is closed primarily. The transfer of the island flap achieves two goals. It isolates the explanted specimen on a vascularized pedicle away from potential cannibalization, as well as facilitates observation and accurate measurement of the specimens. Importantly, this provides an isolated vascular pedicle delivering the blood to the explanted sample and, thus, allowing for direct perfusion of any test agents to the human tissue explant (Kuhn et al. 2001; Polo et al. 1998). Animals with explanted Dupuytren's tissue can be directly perfused with recombinant TGF-B2, anti-TGF-B2 neutralizing antibody, or a control substance.

In addition to placing the pathologic specimens into the "nude" rat flap, sections of the specimens taken directly from patients can be used for in vitro cell culture and proliferation kinetics (Kuhn et al. 2001).

Similarly, biopsies of the explanted tissue can be obtained serially from the sandwich-island flaps and can be used to determine potential treatment agent responses (Hayward et al. 1991). Assessment of DNA synthesis can be determined by ^{3}H-thymidine uptake of a cell lysate, and the amount of total protein synthesized can be determined by the ^{3}H-proline uptake (Kuhn et al. 2001).

22.3 Results Obtained from Use of the Laboratory Models

22.3.1 In Vitro Model

Kuhn et al. demonstrated the usefulness of the FPCL model in evaluating the role of TGF-B2 in Dupuytren's Disease (Kuhn et al. 2002). They compared the activity of fibroblasts from Dupuytren's affected palmar fascia with normal fascial fibroblasts obtained from cases of carpal tunnel syndrome. They also showed the effect of using an agent to downregulate TGF-B2 on the activity of Dupuytren fibroblasts.

22.3.1.1 Baseline TGF-B2 Levels and FPCL Contraction

When comparing the percentage of contraction over a 5-day study period, FPCLs populated with fibroblasts cultured from Dupuytren's affected palmar fascia contracted significantly more at days 1, 2, 3, 4, and 5 compared with the FPCLs populated with fibroblasts from the carpal tunnel controls (Fig. 22.2). From day two onward, the differences were quite marked ($P<0.001$) (Kuhn et al. 2002). There was a significant increase in TGF-B2 expression in the supernatant obtained from FPCLs populated with Dupuytren fibroblasts compared with the supernatant obtained from FPCLs populated from carpal tunnel affected fascia ($P<0.05$) (Kuhn et al. 2002).

22.3.1.2 Effect of Tamoxifen on TGF-B2 Levels and FPCL Contraction

FPCLs populated with Dupuytren fibroblasts that were treated with tamoxifen to downregulate TGF-B2 had significantly decreased contraction rates on days 1, 2, 3, 4, and 5 compared with untreated FPCLs ($P<0.05$) (Fig. 22.3). Although fibroblasts obtained from patients with carpal tunnel syndrome (normal palmar fascia) treated with tamoxifen did affect FPCL contraction on

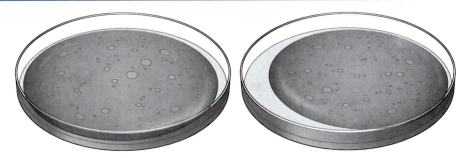

Fig. 22.2 FPCL Contraction. Contraction of the collagen lattice. *Left*: day zero; *Right*: day 3

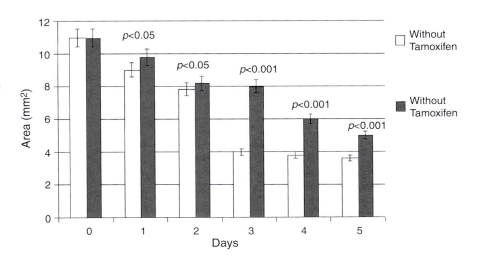

Fig. 22.3 Tamoxifen decreases activity of fibroblasts from a patient with Dupuytren's. Surface area of FPCL seeded with Dupuytren's tissue fibroblasts from Dupuytren's, showing inhibition of contraction by Tamoxifen

days 3, 4, and 5 compared with untreated fibroblasts, the FPCL contraction was to a lesser degree than that of the FPCLs containing Dupuytren fibroblasts (Kuhn et al. 2002).

Tamoxifen treatment of fibroblasts obtained from Dupuytren's affected fascia resulted in a significant downregulation of TGF-B2 expression compared with untreated fibroblasts. Supernatants from FPCLs populated with fibroblasts obtained from carpal tunnel fascia (normal) that were treated with tamoxifen did not show any significant downregulation of TGF-B2 compared with untreated fibroblasts (Kuhn et al. 2002). Just as tamoxifen downregulated TGF-B2 and decreased the activity of the fibroblasts from Dupuytren's Disease, it has been shown to have similar effects with fibroblasts isolated from the fibrosing condition of rhinophyma (Payne et al. 2006). Neutralizing antibodies to TGF-B1 and TGF-B2 have been shown to decrease contraction of keloid and burn hypertrophic scar fibroblast-populated collagen lattices (Smith et al. 1999).

22.3.2 In Vivo Model

Because Dupuytren's Disease does not occur in animals, the in vivo model of explanting human tissue into the "nude" rat serves as a useful tool for study. Kuhn and colleagues reported using the model to study cytokine manipulation of explanted Dupuytren's affected human palmar fascia (Kuhn et al. 2001). The Dupuytren's Disease tissue explanted into the "nude" rats remained viable in this system without any evidence of rejection during a 60-day study. Histological examination of the biopsies obtained at 30 and 60 days following explantation demonstrated maintenance of the parent human Dupuytren's tissue structure (Kuhn et al. 2001).

The report by Kuhn et al. described three groups of explanted tissue into sandwich-island flaps. One group was perfused with TGF-B2, a second group perfused with an antibody to TGF-B2, and a third group perfused with saline as a control (Kuhn et al. 2001). Masson's trichrome stain to demonstrate collagen of biopsies obtained at 30 days showed a higher intensity of staining for the TGF-B2 treated group compared with the control and TGF-B2 antibody-treated groups ($P<0.001$). There was also an increased intensity of staining for the control group compared with the TGF-B2 antibody-treated group ($P<0.001$) (Kuhn et al. 2001).

22.3.2.1 Collagen Assay

The immunohistochemical staining for collagen I or collagen III of biopsies obtained at 30 days demonstrated that the group treated with TGF-B2 had increased intensity of staining compared with controls and the TGF-B2 antibody groups ($P<0.001$). There was also increased intensity of staining for both collagen I and collagen III in the control group compared with the TGF-B2 antibody group ($P<0.001$) (Kuhn et al. 2001).

22.3.2.2 Cell Growth Kinetics

Biopsies of explanted Dupuytren's tissue obtained at 30 days and then grown in tissue culture were compared for the different groups in terms of their cell growth kinetics. TGF-B2 appeared to stimulate the cells to reproduce and proliferate significantly more than cells from explants treated with the control saline or the TGF-B2 antibody. In fact, cells from the 30 day biopsies of TGF-B2 perfused explants demonstrated an increased proliferative potential than the original biopsies of Dupuytren's tissue which had not been explanted or exposed to exogenous TGF-B2 (Kuhn et al. 2001).

These data are similar to previous data demonstrating increased Types I and III collagen production by keloid and burn hypertrophic scar xenografts in the same in vivo model of explanted tissue from fibrotic disorders into "nude" rats (Wang et al. 1999). Tissue cultures developed from explants of TGF-B2-treated keloid and burn hypertrophic scars also displayed increased in vitro cell proliferation kinetics and inhibition of these same biologic effects following treatment of keloid and proliferative scar with a neutralizing TGF-B2 antibody (Smith et al. 1999; Polo et al. 1999).

22.4 Discussion

22.4.1 Role of TGF-B

An abundance of data obtained from the laboratory models described, and other observations, confirms that the fibrogenic isoforms of TGF-B play a key role in the pathobiology of Dupuytren's Disease, burn hypertrophic scar, keloids, rhinophyma, and periprosthetic breast capsules (Border and Noble 1994; Border and Rouslahti 1992; Igarashi et al. 1996; Kuhn et al. 2000, 2001, 2002; Lee et al. 1999; Mancoll et al. 1996; O'Kane and Ferguson 1997; Payne et al. 2002; Pu et al. 2000; Shah et al. 1995; Younai et al. 1994, 1996). All of these conditions have in common excess fibrosis. The effects of TGF-B2 on scar formation may be the modulation of apoptosis or programmed cell death (Robson et al. 2001; Wassermann et al. 1998). It has been shown that the *bcl-2* proto-oncogene known to inhibit apoptosis is elevated markedly in the peripheral blood of patients with proliferative burn scars (Wassermann et al. 1998). Not only is this inhibitor increased in the peripheral blood, but also the fibroblasts in the corresponding scars show a significantly decreased level of interleukin-converting enzyme (ICE), an important effector of apoptosis. Together, these observations suggest that programmed cell death of fibroblasts is decreased markedly in cases of fibrotic scarring and that this may be mediated by the fibrogenic isoforms of the cytokine TGF-B (Robson et al. 2001).

22.4.2 Pharmacologic Manipulation of TGF-B Activity

If overexpression or dysregulated activation of TGF-B results in excessive scarring and fibrosis, then attempts to abrogate or neutralize TGF-B1 or TGF-B2 present potential avenues for novel treatment of fibrotic disorders. There are several ways to decrease or neutralize the TGF-B fibrogenic isoforms. As has been discussed, neutralizing antibodies to TGF-B1 and TGF-B2 have reduced proliferative scarring (Hayward et al. 1991), and decreased FPCL contraction by keloid, burn hypertrophic scar, and Dupuytren fibroblasts (Smith et al. 1999; Kuhn et al. 2002).

These observations have been extended to in vivo demonstrations that explanted human proliferative scar collagen production can be downregulated by TGF-B2 antibody (Kuhn et al. 2001; Wang et al. 1999). A third isoform of TGF-B, TGF-B3, can also be considered as an antifibrotic agent (Shah et al. 1995; Cox 1995; Occleston et al. 2008). There are other ways to attack overproduction of TGF-B1 and TGF-B2. McCallion and Ferguson have used exogenous mannose-6-phosphate to reduce scarring in rodent, porcine, and human wounds (McCallion and Ferguson 1996).

Decorin proteins have been used in the central nervous system to decrease fibrotic scarring known to be secondary to TGF-B1 (Logan et al. 1994). Decorins bind and neutralize all three TGF-B isoforms (Hildebrand et al. 1994).

Interferon gamma and interferon-alpha-2b have been demonstrated to downregulate collagen synthesis (Robson et al. 2001). Systemic use of interferon-alpha-2b has been reported clinically to decrease the volume of burn hypertrophic scars (Hildebrand et al. 1994). Its action on collagen has been postulated to be due to its ability to antagonize TGF-B gene regulation and production, normalizing levels of TGF-B1 and TGF-B2 (Robson 2003; Tredget et al. 1998).

As discussed, tamoxifen has been used to downregulate fibroblast activity and TGF-B2 expression in FPCLs populated with Dupuytren fibroblasts and fibroblasts isolated from rhinophyma (Kuhn et al. 2002; Payne et al. 2006). Tamoxifen inhibits the proliferation of fibroblasts harvested from fibrotic disorders, decreases the rate of collagen synthesis, and decreases production of TGF-B. Although tamoxifen is usually administered systemically and is fairly well tolerated when given orally, Hu et al. have suggested its use topically (Hu et al. 1998). Pujol and colleagues reported a percutaneous gel administration of tamoxifen in a small randomized study (Pujol et al. 1995). A chlorinated tamoxifen analog, toremifene, has been investigated experimentally in a topical methylcellulose formulation (Maenpaa et al. 1993).

Recently, two newer compounds have been suggested as potential treatments for Dupuytren's Disease. Imiquimod is an immune modifier that downregulates TGF-B and basic fibroblast growth factor (bFGF) (Namazi 2006). Finally, N-acetyl-L-cysteine (NAC) has been shown to abrogate TGF-B signaling and subsequent expression of fibrogenesis (Kopp et al. 2006).

The laboratory models discussed in this review can help to evaluate potential treatments with agents to abrogate or neutralize the fibrogenic isoforms of TGF-B, and by extrapolation to treat human fibrotic conditions such as Dupuytren's Disease.

22.5 Conclusions

Although the exact etiology of Dupuytren's Disease remains unclear, it is pathobiologically related to progressing fibrotic disorders. TGF-B plays a role in the pathogenesis of Dupuytren's Disease, as it does with other forms of fibrosis. Realizing that the overexpression or dysregulated activity of the fibrogenic isoforms of TGF-B and its attendant effect on apoptosis may be responsible for proliferative fibrotic scarring opens the route to propose rational molecular/mechanistic manipulations that can be tested for the prevention or treatment of these disorders (Robson 2003).

Proven laboratory models such as the in vitro fibroblast-populated collagen lattices and the in vivo explantation of human tissue into athymic "nude" rats provide a means to evaluate proposed treatments prior to the institution of necessary double-blinded, randomized, placebo-controlled clinical trials.

Acknowledgment Figures 22.1 and 22.2 courtesy of Mark Eaton, MarkEatonIllustration.com.

References

Badalamente MA, Hurst LC (1999) The biochemistry of Dupuytren's disease. Hand Clin 15:35–42

Border WA, Noble NA (1994) Transforming growth factor beta in tissue fibrosis. N Engl J Med 331:1266–1292

Border WA, Rouslahti E (1992) Transforming growth factor beta in disease: the dark side of tissue repair. J Clin Invest 90:1–7

Cox DA (1995) Transforming growth factor beta-3. Cell Biol Int 19:357–370

Dupuytren G (1834) Permanent retraction of the fingers produced by an affection of the palmar fascia. Lancet 2:222

Gonzalez-Martinez R, Marin-Berolin S, Amorrortu-Velayos J (1995) Association between keloids and Dupuytren's disease. Br J Plast Surg 48:47–48

Hayward PG, Linares HA, Evans M, McCauley RL, Robson MC (1991) Human scar in a "nude" rat model. Surg Forum 42: 612–614

Hildebrand A, Romarís M, Rasmussen LM, Heinegård D, Twardzik DR, Border WA, Ruoslahti E (1994) Interaction of the small interstitial proteoglycans biglycan, decorin, and fibromodulin with transforming growth factor beta. Biochem J 302:527–534

Hu D, Hughes MA, Cherry GW (1998) Topical tamoxifen: a potential therapeutic regimen in treating drermal scarring? Br J Plast Surg 51:462–469

Hurst LC, Badalamente MA (1999) Nonoperative treatment of Dupuytren's disease. Hand Clin 15:97–107

Igarashi A, Nashiro K, Kikuchi K, Sato S, Ihn H, Fujimoto M, Grotendorst GR, Takehara K (1996) Connective tissue growth factor gene expression in tissue sections from localized scleroderma, keloid, and other skin disorders. J Invest Dermatol 106:729–733

Ketchum LD, Cohen IK, Masters FW (1974) Hypertrophic scars and keloids: a collective review. Plast Reconstr Surg 53:140–154

Kischer CW, Pindur J, Madden J, Shetlar MR, Shetlar CL (1989) Characterization of implants from Dupuytren's contracture tissue in the nude (athymic) mouse (42859). Proc Soc Exp Biol Med 190:268–274

Kloen P, Jennings CL, Gebhardt MC, Springfield DS, Mankin HJ (1995) Transforming growth factor-beta: possible roles in Dupuytren's contracture. J Hand Surg Am 20:101–108

Kopp J, Seyhan H, Müller B, Lanczak J, Pausch E, Gressner AM, Dooley S, Horch RE (2006) N-acetyl-L-cysteine abrogates fibrogenic properties of fibroblasts isolated from Dupuytren's disease by blunting TGF-B signaling. J Cell Mol Med 10:157–165

Kuhn A, Singh S, Smith PD, Ko F, Falcone R, Lyle WG, Maggi SP, Wells KE, Robson MC (2000) Periprosthetic breast capsules contain the fibrogenic cytokines TGF-beta1 and TGF-beta2, suggesting possible new treatment approaches. Ann Plast Surg 44:387–391

Kuhn MA, Payne WG, Kierney PC, Pu LL, Smith PD, Siegler K, Ko F, Wang X, Robson MC (2001) Cytokine manipulation of explanted Dupuytren's affected human palmar fascia. Int J Surg Investig 2:443–456

Kuhn MA, Wang X, Payne WG, Ko F, Robson MC (2002) Tamoxifen decreases fibroblast function and downregulates TGF beta-2 in Dupuytren's affected palmar fascia. J Surg Res 103:146–152

Larsen R, Tagagishi N, Posch J (1960) The pathogenesis of Dupuytren's contracture. Experimental and further clinical observations. J Bone Joint Surg 42A:993–1007

Lee TY, Chin GS, Kim WJ, Chau D, Gittes GK, Longaker MT (1999) Expression of transforming growth factor beta 1, 2, and 3 proteins in keloids. Ann Plast Surg 43:179–184

Linares HA (1988) Hypertrophic healing: controversies and etiopathogenic review. In: Carvajal HF, Parks DH (eds) Burns in children: pediatric burn management. Year Book Medical Publishers, Chicago, pp 348–362

Logan A, Berry M, Gonzalez AM, Frautschy SA, Sporn MB, Baird A (1994) Effects of transforming growth factor–B1 on scar production in the injured central nervous system of the rat. Eur J Neurosci 6:355–363

Maenpaa J, Dooley T, Wurz G, VandeBerg J, Robinson E, Emshoff V, Sipila P, Wiebe V, Day C, DeGregorio M (1993) Topical toremifene: a new approach for cutaneous melanoma? Cancer Chemother Pharmacol 32(5):392–395

Mancoll JS, Zhao J, McCauley RL, Phillips LG (1996) The inhibitory effect of tamoxifen on keloid fibroblasts. Surg Forum 47:718–720

McCallion RL, Ferguson MWJ (1996) Fetal wound healing and the development of antiscarring therapies for adult wound healing. In: Clark RAF (ed) The Molecular and Cellular Biology of Wound Repair. Plenum Press, New York, pp 561–600

Murray JC, Pinnell SR (1992) Keloids and excessive dermal scarring. In: Cohen IK, Diegelmann RF, Lindblad WJ (eds) Wound Healing: Biochemical and Clinical Aspects. W.B Saunders, Philadelphia, pp 500–509

Namazi H (2006) Imiquimod: a potential weapon against Dupuytren contracture. Med Hypotheses 66:991–992

O'Kane S, Ferguson MWJ (1997) Transforming growth factor Bs and wound healing. Int J Biochem Cell Biol 29:63–78

Occleston NL, Laverty HG, O'Kane S, Ferguson MW (2008) Prevention and reduction of scarring by transforming growth factor beta-3 (TGF-B3) from laboratory discovery to clinical pharmaceutical. J Biomater Sci Polym Ed 19:1047–1063

Payne WG, Wang X, Walusimbi M, Ko F, Wright TE, Robson MC (2002) Further evidence for the role of fibrosis in the pathobiology of rhinophyma. Ann Plast Surg 48:641–645

Payne WG, Ko F, Anspaugh S, Wheeler CK, Wright TE, Robson MC (2006) Downregulating causes of fibrosis with tamoxifen: a possible cellular/molecular approach to treat rhinophyma. Ann Plast Surg 56:301–305

Polo M, Ko F, Busillo F, Cruse CW, Krizek TJ, Robson MC (1997) 1997 Moyer Award: cytokine production in patients with hypertrophic burn scars. J Burn Care Rehabil 18:477–482

Polo M, Kim YJ, Kucukcelebi A, Hayward PG, Ko F, Robson MC (1998) An in vivo model of human proliferative scar. J Surg Res 74:187–195

Polo M, Smith PD, Kim YJ, Wang X, Ko F, Robson MC (1999) Effect of TGF-B2 on proliferative scar fibroblast kinetics. Ann Plast Surg 43:185–190

Pu LL, Smith PD, Payne WG, Kuhn MA, Wang X, Ko F, Robson MC (2000) Overexpression of transforming growth factor beta-2 and its receptor in rhinophyma: an alternative mechanism of pathobiology. Ann Plast Surg 45:515–519

Pujol H, Girault J, Rouanet P, Fournier S, Grenier J, Simony J, Fourtillan JB, Pujol JL (1995) Phase I study of percutaneous 4-hydroxytamoxifen with analysis of 4-hydroxytamoxifen concentrations in breast cancer and normal breast tissue. Cancer Chemother Pharmacol 36(6):493–498

Robson MC (2003) Proliferative scarring. Surg Clin N Am 83:557–569

Robson MC, Barnett RA, Leitch IO, Hayward PG (1992) Prevention and treatment of postburn scars and contracture. World J Surg 16:87–96

Robson MC, Steed DL, Franz MG (2001) Wound healing: biologic features and approaches to maximize healing trajectories. Curr Probl Surg 38:61–140

Shah M, Foreman DM, Ferguson MW (1995) Neutralization of TGF-beta 1 and TGF-beta 2 or exogenous addition of TGF-beta 3 to cutaneous rat wounds reduces scarring. J Cell Sci 108:985–1002

Smith P, Mosiello G, Deluca L, Ko F, Maggi S, Robson MC (1999) TGF-B2 activates proliferative scar fibroblasts. J Surg Res 82:319–323

Tredget EE, Shankowsky HA, Pannu R, Nedelec B, Iwashina T, Ghahary A, Taerum TV, Scott PG (1998) Transforming growth factor-B in thermally injured patients with hypertrophic scars: effect of interferon alpha-2b. Plast Reconstr Surg 102(5):1317–1330

Verheyden CN (1983) The history of Dupuytren's contracture. Clin Plast Surg 10:619–625

Viljanto J, Seppala PO, Lehtonen A (1971) Chemical changes underlying Dupuytren's contracture. Ann Rheum Dis 30:423–427

Wang X, Smith P, Pu LL, Kim YJ, Ko F, Robson MC (1999) Exogenous transforming growth factor B2 modulates collagen I and collagen III synthesis in proliferative scar xenografts in nude rats. J Surg Res 87:194–200

Wassermann RJ, Polo M, Smith P, Wang X, Ko F, Robson MC (1998) Differential production of apoptosis-modulating proteins in patients with hypertrophic burn scar. J Surg Res 75:74–80

Younai S, Nichter LS, Wellisz T, Reinisch J, Nimni ME, Tuan TL (1994) Modulation of collagen synthesis by transforming growth factor-beta in keloid and hypertrophic scar fibroblasts. Ann Plast Surg 33:148–151

Younai S, Venters G, Vu S, Nichter L, Nimni ME, Tuan TL (1996) Role of growth factors in scar contraction: an in vitro analysis. Ann Plast Surg 36:495–501

Part V

Surgical Treatment

Editor: Paul M.N. Werker

Plastic Surgical Management of Scars and Soft Tissue Contractures

23

Paul M.N. Werker

Contents

23.1	**Introduction**	187
23.2	**Wound Healing**	187
23.3	**Scar Formation**	188
23.4	**Skin Scar Treatment**	189
23.5	**Scar Revision**	190
23.6	**Handling Skin Shortage and Skin Replacement in Dupuytren's Disease**	191
23.7	**Conclusions**	191
References		193

23.1 Introduction

In Dupuytren's disease myofibroblasts deposit collagen, giving rise to the formation of nodules and cords. As the disease progresses, the cords, for reasons not completely understood, shorten, giving rise to the development of contractures. These processes are akin to those occurring during scar formation following soft tissue injury, especially in keloid formation. Keloid formation – if it occurs – can be extremely difficult to handle. Generally speaking, a keloid cannot be cured and in this respect the difficulties encountered in keloid

treatment such as recurrence are similar to those for Dupuytren's Disease. The purpose of this chapter is to discuss aspects of wound healing and scar formation (including characteristics of keloids) and both nonsurgical and surgical treatment modalities to set the stage for the discussion of treatment methods of Dupuytren's disease.

23.2 Wound Healing

Any injury to soft tissue including skin will initiate a cascade of events, ultimately resulting in the formation of a scar. There is only one situation in which damage to the soft tissues does not result in a discernable scar, that is, whenever a wound is created and repaired in a fetus (Larson et al. 2010). The discussion of fetal wound healing, however, is beyond the scope of this paper.

Wound healing takes place in stages, which do overlap. Nevertheless, three stages can be discriminated: the inflammatory phase (day 0–5), the proliferative stage (day 3–week 3), and the remodeling phase [week 2-1 year (Lorenz and Longaker 2006)]. During the inflammatory phase bleeding is stopped (hemostasis) and white blood cells are attracted into the area of tissue damage. These white cells make great efforts to clean the wound of cell debris, dirt, and bacteria, and also initiate repair processes by attracting fibroblasts, endothelial cells, and keratinocytes from the surroundings. During this proliferative phase, fibroblasts synthesize and deposit the new tissue scaffold (extracellular matrix), endothelial cells start to create new capillaries, and keratinocytes make new skin. The extracellular matrix is filled with fibrillar collagen, predominantly

P.M.N. Werker
Department of Plastic Surgery,
University Medical Centre Groningen,
Groningen, The Netherlands
e-mail: p.m.n.werker@umcg.nl

C. Eaton et al. (eds.), *Dupuytren's Disease and Related Hyperproliferative Disorders*,
DOI 10.1007/978-3-642-22697-7_23, © Springer-Verlag Berlin Heidelberg 2012

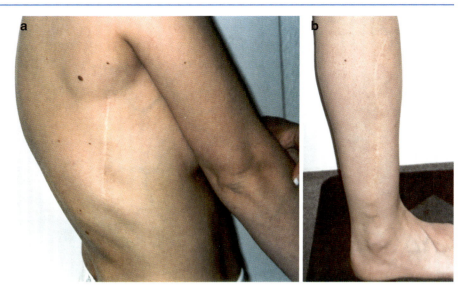

Fig. 23.1 Normal scars (**a**) on the right leg after harvest of a free fibula and (**b**) right side of the back after harvest of a free latissimus dorsi in a patient in whom two free flaps were needed to reconstruct a left lower limb

consisting of Types I and III. During the remodeling phase, a mature scar is formed: redundant collagen is degraded, whereas collagen which is in the right place and direction is strengthened by cross-linking, resulting in a dense package of collagen. Epithelial coverage is created by proliferating keratinocytes. This process, together with wound contracture, will ultimately lead to wound closure and the formation of a scar.

23.3 Scar Formation

The type of scar that is ultimately formed and its behavior in time depends on a great number of variables such as the general condition of the patient (nutritional state and underlying diseases), the age of the patient (young versus old), type of injury (crush versus clean cut), amount of contamination with dirt and bacteria, condition of the soft tissues (healthy versus damaged by radiotherapy, chemotherapy, systemic medication), location of the scar on the body, its position relative to skin tension lines (parallel versus perpendicular), the skin type (Roberts 2009), the amount of tension on the wound, wound management, etc.

A surgically inflicted scar, resulting from a well-planned and placed incision, respecting all the above in a healthy patient, usually remains within the borders of the original wound and may end as a fine line, which is hardly visible (Fig. 23.1).

Nevertheless, there are circumstances in which there is overgrowth within the limits of the original wound, leading to the formation of a so-called hypertrophic scar (Fig. 23.2).

In some cases, the scar tissue even grows beyond the borders of the original wound, giving rise to the formation of a keloid (Fig. 23.3).

These types of overgrowth are the result of ineffective or incomplete "stop" signals, which however are still not completely understood, but are thought to become effective once the dermal defect is closed and the epithelialization is complete.

Hypertrophic scars and keloids are both fibroproliferative disorders of wound repair with excess healing. As such, they share some similarity with the fibroproliferative diseases like Dupuytren's disease (Tredget et al. 1997). Since hypertrophic scars and keloids are unique to mankind, no animal models are available to study them under controlled conditions. Nevertheless, it has become clear from studies in humans that in both types of scars there is an upregulation of collagen synthesis, deposition, and accumulation. Especially keloid fibroblasts have been found to respond more profoundly to stimulation with exogenous TGFβ than normal fibroblasts (Bettinger et al. 1996). Research on myofibroblasts in Dupuytren's disease has revealed a

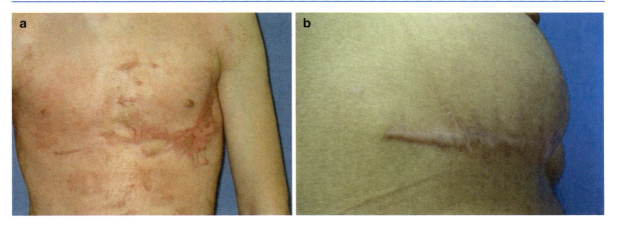

Fig. 23.2 Examples of hypertrophic scars. (**a**) Following healing of a deep dermal burn; (**b**) after breast reduction. (Courtesy Dr. M. Ruettermann)

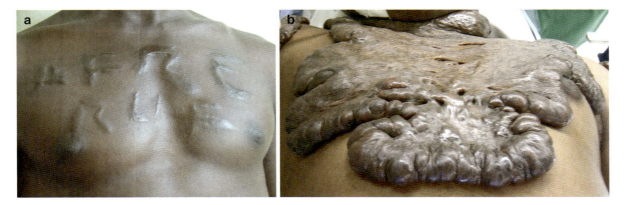

Fig. 23.3 Examples of keloids. (**a**) Following a mutilation by rebels in Africa; (**b**) unknown cause. (Courtesy Dr. M. Ruettermann)

similar response: fibroblasts form both nodules and cords respond to TGFβ-(1) more profoundly than fibroblasts derived from control tissue (flexor retinaculum) (Bisson et al. 2003).

Contracture is a normal aspect of open wound healing and helps to decrease the wound size. Besides, any linear scar has a tendency to contract, which in itself may cause functional or aesthetic problems, necessitating further action. In plastic surgery, we are not only faced with a great variety of skin scars. Scars may also form around tendons or joints and thereby limit function. Scar tissue may even form in response to the implantation of a foreign body such as a breast implant and cause capsular contraction. It can appear at the adaptation site of vessels or nerves hampering the passage of blood or the outgrowth of axons. Last but not least, pathological fibroproliferation may occur in diseases such as Dupuytren's, Ledderhose's, or Peyronie's for unknown reasons.

23.4 Skin Scar Treatment

There are various treatment modalities available for scars of the skin (Mustoe et al. 2002). Their application is dictated by the appearance of the scar, but usually consists of nonsurgical treatment. Widely used are the topical application of silicone gel sheeting, steroid injection and pressure, and 585 nm pulse dye laser, if erythema persists for more than 1 month. Whenever the primary wound conditions have been unfavorable, re-excision can be attempted.

Widespread burn hypertrophic scars can best be treated at burn centers with the earlier mentioned treatments combined with custom-made pressure garments, massage, and ultrasound. Ultimately, skin transpositions and transplantation might be unavoidable.

The treatment of keloid is even more difficult and should take place in specialized centers. Minor, immature keloids can be treated with intralesional steroid injections combined with silicone sheeting. More mature keloids usually do not respond to this treatment and need excision combined with low-dose radiotherapy on the fresh scar to reduce the rate of recurrence.

23.5 Scar Revision

Scar revision is the surgical procedure aimed to ameliorate all aspects of a scar (Parkhouse et al. 2006). This should be done using sharp blades and fine forceps and skin hooks that cause minimal tissue damage during the process of revision. Skin edges should be apposed correctly and everted, using multilayer sutures as appropriate. Transdermal sutures should be removed timely, to prevent the occurrence of stitch marks. Wound stabilizers such as tape or glue have been found to support wound healing (Coulthard et al. 2010).

Three basic types of scar revision can be distinguished (Borges, 1990): Fusiform excision, Z-plasty, and W-plasty (Fig. 23.4). They all aim to reconstitute anatomic landmarks, redirect the scar toward the resting skin tension lines (RSTL), and break the scar into smaller parts, which have fewer tendencies to contract.

An additional benefit of a Z-plasty is the elongation of the scar by a percentage, depending on the angle of the Z chosen. The maximal length gain at 60° is 73%. The extra length that is gained by the application of a Z-plasty is recruited from the skin area on both sides the scar. If the redundancy is limited, a multiple Z-plasty might be an option to achieve lengthening, without borrowing too much tissue from the sides. Any Z-plasty necessitates undermining to allow for the transposition of flaps. If skin conditions are unfavorable and blood supply is at stake, a Y-V transposition might offer a solution (Fig. 23.5).

Whenever the scar is too large to be excised without excessive tension, the scar revision must be staged. As an alternative, tissue expanders can be used to increase

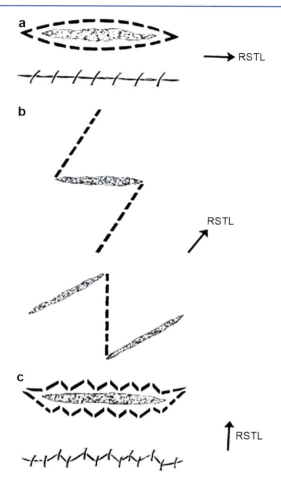

Fig. 23.4 Three methods for scar revision. The choice for each technique is dictated by the direction of the resting skin tension lines (*RSTL*) relative to the direction of the scar. (**a**) Fusiform excision; (**b**) Z-plasty; (**c**) W-plasty. (Reprinted with permission from Parkhouse et al. 2006)

the amount of skin available for closure. This method however carries more risk for complications than serial excision.

If there is skin shortage following scar release, and local skin transposition is no option, skin grafting is the method of choice. Skin grafts can be taken as full thickness skin grafts (FTSG) or split thickness skin grafts (STSG). FTSGs need the best possible wound bed vascularity to take because they are relatively thick, but give the best ultimate aspect of the scar area since they resemble normal skin the closest. They remain more pliable and elastic than split thickness skin grafts and are therefore more sturdy. Following dermofasciectomy in DD this is therefore the skin

23 Plastic Surgical Management of Scars and Soft Tissue Contractures

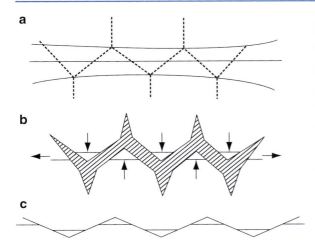

Fig. 23.5 Y-V plasty to increase length of scar. (**a**) Planning of incision (*dotted line*); (**b**) following incision; (**c**) final result. (Reprinted with permission from Parkhouse et al. 2006)

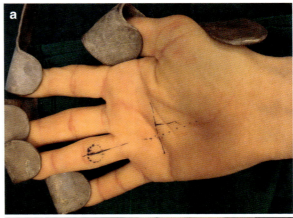

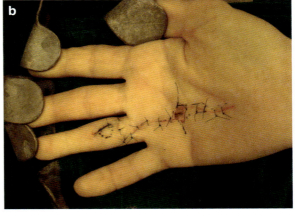

Fig. 23.6 Patient with DD in right ring finger. (**a**) Excision of pathologic tissue is planned using a straight line incision. (**b**) Skin shortage is corrected using a Z-plasty at the level of the proximal phalanx

grafting method of choice. However, the availability of FTSGs is limited, because the wound from which they originate can only heal by contraction and re-epithelialization from the skin edges if not closed primarily. Donor sites of STSGs, in contrast, heal by re-epithelialization from remaining epidermal appendages such as sweat glands and hair follicles. Their disadvantage however is their tendency to contract during the remodeling phase. For major burn contractures however, they frequently are the only option.

If wound bed conditions are poor (i.e., after irradiation) and local tissue is not available, wound closure can only be obtained using tissue from a more remote place that brings its own vascularization into the wound. In these cases, regional or distant pedicled flaps or free flaps are alternatives. In regional or distant pedicled flaps the vascular supply remains intact during and following transfer, whereas in free flaps the vascular pedicle is divided in the donor area and reconnected to recipient vessels in the scar area.

23.6 Handling Skin Shortage and Skin Replacement in Dupuytren's Disease

All wound healing principles and the aforementioned basic plastic surgical techniques also apply in the surgical treatment of Dupuytren's disease (McGrouther, 2005).

Linear incisions to remove pathologic tissue are usually elongated and broken by using Z-plasties (Fig. 23.6).

Zig-zag incisions can be elongated by the use of the V-Y principle (Fig. 23.7).

Skin defects following dermofasciectomy can be closed using full-thickness skin grafts or regional flaps such as the cross-finger flap (Fig. 23.8).

Rarely, if major defects remain, pedicled flaps such as a reversed radial forearm flap or a free skin flap might be options for reconstruction.

23.7 Conclusions

- At cellular level, there appear to be striking similarities between Dupuytren's disease and pathologic scars.

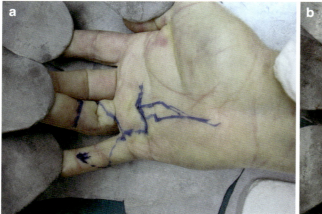
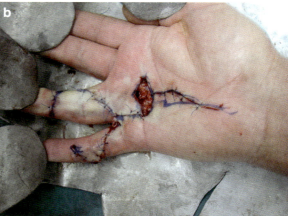

Fig. 23.7 Patient with DD in right ring and little finger. (**a**) Excision of pathologic tissue is planned using a zig-zag incision on the fingers. (**b**) Skin shortage of the fingers is corrected using a YV-plasty at the level of the proximal interphalangeal (PIP-) joint. In the palm, the wound is left open (McCash technique)

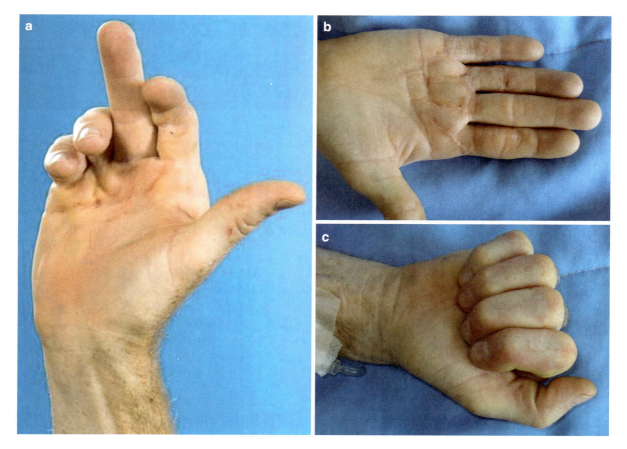

Fig. 23.8 Patient with severe recurrences of DD in both hands, treated by excision of pathologic tissue and affected skin and full thickness skin grafting. (**a**) Prior to surgery. (**b–e**) Functional result 3 months after the operation

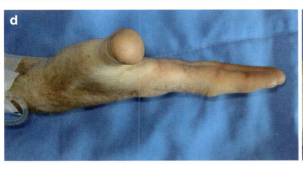
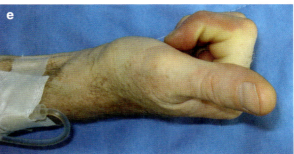

Fig. 23.8 (continued)

- Disturbed wound healing as seen in hypertrophic scars and keloids shows similarities with disease processes observed in Dupuytren's disease.
- Nonsurgical treatment options that are used in the treatment of pathological scars such as intralesional injection of steroids and radiotherapy are also applied in Dupuytren's disease.
- Skin management techniques in surgical scar revision are also routinely applied in skin management in Dupuytren's disease.

References

Bettinger DA, Yager DR, Diegelmann RF, Cohen IK (1996) The effect of TGF-beta on keloid fibroblast proliferation and collagen synthesis. Plast Reconstr Surg 98:827–833

Bisson MA, McGrouther DA, Mudera V, Grobbelaar AO (2003) The different characteristics of Dupuytren's disease fibroblasts derived from either nodule or cord: expression of alpha-smooth muscle actin and the response to stimulation by TGF-beta1. J Hand Surg Br 28B(4):351–6

Borges AF (1990) Timing of scar revision techniques. Clin Plast Surg 17:71–76

Coulthard P, Esposito M, Worthington HV, van der Elst M, van Waes OJ, Darcey J (2010) Tissue adhesives for closure of surgical incisions. Cochrane Database Syst Rev 12:CD004287, review

Larson BJ, Longaker MT, Lorenz HP (2010) Scarless fetal wound healing: a basic science review. Plast Reconstr Surg 126:1172–80

Lorenz HP, Longaker MT (2006) Wound healing: repair biology and wound and scar treatment. In: Mathes SJ (ed) Plastic surgery, 2nd edn. Saunders Elsevier, Philadelphia

McGrouther DA (2005) Dupuytren's contracture. In: Green DP, Hotchkiss RN, Pederson WC, Wolfe SW (eds) Green's operative hand surgery, 5th edn. Elsevier Churchill Livingstone, Philadelphia

Mustoe TA, Cooter RD, Gold MH et al (2002) International clinical recommendations on scar management. Plast Reconstr Surg 110:560–571

Parkhouse N, Cubison TCS, Humzah MD (2006) Scar revision. In: Plastic surgery, 2nd edn. Saunders Elsevier, Philadelphia

Roberts WE (2009) Skin type classification systems old and new. Dermatol Clin 27:529–33

Tredget EE, Nedelec B, Scott PG, Ghahary A (1997) Hypertrophic scars, keloids, and contractures. The cellular and molecular basis for therapy. Surg Clin North Am 77:701–730

Cline's Contracture: Dupuytren Was a Thief – A History of Surgery for Dupuytren's Contracture

24

A. Lee Osterman, Peter M. Murray, and Teresa J. Pianta

Contents

24.1	**Introduction**	195
24.1.1	The Hand of Benediction	195
24.1.2	Early Scandinavian History	195
24.1.3	The Curse of the MacCrimmons	196
24.1.4	Felix Plater	197
24.2	**Discussion**	197
24.2.1	Henry Cline Sr.	197
24.2.2	Sir Astley Paston Cooper	198
24.2.3	Postrevolution Paris	199
24.2.4	Baron Guillaume Dupuytren	200
24.2.5	Dupuytren's Fasciotomy	201
24.2.6	Guérin and Goyrand	202
24.2.7	The Modern Era	204
24.3	**Conclusion**	204
References		204

24.1 Introduction

24.1.1 The Hand of Benediction

There are no records in Greek or Roman literature describing the condition of Dupuytren's disease. The gesture of legality or truth as seen in Roman statues mirrors the classic contracture seen in Dupuytren's (Fig. 24.1).

A.L. Osterman (✉) • T.J. Pianta
Thomas Jefferson University Hospital,
The Philadelphia Hand Center, P.C. 700 South Henderson
Road, Suite 200, King of Prussia, PA 19406, USA
e-mail: alosterman@handcenters.com

P.M. Murray
Department of Orthopaedic Surgery, Mayo Clinic,
Jacksonville, FL, USA

There is also unsubstantiated speculation that the gesture of Benediction used in the early Christian church may be a reference to Dupuytren's disease. This gesture involves extension of the thumb, index, and long fingers with flexion of the ring and small fingers toward the palm (Fig. 24.2).

While the "Hand of Benediction" is thought to be a Christian symbol, it probably represents a superimposition of an earlier Roman gesture on the Christian church. The hand gesture is found on a gold glass in the Museo Sacro at the Vatican depicting Pope Xystus II (257–258 A.D.) indicating that the symbol dates back to that time (Elliot 1988a). The striking resemblance of the hand position portrayed in the Hand of Benediction to that commonly seen in Dupuytren's patients, however, begs the question as to how ancient is this condition?

A recent report suggests that Dupuytren's may be found in ancient Egypt (Garcia-Guixé et al. 2010). The Monthemhat Project analyzed 18 mummies, probably from the Third Intermediate Period (1010–820 B.C.), and reported the diagnosis of Dupuytren's contracture involving the left hand of one of the male mummies. If this is true, this identifies a case of Dupuytren.s nearly 2000 years before the earliest reports of Dupuytren's in Orkney and Iceland in the twelfth and thirteenth centuries.

24.1.2 Early Scandinavian History

As Dupuytren's disease is common among people of Northern European decent, historians have looked toward early Scandinavian written tradition in an attempt to find direct evidence of the disease in the early literature of northern Europe. Four miracle cures in the ancient

C. Eaton et al. (eds.), *Dupuytren's Disease and Related Hyperproliferative Disorders*,
DOI 10.1007/978-3-642-22697-7_24, © Springer-Verlag Berlin Heidelberg 2012

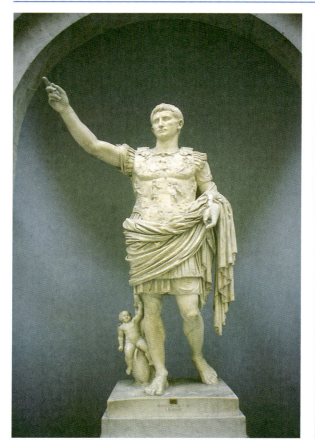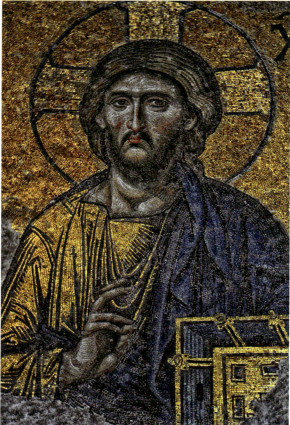

Fig. 24.1 Augustus of the Prima Porta. The Roman symbol for justice and truth in this statue of Augustus Caesar mimics the hand contracture of Dupuytrens. Augustus of the Prima Porta, c. first century A.D., Vatican Museum, Italy. (Photo obtained online from Flikr.com)

Fig. 24.2 Deësis Mosaic, Hagia Sophia. The Hand of Benediction as seen in the Mosaic of the Deësis (1261) basilica Hagia Sophia may be a superimposition of the Roman gesture. Detail from the Mosaic of the Deësis, c. 1261, Hagia Sophia, Istanbul, Turkey. (Photo obtained online from Flickr.com)

Icelandic sagas describe conditions of the hand that resemble Dupuytren's disease. The miracles are set in the twelfth and thirteenth centuries and are recorded in the sagas of the Earls of Orkney and of the Bishops of Iceland (Whaley and Elliot 1993). An interesting account from c. 1200 describes a female servant massaging the feet of priest Guomundr. This woman had "a hand unusable for work, since three fingers lay clenched into the palm," and Guomundr became frustrated that she was working too slowly. Out of frustration, he thrust his foot against the floorboard and her crippled hand got caught under his heel. While painful initially, the servant was rewarded when within a few days those same contracted fingers were quite straight. This may be one of the first historical reports of traumatic rupture of Dupuytren's contracture (Sirotakova and Elliot 1997).

24.1.3 The Curse of the MacCrimmons

Another likely early account of Dupuytren's disease comes from sixteenth century Scotland. The condition was then known as the "Curse of the MacCrimmons," named after members of the MacCrimmon clan, who were bagpipers to the chieftains of the Clan MacLeod of Skye in the sixteenth century. Members of the clan were thought cursed by a condition that led to a bent small finger, making playing the bagpipes nearly impossible (Elliot 1988a). This curse had important social consequences, as accomplished bagpipers held high positions in Scottish society in the 1700s, and loss of hand function was associated with loss of their prestigious positions among the society. It is presumed that this condition of a bent small finger represented Dupuytren's disease and not camptodactyly since it affected mature, accomplished adult pipers. Interestingly, Dupuytren's disease remains common among today's bagpipers, and it is still termed the "Curse of the MacCrimmons" by some Scottish pipers.

24.1.4 Felix Plater

The earliest account of a flexion deformity of the hand in medical literature comes from Felix Plater (1536–1614) of Basel, Switzerland. In his book, *Observationum in Hominis Affectibus* (Plater, 1614), in which autopsy findings were cataloged, Plater described a case of a stonecutter who presented with a fixed flexion contracture of the ring and small digits (Fig. 24.3).

"A certain well-known master mason, on rolling a large stone, caused the tendons to the ring and little fingers in the palm of the left hand to cease to function. They contracted and in doing so were loosed from the bonds by which they are held and became raised up, as two cords forming a ridge under the skin. These two fingers will remain contracted and drawn in forever" (Elliot 1988a). Plater's account that the disease of the hand was caused by shortening and dislocation of the flexor tendons is thought to be due to a misinterpretation of the original Latin text, rather than an erroneous description of the disease process. Plater was an accomplished anatomist, and he used anatomical studies to prove that the subcutaneous ligamentous extensions of the palmar aponeurosis were responsible for the disease, not the flexor tendons. Therefore, it is Plater who realized over 200 years prior to Dupuytren that the palmar aponeurosis was the anatomical substrate of the disease (Belusa et al. 1995).

24.2 Discussion

24.2.1 Henry Cline Sr.

After Plater's description of hand contracture in 1614, the medical literature is sparse on this topic until the time of the great anatomist-surgeons of late eighteenth century Europe. One such anatomist-surgeon was Henry Cline Sr. (1750–1827) (Fig. 24.4).

Cline was a pupil of John Hunter, who is widely known as the father of British surgery. While little-known today, Henry Cline Sr. was a prominent London

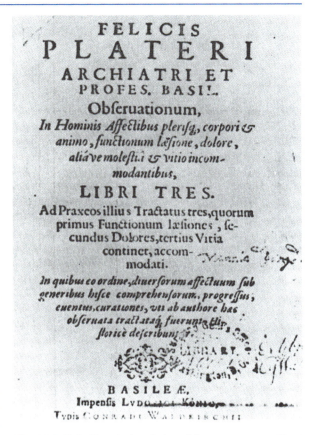

Fig. 24.3 Felix Plater's description of finger contracture. Front page from Felix Plater's book *Observationum in Hominis Affectibus* (Plater 1614)

surgeon in his time. Born in 1750, he was apprenticed at the age of 17 to Thomas Smith and was appointed Lecturer in Anatomy and Surgery to St. Thomas Hospital in 1781. In 1777, the year of Guillaume Dupuytren's birth, Cline dissected two cadaver hands that had contractures of the fingers. An entry from his notebook recorded the involvement of the palmar fascia and the effect of dividing it (Cline Sr. 1777). It was in these notes that Cline recognized the disease as one of "laborious people." Soon after, in 1778, one of Cline's students Richard Whitfield recorded in his lecture notes that Cline proposed an operative cure for the disease by palmar fasciotomy, although the procedure had not yet been performed at the time (Cline Sr. 1787). This is the first known description of surgical treatment for Dupuytren's disease. The same lecture also made reference to the accidental treatment of finger contracture by rupture after a patient let a large book fall on his fingers.

year, he resigned his clinical post to his son, Henry Cline Jr. The notes of student John Windsor describe the state of the art in 1808 as expressed in a lecture by Henry Cline Jr. (1808).

> One or more of these tendinous columns of the aponeurosis palmaris sometimes becomes contracted and thickened; most generally one only is affected, but sometimes more, and proportionably so many fingers are bent into the palm of the hand. The treatment is easy and efficacious; it consists in cutting through the aponeurosis with a common knife. In performing the operation, carefully dissect through, fibre by fibre, the aponeurosis Palmaris, in order to avoid the blood-vessels and nerves beneath; the finger or fingers may be kept extended afterwards by a splint, for the flexor muscle has in some degree become shortened, and without this the disease might be reproduced.

Cline thus had laid out the foundations of Dupuytren's contracture long before Dupuytren.

24.2.2 Sir Astley Paston Cooper

Cline Sr's most lasting influence, however, was not his original description of Dupuytren's disease, but rather the bringing together of John Hunter and Sir Astley Paston Cooper (1768–1841) (Fig. 24.5).

Cooper was born in 1768 at Brooke Hall near Norwich England. In 1784, at the age of 16, the young Cooper was sent by his parents to study with his uncle, William Cooper, then senior surgeon at Guy's Hospital. Guy's Hospital and St. Thomas Hospital were closely associated at that time, and William Cooper sent his young nephew to apprentice with Henry Cline Sr, who was newly appointed to St. Thomas Hospital. Under Cline, Astley Cooper quickly found enthusiasm for surgery, anatomy, and for the teachings of John Hunter. He said "if I laid my head upon my pillow at night without having dissected something in the day, I should think I had lost the day" (Verheyden 1983).

While John Hunter was thought publically as uncouth, and his lectures boring, Cooper was handsome and pleasant and a gifted lecturer. He spoke widely in support of John Hunter in the 5 years he apprenticed with Cline, and in 1789, a 22-year partnership between Cline and Cooper began. This partnership dominated surgical teaching in London for decades to follow until Cline's retirement in 1811. Cooper continued partnership with Cline's son until Cline Jr's untimely death in 1820. Cooper rapidly became well known and wealthy soon after beginning his medical

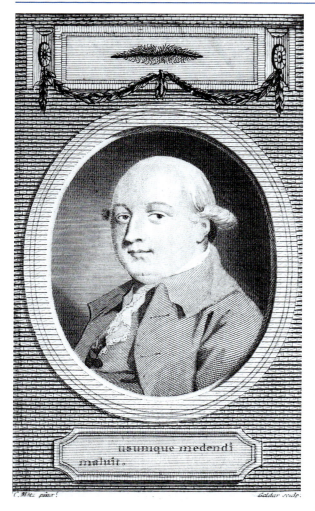

Fig. 24.4 Presumed portrait of Henry Cline Sr. (1750–1827). (Photo reprinted with permission by Wellcome Library, London)

Henry Cline Sr. both anatomically described the condition now known as Dupuytren's disease, and proposed a surgical treatment for the condition. It is unclear why credit is given to Dupuytren, except perhaps because Cline did not publish his finding and surgical practices. He was a devoted family man and did not care for writing. He did, however, teach and lecture and play an important role in spreading the word of the new discipline of surgery throughout England. It is, in fact, from the notes of his teachings recorded by his students that we know of his original description of a disease of the palmar fascia leading to finger contractures. His teaching continued until 1811, when he retired from his teaching appointment. The following

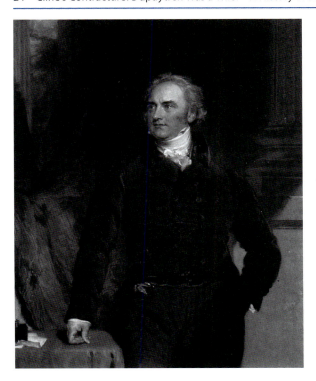

Fig. 24.5 Sir Astley Paston Cooper (1768–1841). (Photo reprinted with permission by Wellcome Library, London)

practice, but he always maintained a commitment to the treatment of the poor.

Cooper was undoubtedly a well-respected anatomist and surgeon in his time, and he also holds an important place in the description of Dupuytren's disease. In a description in his book, *A Treatise on Dislocations and Fractures of the Joints*, 1822, he described the condition of palmar fibromatosis as follows:

> The fingers are sometimes contracted in a similar manner by a chronic inflammation of the thecae, and aponeurosis of the palm of the hand, from excessive use of the hand in the use of the hammer, the oar, ploughing, etc., etc. When the thecae are contracted, nothing should be attempted for the patient's relief, as no operation, or other means, will succeed; but when the palmar aponeurosis is the cause of contraction, and the contracted band is narrow, it may with advantage be divided by a pointed bistoury, introduced through a very small wound in the integument. The finger is then extended, and a splint is applied to preserve it in the straight position.

This statement indicates an understanding of the difference between palmar contractures arising from disorders of the flexor tendon, as opposed to the palmar aponeurosis. Later, Cooper was misquoted by

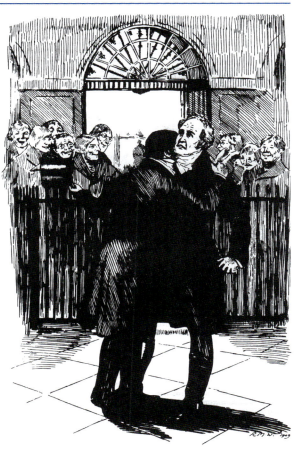

Fig. 24.6 Dupuytren's visit to Guy's Hospital, London, in 1826. (Illustration from Wilks and Bettany's *A Biographical History of Guy's Hospital*, 1892)

Dupuytren, and said to have made an absolute statement that Dupuytren's disease is incurable. There is no record of Cooper ever stating that Dupuytren's disease is incurable. Rather, he recognized that disease affecting the palmar aponeurosis, not the tendons, was amenable to surgical treatment via subcutaneous fasciotomy. Dupuytren visited Cooper in London in 1826 (Fig. 24.6), and on several other occasions. He would have been more than aware of the works of Cline and Cooper on hand contracture.

24.2.3 Postrevolution Paris

While not considered distant lands by today's standards, London and Paris were a world apart in their medical views at the turn of the nineteenth century. By

the name "le paratrime palmaire" (Elliot 1999). Baron Alexis Boyer (1757–1833) referred to earlier descriptions of "crispatura tendinum," a condition where contraction of the fingers was a result of drying, hardening, and stiffening of the flexor tendons and the overlying skin. In 1826, Boyer published his 11th and final volume of the massive works, the *Traité des Maladies Chirurgicales*. In this, he declared that the theory of "crispatura tendinum" was the current French surgical understanding of finger contractures. This was nearly 50 years after Cline's anatomical dissection and description of finger contractures resulting from disease of the palmar fascia, not the flexor tendons.

24.2.4 Baron Guillaume Dupuytren

It was Mailly, one of Boyer's pupils, who in 1831 first involved Baron Guillaume Dupuytren (1777–1835) in the treatment of hand contractures. Dupuytren was born October 5, 1777 the son of a lawyer (Fig. 24.7). His grandfather and two uncles were surgeons before him. Though Dupuytren wanted to join the army, his father instead sent him to Paris to become a surgeon. He was assistant surgeon to Phillippe-Joseph Pelletan at the Hôtel-Dieu in Paris by age 25, and the two had many conflicts. In 1815, at age 38, Dupuytren was named head surgeon at Hôtel-Dieu. This started the "Age of Dupuytren" in Paris medicine.

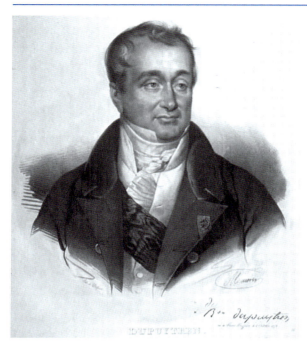

Fig. 24.7 Baron Guillaume Dupuytren (1777–1835). (Image obtained online from http://commons.wikimedia.org, public domain, copyright expired)

1822, Cline and Cooper, in London, had theorized an origin of what is now known as Dupuytren's disease in the palmar aponeurosis. They also supported a surgical treatment with fasciotomy. The fact that little interest mounted for the surgical treatment of palmar contracture is likely a reflection of the times. Without anesthesia and with frequent postoperative sepsis leading to death, there were likely few candidates for elective hand surgery.

In Paris, change in the practice of medicine was mounting in the early 1800s. In the late 1700s with the French Revolution, the old way of medicine was abolished. Under Napoleon Bonaparte, new medical schools were formed and a new generation of thinking men became largely responsible for the creation of modern medicine as we know it today. Contracture of the palmar fascia soon appeared in the new medical texts and journals having a variety of suggested etiologies.

In 1813, Chomel suggested in his graduate thesis that flexion contractures of the fingers were a complaint associated with rheumatism or gout. In 1832, Baron Alibert, the father of dermatology in France, may have described the condition of Dupuytren's disease under

Dupuytren was an accomplished teacher and surgeon with legendary powers of diagnosis. He kept a grueling schedule arriving at the hospital at 6 a.m. for 3 h of morning rounds. He then held a daily lecture for up to 500 medical students and followed lecture with surgery. After surgery, he saw free consultations in clinic and was said to show the same attention to the indigent as the rich. He returned to Hôtel-Dieu by 7–8 p.m. for postoperative rounds, and finally devoted his nights to the laboratory (Gudmundsson et al. 2003). He was a high volume surgeon performing 764 major surgeries in the year 1818. He was said to have told his adjunct surgeon at Hôtel-Dieu "when I am away or ill, I expect you to act as my substitute, but I warn you, I am never away and never ill." Not only did Dupuytren contribute to the field of hand surgery, but he also described congenital dislocation of the hip, fractures of the distal fibula, Madelung's deformity, posttraumatic shock, and the depth of burns.

Dupuytren was dedicated to medicine, but his approach and personality aroused many enemies in the field. He was described by Jacques Lisfranc as an outlaw; the "brigand of Hôtel- Dieu." Percy described him as "the greatest of surgeons and the least of men." He was rumored to have been so cold as to follow a man with hand contractures for years only to obtain his body for dissection at death saying "I had kept my eye on him for some years, and was determined not to lose this opportunity of investigation (Dupuytren 1834)." Dupuytren's medical career was cut short by a stroke in 1833, and his death from pleurisy came 2 years later in 1835.

24.2.5 Dupuytren's Fasciotomy

Dupuytren, while accomplished in many fields of medicine, is best known today for his description of contractures of the hand, and the resulting eponym Dupuytren's disease. Dupuytren's involvement in the description of finger contractures began after referral of a patient from Mailly, one of Boyer's pupils in 1831. The patient (M.L), a wine merchant, presented to Mailly with a complaint of ring and small finger contractures on the left hand. Remembering Boyer's advice that surgery was ill advised for this type of condition, Mailly referred the patient to Dupuytren who was senior surgeon at Hôtel Dieu at the time.

By report, the patient had injured his left hand back in 1811, 20 years prior to his presentation to Dupuytren. While lifting a large cask of wine, he placed his left hand under the heavy object and felt a crack and pain in the palm of his hand. In the following days there was some pain and stiffness. The symptoms disappeared slowly and M.L noticed a gradual contracting of his ring finger toward the palm. Over many years, this progressed to the point that the ring and small finger were completely flexed and bent over the palm. He saw many doctors who thought the problem was with his flexor tendons and the only cure being to cut them. Dupuytren, however, was of the opinion that the problem did not lie with the flexor tendons, but rather with the aponeurosis of the palm. He suggested that several small resections of the aponeurosis would sufficiently restore mobility to the contracted fingers (Alexandre et al. 2005).

On June 12, 1831, Dupuytren, assisted by Mailly and Marx, performed his first fasciotomy for Dupuytren's disease on patient M.L. The ring finger was addressed first. Through a transverse incision over the level of the metacarpalphalangeal joint, the skin and then the palmar aponeurosis were divided with a scalpel, the latter with an audible crack. The ring finger immediately could be straightened. Dupuytren tried to address the small finger subcutaneously though the same incision to avoid inflicting more pain on the patient, but this was in vain. He had to extend the incision over the small MCP joint and make two more incisions to straighten the small finger, one at the level of the mid-proximal phalanx and the other over the proximal interphalangeal joint. The final incision, over the proximal phalanx, resulted in immediate small finger extension. Dupuytren deduced that thus incision was made at the point where the distal extension of the aponeurosis of the palm inserted.

All incisions were left open to heal by secondary intent. Postoperatively, the patient was placed in an extension splint. At first there was little pain, but over the next several days, pain, swelling, and suppuration set in and lead acetate soaks were initiated. The patient was also placed in a splint more skillfully constructed by Lacroix. By July 2, 1831, 20 days after the operation, all the wounds were healed. For the next month, the extension splint was worn followed by night splinting only. His finger flexion returned and by December of that year he was reported to be in perfect health (Alexandre et al. 2005).

It was December 5, 1831, when Dupuytren gave his now famous lecture on finger contracture. It was recorded and published verbatim by three of his assistants, Alexandre, Paillard, and Marx in the *Journal Universel et Hebdomadaire de Médecine et de Chirurgie Pratiques et des Institutions Médicales* in 1831. The article "Concerning finger contracture as a result of a condition affecting the palmar fascia; a description of the illness; a surgical operation that is suitable for it" is an account of the lecture, case presentation, and surgery that was performed by Dupuytren for hundreds of spectators. As was the practice in that time, surgeons would hold lectures in which a patient was presented, a topic discussed, and the surgery performed in front of the crowd to be observed by the students in attendance.

That day, Dupuytren discussed one of his patients, Jean Joseph Demarteau, who was approximately 40 years of age and a coachman. The patient had permanent contractures of the ring and adjacent fingers that developed over years without any known trauma. He demonstrated the subcutaneous bands that crossed the patient's palm and their exaggeration with attempted digital extension. Dupuytren reported having seen 30–40 such cases over the prior 20 years, and he denounced that the condition had any rheumatologic, gouty, or inflammatory cause or that joint pathology was the cause. He also dismissed the so-called crispatura tendinum theory that the condition arose from chronic thickening of the flexor tendons and loosening from their sheaths. Instead, while passing out drawings from one of his dissections, Dupuytren announced his own opinion that this condition resulted from the contracting force of the palmar aponeurosis and its distal prolongations to the sides of the fingers (Elliot 1988b.) Dupuytren firmly believed this disease was associated with chronic local trauma, but admitted there were cases in which this theory failed to fully explain the presence of disease.

After reporting to the audience his opinion of the palmar aponeurosis as the offending agent in finger contractures (which was Cline's observation back in 1777), Dupuytren then introduced his thoughts on surgical treatment. After misquoting Cooper as having previously pronounced the disease "incurable," Dupuytren proposed operation on finger contracture with fasciotomy. He retold the story of the wine merchant from the previous June, where fasciotomy through transverse incisions resulted in complete straightening of the digits. No acknowledgment was given for Cline and Cooper who, years prior, had also treated finger contracture with fasciotomy.

Why didn't these English surgeons get their appropriate credit? Why is it not Cline's or Cooper's disease? We believe Dupuytren consciously claimed the credit for himself. Being the egomaniac and "brigand" that he was, his goal was to further his own ambitions. Therefore, he never acknowledged Cooper except to misquote him. The prestige of the Hôtel de Dieu and the fact that Paris was the medical center of Europe while London was isolated and a less medically cosmopolitan city abetted his goal.

Cline predated medical journalism. By Dupuytren's lecture in 1831, Paris was the publishing capital of the new medical journalism with 3 weekly and 2 monthly medical journals. Dupuytren's lecture was the lead article in *Lecons Orales de Clinique Chirurgicale faites a L'Hotel – Dieu de Paris*. In his 1834 publication in Lancet, he chides previous authors who have "spoken incompletely" on the subject and fails to acknowledge Cline or Cooper for the original description of disease. His efforts paid off and he won the eponym.

24.2.6 Guérin and Goyrand

By 1833, Dupuytren's (and Cline's) theories of palmar contracture began to fall under scrutiny. Guérin wrote of a much younger patient from Dupuytren's clinic, at 22 years of age, with a more severe case involving all five digits of the right hand, including the thumb. Guérin noted that it was difficult to explain the involvement of the thumb based on Dupuytren's theory that the disease was of the aponeurosis alone as the thumb does not have extensions of the aponeurosis (Elliot 1988b). Jean-Gaspard Blaise Goyrand (1803–1866), a surgeon from Aix-en-Provence, also provided criticism of Dupuytren's work. He submitted meticulous dissections to the Académie Royale de Médicine of two hands from the same cadaver that were severely afflicted with finger contractures. He claimed that the skin was involved as it was closely bound to the underlying bands. He also claimed that the tendons and palmar aponeurosis were normal and that contracture was due to bands of new fibrous tissue. He noted some bands to pass from the palmar aponeurosis to the flexor tendon sheath or lateral borders of the phalanges, while others passed only from one point to another along the volar surface of the tendon sheath. A detailed description of each band followed, and from the description, it is clear that Goyrand considered the disease to lie anterior to the palmar aponeurosis (Elliot 1989).

Given that Goyrand's findings neither echoed Boyer's "crispatura tendinum" theory nor Dupuytren's retraction of the palmar aponeurosis, he wondered if he was describing a different disease. He believed strongly, however, that all descriptions were of the same disease, just that the anatomic structure responsible for the disease was not correctly determined. He explained to the Académie that Dupuytren's simple description of the disease being due to prolongations of the palmar aponeurosis could not be the case as this would not result in PIP joint flexion. Goyrand used Dupuytren's own patient, the wine merchant, to support his theory. Dupuytren had stated that to release the PIP joint of the small finger of the wine merchant, a second and third incision beyond the palmar incision was necessary. Goyrand felt that from the description of the location of each incision, the palmar aponeurosis could not have

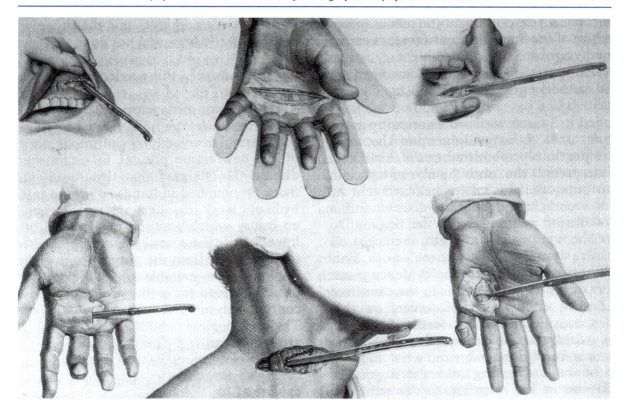

Fig. 24.8 Drawing from a French Atlas of Surgery from 1839. The drawing shows the incisions of Cooper (*bottom right*), Dupuytren (*top center*), and Goyrand (*bottom left*). (From Bougery and Jacob 1839)

been cut with these additional incisions (Elliot 1989). He also called into question Dupuytren's theory of this disease being due to chronic palmar trauma as he had observed the disease in nonlaborious people and in the nondominant hand of laborers.

Goyrand also proposed a variation in surgical approach to the disease, considering that he felt division of the new fibrous bands to be the only way to correct the deformity. He felt the transverse incision of Dupuytren gaped with finger extension and had to close by secondary intention therefore subjecting the finger to an increased risk of infection. Instead, Goyrand suggested the use of a longitudinal skin incision, and that the skin could be carefully detached from the fibrous bands with a bistoury. Each fibrous band should be approached via a separate skin incision, and any loose ends of fascia present in the wound after division of the bands should be excised. This was the first description of a limited fasciectomy (Fig. 24.8). Goyrand also supported the use of postoperative extension splinting, but felt it was important to take the operated fingers through a full range of motion each day to prevent stiffness (Elliot 1989).

Sanson, a member of Dupuytren's staff, proposed a theory of compromise between Goyrand and Dupuytren. He thought the bands described by Goyrand were not actually new tissue, but rather a proliferation of fibrocellular tissues present in a rudimentary state in the normal hand that extend into the fingers from the distal palmar aponeurosis (Elliot 1999). Sanson and Breschet, another of Dupuytren's staff members, presented hands dissected to show these rudimentary tissues to the Académie. Goyrand responded by attempting to prove by experimentation that the palmar aponeurosis could not entirely be to blame for Dupuytren's contracture. He divided the palmar aponeurosis, excised a segment, and resutured the remaining ends. This resulted in contracture of the MP joint, but the PIP joint remained unaffected. He therefore concluded that the disease was caused by bands of abnormal fibrous tissue that he called "the predigital bands." He believed that the palmar aponeurosis and its prolongations had no part in the condition (Elliot 1999).

Earlier, in 1832, Velpeau had concluded on clinical grounds that the disease did not always involve the palmar aponeurosis. Though he came to this conclusion a full year prior to Goyrand and Sanson, this was largely ignored. In his 1833 edition of *Traité Complet d'Anatomie Chirurgicale*, Velpeau stated that the superficial fibers of the palmar aponeurosis sometimes become raised as bands and prevent finger extension. It is very unlikely that Goyrand possessed this most current edition of the anatomy text prior to making his announcement to the Académie regarding the involvement of "predigital bands" rather than the palmar aponeurosis in the pathophysiology of Dupuytren's disease (Elliot 1999).

24.2.7 The Modern Era

The early history and surgery on Dupuytren's disease was about to proceed into the modern era of medicine. By the mid 1840s, the development of anesthesia ushered in the modern era of surgery. Dupuytren's surgery refined the pathophysiology of the contracture and proceeded through such operations as complete fasciectomy to limited fasciectomy as popularized by McIndoe and Beare in 1958 (McIndoe and Beare 1958). In 1964 McCash described the open palm technique to eliminate hematomas (McCash 1964). John Hueston, a student of McIndoe, contributed to our knowledge by defining the genetic predisposition, the prognostic factors of surgery, and dermatofasciectomy and skin grafting (Hueston 1963). Finally, the current popularity of needle fasciotomy harkens back to the type of release advocated by Cline and Cooper.

24.3 Conclusion

- Dupuytren's disease may have been depicted in early art symbols such as the Roman symbol of justice or the "Benediction Sign."
- The first medical writing on finger contractures was by Felix Plater in 1614.
- Cline and Cooper were the first surgeon anatomists to describe the condition now termed Dupuytren's disease in any detail. They also suggested surgical cure via fasciotomy.

- Dupuytren was a master surgeon of his time, but not well regarded by his peers.
- He stole the observations made by Cline and Cooper that the disease of palmar contracture was associated with diseased palmar aponeurosis.
- Dupuytren advocated the open palm transverse fasciotomy, which was meant to heal by secondary intension. He also was a proponent of postoperative extension splinting.
- Goyrand and Velpeau challenged Dupuytren that the disease was more complicated than simply involving the palmar aponeurosis, and Goyrand suggested the disease resulted from bands of abnormal fibrous tissue that he called "the predigital bands."

References

Alexandre, Paillard, Marx (2005) Report on the surgical clinic at the Hôtel-Dieu, 1831. J Hand Surg Br 30(6):546–550

Belusa L, Selzer AM, Partecke BD (1995) Description of Dupuytren disease by the Basel physician and anatomist Felix Plater in 1614. Handchir Mikrochir Plast Chir 27(5): 272–275

Bougery JM, Jacob NH (1839) Traité Complet de l'Anatomie de l'Homme comprenant la Médicine Opératoire, vol 6, Paris, Delaunay, 1839, plate 23

Cline H Jr. (1808) Notes of John Windsor (student) from a lecture by Henry Cline Jr., Manuscript collection. John Rylands University Library of Manchester, Manchester, pp 486–489

Cline H Sr. (1777) Notes on pathology and surgery, Manuscript 28. St. Thomas's Hospital Medical School Library, London: 185

Cline H Sr. (1787) Notes of Richard Whitfield (student) from a lecture by Henry Cline Senior, Manuscript 30. St. Thomas's Hospital Medical School Library, London

Dupuytren G (1834) Permanent retraction of the fingers, produced by an affection of the palmar fascia. Lancet ii:222–225

Elliot D (1988a) The early history of contracture of the palmar fascia (part I). J Hand Surg Br 13B:246–255

Elliot D (1988b) The early history of contracture of the palmar fascia (part 2). J Hand Surg Br 13B:371–378

Elliot D (1989) The early history of contracture of the palmar fascia (part 3). J Hand Surg Br 14B:25–31

Elliot D (1999) The early history of Dupuyten's disease. Hand Clin 15:1–19

Garcia-Guixé E, Fontaine V, Baxariasn J, Núñez M, Dinarès R, Herrerín J (2010) Estudio antropológico, paleopatológico y radiológico de las momias localizadas en el almacen número 4 de la Casa Americana (el Asasif, Luxor, Egypt): proyecto Monthemhat 2009. Studia Antiquitatis et Medii Aevi XIII(20). Ed. esp 3. Published electronically. http://www.hottopos.com/rih20/garciaguixe.pdf. Accessed May 2011

Gudmundsson KG, Jónsson T, Arngrímsson R (2003) Guillaume Dupuytren and finger contractures. Lancet 362:165–168

Hueston JT (1963) Dupuytren's contracture. Churchill Livingstone, London

McCash CR (1964) The open technique in Dupuytren's contracture. Br J Plast Surg 17:271–280

McIndoe A, Beare RLB (1958) The surgical management of Dupuytren's contracture. Am J Surg 95(2):197–205

Plater F (1614) Observationum in Hominis Affectibus. Libri Tres. Konig and Brandmyller, Basel, pp 140–146

Sirotakova M, Elliot D (1997) A historical record of traumatic rupture of Dupuytren's contracture. J Hand Surg Br 22B:198–201

Verheyden CN (1983) The history of Dupuytren's contracture. Clin Plast Surg 10(4):619–625

Whaley DC, Elliot D (1993) Dupuytren's disease: a legacy of the north? J Hand Surg Br 18B:363–367

Wilks S, Bettany GT (1892) A biographical history of Guy's hospital. Ward & Co, London

Cellulose Implants in Dupuytren's Surgery

25

Ilse Degreef and Luc De Smet

Contents

25.1	**Introduction**	207
25.2	**Impact**	207
25.3	**Cellulose Implant**	208
25.3.1	Firebreak Augmentation	208
25.3.2	Surgical Technique	208
25.3.3	Postoperative Regime	209
25.3.4	Outcome	209
25.4	**Discussion**	210
25.5	**Conclusions**	211
References		211

25.1 Introduction

Surgery in Dupuytren's disease is performed to correct contractures in the fingers and to maintain this effect after the operation (Bulstrode et al. 2005). Recurrent contracture is a frequent "complication" in the long term. In some cases, this occurs in a close period after surgery (within weeks), during the healing process. Although not all diseased tissue is removed in minimally invasive surgery, we have seen earlier that segmental fasciectomy does not hold a higher recurrent contracture rate (Degreef et al. 2009a). We concluded that although the surgeon can cut the strands to correct contractures, he cannot cure the disease with the knife.

I. Degreef (✉) • L. De Smet
Department of Orthopaedic Surgery,
Leuven University Hospitals, Weligerveld 1, 3212, Pellenberg, Belgium
e-mail: ilse.degreef@uzleuven.be

It is not the surgical technique that precludes recurrence, but the fibrosis diathesis. Patients at risk can be identified based on clinical parameters (Abe et al. 2004; Degreef et al. 2009b). In high risk patients with a high diathesis for Dupuytren's disease, recurrence can be fast and furious, within weeks after surgery. Myofibroblasts within the scar tissue and extending around the operated areas can initiate rapidly progressing and disabling contractures. Often, the skin is involved and diffusely retracted in these cases. The myofibroblasts align and attach to the deepest layers of the epidermis (Fig. 25.1).

We intended to improve the firebreak effect of segmental fasciectomy and disconnect the skin with the fibroblastic tissue in Dupuytren's surgery with a metabolically inert mechanical barrier. This inspired us to use cellulose implants, a known adhesion barrier (Farquhar et al. 2000).

25.2 Impact

Dupuytren's surgery is an important part of the hand surgeon's practice. At our department alone, we perform about 100 interventions for Dupuytren's disease every year, which is about 8% of the elective hand surgery. With a mean incidence of once a year, an amputation is chosen. This makes Dupuytren's disease a predominant reason for elective finger amputation in adults (Degreef and De Smet. 2009). An amputation in Dupuytren's disease is mostly done after surgery for recurrent disease with a hindering hooked finger deformity. In recurrent disease, surgery is more prone to complications (Coert et al. 2006; Roush and Stern 2000).

The high incidence in hand surgery practice is a direct consequence of the very high prevalence (1 male in 3) of the disease in all stages in people over 50, as

C. Eaton et al. (eds.), *Dupuytren's Disease and Related Hyperproliferative Disorders*,
DOI 10.1007/978-3-642-22697-7_25, © Springer-Verlag Berlin Heidelberg 2012

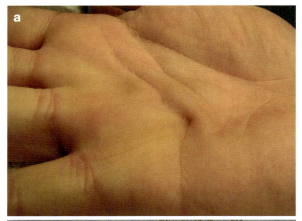

25.3 Cellulose Implant

25.3.1 Firebreak Augmentation

In minimally invasive surgery, the contractures are treated without the intention to cure the patient or to remove all diseased tissue. In fasciotomy, strands are interrupted with a knife or with a needle. In segmental fasciectomy, a small "firebreak" is created by removing a centimeter or less of the strands (or nodules). The intention of this firebreak is to avoid fast recurrent contractures caused by sectioned strands that may reattach if they make a direct contact. However, the hematoma that forms in these firebreaks, which are actually surgically created free spaces, may induce new adhesions that may bridge the interrupted strands in some cases. A collection of new myofibroblasts appears, forming recurrent nodules, skin retraction, and finger contractures in patients with a high fibrosis diathesis. Adhesion barriers are well known from infertility surgery (adhesiolysis). Its use has been extended in neurosurgery and also in hand surgery, where it is used to prevent adhesions and fibrosis after tenolysis (Temiz et al. 2008). This inspired us to use the cellulose implant (we use Divide™, DePuyMitek, Johnson & Johnson Medical Inc, New Brunswick, NJ) in Dupuytren's surgery.

Fig. 25.1 Clinical (**a**) and immunohistological (**b**) picture of the skin retraction in Dupuytren's disease. Skin retractions are often seen in more severe Dupuytren's disease, with the formation of skin "dimples" (**a**). This immunohistological micrograph illustrates the aligned myofibroblasts (stained with alfa-smooth-muscle actin, original magnification, ×400), attached to the deepest edge of the epidermis, actively retracting the skin (**b**)

25.3.2 Surgical Technique

Segmental fasciectomy is performed with small curved incisions overlying the strands on one to three places with intervals of 1 cm (Moermans 1991). Often, it is chosen to take out the most prominent nodules. After dissecting the strands, 5–10 mm of the strand is removed and by gentle manipulation, the fingers are forced to regain full extension. Care is taken not to harm neurovascular bundles.

In case of important skin retraction, we have extended the technique to loosen the skin (Figs. 25.2 and 25.3). The skin is further undermined, in some cases even centimeters from the incision site to loosen the retractions. In case of diffuse fascia retraction, a subcutaneous fasciotomy is performed in the neighboring palmar finger rays, to loosen the fascia palmaris.

After the fasciotomies, segmental fasciectomy and skin releases are all performed, careful hemostasis needs to be done with cauterization to prevent significant

we have seen ourselves in Flanders in a study of random people on market places (Degreef and De Smet 2010). Thus, there are a lot of patients needing advice from a lot of doctors. Since the disease is incurable, it is important that patients are well informed, soundly assisted within their disease, and surgical treatment is limited to the necessary for keeping the fingers mobile. "Doctor shopping" and over-treatment of patients by compromised caretakers with commercial interests is a risk that needs to be avoided. We need to optimize the efficiency of any treatment option.

25 Cellulose Implants in Dupuytren's Surgery

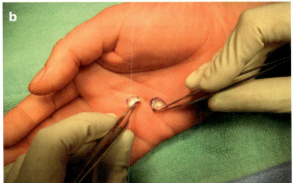

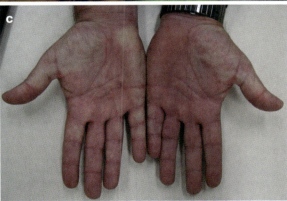

Fig. 25.2 Clinical and intraoperative images of a correction of skin retraction with cellulose implant and clinical results after 7 months. The skin retraction (**a**) is addressed with a curved mini-incision, the skin is dissected off the underlying fascia and a segmental strand resection is performed. After hemostasis, the cellulose implant is sized as needed and implanted in a horizontal single-layer fashion (**b**). Clinical result after 7 months (**c**), the retraction is corrected, skin and fingers are supple

hematoma formation. Then, the cellulose patch is cut into small pieces, to fit the free spaces that were created. The cellulose patch should be implanted in a horizontal single layer and cannot be "overstuffed." This could lead to prolonged wound drainage (as we encountered in the beginning of cellulose use in tenolysis, but until now, we have not seen in Dupuytren's surgery). The cellulose will liquefy within 48 h, forming a 3 dimensional passive adhesion or firebreak barrier. Dissolving skin sutures are used and the hand is wrapped with a firmly compressing softly padded dressing.

25.3.3 Postoperative Regime

Within 5 days after surgery, small band-aids are put on the skin wounds and early mobilization is initiated. An extension splint is manufactured to wear nightly for 8 weeks, the first 4 weeks also during daytime by means of an intermittent mobilization and splinting regime (2 h on – 2 h off).

25.3.4 Outcome

In a randomized controlled trial within 29 patients, segmental fasciectomy was compared with and without a cellulose implant (Degreef et al. 2011, summary reported with permission). All patients had a high fibrosis diathesis with scores of 4 and higher as described by Abe (Abe et al. 2004). They were known with knuckle pads, Peyronie's disease, Ledderhose disease, a young age of onset, multiple ray, bilateral and/or radial side involvement, and a positive family history. Patients were monitored with visual analogs scales for pain and satisfaction, DASH scores, and most importantly with goniometric measuring of the contractures, which was documented with standardized digital photography (Smith et al. 2009).

A significant improvement of the mobility of the fingers was confirmed in the trial (Degreef et al. 2011). A relative correction of 87% with the implant versus 51% without the implant was seen (goniometric coefficient in Tubiana et al. 1968). This reflected in superior satisfaction scores which increased by 27% with cellulose implants. After 3 months, the results remained unchanged (with a follow-up now of over 2 years). Although the correction is complete during the surgical procedure, a short period of rebound is

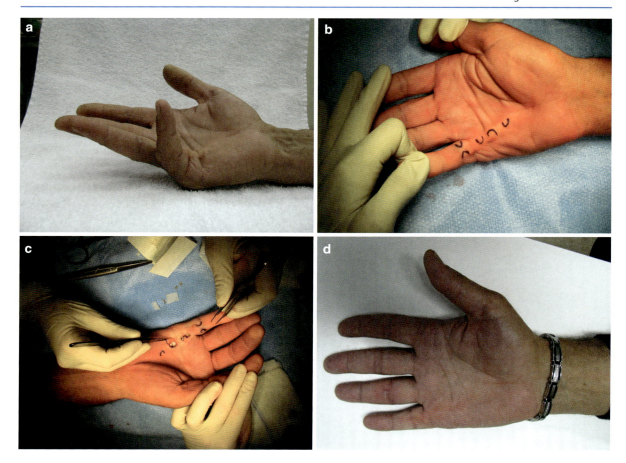

Fig. 25.3 Clinical and intraoperative images of a fifth ray contracture, which is treated with segmental fasciectomy and cellulose implants (**a**). The contracture of both the MCP and PIP joints is addressed with numerous small curved skin incisions (**b**). After segmental strand resection on all levels needed to achieve full finger extension, thorough hemostasis is done and cellulose is implanted in all wounds (**c**). A supple hand is seen days after the operation with a good clinical result after 7 months (**d**)

often seen, in which some of the correction is lost during the initial scar tissue formation during the first 12 weeks. Remember, these are all high-risk patients with a high fibrosis diathesis. This rebound phenomenon was reduced if the cellulose was implanted and no complications were seen.

Although difficult to measure, we saw an impressive quick and easy rehabilitation in the patients with the implants. When the small band-aids were set at 5 days, they all had a supple and painless full range of motion. After 8–10 weeks, the scar tissue did harden again in most cases, as it did in the patients without the implant. However, all patients with the implant had easily regained a normal mobility at that point, contrasting to the patients without.

We now use the cellulose implant at a regular basis at our office and we continue to see easy rehabilitation and good skin mobility after the surgery, without recurrent contraction.

25.4 Discussion

We have stated that surgery is only used in Dupuytren's disease to correct contractures, not to cure the disease. We saw that minimally invasive surgery does not imply higher recurrence risks. Fibrosis diathesis remains the most important way to determine if recurrence is imminent (Degreef et al. 2009c). In severe diathesis, recurrence is often fast within the period of scar tissue formation. In the technique of segmental fasciectomy, firebreaks are created within the strands. To augment this firebreak effect, we have now added the dissolving adhesion barrier and passive fibrosis inhibitor cellulose. We have seen an easy rehabilitation with an improved outcome and high satisfaction rate in high-risk patients with a severe fibrosis diathesis. Our group now uses the implant on a regular basis to improve the results of minimally invasive surgical techniques and to release retracted overlying skin. Future studies are conducted to continue the monitoring of the results of this innovative technique. It looks promising and holds new possible pathways, in which active myofibroblast inhibiting substances may be added to the implant material.

25.5 Conclusions

- Cellulose implants significantly improve surgical outcome in patients with diathesis.
- The firebreak effect is augmented and skin retractions are released.
- Finger extension is improved and satisfaction is high.
- The implant is well-tolerated and rehabilitation is facilitated.
- Future pathways of adding an active substance to the implant are considered.

References

Abe Y, Rokkaku T, Ofuchi S, Tokunaga S, Takahashi K, Moriya H (2004) An objective method to evaluate the risk of recurrence and extension of Dupuytren's disease. J Hand Surg [Br] 29B:427–430

Bulstrode NW, Jemec B, Smith PJ (2005) The complications of Dupuytren's contracture surgery. J Hand Surg [Am] 30A: 1021–1025

Coert JH, Nérin JP, Meek MF (2006) Results of partial fasciectomy for Dupuytren disease in 261 consecutive patients. Ann Plast Surg 57:13–17

Degreef I, De Smet L (2009) Dupuytren's disease: predominant reason for elective finger amputation in adults. Acta Chir Belg 109:494–497

Degreef I, De Smet L (2010) A high prevalence of Dupuytren's disease in Flanders. Acta Orthop Belg 76(3):316–320

Degreef I, Boogmans T, Steeno P, De Smet L (2009a) Surgical outcome of Dupuytren's disease. No higher self-reported recurrence after segmental fasciectomy. Eur J Plast Surg 32:185–188

Degreef I, De Smet L, Sciot R, Cassiman JJ, Tejpar S (2009b) Beta-catenin overexpression in Dupuytren's disease is unrelated to disease recurrence. Clin Orthop Relat Res 467: 838–845

Degreef I, Vererfvre PB, De Smet L (2009c) Effect of severity of Dupuytren contracture on disability. Scand J Plast Reconstr Surg Hand Surg 43:41–42

Degreef I, Tejpar S, De Smet L (2011) Postoperative outcome of segmental fasciectomy in Dupuytren's disease improves by creating firebreaks with an absorbable cellulose implant. J Plast Surg Hand Surg 45(3):157–164

Farquhar C, Vandekerckhove P, Watson A, Vail A, Wiseman D (2000) Barrier agents for preventing adhesions after surgery for subfertility. Cochrane Database Syst Rev 2:CD000475

Moermans JP (1991) Segmental aponeurectomy in Dupuytren's disease. J Hand Surg [Br] 16B:243–254

Roush TF, Stern PJ (2000) Results following surgery for recurrent Dupuytren's disease. J Hand Surg [Am] 25A:291–296

Smith RP, Dias JJ, Ullah A, Bhowal B (2009) Visual and computer software-aided estimates of Dupuytren's contractures: correlation with clinical goniometric measurements. Ann R Coll Surg Engl 91:296–300

Temiz A, Ozturk C, Bakunov A, Kara K, Kaleli T (2008) A new material for prevention of peritendinous fibrotic adhesions after tendon repair: oxidised regenerated cellulose (Interceed), an absorbable adhesion barrier. Int Orthop 32:389–394

Tubiana R, Michon J, Thomine JM (1968) Scheme for the assessment of deformities in Dupuytren's Disease. Surg Clin North Am 48:979–984

Expanded Dermofasciectomies and Full-Thickness Grafts in the Treatment of Dupuytren's Contracture: A 36-Year Experience

26

Lynn D. Ketchum

Contents

26.1	Introduction	213
26.2	Material and Methods	216
26.3	Results	217
26.4	Discussion	218
26.5	Conclusions	219
References		220

26.1 Introduction

In 1967, the author performed a limited fasciectomy on a patient with a 40° contracture of the PIP joint of the left fourth digit (Fig. 26.1).

Full release of the contracture was obtained, but within a year the contracture recurred to the same degree as before the first surgery; at reoperation very

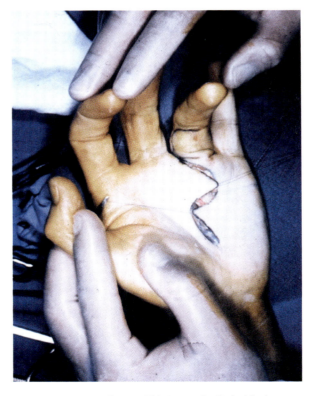

Fig. 26.1 Recurrent disease within 1 year after limited fasciectomy

L.D. Ketchum
11111 Nall Ave., Leawood, Ks., USA, and U. of Kansas Medical Center, 39th and Rainbow, Kansas City, Ks., USA
e-mail: ldkmd5701@aol.com

similar findings were encountered as were seen at the original procedure, which were both frustrating and enigmatic. In 1970, the author attended a symposium in which Richard Gonzalez demonstrated the technique of using multiple incisions to release a cord of a Dupuytren's contracture and then inserted firebreak grafts to resurface the defects, as Berger and Lexer used to release burn scar contractures (Berger 1892; Gonzalez 1985; Lexer 1931) (Fig. 26.2).

Inspired by the potential of this technique, the author performed a series of such firebreak grafts. Although there were no recurrences under the grafts, tantalizing extensions occurred around the edges of the grafts, reproducing the contractures. This was not the answer that had been sought. Not knowing how or why the extensions developed, fortuitously the dermofasciectomies and grafts were expanded so that on the palmar side, the grafts extended from mid-lateral to mid-lateral line in the digit, and from the mid-lateral line on the ulnar side of the hand to the level of the second web space at the distal palmar crease, if the disease was limited to the ulnar side of the hand (Fig. 26.3a, b).

Each graft was at least 2 cm in width from proximal to distal. If the disease also involved the radial side of the hand, the grafts were extended from mid-lateral line ulnarly to mid-lateral line radially (Fig. 26.4c). This did make a significant difference as not only were there no recurrences of disease under the grafts, but extension disease was minimized.

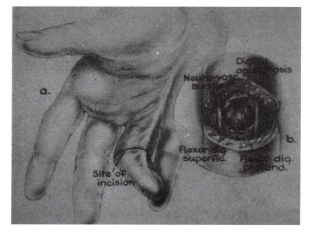

Fig. 26.2 Schematic illustration of Dupuytren's contracture being released by a series of incisions into a cord and insertion of multiple firebreak skin grafts

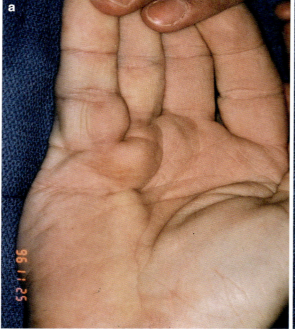
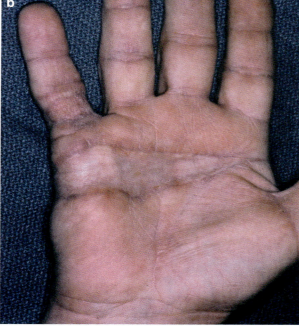

Fig. 26.3 Contracture release of palm and digit with dermofasciectomy. (**a**) Flexion contractures of the right palm and fifth digit from Dupuytren's disease. (**b**) That hand after the contractures were released with dermofasciectomies and the defects were resurfaced with full-thickness skin grafts from the medial aspect of the upper arm

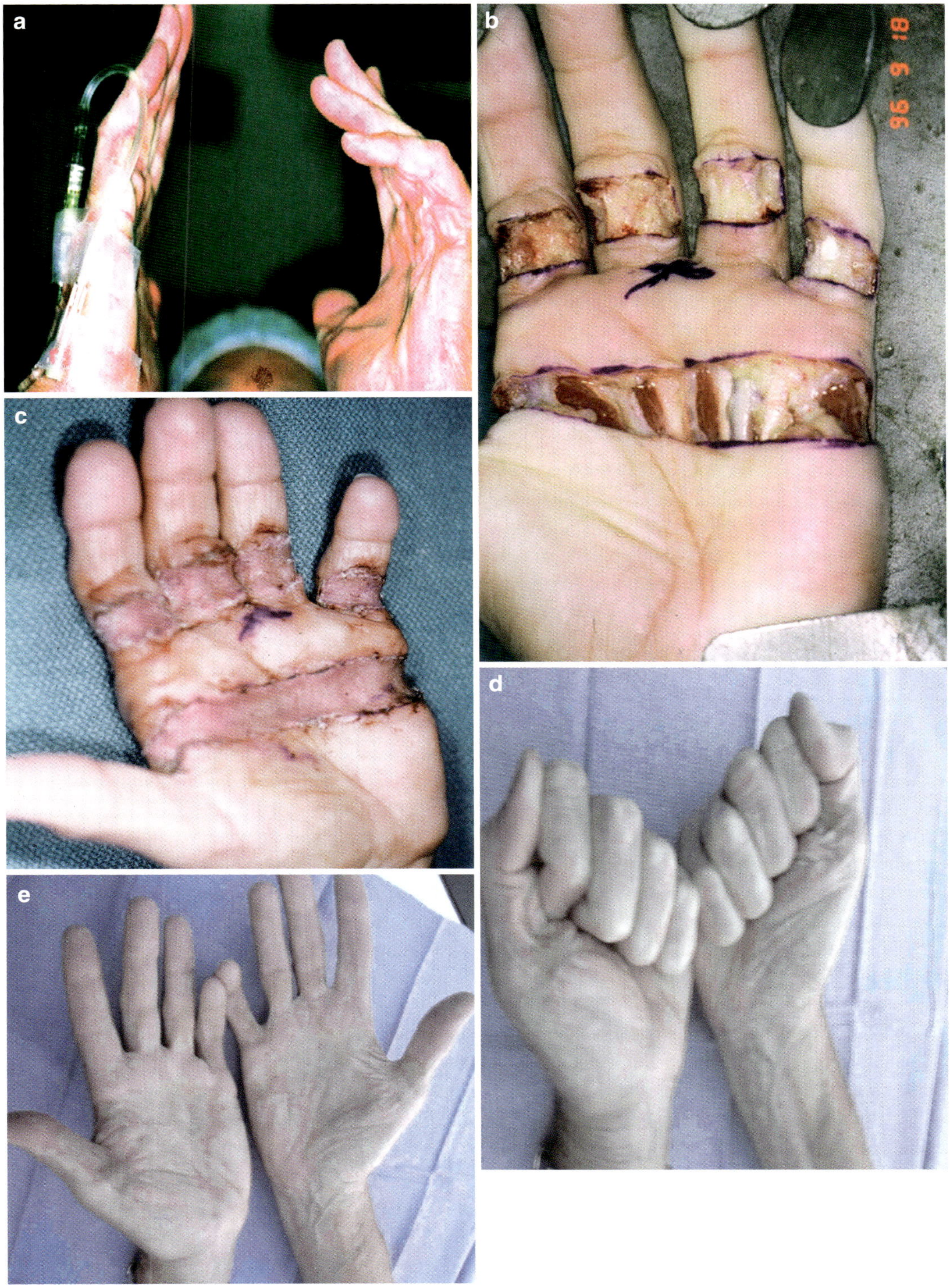

Fig. 26.4 Example of dermofasciectomy. (**a**) Patient is post-op dermofasciectomy and full-thickness grafts on the right hand and pre-op on the left after recurrent contractures bilaterally following limited fasciectomies. (**b**) The left hand immediately after dermofasciectomies of the left palm and digits 2–5. (**c**) The fresh grafts immediately after the bolus dressings were removed at 21 days. (**d, e**) The patient's flexion and extension 12 years post-op

In the last 36 years, the author has used the expanded full-thickness grafts after the release of Dupuytren's contracture with a dermofasciectomy in the palm and/or fingers. An initial study of 36 hands in 24 patients treated with this technique from 1970 to 1984 was published in 1987 (Ketchum and Hixson 1987). In that initial study, there was no recurrence of Dupuytren's disease in the area of the palm and/or fingers covered with the full-thickness grafts, and the extension rate (new disease outside of the parameters of the original surgery) using this technique was 8.3%. Considering the substantially higher percentages of recurrences and extensions reported in the literature (Tubiana 1985), with an average of 50% for limited fasciectomy and a 32% recurrence rate and a 48% extension rate for the McCash technique, as well as flexion loss in one or more digits in 41% of involved hands, as reported by Schneider et al. (1986), the question was, were the recurrence and extension rates for the expanded grafts realistic, or were they an aberration? To answer that question, the second cohort of patients was studied from 1985 to 2005 with an additional 168 hands in 129 patients using the same protocol as in the original study for a total of 204 hands in 153 patients.

26.2 Material and Methods

Patients with the nodular form of Dupuytren's disease, but no contracture, were offered an intranodular injection of triamcinolone at 6 week intervals until softening and/or flattening of the diseased area occurred. The patients with contracture were offered release and graft if they had any of the facets of the Dupuytren's diathesis or any proximal interphalangeal (PIP) joint contracture or any contracture of the fifth digit. The procedure is usually performed in ambulatory surgery with the patient under regional block anesthesia. After the patient is anesthetized, the upper extremity is prepped and draped, and the dermofaciectomies of the palm and fingers, if contracted, are performed (Fig. 26.5a).

The fascia is removed en bloc with involved skin, sparing the transverse fibers of the palmar aponeurosis, which are not involved in the disease process.

No further dissection is done or dead spaces created by this procedure. A digital proximal interphalangeal contracture is released by a mid-lateral to mid-lateral transverse dermofasciectomy on the palmar side of the proximal phalanx. Occasionally, it is necessary to develop short proximally and distally based flaps to sufficiently release a cord or accessory collateral ligaments

that are contributing to a contracted PIP joint. Care is taken not to open the tendon sheath in the area to be covered by the full-thickness graft. The main caveat is prevention of a hematoma under the graft by obtaining absolute hemostasis in the palm and fingers prior to the application of full-thickness skin grafts. The tourniquet is then released and removed after a long-acting local anesthetic is injected around the skin edges; hemostasis is achieved while the graft is being taken and the donor site is being closed.

Whereas Gonzalez reported taking grafts from the groin and Hueston reported a vertical excision of skin from the medial aspect of the upper arm (Hueston 1962), we found that a large swathe of skin that can cover the entire width of the palm can be obtained obliquely from the anteromedial aspect of the upper arm, leaving a relatively obscure scar. The average graft measures 10 by 2 cm, and is harvested after the upper arm is prepped and re-draped, and the area to be excised is marked and injected with 1% Lidocaine, containing 1/100,000 epinephrine.

The grafts are supported by bolster dressings that are left in place for 3 weeks (Fig. 26.5b, c). After this period of compression and elevation, graft survival is assured.

The donor site wound edges are undermined and closed per the surgeon's choice; it is our choice to close such wounds with interrupted subcuticular absorbable sutures and steri-strips on the skin (Fig. 26.6a–d).

Both wounds are covered with compression dressings, including a volar splint on the hand, crossing the wrist, with the PIP joints in extension and the MP joints in enough flexion to permit extension of the interphalangeal joints. In 10 days, the dressings are freshened; the donor site dressing is either eliminated except for the steri-strips, or a very light dressing is applied. The hand wound dressing is lighter, and the splint is worn at night only for the next 6 weeks to 6 months. When the bolster dressing and sutures are removed at 21 days, a light coating of antibiotic ointment is applied to the grafts, which are then covered with a nonadherent light gauze dressing, supported with a layer of self-adherent coban. The grafts can be exposed in the shower and the dressing changed daily for 21 days, at which time all dressing are removed. The grafts mature rapidly, allowing for gripping of sport handles within a week to 10 days thereafter. If the patient has a history of, or tendency to stiffness, hand therapy is started at the first dressing change, or at any appropriate time during the first 6 weeks after surgery.

26.3 Results

In total, 153 patients with contractures from Dupuytren's disease were treated surgically with the above protocol from 1970 to 2005. Two-hundred-and-four hands of 153 patients were reviewed. One hundred and fourteen patients were male, and 39 were female. Twenty-two percent of the patients had plantar involvement; 49% had a positive family history. The average age of onset was 51.6 years. The disease was bilateral in 76.1%, and the individual finger involvement was as follows: thumb 7.5%; index finger 6.4%; long finger 12.0%; ring finger 27.3%; small finger 46.7%. The average follow-up for the last 129 patients was 2.8 years.

In the early part of the series when the bolster dressing over the graft was left in place for 2 weeks only, there had been occasional partial loss of the graft; this occurred because of the inability of the immature capillaries nurturing the graft to withstand the increased hydrostatic pressure created when a hand inadvertently assumed a dependent position. In the middle 1970s, we began leaving the bolster dressing on for 3 weeks and since that time skin graft loss has been a rare occurrence.

There were no infections except for an occasional suture abscess. Patients were able to return to light duty in a mean of 2 weeks after removal of the bolster. Occasionally, a light growth of hair was reported in the grafts, which was easily handled with a depilatory; after a year, hairs were rarely seen, being worn away by regular usage. The color match and general appearance of the graft from the upper arm to the palm was satisfactory in 95% of patients; hyperpigmentation was not uncommon and was mentioned, but was not a complaint. Decreased sensibility in the grafts was tested for and noted by many patients, but because the grafts were not in critical areas for sensibility, it was not a complaint.

There were no instances of a flare reaction. There were no differences in functional results, that is, increased range of motion postoperative, compared to preoperative between the two cohorts. There was a 1% higher incidence of recurrence and extensions associated with re-contractures that occurred in the second part of the study. There was a total absence of recurrence of Dupuytren's disease under the grafted area of the palm. Extension of the disease to areas outside the graft was seen in only 19 of the 204 hands treated, which equated to 9.3% of the total hands treated between 1970 and 2005. These findings validate the conclusion that expanded full-thickness grafts that resurface defects

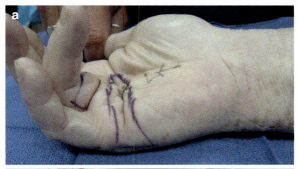
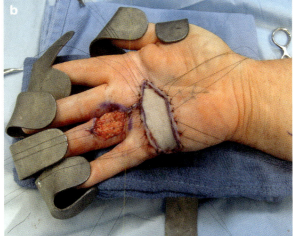
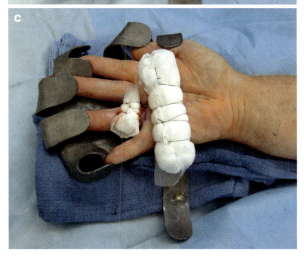

Fig. 26.5 (**a**) Preparing dermofasciectomy. Preoperative markings for release of a Dupuytren's contracture of the right palm and fourth digit by dermofasciectomies and full-thickness grafts. The dermofasciectomies go from the mid-lateral line ulnarly to the level of the second web space at the distal palmar crease, and from mid-lateral line to mid-lateral line in the proximal phalanx. (**b**) The graft is in place in the palm and will be supported with a bolster dressing. (**c**) The bolster dressings are in place and will be covered with a compression dressing of the entire hand that will include a volar splint

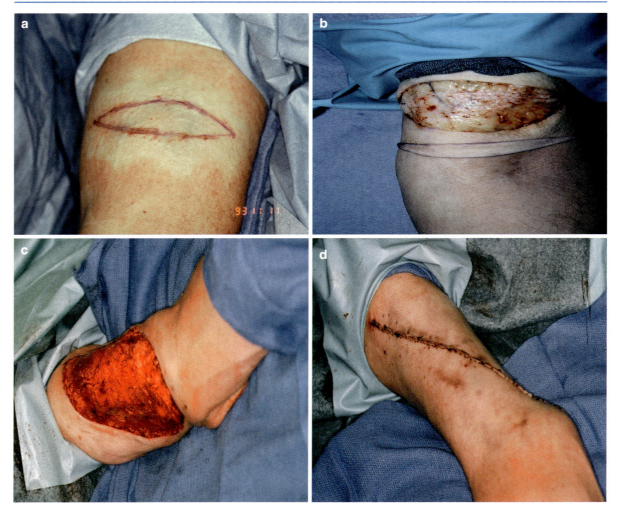

Fig. 26.6 Graft harvesting. (**a**) A full-thickness graft can be harvested using a transverse excision. (**b**) The graft and defect prior closing. (**c**) Larger grafts can be taken obliquely From the medial aspect of the upper arm; here the axilla is to the left. (**d**) The wound edges are undermined and closed with subcuticular sutures.This is the same patient as in (**c**), but it is the closed wound of his right arm. He underwent staged dermofasciectomies and grafts of both palms and digits 6 months apart

following dermofasciectomy are effective in decreasing the postoperative incidence of recurrence and extension in the treatment of Dupuytren's contracture.

26.4 Discussion

Just as the progress of untreated Dupuytren's disease still remains unpredictable, so exists uncertainty concerning its evolution after operation. Is it possible that surgery may aggravate the disease and cause a more rapid development of deformity than would have occurred had it not been performed? This is certainly suggested after seeing numerous hands crippled by contractures in patients with a strong Dupuytren's diathesis who previously had multiple attempts at release and excision of the involved tissue with a limited fasciectomy. The question is why does recurrent and extension disease recur so frequently after limited fasciectomy, and what effect might the expanded grafts exert in modifying this phenomenon?

Fitzgerald and coworkers have demonstrated through the use of picropolychrome differential stains that type III collagen is in greatest concentration in the papillary layer of the dermis of patients with Dupuytren's disease and decreases through the reticular dermis to the subcutaneous tissue and is in minimal concentration in cords (Fitzgerald et al. 1995). McCann et al. (1995) found myofibroblasts in dermis and nodules, but very few in cords. Murrell and Vracko found microangiopathy in skin and subcutaneous tissue and nodules in hands of patients with Dupuytren's disease as well as those of smokers and diabetics (Murrell 1991; Vracko 1974).

In the limited fasciectomy procedure, dermis and subcutaneous tissue that may have been intimately involved in the disease process would be left in place; that disease process involves the degradation of ATP to xanthine and uric acid with the release of free radicals that generate inflammation with the release of cytokines, growth factors, and arachadonic acid metabolites (Badalamente et al. 1983); along with longitudinal skin tension, growth factors, particularly TGFb1 (Transforming growth factor beta) cause differentiation of fibroblasts into myofibroblasts which, through their contraction in nodules, transmit a deforming force through cords to involved digits (Tomasek et al. 1999).

What effect would expanded full-thickness grafts have in modifying this process?

First, a dermofasciectomy interrupts longitudinal mechanical stresses, which along with the growth factor TGFb1 differentiate fibroblasts into myofibroblasts by developing dense bundles of actin microfilaments that are integral to the contractile mechanism; in addition, they develop a transmembrane fibronexus that transmits the force of the actin/myosin contraction to the extracellular milieu (fibrin/fibronectin/collagen) (Tomasek et al. 1999).

Second, a dermofasciectomy removes diseased dermis as well as fascia that contain all the elements mentioned above for the development and progression of the disease process.

Third, full-thickness skin from areas of the body that do not get involved in the Dupuytren's process is applied to a healthy recipient bed of normal tissue.

Fourth, Piulachs and Mir and Mir (1952), Hueston (1962), Gordon (1963), Tonkin et al.(1984), and Ketchum and Hixson (1987) have demonstrated that Dupuytren's disease does not recur under full-thickness skin grafts; expanding the grafts decreases the areas in which recurrent disease can develop.

Hueston established the parameters for the Dupuytren's diathesis, the tendency for the full expression of the disease (Hueston 1986). McFarlane demonstrated that the more elements of the diathesis a person has, the greater tendency there is for that person to have recurrent disease (McFarlane 1995). Hueston reasoned further that if recurrent disease does not occur beneath full-thickness grafts, would it not be feasible to use full-thickness grafts in people with a strong diathesis and tendency to recurrent disease (Hueston 1962)?

Finally, Rudolph et al. demonstrated experimentally in contracting cutaneous wounds that full-thickness grafts cause the myofibroblast population to decrease rapidly, and projected a beneficial effect in the treatment of Dupuytren's contracture (Rudolph et al. 1977).

26.5 Conclusions

Possibly, the cure for the Dupuytren's condition will be in the nature of a biochemical modality similar to the use of collagenase and/or triamcinolone to modify collagen metabolism, fibroblastic proliferation, and contraction of myofibroblasts at the onset of the disease (Badalamente et al. 2003; Watt et al. 2010; Ketchum and Donahue 2000). Once the disease has become established and has advanced to contracture of one or more digits, the contractures must be released in a way that reduces morbidity and the incidence of recurrence and extension of the disease. At this time, the use of full-thickness grafts after release of the contractures appears to be a feasible biological approach to the problem. As Hueston suggested, shutting off the mediating organ, or tissue, that he thought was the skin, may account for the lack of recurrences after full-thickness skin grafting (Fig. 26.5a, b) (Hueston et al. 1976).

Our opinion is that the most benign and physiological approach to this disease process is the minimal dissection required to release contracted joints and the interruption of the disease process with a full-thickness graft or grafts as necessary. The result is less edema, inflammation, stiffness, and reduction of the incidence of recurrence. We believe that the use of expanded full-thickness grafts, particularly over the ulnar aspect of the hand, decreases the incidence of extension of the disease process. This technique is appropriate in the surgical treatment of patients with Dupuytren's disease in whom contracture of one or more digits develops before the age of 40 years, or who have recurrent disease, bilateral disease, a positive family history, or evidence of ectopic disease.

Acknowledgment The author would like to thank Mrs. DeLois McPherson for her invaluable help in preparing this manuscript.

References

Badalamente MA, Sterl L, Hurst LC (1983) The pathogenesis of Dupuytren's contracture: contractile mechanisms of the myofibroblasts. J Hand Surg Am 8:235–242

Badalamente MA, Hurst LC, Hentz VR, Hotchkiss RN, Kaplan TD, Meals RA (2003) Collagen as a chemical target: nonoperative treatment of Dupuytren's disease. J Hand Surg Am 27A: 788–798

Berger P (1892) Traitment de la retraction de l'aponeurose palmaire par une autoplastie. Bull Acad Med 56:608

Fitzgerald AMP, Kirkpatrick JJR, Foo LTH, Naylor IL (1995) A picropolychrome staining technique applied to Dupuytren's tissue. J Hand Surg Am 20B:519–524

Gonzalez R (1985) The use of skin grafts in the treatment of Dupuytren's contracture. Hand Clin 1:641–647

Gordon SD (1963) Dupuytren's contracture. The use of free skin grafts in treatment. In: Transactions of the 3 rd Congress of Plastic Surgery. Excerpta Medica Foundation, Amsterdam, pp 963–967

Hueston JT (1962) Digital Wolfe grafts in recurrent Dupuytren's contracture. Plastic Reconstr Surg Transplant Bull 29: 342–344

Hueston JT (1986) Dupuytren's contracture. Lancet 2:1226

Hueston JT, Hurley JV, Whittingham S (1976) The contracting fibroblast as a clue to Dupuytren's contracture. Hand 8:10–12

Ketchum LD, Donahue TK (2000) The injection of nodules of Dupuytren's disease with triamcinolone Acetonide. J Hand Surg Am 25A:731–733

Ketchum L, Hixson P (1987) Dermofasciectomy and full-thickness grafts in the treatment of Dupuytren's contracture. J Hand Surg Am 12A:659–663

Lexer E (1931) Die gesamte Wiederherstellungschirugie, vol 2, 2nd edn. JA Barth, Leipzig, p 837

McCann L, Belcher W, Warn A, Warn RM (1995) The presence of myofibroblasts in the dermis of patients with Dupuytren's contracture. J Hand Surg Am 18B:656

McFarlane RM (1995) The current status of Dupuytren's disease. J Hand Ther 8:181–184

Murrell GAC (1991) The role of the fibroblast, in Dupuytren's contracture. Hand Clin 7:669–680

Piulachs P, Mir y Mir L (1952) Consideraciones sobre la enfermedad de Dupuytren. Folia Clin Int (Barcelona) 2:8

Rudolph R, Guber S, Suzuki M (1977) The life cycle of the myofibroblast. Surg Gynecol Obstet 145:399

Schneider LH, Hankin FM, Eisenberg T (1986) Surgery of Dupuytren's disease: a review of the open palm method. J Hand Surg Am 11A:23–27

Tomasek JJ, Vaughn MB, Haaksma CJ (1999) Cellular structure and biology of Dupuytren's disease. Hand Clin 15:21–34

Tonkin MA, Burke FD, Varian JPW (1984) Dupuytren's contracture: a comparative study of fasciectomy and dermofasciectomy in one hundred patients. J Hand Surg Am 9B: 156–162

Tubiana R (1985) Recurrent Dupuytren's disease. In: Hueston JT, Tubiana R (eds) Dupuytren's disease, 2nd edn. Churchill Livingstone, Edinburgh

Vracko R (1974) Basal lamina layering in diabetes mellitus: evidence for accelerated rate of cell death and cell regeneration. Diabetes 23:94–104

Watt AJ, Curtin CM, Hentz VR (2010) Collagen injection as nonoperative treatment of Dupuytren's disease: 8 year follow-up. J Hand Surg Am 35A:534–539

Minimizing Skin Necrosis and Delayed Healing After Surgical Treatment for Dupuytren's Contracture: The Mini-Chevrons Incision

27

Michael Papaloïzos

Contents

27.1	**Introduction**	221
27.2	**Material and Methods**	222
27.2.1	Technique	222
27.2.2	Patients	222
27.3	**Results**	222
27.4	**Discussion**	224
27.5	**Conclusion**	225
References		225

27.1 Introduction

Surgical fasciectomy remains the treatment of choice for most patients affected by Dupuytren's contracture (Chick and Lister 1991; Roy et al. 2006). Since the initial open palm technique by Dupuytren himself in 1832 and its renewal by McCash in the 1960s (McCash 1964), this approach has always been in use and has still many defenders (Shaw et al. 1996; Lubahn 1999; Armstrong et al. 2000). It allows fasciectomy in the palm, whereas some kind of flap design and elevation is used for removal of the diseased tissue at the finger level. The main criticism toward this technique is the postoperative prolonged period of daily or near daily dressings, until skin healing is obtained (Shaw et al. 1996).

Therefore, many alternatives which allow for closure of the skin have been introduced (King et al. 1979; Lubahn et al. 1984; Roy et al. 2006). As straight longitudinal incisions are prone to secondary skin contractures, they should be avoided and need to be made with acute angles. For this purpose, the most common designs are the zigzag incision, the V-Y incision, and Z-plasties. They are often associated with a transverse or a T-incision in the palm (Jabaley 1999). Whatever the design, large flaps are elevated to perform an appropriate fasciectomy. These large skin dissections frequently lead to some degree of skin necrosis. The delay in wound healing urges the need for renewed dressings, which may impair early and full mobilization and slow down rehabilitation (Boyer and Gelberman 1999). This may also increase the rate of early complications like persistent edema, local infection, and the likelihood of CRPS (Sennwald 1990).

M. Papaloïzos
Center for Hand Surgery and Therapy,
Charles-Humbert 8, 1205 Geneva, Switzerland
e-mail: mpapaloizos@ch8.ch

C. Eaton et al. (eds.), *Dupuytren's Disease and Related Hyperproliferative Disorders*,
DOI 10.1007/978-3-642-22697-7_27, © Springer-Verlag Berlin Heidelberg 2012

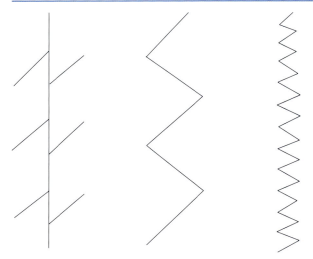

Fig. 27.1 Schematic comparison of Z-plasties, zigzag and mini-chevrons incisions (from left to right)

The objective of this work was to minimize early skin complications, so as to allow early active motion, to reduce edema, to rapidly involve the patient in its own recovery, and overall to improve immediate quality of life.

Our hypothesis was that raising flaps in a classic zigzag fashion but with very short arms could be an advantage regarding primary skin healing, without impairing an open, radical fasciectomy. This technique exhibits similarities to the honeycomb technique, especially when small transverse incisions are used (Bedeschi et al. 1990). However, the arms in our technique are much shorter.

27.2 Material and Methods

27.2.1 Technique

The basic idea underlying the new design proposed here is that a zigzag incision with arms as short as 4–5 mm will behave exactly like those with longer arms regarding skin contracture but will better preserve the blood supply and drainage of the flaps, thus enhancing primary healing (Fig. 27.1). The small flaps are elevated tangentially to the skin and kept as thick as possible. Care is taken to preserve the subdermal layers and their perforating vessels, particularly at the commissural level where deep tissues should be kept intact whenever possible. Usually, one incision is made for each ray or finger, from the palm to the most distal extension as required. One to five distinct incisions can thus be performed. In cases with a broad diseased palmar aponeurosis, the incisions can be coupled at their proximal end with a transverse or T-incision in the palm. V-Y advancement flaps are used as required, if the numerous small transverse incisions by themselves do not elongate the skin enough. Closure is by simple stitches at the tip of each flap, intermediate stitches are usually unnecessary and even not mandatory to allow spontaneous drainage. The basic steps of the operative procedure are illustrated in Fig. 27.2.

27.2.2 Patients

This continuous prospective series contains all patients operated for Dupuytren's contracture between November 2007 and November 2009. There were no exclusion criteria, except unwillingness to surgery. Diabetic patients ($n=3$), smokers ($n=4$) and patients with recurrences ($n=3$) were included. The common approach was: one ray, one incision, implying multiple separate incisions, sometimes even on both sides of the same finger. Suction drainage was applied in three cases. No skin resection nor graft was performed. Severity of the disease was graded according to the number of affected rays, digital extension of the disease (PIP or DIP), and Tubiana's stages (1 – 4) (Table 27.1).

Fifty-five patients (11F/44M, mean age 63.4 years, 29–94) were operated using one or several mini-chevrons incisions (up to five). Fasciectomy was otherwise performed according to standard rules. Z-plasty was used only once to cover a zone of skin resection in the palm. Suction drainage was used in three cases in which dissection had been extensive.

Skin healing was graded as follows: 0 (no necrosis), 1 (one limited point of superficial necrosis), 2 (2–3 points of superficial necrosis or one point of deeper but still dermal necrosis), 3 (multiple points, extended or deep, subdermal necrosis), at day 5 (first dressing), 12–14 days (stitches removal) and 30 days after surgery. Other complications within the follow-up period were recorded. All patients were followed at regular intervals within 1 month and more if required (mean FU 7 weeks, 4–16).

27.3 Results

The outcome regarding skin healing problems is illustrated in Table 27.2.

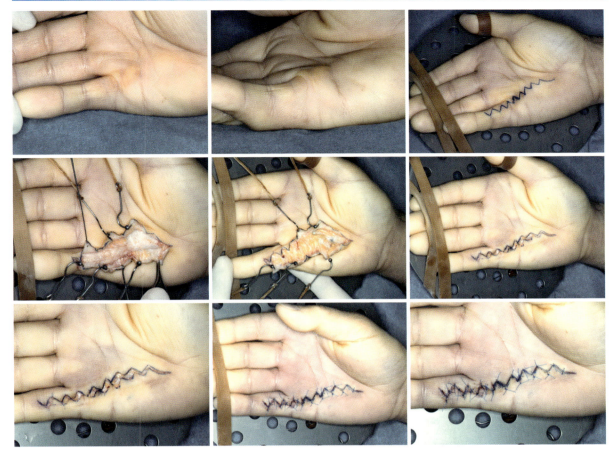

Fig. 27.2 Steps of the operative procedure in a simple case (one ray)

Table 27.1 Severity of the disease according to the number of affected rays, digital extension of the disease, and Tubiana's stages

Number of rays operated	1	2	3	4	5
n =	22	17	9	5	2
Digital extension	to MCP	to PIP	to DIP		
n =	20	23	12		
Tubiana's stages	1	2	3	3+	4
n =	15	27	8	4	1

Table 27.2 Outcome regarding skin healing from day 0 to day 30

		5 days	Stitches removal	1 month
0	No necrosis	48	38	52
1	Limited superficial necrosis	7	13	3
2	Intermediate necrosis	0	4	0
3	Serious deep necrosis	0	0	0

The majority of cases healed primarily with no signs of skin necrosis or limited dermal perfusion (Fig. 27.3). Restricted and superficial spots of suboptimal vascularized skin were observed in 13 cases between days 12 and 14. Two cases are shown in Fig. 27.4. Four of them required more attention and care than simple dry dressings. At 1 month postoperatively, 3 out of the 55 patients had limited residual skin lesions. A serious deep necrosis never occurred. Most of the patients with some degree of healing problems had in retrospect presented with a more severe disease (more affected rays and/or more advanced stages). This was also related to the extent of postoperative hematoma. Smoking and diabetes did not appear to play a role in wound healing. Complications were four self-limiting hematomas which resolved spontaneously

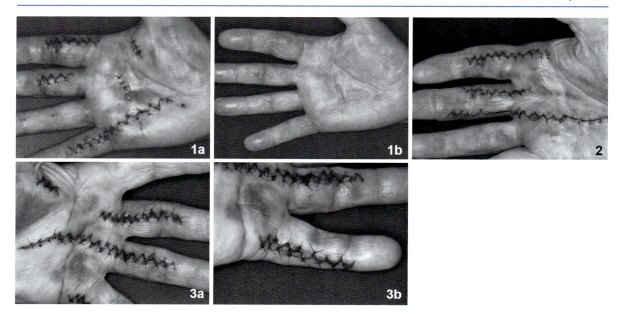

Fig. 27.3 Three postoperative results at different stages. Three patients postoperatively: (**1a**) at 5 days, (**1b**) same at 5 weeks; (**2**) at 5 days; (**3a**) at 12 days, (**3b**) detail (same case)

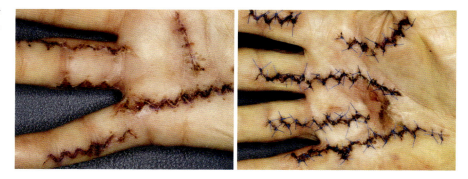

Fig. 27.4 Two examples of stage 2 skin lesions at the time of stitches removal

within 2–3 weeks and one superficial infection in a patient known for furunculosis, which responded well to oral antibiotherapy. No CRPS were seen in this series.

27.4 Discussion

In this short series of 55 patients operated by use of one or several mini-chevrons incisions, interesting results were obtained in terms of skin healing, with very few and easy-to-cope-with problems. Patient satisfaction was high (not quantified) and dressings were usually required no longer than 10–12 days. Return to daily activities was therefore not hampered and full or nearly full mobility was easily recovered without therapy in most cases. The mini-chevrons incision is now my standard approach for almost all patients presenting with Dupuytren's contracture.

Obviously, switching from incisions with large flaps to incisions with small flaps does not solve all the problems related to the surgical treatment of Dupuytren's disease. Advanced and more severe stages remain more difficult to manage and this is also true in this series, where the degree of skin injury appeared to be proportional to the severity of the disease. However, it is a safe and convenient technique for the middle-stage cases, at least regarding the early outcome.

Retrospectively, hematomas may have been better prevented by a more generous use of aspirative drainage in cases requiring extensive dissection, especially in the palm, where all hematomas occurred in this series.

It was not under the scope of this study to evaluate the recurrence rate. This aspect will be evaluated by mid- and long-term studies of the cases operated with the mini-chevrons technique.

27.5 Conclusion

The cutaneous approach of Dupuytren's contracture by the mini-chevrons incisions appears to be a useful addition to the surgeon's toolbox. Thanks to its simple design, further advantages of this technique are its versatility, ubiquity, and easy combination with other local plasties, especially the V-Y design – somewhat reminding of the honeycomb technique (Bedeschi et al. 1990). It is easy to learn and to teach. Benefits for the patient are the promotion of primary skin healing, functional recovery, and immediate postoperative quality of life.

References

Armstrong JR, Hurren JS, Logan AM (2000) Dermofasciectomy in the management of Dupuytren's disease. J Bone Joint Surg Br 82:90–94

Bedeschi P et al (1990) Various views and techniques, management of the skin, honeycomb technique. In: McFarlane RM (ed) Dupuytren's disease. Biology and treatment. Churchill Livingstone, Edinburgh/London/Melbourne, pp 311–315

Boyer MI, Gelberman RH (1999) Complications of the operative treatment of Dupuytren's disease. Hand Clin 15(1):161–166

Chick LR, Lister GD (1991) Surgical alternatives in Dupuytren's contracture. Hand Clin 7(4):715–719

Jabaley ME (1999) Surgical treatment of Dupuytren's disease. Hand Clin 15(1):109–126

King EW, Bass DM, Watson HK (1979) Treatment of Dupuytren's contracture by extensive fasciectomy through multiple Y-V-plasty incisions: short-term evaluation of 170 consecutive operations. J Hand Surg Am 4(3):234–241

Lubahn JD (1999) Open-palm technique and soft-tissue coverage in Dupuytren's disease. Hand Clin 15(1):127–136

Lubahn JD, Lister GD, Wolfe T (1984) Fasciectomy and Dupuytren's disease: a comparison between the open-palm technique and wound closure. J Hand Surg Am 9A(1):53–58

McCash CR (1964) The open palm technique in Dupuytren's contracture. Br J Plast Surg 17:271–280

Roy N, Sharma D, Mirza AH, Fahmy N (2006) Fasciectomy and conservative full thickness skin grafting in Dupuytren's contracture. The fish technique. Acta Orthop Belg 72(6):678–682

Sennwald GR (1990) Fasciectomy for treatment of Dupuytren's disease and early complications. J Hand Surg Am 15(5):755–761

Shaw DL, Wise DI, Holms W (1996) Dupuytren's disease treated by palmar fasciectomy and an open palm technique. J Hand Surg Br 21(4):484–485

Skin Management in Treatment of Severe PIP Contracture by Homo- or Heterodigital Flaps

28

Bernhard Lukas and Moritz Lukas

Contents

28.1	Introduction	227
28.2	Operative Technique	228
28.2.1	Homodigital Flaps	228
28.2.2	Heterodigital Flaps	228
28.2.3	Postoperative Treatment	229
28.3	Patient Characteristics	229
28.4	Results	231
28.4.1	Complications	232
28.5	Discussion	232
28.6	Conclusion	233
References		233

B. Lukas (✉)
Schön-Klinik München-Harlaching, Zentrum für
Handchirurgie, Mikrochirurgie, Plastische Chirurgie,
Harlachingerstr. 51, 81547 Munich, Germany
e-mail: blukas@schoen-kliniken.de

M. Lukas
Klinikum rechts der Isar TUM, cand.med, Studiendekanat,
Munich, Germany
e-mail: moritzlukas@myt.um.de

28.1 Introduction

The classical course of morbus dupuytren is the formation of nodules in the palm, which progresses to the formation of cords and then into the contracture of the finger joints. While metacarpophalangeal joint (MCP-joint) flexion contracture can almost always be corrected at any stage, this is not the case for PIP-joint contractures, especially when seen at an advanced stage (contraction over 30°) when the joints have become fixed. In the classification system of Tubiana and Michon (Tubiana 1985) this difference cannot be appreciated, since it scores the contracture in a complete finger, regardless of the contribution of the MCP-joint or the PIP-joint (Table 28.1).

As a result, whether a finger should be treated conservatively, minimally invasively, or with open surgery cannot be deduced from this classification. For instance, while in Stage 2 a contraction of the MCP-joint of 90°, a needle fasciotomy definitely portrays an alternative to surgical treatment (Foucher et al. 2001), it will be of little success in an exclusive contraction of the PIP-joint of 90°.

The most commonly used incision are the zigzag incision according to Bruner (Bruner 1967), enabling a V-Y Advancement Flap, or the straight line incision, which can subsequently be interrupted using z-plasties (Skoog 1985, Weinzweig 1985). In isolated contractures of the MCP-joint the skin can, in most cases, even with an extended joint, be properly closed by a large area z-plasty. If a moderate degree contracture of the PIP-joint in addition to the contracture of the metacarpophalangeal joint exists, a combination of the Open-Palm-technique in the area of the palm and z-plasties can be carried out over the MCP- and

C. Eaton et al. (eds.), *Dupuytren's Disease and Related Hyperproliferative Disorders*,
DOI 10.1007/978-3-642-22697-7_28, © Springer-Verlag Berlin Heidelberg 2012

Table 28.1 Stage classification according to Tubiana and Michon

Stage N: No contraction
Stage 1: Contraction of 0–45°
Stage 2: Contraction of 46–90°
Stage 3: Contraction of 91–135°
Stage 4: Contraction over 135°

PIP-joint. Considerably, more problematic is skin handling in severe contractures of the PIP-joints. For this joint, it is at best possible to correct contractures up to 30° using z-plasties (Gonzalez 1990).

In all other cases and especially when the PIP-joint is completely extended after an open arthrolysis, it is necessary to cover the missing palmar skin with flap plasties. In these cases, the use of homodigital or heterodigital flap plasty is a possibility. If thereafter a skin deficit remains in the palm, this can be managed using "the Open-Palm-Technique" (McCash 1964).

The purpose of this study is to report on our experience using these flaps in severe PIP contractures and compare the results with those of a historic cohort, in which we used more standard techniques.

28.2 Operative Technique

28.2.1 Homodigital Flaps

The skin over the proximal phalanx is elevated as an ulnarly based right-angle flap and the flap that is ultimately used to close the palmer defect after contracture release is planned and developed on the ulnar side of the midphalanx (Figs. 28.1 and 28.2).

After excision of the pathologic tissue and joint release, the initially planned flap is transposed to the palmer side (Figs. 28.3 and 28.4).

The donor site is closed using a full-thickness skin graft. This can either be taken from the antecubital fossa, the forearm, or from the thenar area (Fig. 28.5).

28.2.1.1 Bilobed Flap

A modification is the so-called bilobed flap: a second flap is taken from the dorsal skin at a 90° angle to the first flap over the midphalanx (Figs. 28.6 and 28.7). This second flap is rotated into the donor site of the first flap (Fig. 28.8). The second donor site is closed primarily (Fig. 28.9). The advantage is that no skin graft is necessary.

28.2.1.2 Combination of Homodigital Flap with Open Palm Technique

The technique of homodigital flap taken from the midphalanx can also be combined well with the open palm technique for severe contractions of the MCP- and PIP-joint (Figs. 28.10 and 28.11).

28.2.2 Heterodigital Flaps

A heterodigital flap plasty offers an alternative to the homodigital transposition flap (Figs. 28.12, 13, 14). This in our eyes allows for a very functional and

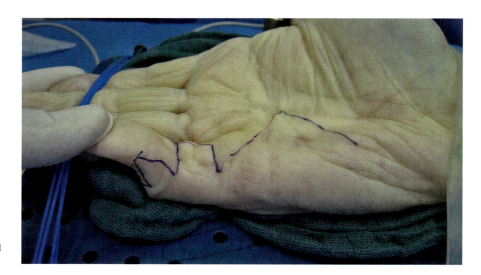

Fig. 28.1 The preoperative planning of the incisions and the homodigital flap

28 Skin Management in Treatment of Severe PIP Contracture by Homo- or Heterodigital Flaps

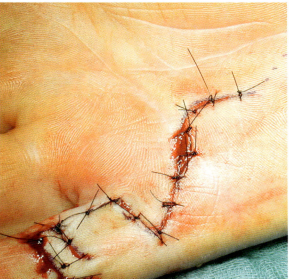

Fig. 28.2 The flaps after excision of the pathology and joint release just prior to closure

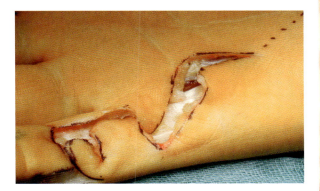

Fig. 28.3 Rotating of the homodigital flap into the defect of the proximal phalanx

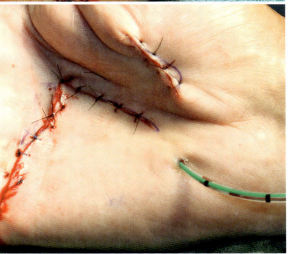

Figs. 28.4 and 28.5 The skin closure of the proximal phalanx and the thenar region

exceptionally nice cosmetic coverage. The donor site also needs to be treated with a full thickness skin graft (Fig. 28.15).

28.2.3 Postoperative Treatment

The postoperative treatment is very important for a good outcome: We advise to apply a daily manual lymphatic drainage for 14 days beginning on the first postoperative day. In addition, after the second postoperative day, 30 min hand therapy everyday plus an individually customized splint to be worn the first 14 days permanently and then for several months at night to avoid a reappearance of the flexion contracture.

After taking out the stitches, which should be done on the 14th postoperative day, it is necessary to treat the at this time often thickened scar with a silicon bandage at night and a scar massage combined with mechanical vibration therapy several times a day.

28.3 Patient Characteristics

Between January 2005 and November 2009 homo- and heterodigital flap plasty was used on a total of 40 patients, 5 of which were women and 35 men. The

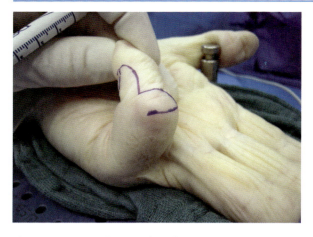

Fig. 28.6 Preoperative planning of a second flap over the dorsal PIP-joint

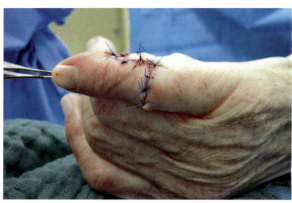

Fig. 28.9 Closing the donor site of the second flap

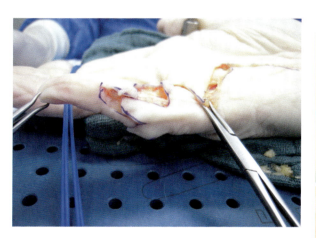

Fig. 28.7 Rotating the first flap to the palmar defect (other patient)

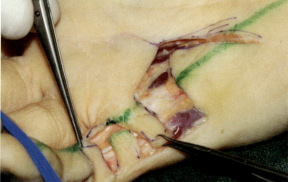

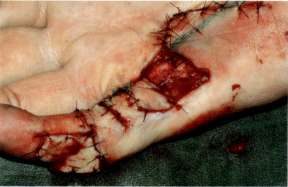

Figs. 28.10 and 28.11 Combination of PIP-joint closure with a homodigital flap and open palm technique

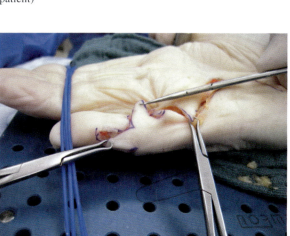

Fig. 28.8 Rotating the second flap to the ulnar-dorsal defect

average age was 62 years, the youngest patient had an age of 35 years, the oldest one was 85 years old. No patient had diabetes mellitus type I, 6 patients had diabetes type II. The patients had no other remarkable diseases.

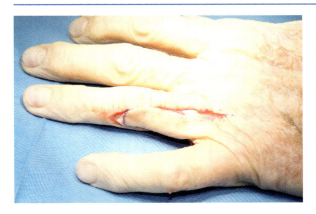

Fig. 28.12 A dorsolateral skin flap is cut on the fourth finger

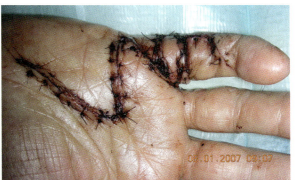

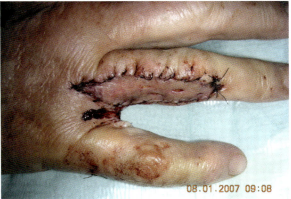

Figs. 28.14 and 28.15 The final result of both fingers

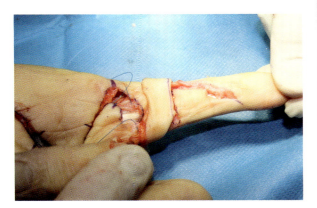

Fig. 28.13 Rotating this flap to the first phalanx of the fifth finger

Details of the preoperative status of the patients, including Tubiana staging and the operative procedure performed is shown in Table 28.2.

Table 28.2 Patients and kind of surgeries

Forty patients
- 25 × finger V
- 10 × finger IV
- 5 × fingers I–III

Preop. contracture PIP	*Operation*
– 15 × 45–60°	30 × primal operation
– 10 × 60–90°	10 × relapse operation
– 15 × more than 90°	
Stage according to Tubiana	*Type of flap plastique*
– 25 × Stage 2	35 × homodigital
– 10 × Stage 3	5 × heterodigital
– 5 × Stage 4	15 × open athrolysis

28.4 Results

In all cases with preoperative PIP-joint contracture of less than 60°, full joint extension could be achieved intraoperatively. However, in these cases, universally, a flexion contracture reappeared after 6 months of up to 15° (Fig. 28.16), which further aggravated after 2 years until up to 30° (Figs. 28.17 and 18).

In cases with a preoperative PIP-joint contracture of over 60°, an extension deficit of between 10 and 30° remained, despite an open arthrolysis. In these cases, the reappearing flexion contracture after 6 months was up to 40°, and worsened after 2 years up to 60°. The residual amount of flexion contracture of the fifth finger and relapse surgeries was 50% higher than for all the other fingers or for first-time surgeries. In 40% of cases, the sensitivity disturbance, as a result of the surgery which was tested with the monofilament test, continuously improved up to 2 years postoperatively,

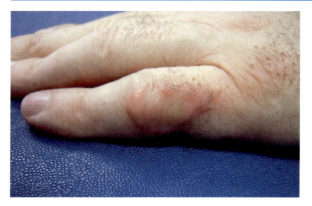

Fig. 28.16 Short-term postoperative result: contracture of 10°

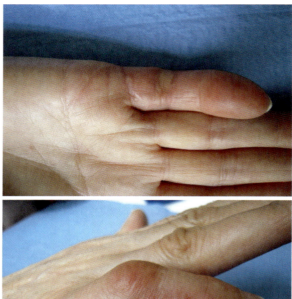

Figs. 28.17 and 28.18 Recurrence of PIP-joint contracture after 2 years: 40°

whereas the transposed sliding flaps remained insensate as expected.

In the donor site, we ultimately did not have any aesthetic or functional problems, whereas in the beginning the skin graft was somewhat bulky.

Twenty-five patients (63%) complained of slight to moderate coldness sensitivity even up to 2 years after surgery. A summary of the results is shown in Table 28.3.

28.4.1 Complications

In four patients, wound healing disorders occurred (Fig. 28.19). These healed without further surgical revision. We had one homodigital flap loss. In three cases, the full-thickness skin graft that was used to close the donor defect was lost partially or completely, which was allowed to heal secondarily.

Two revisional surgeries had to be carried out about 1 year later. In the first case, an arthrodesis of the PIP-joint was carried out because of severe recurring contracture of the joint, in a further case a finger amputation was done because the patient had a severe sensitivity to coldness and wished this option due to the danger of losing his job.

Table 28.3 Summary of results

	Intraop deficit of extension	Flexion contracture after 6 months	Flexion contracture after 2 years
Preop contracture PIP 45–60° (n = 15)	Full extension possible	10–15°	15–30°
Preop contracture PIP 60–90° (n = 10)	10–20° (despite athrolysis)	20–30°	30–45°
Preop contracture PIP >90° (n = 15)	20–30° (despite athrolysis)	30–40°	40–60°

28.5 Discussion

Correction of MP joint contracture in Dupuytren's Disease is rarely a problem. It can almost always be released and skin shortage can be managed by simple Z-plasties or the open palm technique. Management of PIP-joint contracture however, remains a controversial point in literature. The outcome of PIP-joint release is uncertain (Belusa et al. 1997) and there seems to be a general agreement that there is no clear benefit of joint release as addition to fasciectomy (Weinzweig et al. 1996). In our opinion one of the most important

Fig. 28.19 Delayed wound healing

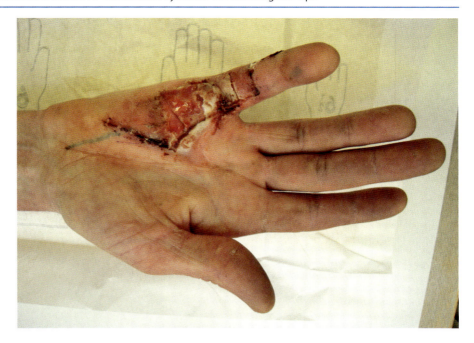

procedures is to combine joint release by skin closure without any tension.

In a former control group of 30 patients (Tubiana 2/3 with severe PIP-involvement), which was treated by conventional Bruner zigzag incisions or z-plasties, the flexion contracture of PIP-joint 2 years later was 30–45° if preoperative contracture had been less than 60°. It was 50–70° if the preoperative contracture had been more than 60°.

By using our technique of homodigital or heterodigital flap plasty, these figures could be reduced by 20–30%: In cases with preoperative flexion contracture of less than 60°, a flexion contracture reappeared after 2 years until up to 30°. In cases with a preoperative PIP-joint contraction of over 60°, the reappearing flexion contracture after 2 years was up to 60°.

The coverage of palmar defects at the PIP-joint with cross finger flaps makes less sense to us. A much longer immobilization period than we strive for is necessary and a second surgery is needed to divide the pedicle of the flap and sometimes a third operation to make final corrections. The alternative for this treatment is dermofasciectomy and full-thickness skin grafting (Hueston 1984). The results of this technique have shown similar results of 30° residual contracture of the PIP-joint of little finger as we have found in our technique. (Gonzalez 1990). The advantage of flaps in comparison to skin grafts is the better healing over flexor tendon sheet, especially once opened and the provision of better padding. We do not think that the coverage of the palmar defect with a full thickened skin graft is a good alternative because of the often insufficient blood circulation of the defect. Therefore, full-thickness skin grafting is from our viewpoint unsafe.

28.6 Conclusion

The primary planning of a homo- or heterodigital flap plasty for contraction of the PIP-joint over 30° clearly increases the short- and medium-term result, because the rate of recurrence of a flexion contracture is 20–30% less than when using other skin incisions.

References

Belusa L, Buck-Gramcko D, Partecke BD (1997) Results of inter-phalangeal joint athrolysis in patients with Dupuytren's disease. Handchir Mikrochir Plast Chir 29:158–163

Bruner JM (1967) The zig-zag volar-digital incision for flexor-tendon surgery. Plast Reconstr Surg 40:571–574

Foucher G, Medina J, Navarro R (2001) Percutaneous needle aponeurectomy. Complications and results. Chir Main 20:206–211

Gonzalez RI (1990) Various views and techniques: management of the skin: IV. Limited fasciectomy and skin graft. In:

McFarlane RM, McGrouther DA, Flint MH (eds) Dupuytren's disease: biology and treatment, vol 5, The hand and upper limb series. Churchill Livingstone, Edinburgh, pp 321–324

Hueston JT (1984) Dermofasciectomy for Dupuytren's disease. Bull Hosp Joint Dis 44:224–232

McCash CR (1964) The open palm technique in Dupuytren's contracture. Br J Plast Surg 17:271–280

Skoog T (1985) Dupuytren's contracture: pathogenesis and surgical treatment. In: Hueston JT, Tubiana R (eds) Dupuytren's disease, 2nd edn. Churchill Livingstone, Edingburgh, pp 184–192

Tubiana R (1985) Overview on surgical treatment of Dupuytren disease. In: Hueston JT, Tubiana R (eds) Dupuytren's disease, 2nd edn. Churchill Livingstone, Edingburgh, pp 129–130

Weinzweig R (1985) Overview on surgical treatment of Dupuytren disease. In: Hueston JT, Tubiana R (eds) Dupuytren's disease. Churchill Livingstone, Edingburgh, pp 129–130

Weinzweig N, Culver JE, Fleegler EJ (1996) Severe contractures of the proximal interphalangeal joint in Dupuytren's disease: combined fasciectomy with capsuloligamentous release versus fasciectomy alone. Plast Reconstr Surg 97: 560–566

The "Jacobsen Flap" for the Treatment of Stage III–IV Dupuytren's Disease at Little Finger: Our Review of 123 Cases

29

Massimiliano Tripoli, Francesco Moschella, and Michel Merle

Contents

29.1	**Introduction**	235
29.2	**Patients and Methods**	236
29.2.1	Flap Design and Operative Technique	237
29.2.2	Rehabilitation	238
29.2.3	Follow-up Investigations	238
29.3	**Results**	238
29.3.1	Surgical Complications and Short-Term Outcome	238
29.3.2	Outcome at Follow-up	239
29.4	**Discussion**	239
29.5	**Conclusion**	242
References		242

M. Tripoli (✉) • F. Moschella
Dipartimento di Discipline Chirurgiche ed Oncologiche
Chirurgia Plastica e Ricostruttiva,
Università degli Studi di Palermo,
Via del Vespro 129, 90127 , Palermo, Italy
e-mail: matripoli@yahoo.it; franzmoschella@libero.it

M. Merle
Institut Européen de la Main of Nancy-France et Luxembourg,
Luxembourg, France
e-mail: mmerle@pt.lu

29.1 Introduction

For selective fasciectomy in patients with Dupuytren's disease at Tubiana Stage I–II, midline longitudinal incisions with serial Z-plasties, Bruner zigzag incisions, and V-Y plasties over the palm and most severely affected fingers are accepted methods. Advantages of these approaches are good intraoperative visualization of the fibrous tissue, rapid dissection, minor tissue trauma, and usually the possibility of a tension-free wound closure (Brenner and Rayan 2003). In cases of Dupuytren's disease at Stage III and IV, with severe digital flexion, inelastic overlying skin, and expected skin shortage after contracture release, these incisions may sometimes be useful, but in our experience, quite often are insufficient, since they may increase the risk of edema, skin necrosis, and wound breakdown. In these cases, dermofasciectomy with full-thickness skin grafting and the McCash technique (McCash 1964) are more often performed (Brenner and Rayan 2003), with different rates of complications and recurrence (Lubahn 1996, 1999).

Correction of the digital deformity without skin incisions and the risk of necrosis can be achieved by percutaneous needle fasciotomy. However, the recurrence rate is high and the technique is less suitable for advanced Tubiana stages (van Rijssen and Werker 2006; van Rijssen et al. 2006). In addition, the technique by some has been associated with a significant risk of neurovascular injury of 3.5% (Foucher et al. 2001) at the metacarpophalangeal joint. Here, the spiral cord is known to displace the neurovascular bundles superficially and medially, where they are prone to injury during the percutaneous needling procedure.

C. Eaton et al. (eds.), *Dupuytren's Disease and Related Hyperproliferative Disorders*,
DOI 10.1007/978-3-642-22697-7_29, © Springer-Verlag Berlin Heidelberg 2012

Dermofasciectomy, the local resection of both the fibrotic skin and digital fascias, with subsequent coverage by a full-thickness skin graft, is advised in young adults with digitopalmar fibromatosis infiltrating the skin, in cases of aggressive progression, Dupuytren's diathesis, or multiple relapses since this technique has a reported lower recurrence risk (Brotherston et al. 1994; Hall et al. 1997). Although clinical studies show good long-term results in respect of graft take and extension gain of the fingers (Abe et al. 2007) with a lower rate of relapse underneath the full-thickness skin grafts (Tonkin et al. 1984; Armstrong et al. 2000), there are potential disadvantages to this procedure. These include hematoma, graft failure, and digital stiffness because of immobilization of the hand while the graft takes. In addition, there is a scar in the skin graft donor site which must be accepted by the patients.

The McCash technique uses only transverse incisions at the distal palm and in digital creases. The transverse incisions in the distal palm is left open, avoiding skin suture under tension, ensuring a good blood supply to the wound margins and permitting the palmar skin defect to heal secondarily (Lubahn et al. 1984). There are two main disadvantage of this technique. First, the digital dissection always ends at the proximal interphalangeal joints. Therefore, if needed, the release of distal interphalangeal joints necessitates a second operation. Second, if primary closure of the digital incisions cannot be achieved without tension, full-thickness skin grafts are required because of the exposed flexor tendons.

In this retrospective study, the authors report on their results in treatment of Dupuytren's disease at Stage III–IV at little finger, using the Jacobsen flap (Jacobsen and Holst-Nielsen 1977), a modification of the McCash procedure, which consist of the creation of an L-shape palmar skin-subcutis flap using two linear incisions (Fig. 29.1a, b).

29.2 Patients and Methods

The indication for the Jacobsen flap is Dupuytren's disease in the palm and the little finger with skin shortage, Stage III or IV according to the Tubiana's classification system (Tubiana 1998). This scoring system categorizes the total passive extension deficit of each ray in 4 stages (Stage I: 0–45°, Stage II: 46–90°, Stage III: 91–135°, Stage IV: 136–180°). Between January 2001 and December 2009, 125 patients, 84 men and 41 women, with severe Dupuytren's disease of the little finger underwent surgery with the Jacobsen flap technique in the Department of Plastic and Reconstructive Surgery of Palermo and in the Institut Européen de la Main of Nancy-France et Luxembourg. Their mean age was 63 years. In 81 patients it was primary surgery, and in 44 patients it was revision surgery because of disease recurrence. None of the patients

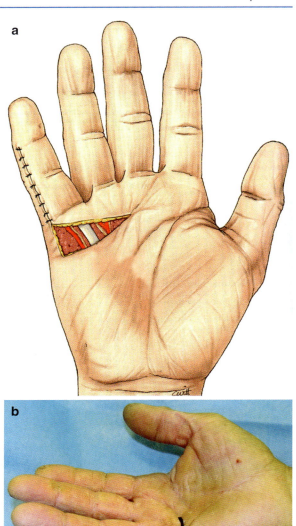

Fig. 29.1 (a, b) The "Jacobsen flap." The L-shaped full-thickness flap is created by performing two linear incisions: the first in the transverse crease of the palm, the second in the midlateral line of the little finger to the distal interphalangeal joint crease

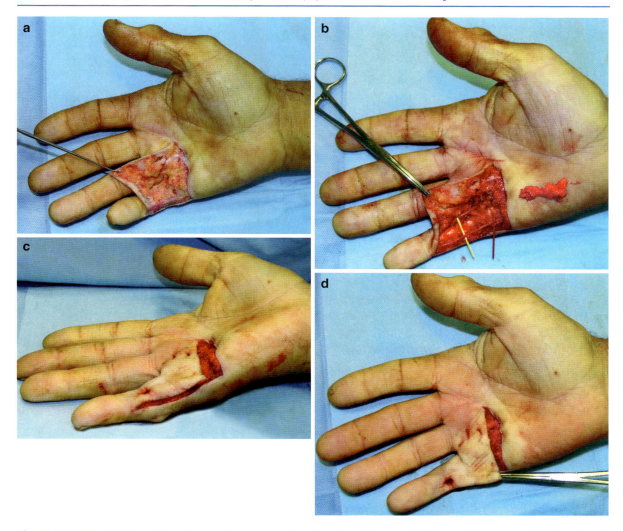

Fig. 29.2 (**a**) The skin flap with its blood supply based on the radial side of the palm. (**b**) Selective fasciectomy (**c-d**) The finger is extended and the flap is transposed distally

had undergone previous Jacobsen flap surgery. At the time of surgery, 37 fingers were at Stage III and 88 at Stage IV. After the operation, all patients were seen at both institutes for follow-up.

29.2.1 Flap Design and Operative Technique

Under brachial plexus block, after application of tourniquet inflated to 300 mmHg, a longitudinal incision was made in the ulnar midlateral line of the little finger, running from the DIP crease to the distal flexor crease of the palm. A transverse incision was then made at the distal palmar crease, thus raising an L-shaped full-thickness skin flap with its blood supply based on the radial side of the small finger (Fig. 29.2a).

A selective fasciectomy is performed, with special attention to preserve the common digital artery and its bifurcation into the proper digital arteries at the level of the metacarpophalangeal joint (Fig. 29.2b). The finger is then fully extended resulting in transposition of the flap distally (Fig. 29.2c-d), and the midaxial arm of the L-shaped incision was closed leaving a mean 15 mm skin defect open in the palm (Fig. 29.3). In 34 cases (21 men, 13 women, 27 at Stage IV, 7 at Stage III) in which more than degrees of flexion persisted in spite of this correction of the contracted finger, an

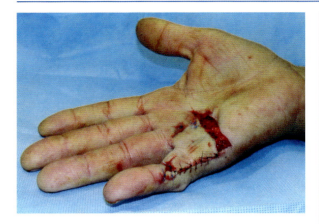

Fig. 29.3 The contracted skin can be stretched and does not prevent full extension of the digits

arthrolysis of the proximal interphalangeal joint with release of the check-rein ligaments of the palmar plate and the collateral ligaments of the proximal interphalangeal was performed as described before (Watson et al. 1979; Beyermann et al. 2004).

29.2.2 Rehabilitation

Forty-eight hours after the operation, the dressings were changed for the first time and thereafter and repeated at intervals of 2–4 days until the wound was healed. A dynamic extension splint was applied for a mean of 6 weeks (range 4–8 weeks), and the healing process was monitored during this period (Fig. 29.4). After the operation, a strict rehabilitation program (physical therapy 3 sessions x 30 min/week, up to an average of 10 weeks with home exercises) was performed.

29.2.3 Follow-up Investigations

The mean follow-up period was 1.8 years (range, 4 months to 3 years). Follow-up included the patient's level of satisfaction and hand mobility. Follow-up was obtained by clinical examination and by the use of a questionnaire which asked for patient satisfaction with the result of the operation. All patients were examined by their surgeons, and results were classified using the Tubiana scale (Fig. 29.5).

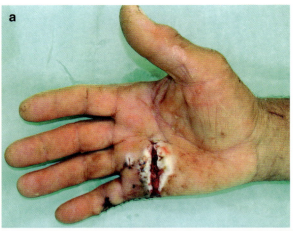
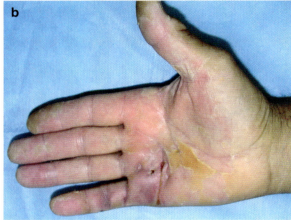

Fig. 29.4 The open wound in the palm heals by secondary intention: postoperative views after 1 week (**a**), 4 weeks (**b**)

29.3 Results

29.3.1 Surgical Complications and Short-Term Outcome

There were some complications as the result of this operation. In one case, a digital nerve injury occurred, and also in one case, a digital artery injury was injured. The nerve was repaired with 9–0 nylon sutures, the artery with 10–0 nylon. Marginal flap necrosis occurred in one case, although both arteries had been preserved, and this was debrided and healed secondarily. There were no hematomas, nor infections.

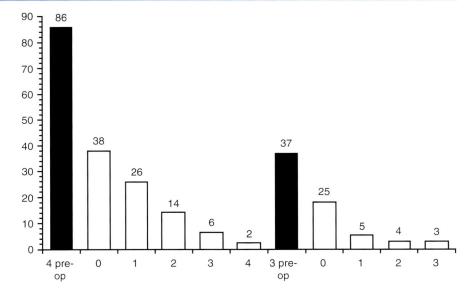

Fig. 29.5 Pre- and postoperative assessment of the patients by the Tubiana classification

Fourteen patients (ten men, four women, 11%) developed recurrent disease after a mean of 10 months after the operations, and ten of them were re-operated using the same technique. In eight, there were no further recurrences during the remaining follow-up period. In two other patients (Stage IV preoperatively), vascular incompetence occurred, probably due to excessive tension on the digital neurovascular bundles, and a little finger amputation was required. Eleven patients (seven men, four women) developed complex regional pain syndrome which was treated with analgesics and physical therapy for a mean of 3 months with complete remission.

One patient, a heavy smoker with type 2 diabetes, had delayed wound healing at the palm. His medication was monitored with scrutiny thrice weekly, and complete wound healing was achieved after 10 weeks.

29.3.2 Outcome at Follow-up

Excluding the two patients with the finger amputation, of the 86 patients who had been Stage IV preoperatively, 38 were converted into Stage 0, 26 into Stage I, 14 into Stage II, and 6 into Stage III at follow-up. Two patients did not improve by the operation and remained in Stage IV. Of the 37 patients with Stage III disease preoperatively, 25 were converted to Stage 0, 5 to Stage I, 4 to Stage II, and 3 to Stage III at follow-up. Thus, 49% improved at least one stage and 49% of 123 patients even achieved Stage 0. Eighty-two percent of the patients scored their outcome as "excellent" (38%) or "good" (44%). Eighteen percent of our patients, all of whom had had complications, considered their outcome "poor." Generally, patients with originally higher Tubiana grading showed poorer outcome and were more likely subject to recurrence. In 34 cases (27 had Stage IV, 7 Stage III), where a 30° flexion defect remained, it had been necessary to release the checkrein ligaments of the palmar plate and the collateral ligaments of the proximal interphalangeal joint to improve the extension of the joint (Fig. 29.6a–c).

29.4 Discussion

Skin closure with Brunner zigzag incisions, V-Y plasties, or Z-plasty closure of a longitudinal midline finger incision can generally only be performed with Stage I and II Dupuytren's contracture. In Stage III and IV disease, which is characterized by contracture of the palmar and finger skin, use of these techniques of closure is associated with a high-risk of edema, marginal necrosis, and wound breakdown.

Dermofasciectomy, using a full-thickness skin graft, is used in cases of recurrences with significant

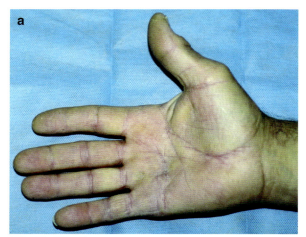

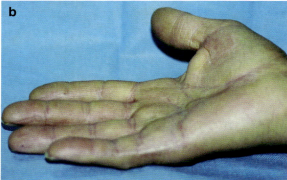

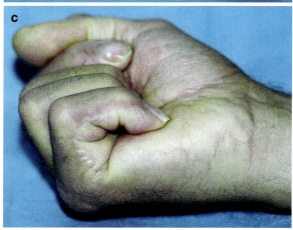

Fig. 29.6 (**a–c**) Two-years postoperative views

(Abe et al. 2007; Brotherston et al. 1994) with a lower rate of recurrence than found with skin preserving surgery (Armstrong et al. 2000), there are potential disadvantages to this procedure. These include hematoma formation, graft failure, and stiffness as a result of immobilization of the hand while the graft takes.

The McCash technique leaves the palmar wound open and avoids skin suture under tension. This ensures a good blood supply to the wound margin (Lubahn et al. 1984). This technique is generally used in conjunction with skin closing techniques in the digits (Lubahn 1999).

The Jacobsen flap technique, a modification of McCash's procedure, permits exposure and removal of the fibrotic tissue in both the palm and in the ring and little fingers. Redistribution of the contracted skin allows for full extension of the digits. In cases in which a 30° flexion defect remains, as described in literature (Watson et al. 1979; Beyermann et al. 2004), it is also possible to release the check-rein ligaments of the palmar plate and the collateral ligaments of the proximal interphalangeal joint to improve the extension of the joint. The open wound in the palm reduces the risk of hematoma and edema. Skin grafting is not required and consequently, there are no donor site scars, and the active mobilization of the hand is immediate with more rapid restoration of hand function. In cases of fibromatosis involving the proximal palmar area and the metacarpophalangeal joint of the fourth finger, it is possible to extend the skin incision at the transverse crease in the palm, and in combination with a zigzag incision proximally, to remove the fibrous tissue at this level (Fig. 29.7a–f). If there is also pathologic tissue in the ring finger distal to the palm, a Jacobsen flap is not indicated.

The Jacobsen technique also has some disadvantages. Careful monitoring of the open wound in the palm is required to avoid infections and delayed healing, especially in patients with metabolic disorders. It is also noted that progressive flexion deformity of the distal interphalangeal joint may occur due to the shortage of the redistributed skin (Merle 2007). The patient must wear a dynamic splint for about 10 weeks and undergo physical therapy three times a week to avoid this flexion deformity.

skin involvement (Tonkin et al. 1984). Although clinical studies show good long-term results in respect of graft take and extension gain of the fingers

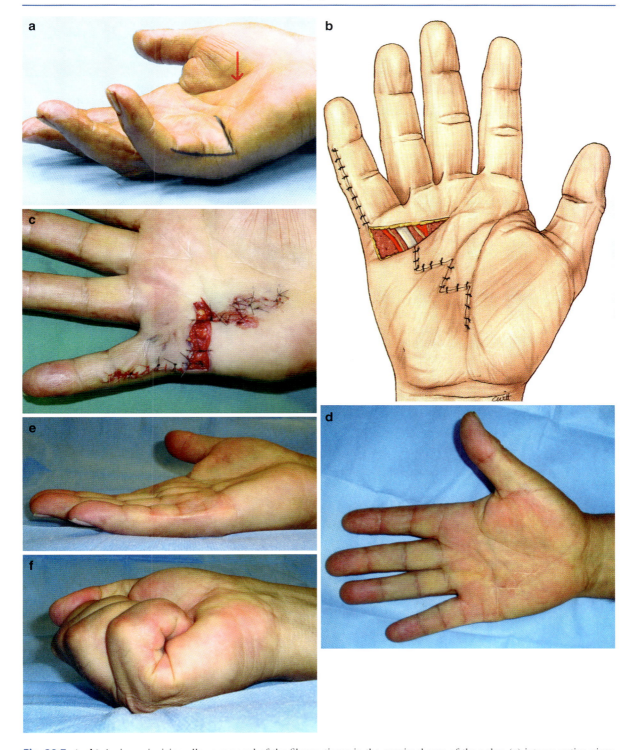

Fig. 29.7 (**a**, **b**) A zigzag incision allows removal of the fibrous tissue in the proximal area of the palm; (**c**) intraoperative view; (**d**–**f**) two-years postoperative result

29.5 Conclusion

The authors consider the Jacobsen flap technique an excellent method for treatment of severe Dupuytren's disease of the little finger (Tripoli and Merle 2008; Tripoli et al. 2010).

References

Abe Y, Rokkaku T, Kuniyoshi K, Matsudo T, Yamada T (2007) Clinical results of dermofasciectomy for Dupuytren's disease in Japanese patients. J Hand Surg Eur 32:407–410

Armstrong JR, Hurren JS, Logan AM (2000) Dermofasciectomy in the management of Dupuytren's disease. J Bone Joint Surg Br 82:90–94

Beyermann K, Prommersberger KJ, Jacobs C, Lanz UB (2004) Severe contracture of the proximal interphalangeal joint in Dupuytren's disease: does capsuloligamentous release improve outcome? Br J Hand Surg 29B:238–241

Brenner P, Rayan GM (2003) Dupuytren's disease, a concept of surgical treatment. Springer Wien, New York

Brotherston TM, Balakrishnan C, Milner RH, Brown HG (1994) Long-term follow-up of dermofasciectomy for Dupuytren's contracture. Br J Plast Surg 47:440–443

Foucher G, Medina J, Malizos K (2001) Percutaneous Needle Fasciotomy in Dupuytren Disease. Tech Hand Up Extrem Surg 5:161–164

Hall PN, Fitzgerald A, Sterne GD, Logan AM (1997) Skin replacement in Dupuytren's disease. J Hand Surg Br 22B:193–197

Jacobsen K, Holst-Nielsen F (1977) A modified McCash operation for Dupuytren's contracture. Scand J Plast Reconstr Surg 11:231–233

Lubahn JD (1996) Dupuytren's fasciectomy: open palm technique. Blair WF, Steyers CM. Techniques in hand surgery. Ed. Williams & Wilkins, Baltimore Philadelphia London, In. pp 508–518

Lubahn JD (1999) Open-palm technique and soft-tissue coverage in Dupuytren's disease. Hand Clin 15:127–136

Lubahn JD, Lister JD, Wolfe T (1984) Fasciectomy and Dupuytren's disease: a comparison between the open-palm technique and wound closure. J Hand Surg Br 9A:53–58

McCash CR (1964) The open palm technique in Dupuytren's contracture. Br J Plast Surg 17:271–280

Merle M (2007) La maladie de Dupuytren. In: Merle M (ed) Chirurgie de la main, vol 3, Affections rhumatismales, dégénératives. Syndromes canalaires. Elsevier Masson, France

Tonkin MA, Burke FD, Varian JPW (1984) Dupuytren's contracture: a comparative study of fasciectomy and dermofasciectomy in one hundred patients. J Hand Surg Br 9B:156–162

Tripoli M, Merle M (2008) The "Jacobsen Flap" for the treatment of stages III-IV Dupuytren's disease: a review of 98 cases. J Hand Surg Eur 33(6):779–782

Tripoli M, Cordova A, Moschella F (2010) The "Jacobsen flap" technique: a safe, simple surgical procedure to treat Dupuytren disease of the little finger in advanced stage. Tech Hand Up Extrem Surg 14(3):173–177

Tubiana R (1998) La maladie de Dupuytren. In: Tubiana R (ed) Traité de chirurgie de la main. Masson, France

van Rijssen AL, Werker PM (2006) Percutaneous needle fasciotomy in Dupuytren's disease. J Hand Surg Eur Vol 31B:498–501

van Rijssen AL, Gerbrandy FS, Ter Linden H, Klip H, Werker PM (2006) A comparison of the direct outcomes of percutaneous needle fasciotomy for Dupuytren's disease: a 6-week follow-up study. J Hand Surg Am 31(5):717–725

Watson HK, Light TR, Johnson S (1979) Check rein resection for flexion contracture of the middle joints. J Hand Surg Br 4:67–71

A Logical Approach to Release of the Contracted Proximal Interphalangeal Joint in Dupuytren's Disease

30

Paul Smith

Contents

30.1 Introduction 243

30.2 Clinical Review 244

30.3 Surgical Release of the PIP Joint 244

30.4 Summary 247

References 247

P. Smith
Bishops Wood Hospital,
Northwood, Middlesex HA6 2JW, UK
e-mail: paul@paulsmithfrcs.co.uk

30.1 Introduction

The PIP joint is at the heart of hand function. A good range of motion at this joint gives good function even in the presence of metacarpophalangeal joint contractures. It is often affected by Dupuytren's contractures due to digital fascial involvement and its correction is the key to good hand function – yet can be most difficult to achieve.

Tonkin et al. (1985) reported a 9% amputation rate for Dupuytren's contractures in patients with a severe diathesis and persistent PIP joint contractures emphasising the difficulty in treating such patients. Inexperienced surgeons may mistake a flexion deformity for a flexion contracture. In PIP-flexion deformity the PIP joint can be fully extended by flexing the wrist, metacarpophalangeal (MP) and distal interphalangeal (DIP) joints. There is no actual joint contracture – only a contraction of the soft tissues. This condition is easily correctable, however if such testing reveals a fixed flexion contracture at the PIP joint – this is much more challenging. These can be referred to as composite flexion deformity versus an isolated joint contracture. It is the isolated PIP joint contractures we are concerned with.

Dupuytren's contracture primarily affects the fascial structures of the hand in the manner described by McFarlane (1974). Fascial contracture then leads to secondary changes in the skin (shortening), joints (peri-articular adhesion) and dorsal apparatus (attenuation and adhesions). It is the author's opinion that joint contractures are secondary and do not represent involvement of Dupuytren's disease of the ligamentous structures of the joint. The logic of the author's

C. Eaton et al. (eds.), *Dupuytren's Disease and Related Hyperproliferative Disorders*,
DOI 10.1007/978-3-642-22697-7_30, © Springer-Verlag Berlin Heidelberg 2012

Fig. 30.1 Pie chart showing surgical and other approaches to PIP joint release in 188 cases

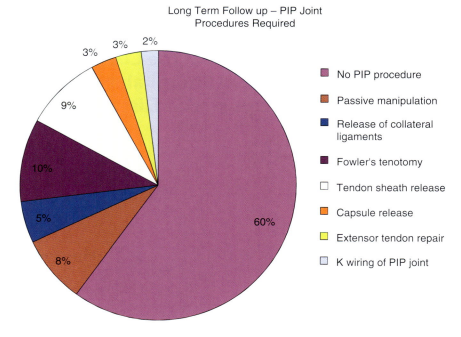

approach is based on this premise and experience of 188 PIP joint contractures as previously reported (Breed and Smith 1996).

30.2 Clinical Review

In this series of 188 PIP joint contractures, digital fasciectomy only resulted in full correction of the PIP joint in 113 cases (60%), leaving 75 cases (40%) requiring a further PIP joint procedure. Fifty-four patients (72%), when tested intra-operatively after fasciectomy, were positive for central slip attenuation (CSA). Review of these patients showed that 80% of them had had a preoperative PIP joint extension deficit in excess of 60°. In this series of the 40% requiring a further PIP procedure 10% required a Fowler's tenotomy to correct DIP joint hyperextension, 9% tendon sheath release, 8% gentle passive manipulation and 5% release of the accessory collateral ligaments. Only 3% required a volar plate release and at that time 3% extensive tendon repair for CSA and 2% were K wired – neither technique would we use today. An analysis of the various treatments regimes showed that a less aggressive approach to the PIP joint yielded better results (Figs. 30.1 and 30.2).

30.3 Surgical Release of the PIP Joint

As a result of these experiences we developed a logical approach to the release of the PIP joint contracture in Dupuytren's disease. We agree with Watson and Fong's (1991) sequential volar to dorsal approach, and want to stress that it is essential to passively test the function of the dorsal apparatus once the contracture is released. Extension at the PIP joint depends on the integrity of the central slip and the lateral bands. If central slip attenuation is present (Smith and Ross 1994) a different postoperative splinting regime is essential. All our patients in this series underwent Skoog's (1948) procedure with McFarlane's (1974) emphasis on extensive digital fasciectomy, combined with the use of the open palm technique (McCash 1964). In regard to the PIP joint our approach is as follows and in the order presented.
1. Skin
   Utilizing the open palm technique allows for up to 1.5 cm of palmar skin lengthening, thereby reducing skin shortage in the digits. In addition, within the digit a linear approach, converted using multiple z plasties with the transverse limbs placed in the digital flexion creases, allows for yet another correction of shortage. Using this approach, skin grafting or local flaps have not been required in this series.

Fig. 30.2 Gentle passive manipulation versus more aggressive surgeries to PIP joint contractures. Graph showing gentle passive manipulation versus more aggressive surgeries to PIP joint contractures. The gentler approach shows better results even for more severe contractures

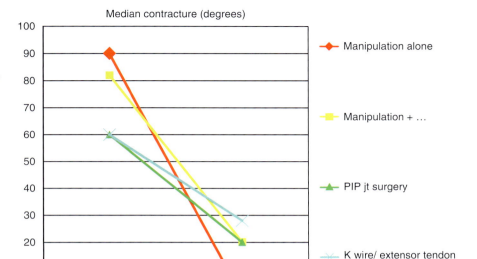

We reserve those techniques for cases with diffuse digital disease.

2. Digital Fasciectomy

   We are aggressive in the resection of the Dupuytren's tissue in the fingers. Care must be taken when there is spiral band. This is often indicated by the preoperative Allen's test which when *positive* indicates vascular compression by Dupuytren's disease – also suggesting that the nerve will be closely surrounded by Dupuytren's tissue. Short and Watson (1982) found the presence of fat in between the cord and the skin in the distal palm also indicative of a spiral band. Care should be taken to remove the retrovascular band of Thomine – if involved, as well as the lateral digital sheet. Fasciectomy may correct the contracture in up to 60% of cases. In all cases with residual flexion contracture we move on to

3. Gentle passive manipulation (Smith 2002)

   This is undertaken with the MP joint in flexion by applying gentle extension on the PIP joint. The premise is that this will correct any secondary periarticular joint adhesions which have developed as a result of prolonged postural flexion deformity, becoming structural over time. Full correction may often be achieved – if not, the next step is

4. Release the flexor sheath

   In this series this was more frequently required than volar plate release and involves resection of the sheath between the A2 and the A4 pulley. This often leads to the desired full extension. If not, this is followed by

5. Release the volar plate

   Watson and Fong (1991) achieved correction in 110 out of 115 PIP joint contractures by releasing of the "checkrein ligaments." This is a neologism, not an anatomical term but is has become commonly used in clinical practice.

   There are no other structures on the volar surface of the PIP joint which can be involved in producing a flexion contracture – unless the flexion tendons exhibit adhesions as a result of previous surgery. If so, we progress to

6. Flexion tenolysis

   It should now be possible to fully extend the PIP joint. However if there has been extensive Dupuytren's tissue around the neurovascular bundles, these may have lost their elasticity and be incapable of allowing PIP extension without producing ischaemia. In such cases a flexed position must be accepted and gradual postoperative splintage is utilized to increase extension. These cases however have a very poor prognosis.

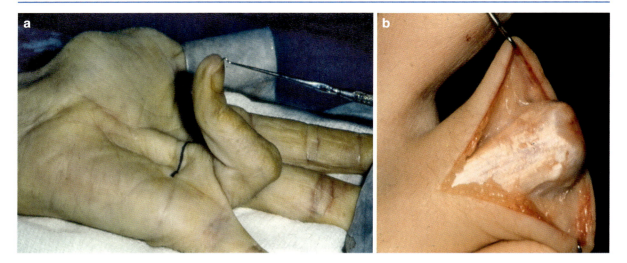

Fig. 30.3 (**a**) A typical patient who is likely to have a central slip attenuation. (**b**) Exposure of a dorsum finger with central slip attenuation over the PIP joint

Once full PIP joint extension has been accomplished, the joint may be found to be stable in full extension or flexion but snap (Smith 2002) from one position to the other. This snapping is usually due to tightness of the accessory collateral ligaments (ACL) which are at the tightest at 15° of flexion. In such cases following release of all contracted structures gentle movement in either direction may push the finger into flexion or extension. This instability in flexion or extension or snapping finger is corrected by

7. Release of the ACL
  Thereafter, no obstruction remains and the digit will be stable both in flexion and extension. Finally, we need to ensure that active extension is possible.
8. Central Slip Attenuation
  This should now be tested for by undertaking the central slip test (Smith and Ross 1994). To this aim, the wrist and MP joint are flexed and, if the central slip is intact the tenodesis effect will tighten the central slip to produce PIP extension. If the central slip is attenuated it will not be able to extend the PIP joint (Figs. 30.3 and 30.4).

  Central slip attenuation requires a specific postoperative splintage regime. The use of the open palm techniques makes it difficult to utilize a Capener splint because the proximal end of the splint would press on the open wound and thus cannot be used for several weeks. However, in these cases immediate commencement of splintage is essential. Our current regime is therefore to immediately fit the patient with a static day and night splint in full MP and PIP extension for 2 weeks, after which they are allowed to remove the splint to exercise for 10 min every hour.

  The splint may be required during the daytime for between 2 and 6 weeks.
9. Release Adhesions of the lateral bands
  There are always adhesions around the dorsal apparatus. These should be freed deep to the dorsal apparatus and superficial to it, clearly defining its edge – the lateral bands. This can be done through a volar approach. Once released gentle pulling on the lateral bands must produce PIP extension – or further release is necessary.

  We should now have a digit which extends fully at the PIP joint – but on occasion there may be DIP joint hyperextension, a boutonniere type deformity which cannot happen without central slip attenuation and tightness of the conjoined lateral bands. In order to allow full DIP joint flexion – we need to
10. Release tightness of the conjoined lateral bands and oblique retinacular ligaments of Landsmeer.
  The conjoined lateral bands act as DIP joint extensors and so when there is hyperextension they can be asymmetrically divided and rejoined at a longer length. The oblique retinacular ligaments of Landsmeer acts to maintain maximum extension at the DIP joint for every degree of flexion. In other words it acts in a similar manner to the lumbricals action on the PIP joint but it differs in that its proximal attachment is fixed to the proximal phalanx unlike the lumbrical which is a mobile moderator band between the flexion and

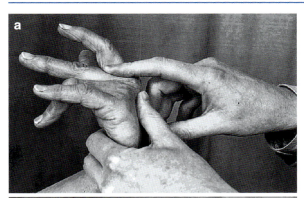

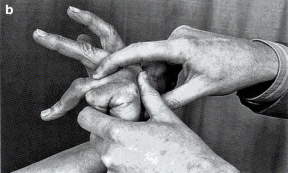

Fig. 30.4 Central slip tenodesis test. Following fasciectomy and correction of all volar contractures the central slip tenodesis test is performed. (**a**) The wrist is held in flexion. The MP joint of the finger being tested is fully flexed. In the middle finger the central slip is intact and the passive tenodesis effect produces automatic extension of the PIP joint. (**b**) The ring finger undergoing the same test shows lack of PIP extension displaying central slip attenuation

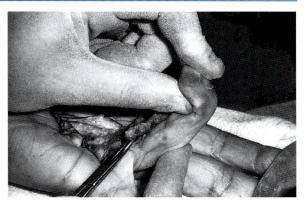

Fig. 30.5 Testing tightness of the lateral bands. Tightness of the conjoined lateral bands and oblique retinacular ligaments can be tested by extending the PIP joint and attempting to flex the DIP joint. The degree to which it cannot be flexed indicates the severity of the tightness of these structures. If there is hyperextension of the DIP joint then they are very tight and may require a Fowler's tenotomy

extension systems. These two mechanisms ensure that the digits close in a Fibonacci curve maintaining maximum extension until the digits are fully flexed. An alternative to surgical release of the hyperextended DIP joint is gentle passive manipulation of the DIP joint into flexion with the PIP joint held in extension (Fig. 30.5).

Despite this comprehensive approach to PIP joint contractures in Dupuytren's disease, there will be many cases where correction cannot be achieved due to: (1) diffuse disease; (2) neurovascular bundle involvement even to the extent of causing ischaemia; (3) previous surgery leading to scar formation, vessel or nerve injury; and (4) prolonged flexion contracture with secondary bone changes and articular cartilage destruction (Field and Hueston 1970).

In such cases one must either accept the residual contracture or consider fusion, arthroplasty or amputation. Loss of flexion in exchange for a gain in extension must be avoided.

30.4 Summary

In summary we can do no better than to quote Kirk Watson (1991) "Persistent flexion deformities are the result of inadequate surgeries. After the resection of the diseased fascia, there may still be persistent joint contractures. This result is due to secondary changes in the joint from longstanding contractures. These should be fully evaluated and corrected at the initial operation." We present a logical approach to their correction. The crucial steps involved are

1. To release all volar contracted structures
2. To ensure flexion and extension stability
3. To guarantee active PIP joint extension
4. Ensure full flexion

References

Breed PM, Smith PJ (1996) A comparison of methods of treatment of PIP joint contractures in Dupuytrens disease. J Hand Surg [Br] 21(2):246–251

Field PL, Hueston JT (1970) Articular cartilage loss in longstanding flexion deformity of the proximal interphalangeal joint. Aust NZ J Surg 40:70–74

McCash CR (1964) The open palm technique in Dupuytrens contracture. Br J Plast Surg 17:21

McFarlane RM (1974) Pattern of the diseased fascia in the fingers in Dupuytrens contracture. Plast Reconstr Surg 54: 31–37

Short WH, Watson HK (1982) Prediction of the spiral nerve in Dupuytren's contracture. J Hand Surg Am 7:84

Skoog T (1948) Dupuytrens contraction with special reference to aetiology and improved surgical treatments, its occurrence in epileptics. Note on knuckle pads. Acta Chir Scand 96(suppl 139):1–190

Smith PJ (2002) Dupuytren's disease. In: Smith PJ (ed) Lister's the hand, 4th edn. Churchill Livingston, London

Smith PJ, Ross DA (1994) The central slip tendosis test for early diagnosis of potential boutonniere deformities. J Hand Surg Br 19(1):88–90

Tonkin MA, Burke FD, Varian JPW (1985) The proximal interphalangeal joint in Dupuytrens disease. J Hand Surg 10B:358–364

Watson HK, Fong D (1991) Dystrophy, recurrence, and salvage procedures in Dupuytren's contracture. Hand Clin 7(4): 745–755

The Influence of Dupuytren's Disease on Trigger Fingers and Vice Versa

31

Bernd Kuehlein

Contents

31.1	Introduction	249
31.2	Diagnosis and Treatment	249
31.3	Patients Characteristics and Incidence of Concurrent Disease	250
31.4	Treatment Outcome	250
31.5	Discussion	250
31.5.1	Why Is DD Concurring with TF?	251
31.5.2	General Considerations for the Treatment of TF of the Middle and Ring Finger	252
31.5.3	Surgical Strategies and Recommendations	252
References		252

B. Kuehlein
Gottfried-Keller Str. 20,
81245 Munich, Germany
e-mail: kuehlein@plastische-praxis.de

31.1 Introduction

Trigger finger release is one of the most frequently performed operations in a hand surgery (Wildin et al. 2006). Trigger finger (TF) is sometimes seen in combination with other hand affections such as Dupuytren's disease (DD). It has been our impression that DD and TF somehow are linked and interact upon each other. Surprisingly enough this problem has hardly received attention in the literature. Speculations on a common root cause (Perry 1994) have not been scrutinized, except maybe for specific cases where diabetes is involved (Papanas and Maltezos 2010; Chammas et al. 1995).

31.2 Diagnosis and Treatment

Dupuytren's Disease is usually diagnosed by the presence of skin pits together with nodules and/or cords in the palmar fascia, with or without related and slowly developing extension deficits of the corresponding finger. In contrast, trigger finger is diagnosed either by circumscriptive pain when pressing on the A1 pulley area or by a triggering phenomenon while bending the finger (Saldana 2001). This examination is daily routine for everyone dealing with hand problems. When both problems are present at the same time, tenderness over the A1 pulley is the prevailing symptom of trigger finger, rather than triggering.

Our standard treatment for TF is decompression of the A1 pulley under local anesthesia in a bloodless field, using a small transverse skin incision (Lange-Riess et al. 2009). In addition and similar to approaches in other clinics (Hoffmann 1999), just before skin closure, we apply 5 mg of Dexamethasonacetonate combined with 30 mg Lidocainhydrochloride (Supertendin®, Schwarz

C. Eaton et al. (eds.), *Dupuytren's Disease and Related Hyperproliferative Disorders*,
DOI 10.1007/978-3-642-22697-7_31, © Springer-Verlag Berlin Heidelberg 2012

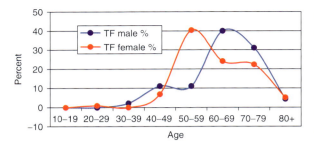

Fig. 31.1 Age distribution of patients with trigger finger ($n=161$)

Pharma AG, Monheim, Germany, catalogue number: PZN −1690426), since this has been found to smoothen the postoperative course. Postoperatively, the finger is mobilized immediately to prevent tendon adhesions. Whenever DD is also present it is uncertain what the best approach is. The purpose of this chapter is to elaborate on this issue.

31.3 Patients Characteristics and Incidence of Concurrent Disease

Between November 2008 and November 2010, we operated 177 trigger fingers in all rays in 161 patients. Sixteen patients had two trigger fingers operated on at the same time. Congenital trigger fingers were excluded. There were 45 males and 116 females in this subgroup. The average age of female patients was 62 years and of the male patients 64.5 years (Fig. 31.1).

Concurrent appearance of Dupuytren's disease and trigger finger was observed in 28 cases in 23 patients: 8 middle fingers (4 male, 4 female), 20 ring fingers (11 male, 9 female). In 5 patients both the middle and ring finger were affected by DD and TF (3 male, 2 female). So in total DD was present in 16% of our trigger finger cases. When considering middle and ring fingers only DD and TF were present in 25%. If three additional cases were included, where within 1 year after surgery for TF Dupuytren's disease developed, the incidence would be 28% and this illustrates the relevance of the issue for TF of middle and ring fingers.

31.4 Treatment Outcome

The outcome of the treatment of 13 cases was analyzed in more detail, since these had a minimal follow-up of 1 year (operated between 11/2008 and 11/2009) after combined surgery for TF and DD. None of these cases exhibited more than 45° extension deficit preoperatively (Tubiana Stages N or I) (Tubiana and Micron 1961).

Within 1 year DD recurred in seven patients (54%) as nodules at the operation site, but without signs of contracture. All seven patients and one that had no clinical signs of DD recurrence reported pain and sourness at the operation site and were unable to completely bend the finger into the palm. Two of them developed clear signs and symptoms of TF again, one needing reoperation. None of the remaining 164 TF cases had persistent or recurrent TF.

31.5 Discussion

The purpose of this study was to report on our experiences in the treatment of combined TF and DD. The major limitation is the number of cases in this study. Nevertheless, the incidence and treatment outcome of cases in which TF occurred in conjunction with DD was so different and appeared less predictable than that of ordinary TF, that we wanted to report this and give some thoughts about this.

The demographics of our trigger finger patients (affected fingers, sex, and age distribution) resemble those reported earlier (Makkouk et al. 2008; Trezies et al. 1998).

We observed a high percentage of concurrent TF and DD in the middle and ring finger (25%) and the following calculation reveals that this percentage is much higher than expected from mere statistical coincidence; if we assume a DD prevalence of 32% (Degreef and de Smet 2010), the average probability to develop a nodule specifically in the fourth ray of 70% (Moermans 1997, Fig. 31.2), and accommodate for two hands (50%), this gives a probability of accidental coincidence of 11% for the ring finger and of 5% for the middle finger. This is an upper limit estimation, ignoring age dependence and timing.

Until now we presumed that TF occurs together with DD just by accident in the same ray. Figure 31.2 shows the distribution of DD involvement of each finger with or without TF. The DD figures are derived from Moermans (1997). Results are nearly identical in both data sets, which might indicate that Dupuytren's disease is the driving force for the development of TF.

31 The Influence of Dupuytren's Disease on Trigger Fingers and Vice Versa 251

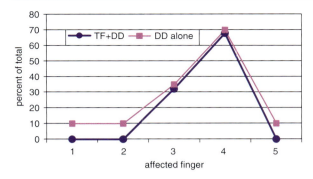

Fig. 31.2 Affected trigger fingers of patients with Dupuytren's disease. The "DD alone" percentages (*purple line*) are the probability figures to develop DD in a specific finger and are taken from Moermans (1997). The TF + DD percentages are those found by the author by ray

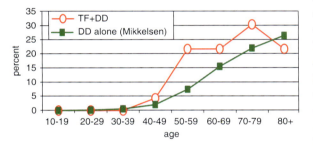

Fig. 31.3 Age dependence of TF+DD combination. The *red data* (TF+DD) is the distribution of the prevalence of TF+DD cases by age group. That distribution qualitatively follows the age distribution of Dupuytren patients (DD alone) which was interpolated from Mikkelsen's data (1972), merging his male and female data in a 1:1 relation to better match the gender relation of our TF+DD data

So far we ignored the effect of age but Fig. 31.3 shows that the percentage of patients with combined trigger finger and DD strongly increases with age.

It is obvious that the percentage of patients suffering from both diseases increases with age. We found that 50% in the "80+" age group (5/10) of our TF patients are suffering from both diseases. While according to Fig. 31.1 the probability to develop trigger finger diminishes quickly with 80+, the probability to develop DD is still increasing. From our data we cannot deduce to what extent both diseases exactly influence each other.

31.5.1 Why Is DD Concurring with TF?

Smith (2001) considers trigger finger as an early indication of Dupuytren's disease and our findings

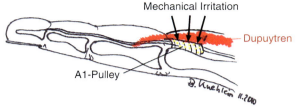

Fig. 31.4 Anatomy of the finger with stage I Dupuytren's disease

(Fig. 31.2) do corroborate with this assumption to some extent. In concordance with McGrouther he believes that the deepest layer of the pretendinous fibers (layer three) play a role in causing trigger finger symptoms in Dupuytren's disease (1999). However, in our cases, we have observed only few relatively strong but very thin fibers in the subcutaneous area over the A1 pulley, which might have corresponded to layer 1 fibers of the pretendinous cord and as such forerunners of DD. No other signs of an onset of Dupuytren's disease were detected, although we must admit that full dissection of layer three might not have been possible, because we used a small transverse incision. Therefore, our findings do not contradict Smith's considerations. One would expect, however, that with increasing DD the layer three fibers named by Smith would aggravate triggering. Yet we have not seen this; with progressing Dupuytren's contracture trigger finger does not seem to be an issue. This requires further investigation and more extensive dissection.

We believe that other factors might play a role: in the extended finger position thickening of the pulley wall leads to narrowing of the A1 pulley and synovial congestion (Makkouk et al. 2008). The additional mechanical irritation of the Dupuytren's cord above it may provoke an aggravation of the irritation (Fig. 31.4).

In more progressed stages of Dupuytren's contracture, e.g. Stages II or III, the concomitant appearance of trigger finger and Dupuytren's contracture is rarely seen (Fig. 31.5). This may be explained by the fact that the DD cord that causes a flexed position of the finger is not in such an intimate relation with A1, resulting in relief of pressure off the affected tendon at the A1 pulley area. This may thus resolve the additional irritation of this part of the tendon that we anticipated is present in Stage N or I. Absence of occurrence of TF in these more advanced DD cases could then be explained as

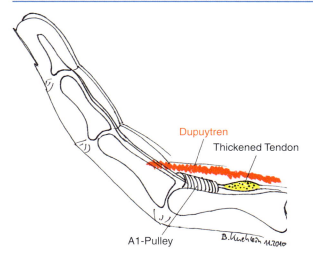

Fig. 31.5 Anatomy of the finger with stage II of Dupuytren's contracture

follows: advanced extension deficit reduces the range of motion of the tendon and thus causes less mechanical irritation at A1. Another explanation would be that the tendon becomes slightly thinner distal to the chiasm of the deep and superficial flexor tendon.

31.5.2 General Considerations for the Treatment of TF of the Middle and Ring Finger

An induration that develops at the very site of pulley release, which shortly after surgery progresses into a DD nodule, may seriously disturb the physician–patient relation, since the patient may feel not to be treated properly (Smith 2001). In these cases a good doctor–patient relation based on confidence is essential for the patient to understand and accept this unforeseen slowly progressing development. Therefore, particularly in operations on the middle and ring fingers, a meticulous examination and search for the slightest hints of Dupuytren's disease in an early stage, e.g. mere hardening of the palmar fascia, is important. A thorough (family) history for risk factors for DD and examination for ectopic lesions such as Ledderhose's disease, Peyronie's diease, and Garrod's knuckle pads is required. If we find any indication of a possible Dupuytren's disease the patient should be warned for a possibly extended healing process. Besides, an even more conservative approach by repeated applications of corticosteroids to postpone surgery is recommended, although the effectiveness of steroids may be limited in these patients.

31.5.3 Surgical Strategies and Recommendations

Initially and for a long time our approach of choice for combined TF and DD had been selective opening of the pulley using a small (transverse) incision without touching the Dupuytren tissue and without additional intraoperative steroids application. Very often this resulted in postoperative sourness and slight flexion deformities at the proximal interphalangeal joint. Longer recovery periods, extending over months, were not rare.

The obvious next approach was to resect the Dupuytren's tissue as well. Yet, of these cases 58% developed a recurrence with induration in the operated area – almost as strong as preoperatively – within 1 year. This recurrence rate was a lot higher than in DD cases without concomitant trigger finger and higher than previously reported (Becker and Davis 2010). In addition, the same patients reported problems in flexion of the fingers with permanent tension in the finger as a result of ongoing irritation reactions for months after the operation, while a deficiency in extension did not occur.

In the last 6 months we have changed our strategy to the following: in case of TF combined with DD we perform an isolated opening of the pulley without touching the Dupuytren tissue. At the end of the procedure we apply corticosteroids (e.g. Dexamethasonacetat, Supertendin®) in the area of the opened pulley. Although follow-up is very limited it is our impression that this is a good strategy: so far we observed no or very little progression of the Dupuytren's disease. Furthermore, postoperative recovery seems a lot faster. Longer follow-up is necessary to find out if this strategy indeed is the best.

References

Becker GW, Davis TR (2010) The outcome of surgical treatments for primary Dupuytren's disease – a systematic review. J Hand Surg Eur 35(8):623–626

Chammas M, Bousquet P, Renard E, Poirier JL, Jaffiol C, Allieu Y (1995) Dupuytren´s disease, carpal tunnel syndrome, trigger finger, and diabetes mellitus. J Hand Surg Am 20(1): 109–114

Degreef I, De Smet L (2010) A high prevalence of Dupuytren's disease in Flanders. Acta Orthop Belg 76(3):316–320

Hoffmann R (1999) Checkliste handchirurgie, 2nd edn. Thieme, Stuttgart, pp 377–378

Lange-Riess D, Schuh R, Hönle W, Schuh A (2009) Long-term results of surgical release of trigger finger and trigger thumbs in adults. Arch Orth Trauma Surg 129(12): 1617–1619

Makkouk AH, Oetgen ME, Swigart CR, Dodds SD (2008) Trigger finger: etiology, evaluation, and treatment. Curr Rev Musculoskelet Med 1(2):92–96

McGrouther D (1999) Dupuytren's contracture. In: Green D et al (eds) Green's Operative hand surgery. Churchill Livingstone, New York

Mikkelsen OA (1972) The prevalence of Dupuytren's disease in Norway. Acta Chir Scand 138:695–700

Moermans JP (1997) Place of segmental aponeurectomy in the treatment of Dupuytren's disease. PhD thesis, University of Brussels, Belgium. http://www.ccmbel.org/These.html. Accessed 20 Dec 2010

Papanas N, Maltezos E (2010) The diabetic hand: a forgotten complication? J Diabetes Complications 24(3):154–162

Perry GF (1994) Why do some people develop two or more inflammatory conditions (ie, carpal tunnel syndrome, Dupuytren's contracture, trigger finger, etc) without any clear-cut etiologic factor(s) being present? J Occup Med 36(3):295–296

Saldana MJ (2001) Trigger digits: diagnosis and treatment. J Am Acad Orthop Surg 9(4):246–252

Smith PJ (2001) Lister´s the hand diagnosis and indications, 4th edn. Churchill Livingston, New York, p 523

Trezies AJH, Lyons AR, Fielding K, Davies TRC (1998) Is occupation an aetiological factor in the development of trigger finger? J Hand Surg Br 23B:539–540

Tubiana R, Micron J (1961) Evaluation chiffree de la deformation dans la maladie de Dupuytren. Mem Acad Chir 87:887–888

Wildin C, Dias JJ, Heras-Palou C, Bradley MJ, Burke FD (2006) Trends in elective hand surgery referrals from primary care. Ann R Coll Surg Engl 88(6):543–546

No Higher Self-Reported Recurrence in Segmental Fasciectomy

32

Ilse Degreef

Contents

32.1	**Introduction**	255
32.1.1	Treatment Options	255
32.1.2	Outcome	256
32.1.3	Questions	256
32.2	**Material and Methods**	256
32.2.1	Segmental Fasciectomy	259
32.2.2	Limited Fasciectomy	259
32.2.3	Dermatofasciectomy	259
32.3	**Results**	259
32.4	**Discussion**	260
32.5	**Conclusions**	260
References		260

I. Degreef
Department of Orthopaedic Surgery,
Leuven University Hospitals,
Weligerveld 1, 3212 Pellenberg, Belgium
e-mail: ilse.degreef@uzleuven.be

32.1 Introduction

In Dupuytren's disease, the primary treatment goal is to regain and maintain a normal range of motion of the patient's fingers and hands. Surgery is performed to correct finger contractures and to maintain this correction as long as possible afterwards. The finger contractures reflect the patient's hand function. Since Dupuytren's disease is painless in almost all patients, the contractures are the first reason most patients present to the hand surgeon. Therefore, the patient will judge the surgical outcome based on the correction of these contractures (Dias and Braybrooke 2006). Recurrence of contractures means recurrence of the original complaint of the patient. Up to this day, there is no known 'cure' for Dupuytren's disease. If the patient shows no symptoms of the disease after surgery, we can only conclude that this patient is in a state of 'remission' as compared to patients successfully treated for systemic cancers.

Smith even stated that 'disease recurrence is an inevitable consequence in Dupuytren's disease, if only the patient lives long enough' (Bulstrode et al. 2005).

32.1.1 Treatment Options

Current treatment options in Dupuytren's disease are numerous. The reason for this is that there are a lot of patients and the disease prevalence is high, as we have shown in Flanders with a prevalence as high as 30% in male over 50 years old (Degreef and de Smet 2010). On the other hand, there is guarantee for indefinite success to any treatment option. Although many nonsurgical treatment methods have been suggested

C. Eaton et al. (eds.), *Dupuytren's Disease and Related Hyperproliferative Disorders*,
DOI 10.1007/978-3-642-22697-7_32, © Springer-Verlag Berlin Heidelberg 2012

in the past, Rayan recently stated that surgery is currently the only reliable treatment option in Dupuytren's disease (Rayan 2008). If all reported surgical options are considered in Dupuytren's disease, a treatment ladder with increasingly extensive techniques becomes obvious (Fig. 32.1). In any surgical procedure, the basic requirements are obviously a good outcome, but also a minimal morbidity for the patient. This is exactly the basis of a very long-lasting discussion in the choice for a surgical technique in Dupuytren's disease. On the bottom of the ladder, minimal to almost noninvasive corrective procedures have been introduced, such as needle aponeurotomy and segmental cord resections. The aim of minimally invasive surgery is to correct the cords with as minimal morbidity to the patient as possible. On the top of the ladder, more drastic procedures have been advocated. Here, the aim of surgery is to remove all diseased tissue, in some techniques even surrounding healthy palmar fascia and overlying skin.

In minimally invasive surgery, the most important complaint of the patient is addressed, namely the correction of the contracture. The morbidity of the patient is minimal. However, in total cord resection, all diseased tissue is removed. Although the patient's morbidity is more profound, the choice for more invasive techniques is supported by the idea that Dupuytren's disease is a tumor-like process and a thorough resection may prevent disease recurrence.

How is one to choose between all these surgical options? Few studies have been performed, to compare the outcome in a standardized manner. There are only few true randomized trials reported and different techniques are almost never compared in similar patient groups. A short-term follow-up study on percutaneous needle fasciotomy versus segmental cord resection was reported and showed no significant different outcome between these techniques (van Rijssen et al. 2006). As Dias recently stated, there is an urgent need for extended research on the outcomes of surgery in Dupuytren's contracture (Dias and Braybrooke 2006).

32.1.2 Outcome

But how can we compare outcome? How do we need to judge if outcome is good, better, or worse in a way that is easy and represents what really matters to the patients? In surgery for Dupuytren's disease, we can look at the correction of the contracture, patient's satisfaction, disability, complication rates, healing time, and so on. The severity of Dupuytren's contracture, however, appears to have no significant influence on current disability scores (Degreef et al. 2009b). Furthermore, essentially all publications describing specific surgical techniques report reasonably good and reliable (short-term) results. However, most studies have been performed in mixed populations with patients with low and high-risk Dupuytren's disease, meaning with low and high diathesis. Patients with a high diathesis for fibrosis carry a higher risk for recurrent contractures. Recurrence is the debate in any surgical procedure for Dupuytren's disease. If we look at recurrence reports, the variability is high and results depend on the time of follow-up and the definition of recurrence (Dias and Braybrooke 2006). Does recurrence mean recurrent disease underneath the skin scar or is extension of the disease included? Is it defined as recurrence of nodules or contractures? Although many definitions have been proposed, the Hueston table top test illustrates the essence of recurrence for the patient (Hueston 1982). Since the disease at its own is never cured, judging recurrence of contractures (not of 'disease') is essential in outcome evaluation, since it will reflect the patient's hand function and it is how the patient judges the outcome of surgery.

32.1.3 Questions

If we consider the parameter 'recurrence' in the outcome of surgery for Dupuytren's disease, there are three basic questions. Is there a 'better' procedure? Is it true that incomplete removal of diseased tissue, as is done in segmental fasciectomy, will lead to a higher recurrence? On the other hand, does an extended surgical approach, with resection of all pathological tissue including the overlying skin, lower recurrence rates? In other words, do we need to fight the disease (full thickness grafting) or can we fight the contractures (minimally invasive surgery, cord interruptions) (Degreef et al. 2009a)?

32.2 Material and Methods

In a retrospective study on 721 files of patients operated on between 1992 and 2005 at a single center, the patients were asked to give their perception on

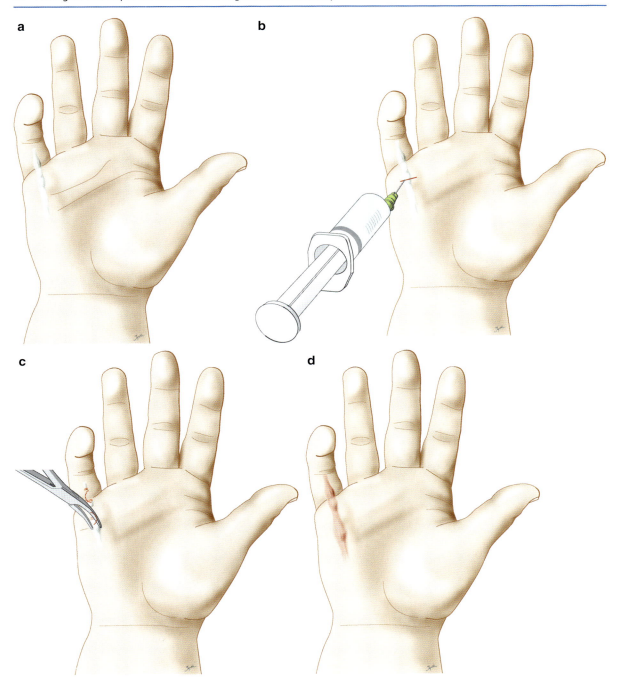

Fig. 32.1 The 'treatment ladder': illustration of the spectrum in surgical treatment methods applied in Dupuytren's disease (**a**) with increasing invasiveness of the techniques. Strand interruptions or fasciotomy (**b**) segmental strand resection (**c**) fasciectomy (**d**) total fasciectomy (**e**) Hueston procedure or subtotal preaxial amputation with skin resection and full thickness grafting (**f**) flap surgery (**g**) and amputation (**h**)

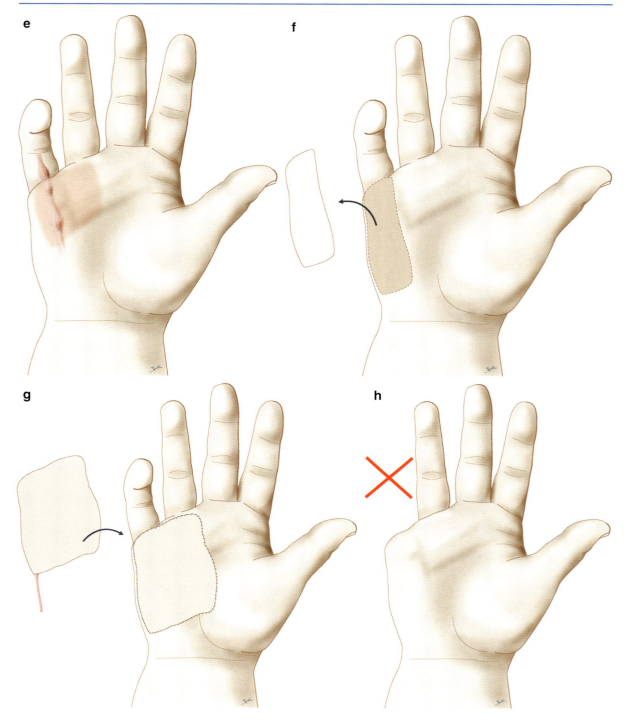

Fig. 32.1 (continued)

recurrence. Surgical techniques were categorized and compared with self-reported recurrence rates. Risk scores on fibrosis diathesis were compared by using the score as was introduced by Abe (Abe et al. 2004).

All patients underwent first-time surgery and there was a minimal follow-up of 2 years, with a mean of over 5 years. The central question was 'did the contracture reoccur after the operation?' Surgical techniques (all performed using loupe magnification) are shortly described as follows:

32.2.1 Segmental Fasciectomy

Small curved incisions of about 1 cm are placed over the cord with a minimal 1 cm interval. A segment of the cord is resected over 5–10 mm to straighten the finger. A total of 1–3 incisions were made per contracted finger. A proximal section of the cord is done within the operation field with the finger in extension and a distal cut of the cord is done with the finger in flexion, to guarantee a maximal cord interruption and firebreak through a minimal incision. The skin is not undermined and nodules or cords between the interruptions remain untouched. In the fingers, the neurovascular bundles are divided from the cords and protected throughout the minimally invasive surgical procedure.

32.2.2 Limited Fasciectomy

Using Brunner zig-zag incisions, the total cord is dissected free and the neurovascular bundles are retracted. The nodules and cords (all fibronodular tissue macroscopically present) are fully resected to achieve a full range of motion of the affected fingers. If needed, a Z plasty of the skin is performed.

32.2.3 Dermatofasciectomy

A Brunner incision is made and the retracted skin overlying the fibrous tissue is removed along with it 'en bloc', mostly over the palmar finger basis. The full thickness skin graft is harvested from the medial side of the proximal forearm using a longitudinal incision with primary closure of the donor site. The graft is perforated to release hematoma formation and fixed to the surrounding skin and pulley to minimize dead space and possible blood collection. A compressive bandage is left in place for 1 week and then active mobilization is started.

32.3 Results

With a response rate of 55%, a global recurrence was reported in over half of the patients (57%). Total cord resection was performed in 46%, segmental cord resection

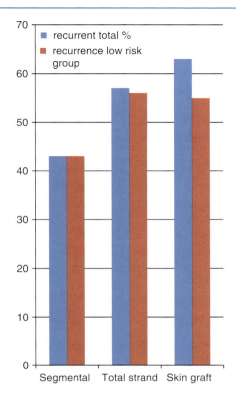

Fig. 32.2 Illustration showing the total recurrence rates and the recurrence rate in the group with a low fibrosis diathesis

in 40% and full thickness grafting in 14%. Recurrence was mentioned in 57%, 43%, and 51%, respectively (Degreef et al. 2009a). The reported recurrence rates were significantly lower in segmental fasciectomy if all patients were included and fibrosis diathesis was not considered. However, if the diathesis is included, by using the score of Abe, it became obvious that the surgeon's decision to use an operation technique was biased by the severity of the diathesis for Dupuytren's disease (Abe et al. 2004). More extensive surgery was chosen in more severely affected patients. However, if patients with the high-risk scores were excluded, there was still no higher reported recurrence in segmental cord resection and although due to the lower numbers, statistical significance was lost, recurrence reports remained even somewhat lower (Fig. 32.2).

The cords can be transected, currently often done blindly with a needle. In the segmental fasciectomy, firebreaks are created by taking out small pieces of the cords. A full cord resection is done through larger incisions, often with a Z-plasty of the overlying skin. In a total fasciectomy, all of the fascia palmaris is removed, in the hope recurrent disease can be avoided. In some cases, the overlying skin is also removed and in some cases, it is replaced by a skin flap (sometimes a pedicle flap). When the battle is lost or in serious complications, the hand is partially amputated.

32.4 Discussion

Segmental fasciectomy has a lot of advantages for the patients. It is a less extensile procedure compared to total cord resections or skin replacement techniques. No wide dissections are needed, wound complications are low, fingers are not stiff after surgery, and rehabilitation is fast (Moermans 1996). Now, we have seen that the reported recurrence is not higher and even somewhat lower than in more invasive surgical techniques. This may be subscribed to the fact that Dupuytren's disease after all is a fibroproliferative process and is comparable with scar tissue formation. The amount of scar tissue is related to the surgical techniques used. In minimally invasive techniques, less scar tissue is induced and this may very well influence postoperative recurrence of contractures. Weaknesses of the study are its retrospective nature, the reporting by patients, and the lack of data on the exact recurrence of the contractures.

However, we conclude that although not all diseased tissue is removed in segmental fasciectomy, this surgical technique appears to have no higher recurrence and even has the lowest patient-reported recurrence rate. Still, it is 40% after a long follow-up period, what does point to the fact that recurrent contractures are immanent in Dupuytren's disease, if only the patient lives long enough (Bulstrode et al. 2005).

On the other hand, full thickness grafting after skin resection does not guarantee a permanent remission state, since here also, over 50% recurrence is reported. A full thickness graft does not appear to lower recurrence of contracture (Ullah et al. 2009). We have seen later on even that if full thickness grafting was performed in recurrent Dupuytren's disease (this means that the surgeon was more radical than the first surgical attempt in the idea that a more radical approach may prevent recurrence), recurrent disease was reported in over 90% (unpublished data).

We therefore advise to confine surgery to a minimally invasive procedure whenever feasible. Surgery is only done to correct the finger contractures, not to remove all diseased tissue. The surgeon should always bear in mind that he can cut out the cords, but not the disease itself (Degreef et al. 2009a).

32.5 Conclusions

- Surgery is performed to correct contractures, not to cure.
- If the patient has no symptoms after surgery, he is in a remission state.
- Segmental cord resection does not have higher recurrence reports.
- Full thickness grafting does not guarantee indefinite results.
- The surgeon can cut the cords but cannot cut out the disease itself.

References

Abe Y, Rokkaku T, Ofuchi S, Tokunaga S, Takahashi K, Moriya H (2004) An objective method to evaluate the risk of recurrence and extension of Dupuytren's disease. J Hand Surg 29B:427–430

Bulstrode NW, Jemec B, Smith PJ (2005) The complications of Dupuytren's contracture surgery. J Hand Surg Am 30A: 1021–1025

Degreef I, De Smet L (2010) A high prevalence of Dupuytren's disease in Flanders. Acta Orthop Belg 76(3):316–320

Degreef I, Boogmans T, Steeno P, De Smet L (2009a) Segmental fasciectomy in Dupuytren disease. Lowest recurrence rates in patient's perception. Eur J Plast Surg 32:185–188

Degreef I, Vererfvre PB, De Smet L (2009b) Effect of severity of Dupuytren contracture on disability. Scand J Plast Reconstr Surg Hand Surg 43:41–42

Dias JJ, Braybrooke J (2006) Dupuytren's contracture: an audit of the outcomes of surgery. J Hand Surg Br 31(5): 514–521

Hueston JT (1982) The table top test. Hand 14(1):100–103

Moermans JP (1996) Long-term results after segmental aponeurectomy for Dupuytren's disease. J Hand Surg 21B: 797–800

Rayan GM (2008) Nonoperative treatment of Dupuytren's disease. J Hand Surg Am 33(7):1208–1210

Ullah AS, Dias JJ, Bhowal B (2009) Does a 'firebreak' full-thickness skin graft prevent recurrence after surgery for Dupuytren's contracture? A prospective, randomised trial. J Bone Joint Surg Br 91(3):374–378

van Rijssen AL, Gerbrandy FS, Ter Linden H, Klip H, Werker PM (2006) A comparison of the direct outcomes of percutaneous needle fasciotomy and limited fasciectomy for Dupuytren's disease: a 6-week follow-up study. J Hand Surg Am 31:717–725

Palmar Cutaneous Branches of the Proper Digital Nerves Encountered in Dupuytren's Surgery: A Cadaveric Study

33

Robert M. Choa, Andrew F.M. McKee, and Ian S.H. McNab

Contents

33.1	Introduction	261
33.2	Materials and Methods	261
33.3	Results	262
33.4	Discussion	262
References		264

33.1 Introduction

Limited fasciectomy is a procedure commonly performed by hand surgeons, for patients with varying degrees of digital contracture due to Dupuytren's Disease. A possible complication of the procedure is injury to the common or proper digital nerves, with rates of nerve injury between 1.5% and 7.8% reported in the literature (McFarlane and McGrouther 1990; Sennwald 1990). Nerves are identified within healthy tissue either proximally or distally and traced carefully through the diseased tissue which is removed.

The senior author had observed palmar cutaneous nerve branches intraoperatively, diverging from the proper digital nerves towards the midline of the fingers, palmar to the metacarpophalangeal joint. These branches on occasion had the appearance of the proper digital nerve. The purpose of this study was to investigate whether these branches are a constant anatomical feature not previously described and to predict the location of these nerve branches, in order to aid the surgeon performing fasciectomy.

33.2 Materials and Methods

Five pairs of fresh frozen cadaveric specimens (four males, one female) severed at the mid-forearm level were used and 40 fingers were thus dissected. None of the specimens had evidence of hand or wrist pathology, including Dupuytren's contractures.

Under loupe magnification, a superficial midline longitudinal palmar incision was made on each finger, extending from the distal interphalangeal joint crease to the proximal transverse palmar crease. The skin was

R.M. Choa (✉) • A.F.M. McKee • I.S.H. McNab
Nuffield Orthopaedic Centre, Windmill Road, Headington,
Oxford OX3 7LD, UK
e-mail: rob_choa@hotmail.com; aandkmckee@mac.com;
ian.mcnab@ntlworld.com

C. Eaton et al. (eds.), *Dupuytren's Disease and Related Hyperproliferative Disorders*,
DOI 10.1007/978-3-642-22697-7_33, © Springer-Verlag Berlin Heidelberg 2012

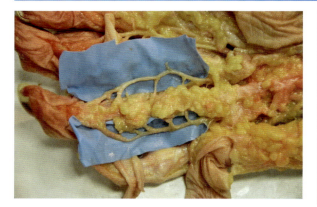

Fig. 33.1 Palmar cutaneous nerve branches

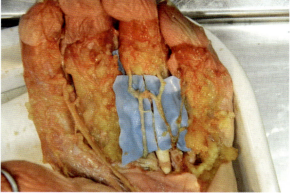

Fig. 33.2 Nerve branches meeting in midline forming 'chevron shape'

dissected off the palmar aspect of each finger superficial to the subcutaneous fat. The A1 pulley and common digital nerves to each finger were identified distal to the transverse palmar fascia. The neurovascular bundles were then dissected distally, identifying and carefully preserving any branches diverging towards the midline, up to the distal interphalangeal joint. To identify the proximal end of the A1 pulley the dissection was extended. The midpoint of the proximal end of the A1 pulley formed the landmark from which distances to the origin of nerve branches were measured to the nearest millimetre. All nerves were then categorised into groups of increasing 5 mm increments i.e. 0–5 mm, 6–10 mm etc. Second, the distance from the midpoint of the proximal end of the A1 pulley to the tip of the finger was measured (Fig. 33.1) to calculate the percentage of nerve branch origin to finger length.

33.3 Results

There were variable numbers of nerve branches in the 0–5 mm and 6–10 mm categories without consistent representation in each finger. However, all the proper digital nerves had one or more branches in either the 11–15 mm or 16–20 mm categories on both the radial and ulnar sides of the finger. Distal to 20 mm there was again inconsistent representation in each 5 mm category of nerve branches, which were seen in categories up to 45 mm in different fingers. Therefore, we concentrated on the nerves in the 11–15 mm and 16–20 mm groups. The branches originating at these distances were found to extend over the palmar aspect of the metacarpophalangeal joint.

Each branch normally had a corresponding branch from the proper digital nerve on the contralateral side of the finger. These pairs of nerve branches were seen to converge to form a "chevron shape" and appeared to serve a dense concentration of Pacinian corpuscles (Fig. 33.2). They were also found to be distinct from the dorsal digital nerves. Distally, each proper digital nerve was found to have multiple smaller palmar cutaneous branches diverging towards the midline of the finger. Of note, the radial border of the index finger was found to have the greatest numbers of these.

A range of values were obtained, allowing both the mean and median distances that the nerves originated at to be calculated in each finger type. Furthermore the mean finger lengths were also calculated allowing both a ratio and percentage of finger length at which the branches originated to be calculated (Table 33.1).

33.4 Discussion

This study specifically sought to identify palmar cutaneous nerve branches at the metacarpophalangeal joint level which could be encountered in Dupuytren's surgery, and potentially mistaken for a proper digital nerve. There are relatively few anatomical studies of the digital nerves, which is surprising due to the frequency of digital nerve injuries, both accidental and iatrogenic. Bas and Kleinert performed a detailed study of 30 cadaveric hands to depict the course and interconnections of the sensory nerves to the digits (Bas and Kleinert 1999). Despite documenting communications between the dorsal and palmar branches of the digits in great detail, no

Table 33.1 Results

Finger	Mean distance of branch from A1 pulley (mm)	Median distance of branch from A1 pulley (mm)	Mean length of finger (mm)	% Length of finger	Ratio of finger length	Range of first chevron branch distances from A1 pulley (mm)
Index	16	18	83	19	1:5	11–20
Middle	15.5	16	88	18	1:6	11–20
Ring	15	15	84	18	1:6	11–20
Little	15	15	73	21	1:5	11–20

mention was made of branches similar to those in this study. Zenn et al. investigated the variations in digital nerve anatomy in ten cadaveric hands (Zenn et al. 1992). They reported on terminal branching of the digital nerves, and branching patterns, but again with no mention of the branches we encountered.

Don Griot et al. have investigated the ramus communicans between the ulnar and median nerves and the associated variations in sensation of the ring finger in great detail (Don Griot et al. 2000). They found this feature in 94% of cadaveric specimens they investigated, suggesting this is a constant anatomical feature rather than an anatomic variation.

Although our findings are somewhat limited due to the relatively small number of specimens, the nerve branches we described appear to be a constant anatomical feature. The exact function is yet unknown. In our experience, these branches can be mistaken for the proper digital nerve, especially when they are of a similar calibre. This could lead to an inadvertent injury of the proper digital nerve, if the surgeon believes this structure has already been protected. Diameters of the proper digital nerves and their associated branches were not measured in this study, as this would have required more accurate digital callipers than were available to us. It is acknowledged that this is an important factor to consider and will be the subject of a future study.

One aim of this study was to try and predict where these branches arise in order to aid the hand surgeon performing fasciectomy. The data suggest that on average the first branches arise at 19% of the distance from the A1 pulley base to the tip of the finger – or in the clinical setting, approximately one fifth of the distance. This is similar when assessing the ratios of nerve branch origin to finger length which are approximately 1:5. The A1 pulley bases were chosen as landmarks, as

they are a fixed point and found in each ray. However, the A1 pulley is not always exposed during fasciectomy which could make prediction of the nerve branches difficult according to our technique. One study used surface landmarks to predict the location of the proximal edge of the A1 pulley with reasonable accuracy (Wilhelmi et al. 2001). We therefore propose that this landmark technique is employed to mark the proximal end of the A1 pulley. Once this has been done the distance to the tip of the finger can be divided into five equal distances. The junction between the two proximal fifths is where the first nerve branches would be expected to be found, thereby facilitating safer surgical dissection.

Acknowledgements We acknowledge Professor John Morris, Martin Barker and Ryan Green in the Oxford University Department of Physiology, Anatomy and Genetics.

References

Bas H, Kleinert JM (1999) Anatomic variations in sensory innervation of the hand and digits. J Hand Surg Am 24(6):1171–1184

Don Griot JP, Zuidam JM, van Kooten EO, Prosé LP, Hage JJ (2000) Anatomic study of the ramus communicans between the ulnar and median nerves. J Hand Surg Am 25(5): 948–954

McFarlane RM, McGrouther DA (1990) Complications and their management. In: McFarlane RM, Flint DA (eds) Dupuytren's disease. Churchill Livingstone, Edinburgh, pp 348–364

Sennwald GR (1990) Fasciectomy for treatment of Dupuytren's disease and early complications. J Hand Surg 15A:755–761

Wilhelmi BJ, Snyder N 4th, Verbesey JE, Ganchi PA, Lee WP (2001) Trigger finger release with hand surface landmark ratios: an anatomic and clinical study. Plast Reconstr Surg 108(4):908–915

Zenn MR, Hoffman L, Latrenta G, Hotchkiss R (1992) Variations in digital nerve anatomy. J Hand Surg Am 17(6):1033–1036

Part VI

Needle Release and Hand Therapy

Editor: Paul M.N. Werker

A Technique of Needle Aponeurotomy for Dupuytren's Contracture

34

Charles Eaton

Contents

34.1   **Introduction** 267

34.2   **History** 267

34.3   **Indications and Contraindications** 268

34.4   **Surgical Anatomy** 268

34.5   **Technique** 269
34.5.1 Setting 269
34.5.2 Instruction 269
34.5.3 Portal Planning 269
34.5.4 Surgical Field Preparation 270
34.5.5 Anesthesia 270
34.5.6 Sequence and Monitoring 271
34.5.7 Maneuvers 271
34.5.8 Bandaging 273

34.7   **Rehabilitation** 273

34.8   **Clinical Case** 273

34.9   **Common Questions** 273

34.10 **Learning Curve Pitfalls** 279

References 279

34.1 Introduction

Needle aponeurotomy (NA) is a method of percutaneous fasciotomy using a small hypodermic needle as a scalpel blade. Compared to fasciectomy, there is a lower incidence of prolonged recovery, nerve injury, flare reaction, or RSD (Cheng et al. 2008; Foucher et al. 2003; van Rijssen and Werker 2006). Nerve injuries are avoided with intradermal anesthesia and distal sensibility monitoring during the procedure. The chance of tendon injury is minimized by monitoring active finger motion while the needle tip position is in proximity of flexor tendons. NA can be performed in the office, usually permits return to normal manual activities 1 week after the procedure, allows both hands to be treated on consecutive days, and is safe in poor-risk patients, including patients on anticoagulants. Disadvantages include recurrences occurring more rapidly than open surgery and an inability to correct either skin shortage or capsular contractures of the proximal interphalangeal joint. The following technique is based on the author's experience with NA on over 8,000 hands.

34.2 History

Percutaneous fasciotomy for Dupuytren's contracture is the first recorded procedure for the treatment of Dupuytren's contracture (Cooper 1822). At that time, percutaneous procedures were common, referred to as "subcutaneous surgery". Dupuytren later introduced open fasciotomy (Dupuytren 1831) and Goyrand fasciectomy (Goyrand 1835). Percutaneous release of Dupuytren's contracture was reported by many surgeons of the time, including Guérin, Fergusson, Little,

C. Eaton
The Hand Center,
1002 S Old Dixie Hwy Suite 105, Jupiter,
FL, 33458, USA
e-mail: eaton@bellsouth.net

C. Eaton et al. (eds.), *Dupuytren's Disease and Related Hyperproliferative Disorders*,
DOI 10.1007/978-3-642-22697-7_34, © Springer-Verlag Berlin Heidelberg 2012

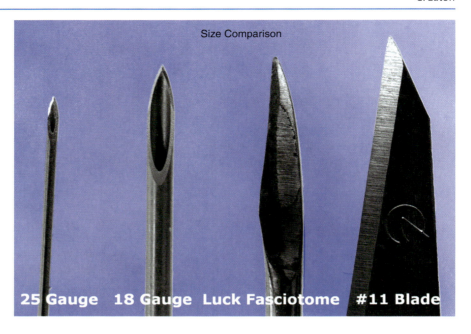

Fig. 34.1 Size comparison of percutaneous fasciotomy instruments. A 25 gauge needle is 0.5 mm in diameter and has a cutting edge length of 0.8 mm

Erichsen, Gant, Druitt, and Adams (Adams 1879). In the nineteen hundreds, following the general trend of open over percutaneous surgery, open procedures for Dupuytren's gained popularity over percutaneous fasciotomy. In the mid 1950s, Luck (1959) revisited percutaneous fasciotomy, using custom fasciotome blades (Fig. 34.1), but Luck's technique never achieved mainstream popularity. In the 1970s, Lermusiaux began performing percutaneous fasciotomy for Dupuytren's using a 25 gauge needle (Lermusiaux and Debeyre 1979). After release, his first patient "…was so happy, she jumped up and kissed me" (Lermusiaux JL, 2004, personal communication). With the Lermusiaux technique, cords are injected with a mixture of lidocaine and methylpredinsone using a 25 gauge needle mounted on a 3 cc syringe. The needle used for injection is then moved in place to cut the cord, and the finger is straightened with manipulation. A minimum number of fasciotomy sites are used – one to three; multiple fingers are treated on multiple visits. Needle release for Dupuytren's has since gained increasing popularity as a practical and effective option (Lermusiaux 2000; Foucher et al. 2003; van Rijssen and Werker 2006; Cheng et al. 2008). The technique presented in this chapter is based on the Lermusiaux technique with modifications including intradermal skin wheal anesthesia, multiple portals, multiple fingers, safety monitoring, and standard documentation.

34.3 Indications and Contraindications

The requirements for NA for Dupuytren's are *contracture* due to a *palpable cord* lying beneath *redundant skin* in a *cooperative patient*. NA will not correct longitudinally inadequate skin or scar and should not be attempted in the absence of a palpable cord. NA will not correct contractures not due to Dupuytren's. Patients with constitutionally treatment-resistant Dupuytren's (Abe et al. 2004; Degreef and de Smet 2011; Hindocha 2006) will just as likely have rapid recurrence after NA as they will after simple fasciectomy and should be considered for arthrodesis or dermofasciectomy and skin graft.

34.4 Surgical Anatomy

Cords are insensate; other structures are not, which allows NA to be performed safely with intradermal anesthesia. Sensory end organs of the skin are in the deep dermis, but the subdermal fat and palmar aponeurosis have no sensory innervation. Joint capsules are innervated (Schultz et al. 1984), digital nerves are sensitive to pressure, and clinical experience is that there is sensory innervation of flexor tendon sheaths.

Dupuytren's transforms and shortens fascia and subdermal fat into cords. Vertical septal fiber anatomy

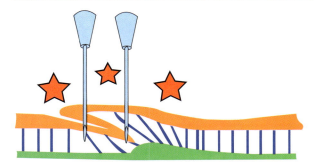

Fig. 34.2 Dimple issues with needle release. Dimples may be deeper than they appear, and if there is a question, a small probe should be used to measure depth. *Left*: without caution, deep dimples may be inadvertently entered or transected. *Right*: innervated deep dermis extends beyond the apparent depth, resulting in unexpected tenderness

is distorted, bunching and dimpling the skin by oblique tethering between the dermis and cord (Fig. 34.2). Secondary contractures may develop from immobilization (PIP joint capsule, intrinsic muscle) and position-related attrition (boutonniere, sagittal band rupture).

34.5 Technique

34.5.1 Setting

NA can be performed in an office setting using local antiseptic prep without either sedation or tourniquet. Alternatively, a formal operating room environment and light sedation may be used as long as the patient remains responsive to mild pain. The patient should be recumbent to prevent vasovagal issues. A 2″ thick pad of folded towels is used as a support behind the metacarpus to facilitate MCP extension.

34.5.2 Instruction

Expectations are explained as possible improvement up to 90° of composite MCP+PIP contracture and/or 50% improvement in PIP contracture. The technique is reviewed, including the importance of reporting paresthesias or numbness and of avoiding sudden movements. Short arc fingertip flexion and extension is demonstrated to and then repeated by the patient. The possibility of skin tear, nerve or tendon injury is reviewed as well as the postoperative care protocol.

Bilateral releases should be staged at least 1 day apart to reduce the likelihood of postprocedure inflammation; bilateral simultaneous releases are not recommended.

34.5.3 Portal Planning

Fasciotomy portals are best planned in areas where the skin is soft and the cord is well defined. Planned portals are marked with a surgical marking pen. Portals are usually spaced longitudinally a minimum of 5 mm apart, directly over the cord. Side by side portals may be used for broad cords over 8 mm wide, connecting the dots transversely under the skin.

34.5.3.1 Cords, Nodules, and Nodular Cords

Pure cords are palpable only under tension, have well-defined lateral margins, and have a distinct plane of separation from the mobile overlying normal skin. If not visible, cords may be identified entirely by palpation while passively flexing and extending the adjacent joint. Pure cords are ideal locations for portals. *Pure nodules feel firm, independent of joint position* and are tethered to the overlying dermis. The dermal papillary ridges are raised and prominent over nodules compared to adjacent normal skin, different than the type of stretching and flattening which develops over a slowly growing palmar soft tissue tumor. Skin texture helps distinguish nodules from areas of skin bunching or prominences overlying dimples or tumors such as sebaceous cysts. Ideally, portals are not planned over pure nodules because they release unpredictably, are prone to skin tears, and for reasons unknown may be painful to needle. *Nodular cords have features of both* cords and nodules. Portals are used over nodular cords if there are not enough available pure cord choices.

34.5.3.2 Skin Deformation

Skin deformation is a useful guide: *releases which restore normal skin contour are usually also effective at contracture release*. Skin creases are not used for portals because of the proximity of the flexor sheath and the likelihood of skin tear. If skin creases are curved or eccentrically bunched up, portals are planned on the convex side of the curve ("*Convex points to the portal*") (Figs. 34.3 and 34.4). PIP joint skin crease deformation to a convex distal shape points to the use of a portal distal to the PIP flexion crease, releasing the

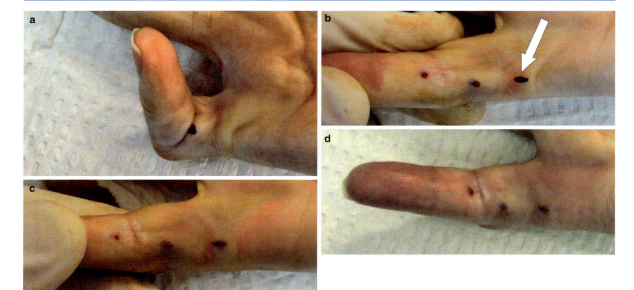

Fig. 34.3 Blanching and skin crease deformation as guides to portal placement. Blanching and skin crease deformation can be used to plan portals and assess adequacy of release. (**a**) Before release. (**b**) Portal planned at an area of loss of blanching (*arrow*). The flexion crease adjacent to this has become curved, convex distally. Both findings suggest cord tethering at the area of the most proximally marked portals. (**c**) after release, normal flexion crease contour; blanching crosses the portal, indicating adequate cord release. (**d**) after release, showing exposure of macerated skin and the use of a distal PIP portal as shown in Fig. 34.4

cord proximal to the portal beneath the flexion crease (Fig. 34.4). *Dimples* are evaluated with a small probe to avoid portals which might transect a dimple sinus or cause pain from contacting the dermis at the depths of the dimple (Fig. 34.2).

34.5.3.3 Blanching

If the underlying cord is tighter than the skin, the skin will not blanch with traction due to stress shielding (Fig. 34.3). An area with soft skin which does not blanch is usually a good site for a portal ("*Pink = Portal*"). Portals are avoided in areas of skin which blanch with traction: unless due to obvious cord bowstringing, blanching indicates that the skin has no residual elastic reserve and that there is nothing deeper to release.

34.5.3.4 Spiral Cords

Doppler examination (Fig. 34.5) should be performed when there is a question of a spiral cord, based on soft tissue prominence in the distal palm or proximal digit (Short and Watson 1982). Areas of identified Doppler tones indicating spiral cords are marked with a surgical marking pen. Portals are avoided at these sites, but may be used with caution 6–8 mm proximal or distal.

34.5.4 Surgical Field Preparation

NA may be performed with local field sterility similar to that for intravenous needle insertion. The patient washes and dries their hands and the palm is painted with antiseptic solution. Sterile needles are used. Gloves are used, but sterile gloves and drapes are not required.

34.5.5 Anesthesia

Pinpoint surface anesthesia is obtained by injecting each portal area intradermally with 0.05–0.1 cc of local anesthetic using a 30 gauge needle, avoiding subcutaneous injection. Injection pain is reduced by buffering the local anesthetic with sodium bicarbonate, using a personal massager to vibrate the adjacent skin during injection, lightly touching the injection site with the needle tip 1–2 s prior to penetration and using a verbal countdown,

34 A Technique of Needle Aponeurotomy for Dupuytren's Contracture

digital nerve conduction block: frequent sensibility checking is mandatory throughout the procedure. If sensitivity to light gauze touch remains, the nerve is considered "live" even if the patient reports a subjective change, and NA may be continued, following the decision tree of Fig. 34.6.

34.5.6.2 Tendon Monitoring

Tendon proximity is repeatedly checked during the procedure. With the needle in place, the patient is asked to lightly flex and extend their PIP and DIP joints to demonstrate presence or absence of needle motion with active tendon excursion. Flexor tendons are close to the skin not only at skin flexion creases, but also just distal to the distal palmar crease (metacarpal head) and just proximal to the PIP flexion crease (proximal phalanx head). Tendon sheath incursion is also possible through a lateral digital portal. All of these areas require repeated monitoring with active finger motion.

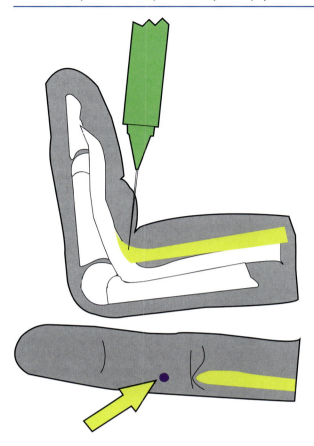

Fig. 34.4 PIP release using portals distal to the PIP flexion crease. Portals distal to the PIP flexion crease may be used to release the insertion of proximal phalanx cords as in Fig. 34.3. This is guided by convex distal deformation of the skin flexion crease

penetrating the skin ¼ second *before* the final count. Penetrate just the surface of the dermis and inject during needle withdrawal: this produces immediate anesthesia.

34.5.6 Sequence and Monitoring

Releases are begun at distal portals, progressing proximally. In the event of an inadvertent anesthetic conduction block at one level, a more proximal portal may still be used, where the nerve should still be sensitive. For the same reason, releases are completed in all fingers before proceeding to palm portals.

34.5.6.1 Nerve Monitoring

Fingertip sensitivity is repeatedly checked through the procedure. Despite careful technique, anesthetic diffusion or mild nerve contusion may rapidly produce

34.5.7 Maneuvers

A 5/8″ 25 gauge needle is used as a scalpel. The needle tip has two cutting edges, which are identified visually (loupes are helpful) and maintained with needle bevel perpendicular to cord fibers after insertion. The goal is to perform a transverse fasciotomy deep to the skin. There are three basic moves: *clear*, *perforate*, *sweep*. Once the needle is through the dermis, the needle is oriented tangentially and a plane between dermis and cord is developed (*cleared*) transversely at the level of the portal at least as wide as the palpable cord width. The needle is reoriented vertically, bevel transverse, and a light reciprocating (*perforating*) motion is used to define the extent and surface geometry of the cord. Once the cord geometry is defined, the needle tip bevel is used to repeatedly *sweep* or graze the surface of the cord, dividing it incrementally from superficial to deep.

34.5.7.1 Traction

Cords must be held under tension, both to allow the needle to cut and to pull the cord up and away from deeper structures. *The safest traction is pulling on the skin or a nodule distal to the portal in distal direction.* The flexor tendons should be slack, reducing the risk of inadvertent tendon injury: *don't pull on the fingertips; remind the patient to relax their fingers.*

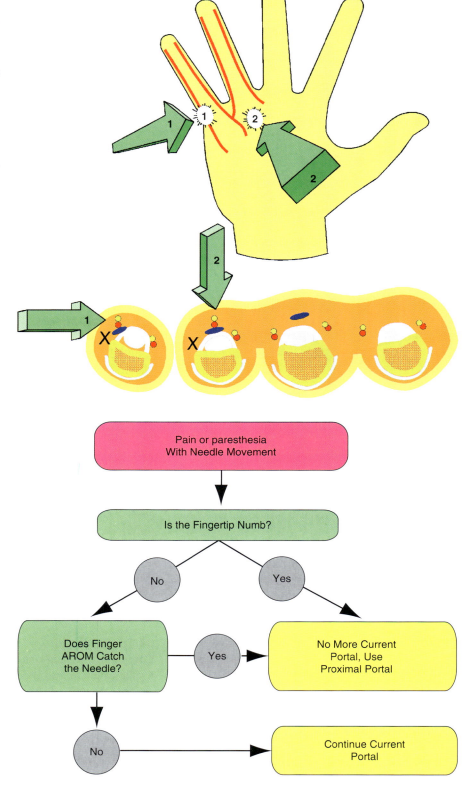

Fig. 34.5 Doppler examination for spiral cords. *Top*: In areas where a fleshy prominence suggests a spiral cord, the Doppler probe tip should be placed at the planned skin portal, but pointed toward areas where a digital artery should *not* be heard: (*1*): superficial and tangential to the palm for prevascular prominences; (*2*): perpendicular to the palm for pretendinous bulges. *Bottom*: cross section of the same with Dupuytren cords shown in blue and "*X*" showing the expected location to hear Doppler tones with normal anatomy

Fig. 34.6 Algorithm to manage pain or paresthesia during NA. Digital nerves in proximity of the current portal are assessed with fingertip sensitivity before and after anesthesia and frequently during instrumentation. Pain may represent nerve or tendon sheath incursion and prompts the need to check each

34.5.7.2 Cord Palpation

Use fingertips to palpate cords, which should be felt to tighten as the finger is passively moved from flexion to extension. In areas of diffuse skin involvement or in the thenar or first web space zones cords can be demonstrated by "trampoline" fingertip bouncing helpful to assess adequacy of cord rupture.

34.5.7.3 Blanching

Blanching will advance across a portal when the underlying fascia has been adequately released (Fig. 34.3).

34.5.7.4 Needle Feel

The fascia should feel crisp or crunchy when being cut. When the needle meets rubbery resistance to insertion or withdrawal, it is dull and should be replaced.

34.5.7.5 Manipulation

Passive stretching may be done after each portal release. *Skin tears* are most common in and adjacent to flexion creases. Once a tear develops, further attempts at passive extension are likely to propagate the tear rather than separate a cord at a different portal. If a portal looks suspicious for tearing, defer definitive pull until several proximal portals have been released to reduce the chance of a skin tear. Flexor tendon tension is reduced by flexing the wrist and having the patient actively extend their fingers at the time of manipulation. MCP and DIP joints passively extend past neutral, but PIP manipulation is limited by lack of passive hyperextension. This can be compensated for using four PIP maneuvers: isolated PIP stretch with MP flexed; dorsal-radial stretch; dorsal-ulnar stretch; composite PIP+MCP stretch. Intraarticular local anesthetic injection of the PIP and MCP joints is helpful as well as axial traction to reduce pain from joint surface compression during manipulation. Manipulation under anesthetic wrist block may also help.

34.5.7.6 Steroid Injection

After releases, portals and nodules may be injected with depot corticosteroid such as triamcinolone acetate or its equivalent, 2 and 20 mg, respectively.

34.5.8 Bandaging

Bandaging should be light, allowing immediate motion and postprocedure icing: small adhesive bandages or a light gauze wrap.

34.6 Documentation

Location of cords, nodules, ROM, portal, and nodule injection sites are documented as in Figs. 34.7 and 34.8. Forms for this are available at http://DocsNA.com.

34.7 Rehabilitation

Rehabilitation therapy is not usually needed. Bandages may be removed the day of the procedure. Ice and elevation are recommended for the first 2 days. Strenuous gripping is strictly avoided for 1 week. Patients must be cautioned that because the fascia is insensate, postoperative gripping may not be painful, but may still provoke a delayed inflammatory reaction resembling infection. After 1 week, activities are resumed as tolerated.

34.8 Clinical Case

This 68-year-old right handed man developed Dupuytren's at the age of 47 years. History is positive for Ledderhose, Peyronie's, and knuckle pads. He underwent left thumb and small fasciectomy 8 years ago. He now has recurrence and extension in the left ring and small finger and new involvement of the right thumb, ring, and small fingers. His hands were treated with NA on consecutive days (Figs. 34.7 and 34.8).

34.9 Common Questions

- *How do you know where the nerves are, especially when using lateral digital portals?* You don't, which is the reason for using a small diameter needle, short arc movements, and frequent sensory checks. Neurovascular bundles are displaced by both cord tension and cord bulk, and are more often shifted dorsally than palmarly. Soft areas between the cord and dermis should have Doppler evaluation for spiral cords, but there is no substitute for frequent sensory testing.
- *What about repeat NA?* This is a common issue because on the average, recurrences occur earlier after NA than after fasciectomy. If there is skin reserve over a palpable cord in a willing patient who had a satisfactory release which lasted a reasonable period of time, repeat NA is a consideration

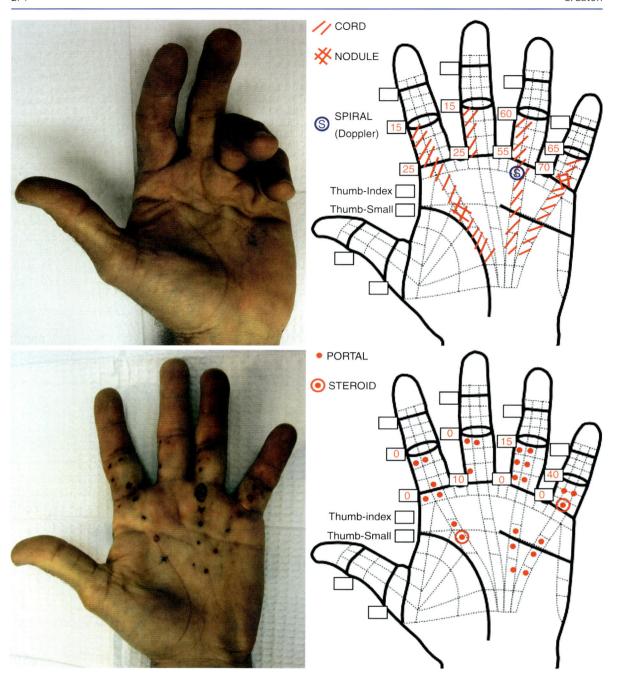

Fig. 34.7 Needle release of multiple fingers. *Top*: Preoperative appearance and documentation of angles, cords, nodules and Doppler identification of a spiral cord. *Bottom*: Immediately after needle aponeurotomy: portals, nodule injections, and active extension. General expectations are up to 50% improvement of PIP contracture and improvement of up to 90° of composite (MCP+PIP) contracture

34 A Technique of Needle Aponeurotomy for Dupuytren's Contracture

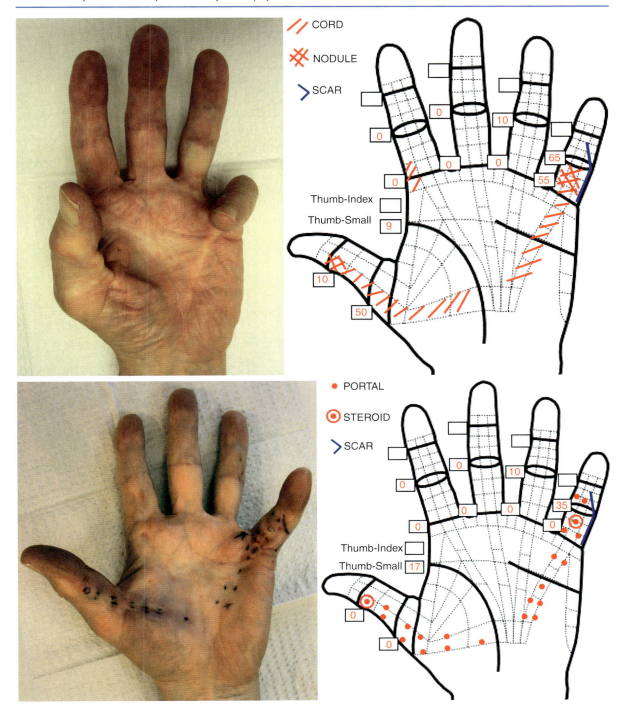

Fig. 34.8 Needle release of thumb and postfasciectomy small finger. The combination of a radial lateral thumb cord and a small finger cord can dramatically narrow the hand span. *Top*: Preoperative appearance and documentation of angles, cords, nodules, and lateral hockey stick fasciectomy scar of small finger. Thumb-small span is measured in centimeters. *Bottom*: Immediately after needle aponeurotomy: portals, nodule injections, and active extension

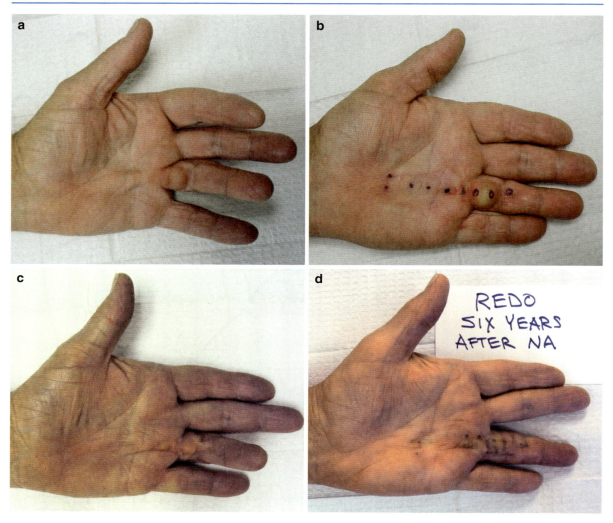

Fig. 34.9 Repeat NA for recurrence after NA. *Top*: First release: Ring finger contractures MCP 40, PIP 20, with nodular finger disease: correction to MCP 0 and PIP 0; nodules injected with steroid. *Bottom*: Second release for recurrence 6 years later with MCP 0, PIP 60: correction to MCP 0 and PIP 0

(Fig. 34.9). These are obviously subjective guidelines. As for fasciectomy, repeated rapid recurrences indicate aggressive treatment-resistant disease.

- *What about NA for recurrence after open surgery?* NA is an option if local conditions are favorable: palpable cord beneath extendible skin (Fig. 34.10). NA is not suitable for tight scars or skin which blanches prominently with extension. Prior skin flap elevation may result in sensitivity of subcutaneous tissues with deep needle tenderness, as discussed below.
- *Your finger portals are sometimes on the side, sometimes on the palm. Why?* Portals are best placed directly over the most palpable area of the cord. Cords just proximal to the PIP flexion crease which fan out to span from midlateral to midline palmar are most safely released with two portals which allows a curved, superficial fasciotomy plane.
- *When do you splint after NA?* Three situations may benefit from nighttime splinting: Composite contractures over 90° before release; contractures for which passive extension exceeds active by more than 20° after release; isolated PIP joint contracture releases. Splinting may be continued indefinitely if tolerated. This topic clearly needs more study and evidence.

34 A Technique of Needle Aponeurotomy for Dupuytren's Contracture

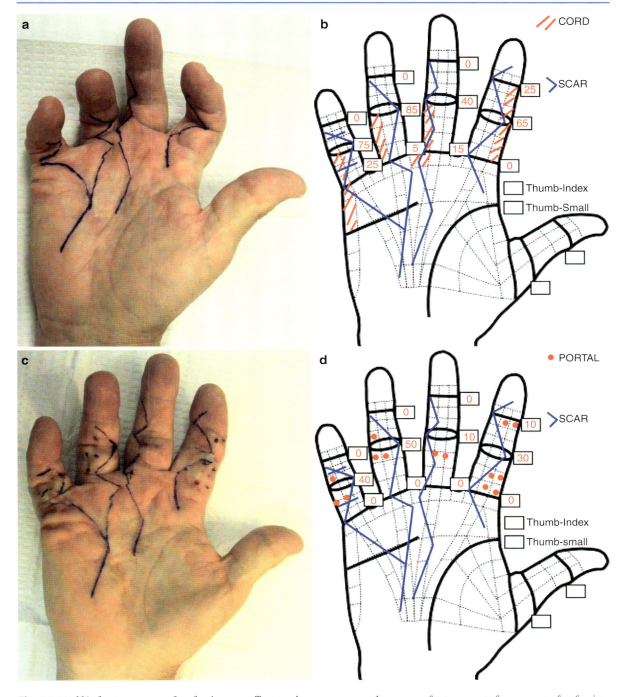

Fig. 34.10 NA for recurrence after fasciectomy. *Top*: cords, scars, angle measurements of recurrence 5 years after fasciectomy. *Bottom*: portals and angles after needle release. As with any approach, outcome for treatment of recurrence after fasciectomy is somewhat unpredictable

- *What to do with a PIP which seems completely stuck and you've released all palpable cords?* As of this writing, there is no safe percutaneous approach to release PIP collateral ligament, volar plate or check rein. Gentle manipulation under anesthetic block may help. The flexor tendon sheath may be the culprit, and this may be released by lightly grazing with the needle tip, passively extending only the PIP while checking active DIP flexion. This risks tendon injury, and should not be used if there is palmar skin tightness because of the risk of a skin tear exposing flexor tendon.

- *What is the approach for releasing a natatory cord?* Put the cord under tension and plan the portal directly over the most palpable area of the cord. Move to face the fingertips, angle the needle nearly tangential to the skin aiming directly proximal and working deep from there. Natatory involvement is surprisingly variable, sometimes a centimeter proximal to the web, sometimes both palmar and dorsal in the web space. Watch to avoid buttonholing dorsally. Scissor the fingers for the final manipulation: flex the MCP of one while extending the other, and then reverse.
- *In the case of a suspected spiral cord, if there are no Doppler tones, is the portal safe?* Probably, but never let up the routine of checking for distal sensation.
- *What if the skin just seems hard or tight?* There are two skin issues – adherent skin vs. inadequate skin from shrinking. The former is approachable with NA but the latter needs an open procedure. One technique for adherent skin is to use more portals and to use the tip of the needle deep to and tangential to the dermis, sweeping around the perimeter of the portal, separating the cord from the dermis (Khouri, 2010, personal communication). In some of these adherent cases, the tissue shortening seems to be in the attachments of the cord to the dermis with oblique fibrous attachments, and once these are freed, all of the tissues soften up and give.
- *How do you handle a numb finger?* As in Fig. 34.6.
- *What should be done for nodules?* Palmar nodules without contracture injected with depot corticosteroid may regress (Ketchum and Donahue 2000). Nodules in continuity with released cords often soften 2 or 3 weeks after release. This change may be augmented by injecting nodules at the time of release with depot corticosteroid. If no release of adjacent cords is performed, nodules in the fingers associated with contractures are not injected as this may be followed by accelerated contracture. (Ketchum, 2008, personal communication).

- *Tips for isolated PIP contractures?* Consider not releasing an associated minimal proximal palmar cord, because the additional MCP hyperextension this allows may result in greater PIP extension lag. Portals distal to the PIP flexion crease (Figs. 34.3 and 34.4) may allow release even if the proximal phalanx skin is nodular or tethered distally. PIP anesthetic before manipulation, composite PIP+MCP manipulation, and nighttime splinting after release are helpful.
- *The cord is painful to needle even though there is good overlying dermal anesthesia. What do I do?* Pure cords are usually insensate, but nodules and nodular cords may have tenderness to needle penetration. Prior needle release and prior local flap elevation may render subcutaneous tissues sensitive. Skin dimples may be deeper than they appear and may lead to deep tenderness and risk of dimple transection (Fig. 34.2). If there is no other option, sensitive deep areas may be injected with local anesthetic before release, and as long as distal sensitivity is monitored at least once a minute during release.
- *What about using a larger needle?* Smaller needles require more passes and more time, but may be safer than larger needles in the event of inadvertent nerve contact. A 25 gauge needle has a cutting edge width of 0.5 mm and a cutting edge length is less than 1 mm, making it difficult to completely transect a digital nerve with a single pass. The corresponding measurements are 0.7 and 1.4 for a 21 gauge needle, 1.3 and 2.6 for an 18 gauge needle, respectively (Fig. 34.1).
- *How do you avoid skin tears?* It's not always possible. Avoid areas of nodular skin involvement, particularly where the fingerprints are raised or prominent. If you do use areas of firm skin:
  - Use more portals to disperse the areas of maximum tension.
  - Sweep the needle tip just deep and tangential to the dermis to release the vertical septa attachments on each side of the portal.
  - Hold off on much stretching until you've released at multiple levels to disperse the areas of maximum tension.

When manipulating, you can use your fingertips to *push on the adjacent skin toward the risky area to shield it from the overall stretch*. Stretch slowly, watching the portals so that if a tear begins, you can stop before you propagate it more. If you get a superficial/epidermal tear, warn the patient that it will look more red the following day and that it may continue to open up over the next few days, but does not change their final expectations.

34.10 Learning Curve Pitfalls

- Not emphasizing enough to avoid strenuous gripping/golf/tennis/gardening/fishing/weight training etc. for a full week postrelease – even if they have no pain or tenderness, because the fasciotomy sites are insensate. Early shearing stress of the portals may provoke a delayed local inflammatory reaction.
- Not clearly warning patients preoperatively that they may have a skin tear which may require bandaging for a few weeks if it is full thickness.
- Not repeatedly checking for distal anesthesia when near a nerve or checking active flexion when near a tendon.
- Not changing to a fresh needle when the entry feels rubbery or the cord just won't cut.

References

Abe Y, Rokkaku T, Ofuchi S, Tokunaga S, Takahashi K, Moriya H (2004) An objective method to evaluate the risk of recurrence and extension of Dupuytren's disease. J Hand Surg Br 29(5):427–430

Adams W (1879) On contraction of the fingers (Dupuytren's contraction). also on the obliteration of depressed cicatrices. J and A Churchill, London, pp 40–48

Cheng HS, Hung LK, Tse WL, Ho PC (2008) Needle aponeurotomy for Dupuytren's contracture. J Orthop Surg (Hong Kong) 16(1):88–90

Cooper AP (1822) On dislocations of the fingers and toes - dislocation from contraction of the tendon. In: A treatise on dislocations and fractures of the joints. Longman, London, pp 524–525

Degreef I, De Smet L (2011) Risk factors in Dupuytren's diathesis: Is recurrence after surgery predictable? Acta Orthop Belg 77(1):27–32

Dupuytren G (1831) De la rétraction des doigts par suite d'une affection de l'aponévrose palmaire - description de la maladie - operation chirurgicale qui convient dans ce cas. Compte rendu de la clinique chirurgicale de l'Hôtel Dieu par MM les docteurs Alexandre Paillard et Marx. J Universel et Hebdomadaire de Médicine et de Chirurgie Pratiques et des Institutions Médicales 5: 349–365

Foucher G, Medina J, Navarro R (2003) Percutaneous needle aponeurotomy: complications and results. J Hand Surg Br 28(5):427–431

Goyrand G (1835) De la rétraction permanente de doigts. Gazette Med Paris 3:481–486

Hindocha S, Stanley JK, Watson S, Bayat A (2006) Dupuytren's diathesis revisited: Evaluation of prognostic indicators for risk of disease recurrence. J Hand Surg 31A(10):1626-34.

Ketchum LD, Donahue TK (2000) The injection of nodules of Dupuytren's disease with triamcinolone acetonide. J Hand Surg 25A:1157–1162

Lermusiaux JL (2000) Le traitement médical de la maladie de Dupuytren. Rhumatologie 52(4):15–17

Lermusiaux JL, Debeyre N (1979) le traitement médical de la maladie de Dupuytren. In: De Sèze S, Ryckewaert A, Kahn MF et al (eds) L'actualité rhumatologique. Expansion Scientifique, Paris, pp 338–343

Luck JV (1959) Dupuytren's contracture: a new concept of the pathogenesis correlated with surgical management. J Bone Joint Surg 4:635–664

Schultz RJ, Krishnamurthy S, Johnston AD (1984) A gross anatomic and histologic study of the innervation of the proximal interphalangeal joint. J Hand Surg Am 9(5):669–674

Short WH, Watson HK (1982) Prediction of the spiral nerve in Dupuytren's contracture. J Hand Surg Am 7(1):84–86

van Rijssen AL, Werker PM (2006) Percutaneous needle fasciotomy in Dupuytren's disease. J Hand Surg Br 31(5): 498–501

Three-Year Results of First-Ever Randomized Clinical Trial on Treatment in Dupuytren's Disease: Percutaneous Needle Fasciotomy Versus Limited Fasciectomy

35

Annet L. van Rijssen, Hein ter Linden, and Paul M.N. Werker

Contents

35.1	**Introduction**	281
35.2	**Methods**	282
35.2.1	Study Design	282
35.2.2	Randomization	282
35.2.3	Surgical Technique	282
35.2.4	Follow-up	282
35.2.5	Definition of Recurrence	282
35.3	**Statistics**	283
35.4	**Results**	283
35.4.1	Recurrence after LF	283
35.4.2	Recurrence after PNF	283
35.4.3	LF Versus PNF	283
35.4.4	Treatment for Recurrent Disease	283
35.4.5	Sensibility Recovery	283
35.4.6	Satisfaction	284
35.4.7	Recurrence Versus Age at Time of Treatment	285
35.5	**Discussion**	285
35.5.1	Recurrence after LF	285
35.5.2	Recurrence after PNF	287
35.5.3	Age Versus Recurrence	287
35.5.4	Treatment of Recurring Disease	287
35.5.5	Satisfaction	287
35.5.6	Future Implications	287
35.6	**Conclusions**	287
References		288

A.L. van Rijssen (✉) • H. ter Linden
Department of Plastic Surgery, Isala Clinics,
Dokter van Heesweg 2, 8025 AB,
Zwolle, The Netherlands
e-mail: annetvanrijssen@hotmail.com

P.M.N. Werker
University Medical Centre Groningen,
University of Groningen, Groningen, The Netherlands
e-mail: p.m.n.werker@umcg.nl

35.1 Introduction

Percutaneous needle fasciotomy (PNF) is a treatment for Dupuytren's disease that exists in its current form since the late 1970s. This treatment was invented by French rheumatologists but is essentially a modification of the first treatment for Dupuytren's disease ever: aponeurotomy or fasciotomy, described by Sir Henry Cline in 1777, the year Baron Guillaume Dupuytren was born (Cline 1777). Recently, this treatment regained popularity because of the growing demand for fast recovery, low complication rate, and minimal invasiveness (Lermusiaux and Debeyre 1980). Disadvantages of this technique are its lower effectiveness for moderately severe and severe forms of the disease (Tubiana stages 3 and 4) and its reported high recurrence rate (Citron and Nunez 2005; Ullah et al. 2009; Jurisić et al. 2008; Foucher et al. 2001; Van Rijssen and Werker 2006).

Limited fasciectomy (LF) still is the most frequently performed treatment by hand surgeons around the globe. It is hampered by a relatively longer recovery period and reasonably high complication rates, especially in recurrent cases (McFarlane and McGrouther 1990; Rodrigo et al. 1976; Tubiana 1999; Coert et al. 2006). In our first report of our ongoing randomized clinical trial on the comparison of LF and PNF, we showed that results in the lower Tubiana stages I and II were similar, but that LF was slightly more effective than PNF for higher Tubiana stages in Dupuytren's disease. Importantly, functional recovery following treatment was significantly faster following PNF (Van Rijssen et al. 2006). In a pilot study, we had found that recurrence rates following PNF after a mean of

C. Eaton et al. (eds.), *Dupuytren's Disease and Related Hyperproliferative Disorders*,
DOI 10.1007/978-3-642-22697-7_35, © Springer-Verlag Berlin Heidelberg 2012

33 months were similar to those reported by others (Van Rijssen and Werker 2006).

To this date, no long-term results of randomized trials on PNF and LF have been published. The aim of this study was to fill this gap. We studied the effect on total passive extension deficit (TPED), patient satisfaction, and recurrence rates up to 3-year follow-up in two groups of patients that had been randomly assigned to both treatment arms.

35.2 Methods

35.2.1 Study Design

This study was designed according to and approved by the Medisch Ethische Toetsings Commissie, the local Medical Ethics Committee, in January 2002.

From August 2002 to January 2005, we considered every patient with primary Dupuytren's disease who presented at our department for this study. Written consent was obtained from all patients.

Inclusion criteria were a total passive extension deficit (TPED) of at least $30°$ in the MCP joint, PIP joint, or DIP joint; the existence of a clearly defined cord; and willingness to participate in this trial.

Exclusion criteria were patients who received previous surgery for Dupuytren's disease on the hand they presented with, patients who were not allowed to stop their anticoagulants, patients generally unfit for surgery, and patients with a specific treatment modality wish.

Study candidates were examined by either PMNW or HTL. During examination, TPED of MCPJ + PIPJ + DIPJ was measured, as well as flexion deficit using a goniometer and sensibility using the Semmes–Weinstein monofilaments. Patients were asked to fill out a questionnaire about their health status, functional recovery, satisfaction with the treatment, and demographics.

35.2.2 Randomization

Randomization was carried out by a secretary by means of pulling a sealed envelope from a box, which contained a note, stating either PNF or LF. This determined which treatment the patient was to receive. For elaborate patient demographics, we refer to our previous study (Van Rijssen et al. 2006). In the article we published on this issue in 2006, we showed that groups

were equally divided over all Tubiana stages and that the majority of the patients were in stages I, II, and III. In the same article, we proved that LF and PNF are equally effective in stage I and II.

35.2.3 Surgical Technique

Treatment was performed by HTL or PMNW in random order. Patients were treated within 1 month after inclusion in this study.

PNF was performed as an outpatient procedure in the same way as previously described by Lermusiaux and Debeyre (1980). Under local anesthesia for the skin only, the cords were divided using a 25-gauge needle at as many places along the cord as necessary to achieve maximal passive extension. A small dressing was applied for 24 h. Patients were encouraged to start practicing the hand immediately after the procedure. They did not receive formal hand therapy. All hands were treated only once.

LF was performed under general or regional anesthesia using a palmar Skoog incision in combination with Bruner-type incision in the digits, which allowed skin transposition if necessary. A compressive bandage was applied which the patient was instructed to wear for 7 days until the first visit to the outpatient clinic. Patients were encouraged to practice extension and flexion of the fingers immediately after the anesthesia had worn off. Hand therapy was not standard but available if indicated.

35.2.4 Follow-up

Following the 6-week interval, patients were seen in the outpatient clinic at 6 months and then yearly after treatment. During this visit, we recorded the amount of passive extension deficit of each joint and calculated the TPED, sensibility, flexion deficit, and signs of recurrence or extension of the disease. Patients were asked to fill out a questionnaire concerning their satisfaction with the treatment. Every follow-up for this study was performed by one of the authors.

35.2.5 Definition of Recurrence

Recurrence was defined as an increase of extension deficit of at least $30°$ compared to the 6-week values as

35 Three-Year Results of First-Ever Randomized Clinical Trial on Treatment in Dupuytren's Disease

the result of disease activity in the area previously treated. Extension was defined as an increase of extension deficit of at least 30° compared to the 6-week values due to disease activity outside the area previously treated. Remaining extension deficit was judged at 6 weeks, because in this postoperative period, improvement in extension was still noticeable. All results were therefore compared to the measurements taken at 6 weeks. In case patients suffered extension or recurrence, the study was terminated.

35.3 Statistics

Statistical analysis was performed using statistical software (SPSS software, SPSS Inc. Chicago, IL). We used the chi-square test for categorical data. The student's t-test was used for recurrence and patient satisfaction. Data were normally distributed. Linear-by-linear association tests were used to define age versus recurrence differences. Patients were stratified into the following groups for this purpose: 0–35, 36–45, 46–55, 56–65, 66–75, >75 years. We used Kaplan–Meier curves for survival. Significance was set at a p-value of less than 0.05.

35.4 Results

At 6 weeks posttreatment, 111 patients were still in the study and had complete data sets. In these patients in total, 115 hands were treated since four patients were treated bilaterally. Ninety-four of these patients were men. Distribution of sexes was equal in both treatment arms, $p = 0.529$. The mean age of patients at follow-up was 63 years in both groups, $p = 0.972$. Fifty-four limited fasciectomies had been performed and 61 percutaneous needle fasciotomies.

Of the four bilaterally included patients, one was lost to follow-up; the others did not develop recurrences in this period.

35.4.1 Recurrence after LF

Three years after surgery, eight patients with eight treated hands were lost to follow-up due to severe disease or death. Forty-two hands showed no signs of recurrence (91.3%), and four had recurrence (8.7%).

35.4.2 Recurrence after PNF

In the PNF group, five patients with six treated hands were lost to follow-up; 35 hands showed signs of recurrence (63.6%), and 20 hands showed no signs of recurrence (36.4%).

35.4.3 LF Versus PNF

The recurrence rate in the LF group is significantly smaller, $p = 0.000$.

Because we did not know if the patients that had been lost to follow-up had recurrent disease or not, we calculated worst-case and best-case scenarios. These are illustrated in Figs. 35.1 and 35.2. They show that even if all lost-to-follow-up patients would have had recurring disease, the difference between LF and PNF was still striking.

Figure 35.3 illustrates differences in recurrences and percentages of patients lost to follow-up.

35.4.4 Treatment for Recurrent Disease

In the LF group, one patient chose to have his recurrence treated by PNF. Three chose not to be treated for their recurrence. Therefore, none of the patients in the LF group who had recurrent disease chose to undergo LF again.

In the PNF group, of 35 patients with recurrent disease, 21 (60%) chose to undergo a second PNF treatment. Six patients (17%) wanted to be treated by LF, and the remaining eight (23%) chose not to undergo treatment for their recurrent disease. In these patients, the increase in extension deficit did not impair their hand function.

There was just one patient who had extension; the study was therefore terminated. He chose not to undergo treatment. We do not have data on whether this patient also suffered from recurrence at a later date.

35.4.5 Sensibility Recovery

During LF, one patient suffered from iatrogenic digital nerve injury. This was recognized immediately, and the nerve was repaired microsurgically in the same session. His preoperative Semmes–Weinstein test was

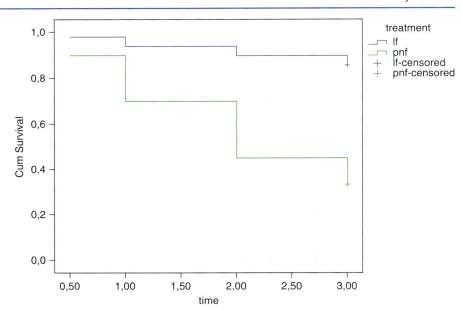

Fig. 35.1 Worst-case scenario. Kaplan–Meier survival curves with both treatment modalities. On the x-axis, time is shown in years posttreatment. On the y-axis, cumulative survival is shown, in which 1.0 means 100% of patients were still included in the study (not lost to follow-up or having recurrent disease). In this case, all "lost-to-follow-up" patients were allocated as having recurrent disease

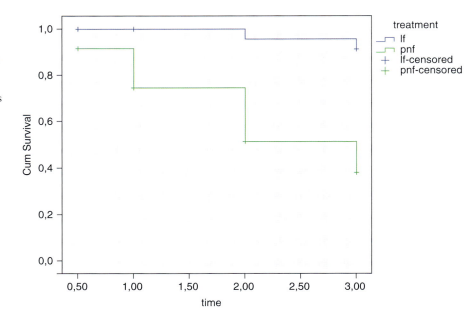

Fig. 35.2 Best-case scenario. Kaplan–Meier survival curves with both treatment modalities. On the x-axis, time is shown in years posttreatment. On the y-axis, cumulative survival is shown, in which 1.0 means 100% of patients were still included in the study (not lost to follow-up or having recurrent disease). In this case, all "lost-to-follow-up" patients were allocated as having NO recurrence

2.83 on the affected side of the finger. Postoperatively this dropped to 4.93 to turn back to the preoperative level of 2.83 after 6 months.

35.4.6 Satisfaction

Patients were asked the following questions:
Q1: Are you satisfied with the results of your treatment? (0 = not at all, 10 = excellent)

Q2: Would you choose this treatment modality again? (0 = no, 10 = yes, definitely)

The results show that although patients are significantly less satisfied with the results of their treatment after PNF, they are still considering undergoing the same treatment modality again. These figures display satisfaction either at time of recurrence (when the study is terminated for the specific patient) or at the time of the 3-year interval (at the end point taken in this study) (Table 35.1).

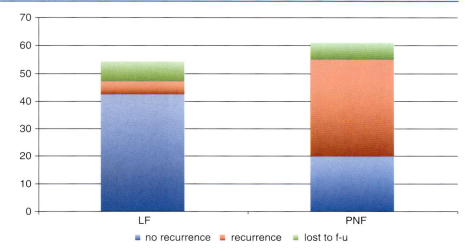

Fig. 35.3 Recurrence rates in the LF group and in the PNF group at 3 years. On the x-axis, the two different treatment modalities are shown, on the y-axis the number of hands treated

Table 35.1 Results of patient survey

	PNF	LF	*p*-value
Q1: results	6.0	8.2	0.007
Q2: treatment modality	7.3	8.0	0.165

35.4.7 Recurrence Versus Age at Time of Treatment

Due to small numbers of recurrence in the LF group, we were not able to draw conclusions on the age effect on recurrence between groups. However, we were able to prove that the higher the age at time of treatment, the lower the chance of getting recurrent disease for both groups together, $p=0.005$. As shown in Figs. 35.4 and 35.5, 3 years after either treatment, the majority of patients 55 and younger had recurrence, whereas the majority of those older than 55 remained disease free. It also shows that the highest age groups have the lowest recurrence rates. Three-year recurrence was 100% in those treated under the age of 46.

35.5 Discussion

This study focuses on recurrence rates in the first 3 years after PNF or LF. We randomized our patients into two groups. Patient demographics and contractures were equally distributed as we have shown before and were comparable to groups in other studies (Van Rijssen et al. 2006). Our direct postoperative results and results at 6 weeks posttreatment were comparable to those reported in literature.

"Recurrence" after treatment for Dupuytren's disease, however, is an ill-defined entity in current literature. The most commonly used definition is "reappearance of Dupuytren's tissue in a previously operated zone" (Tubiana 1999; Becker and Davis 2010). Reported recurrence rates differ enormously: from 0 to 73% for all different techniques combined. Comparison is difficult because of lack of standardized definitions of recurrence and follow-up duration.

We defined recurrence as a worsening of 30° or more compared to the postoperative result after 6 weeks. Our definition deviates somewhat from the definition mentioned above. This definition of recurrence could not be used in this study, however. The reason for this is that after PNF, the diseased tissue is still present in the palm. Nodules that are present before the procedure often remain unchanged or soften. The cords are divided, but over time they seem to reconnect.

We feel that we used a reproducible and clinically important definition of recurrence. Reappearance of Dupuytren's tissue does not have to impair one's hand function. We chose a worsening of 30° because this corresponds to Hueston's tabletop test and is an indication for surgery in our treatment center.

35.5.1 Recurrence after LF

In our study, the recurrence rate after 3 years was 9%.

Citron and Nunez reported their results on a randomized study in which they studied the differences

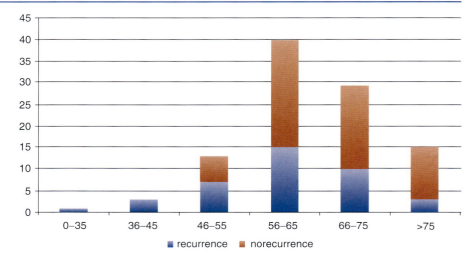

Fig. 35.4 Numbers of patients who are disease-free and have recurrent disease at different age groups. On the *x*-axis, different age-groups are shown in years at time of treatment. On the *y*-axis, numbers of patients are shown (LF and PNF combined)

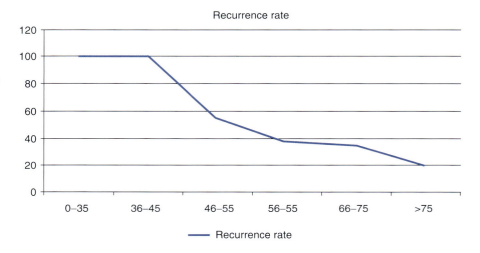

Fig. 35.5 Recurrence rates at different age groups. On the *x*-axis, different age-groups are shown in years at time of treatment. On the *y*-axis, the percentage of these patients that had a recurrence is shown (LF and PNF combined)

between longitudinal incisions closed with Z-plasty or Bruner's incision closed with V-Y plasties (Citron and Nunez 2005). Only one ray was treated in every patient. Recurrence was defined as the reappearance of Dupuytren's tissue in previously operated field. The demographics of their patients were comparable to those of ours. They found 33% recurrence for the former and 18% for the latter after a period of 2 years.

Jurisić retrospectively studied the population of Primorsko-Goranska County, Croatia, and found a 73% recurrence rate after partial fasciectomy after a mean follow-up of 7 years (Jurisić et al. 2008). Recurrence was defined as the development of new Dupuytren's disease lesions including the smallest palpable nodule irrespective if it caused a contracture in the same area where fasciectomy had been performed. Thirty-four percent of those required further surgery.

Degreef reports in a previously unpublished study a recurrence rate of 43% after segmental fasciectomy with a minimum follow-up of 2 years (Degreef 2012).

Ullah et al. performed a prospective study on limited fasciectomy in which they compared direct closure with the use of a "firewall" full-thickness skin graft (Ullah et al. 2009). They found no significant difference in recurrence, which was 13.6% average after a follow-up of 3 years for the group treated by fasciectomy alone. The definition of recurrence in this article is not clear, but the text says "progressive recurrence of contracture."

At this point in our study, our recurrence rates after LF are low. When we compare them to other studies, it seems our recurrence rate is lower than those reported in literature. This can partly be explained by the variations in definitions of recurrence. It is anticipated that recurrence rates will increase in time.

35.5.2 Recurrence after PNF

Compared to studies on LF, recurrences following PNF are even more ill-defined and hard to balance. In our study, the recurrence rate as defined by an increase in TPED compared to the 6-week results was 63% after 3 years follow-up. This figure is very similar to that of previously published series. In a pilot for this study, we found 65% recurrence after a mean of 33 months (Van Rijssen et al. 2006). Foucher reviewed 100 rays after a mean of 3.2 years (Foucher et al. 2001) and found a recurrence rate of 58%. These similar data indicates that we executed PNF well. Therefore, we are confident that the longer term results, which we expect to publish within the near future, will be reliable too. And this is even more so, since we are the first to publish a prospective randomized study on the results of PNF versus LF and therefore there has not been selection bias.

35.5.3 Age Versus Recurrence

Hindocha et al. pointed out that age of onset less than 50 years old will increase chances of recurrent disease (Hindocha et al. 2006). To our knowledge, this is the first study that proves that there is an overall relationship between age at treatment and chance for recurrence. The higher the age of the patient at time of treatment, the lower the chances of getting recurrent disease.

35.5.4 Treatment of Recurring Disease

Recurrence does not necessarily mean that there is a need for reoperation. Twenty-eight percent of the patients who had a recurrence according to our definition chose not to undergo further treatment at that moment. This is probably because the extension deficit was less severe than the preoperative disease and did not impair hand function as it initially did.

35.5.5 Satisfaction

Satisfaction was high for both PNF and LF. Patients receiving LF were at 3 years significantly more satisfied with the results of their treatment than those who underwent PNF. However, many patients who suffered recurrent disease chose to undergo PNF again. This indicates that many patients prefer a minor procedure with fast recovery at the expense of the increased chance of an early recurrence.

35.5.6 Future Implications

Although PNF is equally effective for mild to moderate Dupuytren's disease (Tubiana I and II), as we have shown in previous studies, recurrence rates are significantly higher than after LF. A higher age at disease presentation correlates with less tendency to recurrence. For this reason, we believe that PNF treatment is best suitable for well-informed elderly patients with relatively mild contractures and for those who are willing to accept a higher recurrence risk in the context of a lower complication rate, fast recovery, and minimal invasiveness. PNF could also be used to postpone future surgery.

However, it remains unclear in which way age has its effect on recurrence rate. Hopefully, future studies will elucidate the cause of this correlation, especially if this is a mere issue of biologic aggressiveness or that age at time of onset has any effect on the recurrence rate.

Furthermore, larger studies would be useful to clarify relative (contra) indications for LF and PNF as to which subgroup would be suited best with either treatment modality. Age, age at onset, bilateral disease, ectopic lesions, radial-sided disease, and other individual differences will possibly have their influence on recurrence rates in large studies.

35.6 Conclusions

- Recurrences after PNF are far more frequent and occur sooner than after LF.
- Recurrence after PNF at 3 years is 63% and after LF 9%.
- Satisfaction is high for both treatment modalities, but 3 years after treatment, patients treated by LF are significantly more satisfied with their results than those patients treated by PNF.
- Many patients choose to undergo PNF as their secondary treatment in spite of the disadvantages named above.
- No matter which treatment modality, recurrences occur more frequently in the younger patients than in the older patients.

References

Becker GW, Davis TR (2010) The outcome of surgical treatments for primary Dupuytren's disease–a systematic review. Hand Surg Eur 35(8):623–626

Citron ND, Nunez V (2005) Recurrence after surgery for Dupuytren's disease: a randomized trial of two skin incisions. Hand Surg Br 30(6):563–566

Cline H (1777) Notes on pathology. St Thomas Hospital Medical School Library, London

Coert JH, Nérin JP, Meek MF (2006) Results of partial fasciectomy for Dupuytren disease in 261 consecutive patients. Ann Plast Surg 57(1):13–17

Degreef I (2012) No higher self-reported recurrence in segmental fasciectomy. In: Dupuytren's disease and related hyperproliferative disorders, pp 255–260

Foucher G, Medina J, Navarro R (2001) Percutaneous needle aponeurotomy. Complications and results. Chir Main 20(3):206–211

Hindocha S, Stanley JK, Watson S, Bayat A (2006) Dupuytren's diathesis revisited: evaluation of prognostic indicators for risk of disease recurrence. J Hand Surg Am 31(10):1626–1634

Jurisić D, Ković I, Lulić I, Stanec Z, Kapović M, Uravić M (2008) Dupuytren's disease characteristics in primorsko-goranska county, Croatia. Coll Antropol 32(4):1209–1213

Lermusiaux JL, Debeyre N (1980) In: de Sèze S, Ryckeawaert A, Kahn M-F, Guérin CI (eds) L'actualité rhumatologique. Expansion Scientifique Française, Paris, pp 338–343

McFarlane RM, McGrouther DA (1990) Complications and their management. In: McFarlane RM, McGrouther DA, Flint M (eds) Dupuytren's disease: biology and treatment. Churchill Livingstone, Edinburgh, pp 377–382

Rodrigo JJ, Niebauer JJ, Brown RL, Doyle JR (1976) Treatment of Dupuytren's contracture. Long-term results after fasciotomy and fascial excision. J Bone Joint Surg Am 58(3):380–387

Tubiana R (1999) Surgical management. In: Tubiana R (ed) The hand. WB Saunders Company, Paris, p 480

Ullah AS, Dias JJ, Bhowal B (2009) Does a 'firebreak' full-thickness skin graft prevent recurrence after surgery for Dupuytren's contracture? – a prospective, randomised trial. J Bone Joint Surg Br 91(3):374–378

Van Rijssen AL, Werker PMN (2006) Percutaneous needle fasciotomy in Dupuytren's disease. J Hand Surg Br 31(5):498–501

Van Rijssen AL, Gerbrandy FS, Ter Linden H, Klip H, Werker PMN (2006) A comparison of the direct outcomes of percutaneous needle fasciotomy and limited fasciectomy for Dupuytren's disease: a 6-week follow-up study. J Hand Surg Am 31(5):717–725

Management of Dupuytren's Disease with Needle Aponeurotomy: The Experience at the Hand and Upper Limb Centre, Canada

36

Aaron Grant, David B. O'Gorman, and Bing Siang Gan

Contents

36.1	**Introduction**	289
36.1.1	Needle Aponeurotomy: Literature Summary	290
36.2	**Material and Methods**	290
36.2.1	Needle Aponeurotomy Procedure	291
36.3	**Results**	291
36.4	**Discussion**	291
36.5	**Conclusions**	292
References		292

A. Grant • D.B. O'Gorman • B.S. Gan (✉)
The Hand and Upper Limb Centre, St. Joseph's Health Care
London, University of Western Ontario, 268 Grosvenor Street,
London, Ontario N6A 4L6, Canada
e-mail: bsgan@rogers.com

36.1 Introduction

Dupuytren's disease is a common problem encountered by hand surgeons worldwide, and despite a significant amount of research the exact aetiology remains unclear. There is a genetic component to the disease, and a natural history that results in progressive digital contraction and loss of dexterity. Since the seventeenth-century physician Felix Plater first described the affliction there has been a multitude of reported treatment options. These range from minor limited procedures to radical palmar dermo-fasciectomy. These techniques have very different associated morbidities, and seem to be equally effective in the short term (McGrouther 2005).

One of the pioneers who described the disease and its management, Henry Cline, first suggested a simple percutaneous release of the affected cords with a bistoury knife as a treatment in 1777 (Elliot 1988). This technique fell out of favor and was followed by a movement toward an open approach with wide resection of diseased tissue. Unfortunately, even with open approach the 10-year recurrence rate has been reported to be as high as 66% (Leclercq and Tubiana 2000). This has led certain groups in Europe to return to the use of the percutaneous approach and in particular a modification of Cline's original technique using a needle. This percutaneous needle fasciotomy was subsequently named the needle aponeurotomy NA (Badois et al. 1993; Foucher et al. 2003). There are currently guidelines on the use of this approach published by the United Kingdom's National Institute for Clinical Excellence (NICE 2004). The technique, however, is not routinely practiced in North America, perhaps

C. Eaton et al. (eds.), *Dupuytren's Disease and Related Hyperproliferative Disorders*,
DOI 10.1007/978-3-642-22697-7_36, © Springer-Verlag Berlin Heidelberg 2012

because North American teachings have been influenced by the late Dr. Robert McFarlane, a pioneer in the descriptions of Dupuytren's disease, who himself felt that NA was a blind procedure that put the neurovascular bundles at high risk of division.

36.1.1 Needle Aponeurotomy: Literature Summary

The majority of hand surgeons still rely on palmar fasciectomy in the treatment of Dupuytren's disease, despite multiple reports of complications, including neurovascular injuries, skin necrosis, infections, postoperative stiffness, and prolonged recovery time. In the 1970s, a group in Europe revived the simple technique of limited fasciotomy with a needle tip, and had some success (Lermusiaux and Debeyre 1979). In 1984 a study of NA completed on 107 digits showed an extension deficit reduction EDR of 36° and 7° at 3 months for MCP and PIP joints, respectively. Follow-up at 15 months showed near-complete recurrence at the PIP joints while MCP joints were relatively maintained and there were no reported complications (Rowley et al. 1984). A study in 1993 of NA of 123 hands showed "excellent results" for 81% of patients immediately following the procedure, as defined by extension deficit of less than 45°. At 5 year follow-up 69% maintained these results. Complications were limited to three nerve injuries and three postoperative infections (Badois et al. 1993). The authors of this last study have also published results on the internet from NA completed on 992 hands; however, limited information is available and the results will not be included here. A prospective study in 1997 looked at 110 digits treated with NA. The study reported that 61% of digits had an improvement of more than 50% (Bleton et al. 1997). NA completed on 82 patients followed for 10 years showed a gain of 49° from a preoperative deficit of 71°. Sixty-six percent of these patients required fasciectomy (Duthie and Chesney 1997). NA was performed on 311 digits with immediate EDR of 38° and 24° for MCP and PIP joints. One hundred of these patients were followed for 2.5 years; 59% had recurrence, with 24% requiring reoperation. There was one reported neuroma and one case of possible reflex sympathetic dystrophy (Foucher et al. 2001, 2003). A recent study in 2006 followed 74 digits treated with NA. A 44° 77% immediate improvement in total passive extension deficit was reported. Follow-up at 9 months did not show any significant recurrence; however, at 33 months 42% required treatment for recurrence, and the remainder of patients showed an average increase in extension deficit of 8° compared to immediate post NA (van Rijssen and Werker 2006). A randomized controlled trial conducted in 2006 compared the results of NA and limited fasciectomy LF in 166 digits. It showed better outcomes for LF, especially for contractures at the PIP joint; however, patient satisfaction was greater and postoperative pain was less in the NA group (van Rijssen et al. 2006). A study looking specifically at Chinese patients treated with NA was conducted by Cheng in 2008. Thirteen digits were released with an immediate EDR of 50° and 35° for MCP and PIP joints. The long-term improvement at 22 month follow-up was 70% MCP joints and 41% PIP joints with no complications reported (Cheng et al. 2008).

36.2 Material and Methods

Between September 2009 and April 2010, 35 patients with symptomatic Dupuytren's disease consented to NA. Patients were prospectively enrolled in the study and were included if there was MCP involvement with palpable pretendinous cord. The study group included 26 males and 7 females, and the mean age was 64 years, SD 8.5 years. A total of 35 diseased hands and 62 digits consisting of 22 small, 28 ring, and 12 long digits were treated during this period. Of the 14 hands with a single involved ray, three aponeurotomy sites were required on average to achieve the desired effect. A total of 21 hands had multiple involved digits, and were treated with on average four aponeurotomy sites.

The preoperative assessment consisted of a history and physical exam with measurements of active range of motion for MCP, PIP, and DIP joints. The degrees of flexion contracture at each joint were added cumulatively to determine the total digital extension deficit TDED in each involved digit. DIP contracture was noted to be absent in all patients.

Patients were assessed again immediately following NA and active ranges of motion documented. Follow-up was arranged at 6–8 weeks and the measurements repeated.

36 Management of Dupuytren's Disease with Needle Aponeurotomy

Table 36.1 Digital extension deficit pre- and postoperatively

	Preoperative	Immediate	Six weeks postoperative	Percent improvement
Total $n=62$	46° SD 35°	14° SD 23°	14° SD 20°	69.5
MCP $n=62$	29° SD 15°	5° SD 10°	4° SD 8°	82.8
PIP $n=23$	41° SD 30°	18° SD 24°	19° SD 23°	53.7

36.2.1 Needle Aponeurotomy Procedure

NA was performed in the following manner: the affected hand was cleansed with 0.5% chlorhexidine and 70% isopropyl alcohol and positioned supine on a table. The affected digit was passively extended and palpated to determine the points where the affected cord was most superficial and under maximal tension. These points were then infiltrated with 0.1–0.5 cc of 1% lidocaine with 1:100,000 epinephrine, ensuring the local anesthetic remained dermal/subdermal and volar to the cord. Effort was made not to infiltrate around the neurovascular bundles so as not to affect Tinel's sign. An 18 gauge needle was then inserted through the skin until the cord was palpable with the needle tip. The needle was stroked over the cord in a transverse direction. With sustained passive extension, cord release gives a distinct tactile sensation and audible feedback. The release was stopped when no further extension was appreciated or when the digital nerves were felt to be at risk. Depending on disease severity, single or multiple sites were used for release of an individual digit. Postoperatively, mupirocin ointment and a simple bandage were applied for 24 h. Patients were encouraged to use the hand immediately and perform simple stretching exercises to maintain range of motion.

36.3 Results

The mean preoperative TPED was 46° SD 35°. The immediate postoperative TPED was 14° SD 23°. Forty-two digits were assessed at 6–8 weeks postoperatively and showed a TPED of 14° SD 20°. The observed differences between preoperative and postoperative measurements were compared using a paired t-test. The results were found to be statistically significant $p=0.0001$ and remained so at 6 weeks postoperatively. The immediate extension deficit reduction EDR for MCP joints was 24° and 23° for PIP joints. The EDR 6 weeks post op was maintained at 25° MCP joints and

22° PIP joints. The average total EDR per digit was 32°. A subgroup analysis of the percent improvement at the MCP versus the PIP joint showed that needle aponeurotomy is significantly more effective at the MCP joint. The mean percent improvement for the MCP joint was 83% and significantly less for the PIP at 54% $p=0.002$ (Table 36.1).

Overall, patients were satisfied with their hand function postoperatively. There were no reported neurovascular injuries in this series. Unfortunately, there was a single incidence of flexor tendon laceration. This patient presented to clinic with absent flexion at both PIP and DIP joints. The patient noted this approximately 4 or 5 days post NA, but did not bring this to our attention until the 6 week follow-up appointment. Subsequent exploration in the operating room revealed a zone 3 flexor digitorum superficialis and profundus transection, which was subsequently repaired.

36.4 Discussion

There are many options available for the treatment of Dupuytren's disease. The accepted gold standard therapy is currently limited palmar fasciectomy and is likely to remain so in the foreseeable future. This technique, however, has a high complication rate and a relatively long recovery period and may not be the optimal treatment for all patients (van Rijssen et al. 2006). NA offers a simple alternative, and often patients can use their hands optimally in 1 week.

Our centre began using the technique of NA over 4 years ago. This was the result of multiple requests by patients aware of the procedure's use in Europe. During this time we have found the technique to be successful, and there has been a high degree of patient satisfaction.

In this study we prospectively enrolled patients in order to critically analyze our results. An average improvement of 32° was demonstrated in the 62 digits, which is comparable to that in the literature 34–49° (Duthie and Chesney 1997; Foucher et al. 2003).

At 6 week follow-up this improvement was maintained, with an average residual extension deficit of 14°. Three patients required fasciectomy due to inadequate release; however, we believe that the preoperative NA improved operative exposure. We do not currently have long-term results, but previous reports suggest a 50% recurrence rate at 3–5 years (National Institute for Clinical Excellence, NICE 2004). A subset analysis comparing improvement at the MCP and PIP joints showed significantly better results when NA is used for MCP contractures. This has been documented by others in the literature (Foucher et al. 2003; Rowley et al. 1984).

We agree that only midline and superficial cords are safely amenable to NA. The risk of neurovascular injury increases distal to the distal palmar crease due to the potential presence of spiral cords. Central cords between the distal palmar crease and the proximal digital crease are released only if they are very superficial and tethered to the overlying skin. By taking these precautions we have not had any neurovascular injuries. The one incidence of flexor tendon laceration in this series was our first serious complication in 4 years and was fortunately recognized and rectified. Tendon lacerations and neurovascular injuries are recognized risks of the procedure; however, literature suggests that the overall complication rate for NA is low at approximately 1% (NICE 2004).

We believe NA may have a role in the treatment of Dupuytren's disease for specific patients with MCP involvement. It may also have a role as an adjuvant therapy in select cases prior to fasciectomy. While the technique is relatively simple it has inherent risks, and should only be performed by specialists with an in-depth knowledge of hand anatomy and the anatomic pathology of Dupuytren's disease. Our results underscore the continued need for further molecular studies to elucidate the underlying pathophysiology enabling us to design rational curative methods for this disease.

36.5 Conclusions

- Dupuytren's contracture remains a surgical disease.
- Needle Aponeurotomy may be a useful adjunct in MPJ contractures with a palpable cord.

References

Badois FJ, Lermusiaux JL, Masse C, Kuntz D (1993) Non-surgical treatment of Dupuytren disease using needle fasciotomy. Rev Rhum Ed Fr 60(11):808–813

Bleton R, Marcireau D, Alnot JY (1997) Treatment of Dupuytren's disease by percutaneous needle fasciotomy. In: Saffar P, Amadio PC, Foucher G (eds) Current practice in hand surgery. Martin Dunitz, London, pp 187–193

Cheng HS, Hung LK, Tse WL, Ho PC (2008) Needle aponeurotomy for Dupuytren's contracture. J Orthop Surg (Hong Kong) 16(1):88–90

Duthie RA, Chesney RB (1997) Percutaneous fasciotomy for Dupuytren's contracture. J Hand Surg Br 22B:521–522

Elliot D (1988) The early history of contracture of the palmar fascia. Part 1: the origin of the disease: the curse of the MacCrimmons: the hand of benediction: Cline's contracture. J Hand Surg Br 13(3):246–253

Foucher G, Medina J, Malizos K (2001) Percutaneous needle fasciotomy in dupuytren disease. Tech Hand Up Extrem Surg 5(3):161–164

Foucher G, Medina J, Navarro R (2003) Percutaneous needle aponeurotomy: complications and results. J Hand Surg Br 28(5):427–431

Leclercq C, Tubiana R (2000) Results of surgical treatment. In: Tubiana R, Leclercq C, Hurst LC, Badalamente MA, Mackin EJ (eds) Dupuytren's disease. Martin Dunitz, London, pp 239–250

Lermusiaux JL, Debeyre N (1979) Medical treatment of Dupuytren's disease. In: De Seze S, Ryckewaert A, Kahn MF, Geurin CI (eds) L'Actualite rhumatologique. Expansion Scientifique Francaise, Paris, pp 338–343

McGrouther DA (2005) Dupuytren's contracture. In: Green DP (ed) Green's operative hand surgery, 5th edn. Elsevier, Philadelphia, pp 159–185

NICE (2004) Needle fasciotomy for Dupuytren's contracture, guidance 2004. National Institute for Clinical Excellence. http://guidance.nice.org.uk/IPG43/guidance/pdf/english. Accessed Dec 2010

Rowley DI, Couch M, Chesney RB, Norris SH (1984) Assessment of percutaneous fasciotomy in the management of Dupuytren's contracture. J Hand Surg Br 9(2):163–164

van Rijssen AL, Werker PMN (2006) Percutaneous needle fasciotomy in Dupuytren's disease. J Hand Surg Br 31(5):498–501

van Rijssen AL, Gerbrandy FS, Ter Linden H, Klip H, Werker PMN (2006) A comparison of the direct outcomes of percutaneous needle fasciotomy and limited fasciectomy for Dupuytren's disease: a 6-week follow-up study. J Hand Surg Am 31(5):717–725

Percutaneous Needle Fasciotomy: A Serious Alternative?

37

Holger C. Erne, Ahmed El Gammal, and Bernhard Lukas

Contents

37.1	Introduction	293
37.2	Materials and Methods	293
37.3	Surgical Technique	294
37.4	Results	294
37.5	Discussion	294
37.6	Conclusion	295
References		295

37.1 Introduction

The treatment of Dupuytren's contracture has been controversial since Felix Platter (1614) first described the condition (Dahmen and Kerckhoff 1967). The first fasciotomy was done most likely by Henry Cline in 1808 (Elliot 1988) and the first results of needle fasciotomy were published by Lermusiaux and Debeyre 1980 (Foucher et al. 2003).

The conventional fasciectomy represents a laborious procedure regarding the operation as well as the period of recovery. Additionally the patient has the risk of serious complications such as infection (2.4%), nerve and artery lesions (5.4%), complex regional pain syndrome (5.5%), diminished blood flow of the finger, intolerance to cold temperatures and reduced range of motion (3.6%) (Denkler 2010).

The present study reconsiders the less invasive procedure 'Percutaneous Needle Fasciotomy' as a serious alternative to fasciectomy.

37.2 Materials and Methods

In 2008 and 2009 63 rays in 47 patients with Dupuytren's Disease were treated using the technique of the 'Percutaneous Needle Fasciotomy'. The mean age was 60.3 years (range, 37–79 years). The right hand was affected in 64%. Most often treated was the fourth finger in 59.7% of all cases. The fifth finger was affected in 35.8%, the third in 3%, and the thumb in 1.5%. Almost three quarters of the patients have had a positive family

H.C. Erne (✉) • A. E. Gammal • B. Lukas
Center for Hand Surgery, Microsurgery,
Plastic Surgery, Harlachinger Straße 51, 81547 Munich,
Germany
e-mail: h_erne@hotmail.com

C. Eaton et al. (eds.), *Dupuytren's Disease and Related Hyperproliferative Disorders*,
DOI 10.1007/978-3-642-22697-7_37, © Springer-Verlag Berlin Heidelberg 2012

37.3 Surgical Technique

All patients were treated in an outpatient setting. Patients were instructed about the pain of initial needle penetration of the skin, the possibility of an incomplete outcome and the risk of nerve injury. The upper arm tourniquet was inflated after preparing and draping the operative field. Initially without local anesthesia the affected ray was held in an extended position in order to have the cord prominent and tight. A 20 gauge needle placed on a syringe and filled with local anesthesia (Mepivacaine 1%) was used. Needle entry sites used were only in the palm, not in the digits. The first needle entry site was usually distal to the distal palmar crease, followed by release at a more proximal level. Two palm levels were used on average. The bevel was used to penetrate and cut the cord successively from different angles. After having the feeling the cord was cut or almost cut the ray was hyperextended with little force to tear the remaining fibers. Once the ray was finished, approximately 1 ml local anesthesia was injected. The cutting maneuver was initially performed without any anesthesia to prevent nerve damages. The patients were instructed to inform if there was any prick in order to retract the needle before seriously damaging the nerve. After finishing the procedure the dressing was placed and a splint was fitted in fully extended position to be worn at night for 3 months. Unrestrictive hand and finger movement was recommended throughout the day.

37.4 Results

Within the retrospective study 43 patients (58 rays) have been reviewed with a mean follow-up of 11.1 months. The mean age of the patients was 60.3 years. The flexion contractures were classified with the Classification of Tubiana: Stage I: 34, Stage II: 20, Stage III: 4, Stage IV: 0.

The mean operation time was 9 min. Thirty-nine patients with 52 rays returned to full extension in the follow-up and had no recurrence (89.7%). Four patients (6 rays) showed a mild residual flexion contracture between 5 and 10°. Two of 6 rays retained each 10° flexion contracture postoperatively and increased to 15° each. The recurrence rate was 10.3%. These patients were classified as: Tubiana I: 1 patient, Tubiana II: 2 patients and Tubiana III: 1 patient.

The mean improvement of range of motion was 39.4° overall. The mean improvement of range of motion according to Tubiana's classification was: Tubiana I: 29°, Tubiana II: 47° and Tubiana III: 90°.

There was no hematoma, neither infection nor injury of nerve, vessel, or tendon. There were three patients with minor skin lesions between 0.5 and 2 cm within the palmar crease. 93% of all patients would undergo the procedure again, if necessary.

All patients, except one who was jobless were able to return to their job in an average of 11 days.

37.5 Discussion

Badois et al. 1993 reviewed his patients after performing 'Percutanous Needle Fasciotomy' plus steroid injection. 81% had good or excellent primary results. After 5 years he reported 69% had good or excellent results (Badois et al. 1993). Foucher et al. (2003) reported about an immediate improvement of 76% in his study. Excellent and good primary results reported by those and others influenced us to start the promising 'Percutanous Needle Fasciotomy'. The present study has 89.7% of excellent results after 11 months. This reflects a high number of very satisfied patients of 93% who would undergo the procedure again, if necessary. However data in literature show the decreasing number of satisfied patients with time. The follow-up of the current study was 11 months, thus shorter than the above-cited studies.

When starting to perform the 'Percutanous Needle Fasciotomy' there were reasonable doubts if the procedure would lead to a higher number of nerve and artery lesions. In 58 treated rays which were performed by different surgeons with different levels of education, there was neither nerve nor artery lesion. Other authors like Van Rijssen, Foucher and others report about a nerve lesion rate between 0 and 5% (Foucher et al. 2003; Lermusiaux 1997; Van Rijssen et al. 2006).

The level of needle penetration must also be carefully considered. Newer studies report about using palm- and finger levels, respectively, as many levels as possible in the palm and fingers (Foucher et al. 2003; Van Rijssen et al. 2006) The current study used almost solely palm levels in order to avoid nerve and artery lesions. It appears that the tactic to stay at palm level is still safer than using finger levels. Additionally the patients of the current study were mainly categorized in Tubiana's Stages I and II, whereas other authors treated more patients in higher stages.

Regarding complications it is to add that the current study had three minor skin lesions which resulted from the described hyperextension manoeuvre when the cord is still adherent to the skin. Other authors report the same issue although partially in higher numbers (Badois et al. 1993).

Another reasonable concern with the 'Percutanous Needle Fasciotomy' technique is its rate of recurrence. The recurrence rate in the present study was 10.3% after 11.1 months. Other authors report recurrence rates between 24 and 65% with a time of observation up to 60 months. (Badois et al. 1993) Therefore it is expected that the recurrence rate of the present study will increase once the time period of observation is extended.

The tourniquet was used in order to have the possibility to convert quickly to an open procedure in the case of an artery – or nerve lesion. There was no conversion necessary; insofar we conclude that the tourniquet is not an imperative. The needle size of 20 gauge was chosen to have an instrument which has a large enough edge length of the bevel, but which is small enough not to damage the skin too much.

Since jobless patients around the age of 60 years often struggle to return to the job market, the duration of the recovery period or the time interval to return to work after the operation becomes even more important. The current study shows a very short time period to return to work. Unfortunately there are no comparison figures in the present literature.

The most promising and reasonable conditions to indicate the 'Percutaneous Needle Fasciotomy' have been assessed herewith. To have a good visible and definable cord is important. Multiple cords, broad cords, diffuse skin involvement and scar tissue postoperatively are situations which are not favourable to the technique. Furthermore the flexion contracture should be solely caused by the cord itself. Arthrogenic contractures are likewise not accessible by the described technique.

Though being statistically not verifiable (through the small numbers stage III and IV), Tubiana's stage I and II have had a better outcome than higher stages. This is in concordance with the findings of Van Rijssen et al. (2006). The ideal conditions are Dupuytren's flexion contracture Tubiana stage I and II, a good definable cord, no arthrogenic contractures and a patient who needs to return to work/activity within 1–2 weeks and accepts well the increased recurrence rate.

37.6 Conclusion

'Percutaneous Needle Fasciotomy' is a reliable and relatively simple to perform technique. There is a short time of operation and a short period of recovery combined with a low complication rate. The vast majority of patients have been very satisfied.

The penetration of the skin is indeed painful. The cord remains, which could be the reason for the increased recurrence rates of the described technique. However the procedure allows uncomplicated further interventions since only marginal scar tissue is expected.

Based upon these facts 'Percutaneous Needle Fasciotomy' can be regarded as a serious alternative. The ideal indication is Dupuytren's flexion contracture Tubiana stage I and II, a good definable cord, no arthrogenic contractures and a patient who needs to return to work/activities within 1 or 2 weeks and is well informed about the increased recurrence rate.

References

Badois FJ, Lermusiaux JL, Masse C, Kuntz D (1993) Traitement non chirurgical de la maladie de Dupuytren par aponévrotomie à l'aiguille. Rev Rhum Ed Fr 60:808–813

Dahmen G, Kerckhoff F (1967) Langzeitbeobachtungen operativ und konservativ behandelter Dupuytrenscher Kontrakturen. Arch Orthop Unfallchir 61:187–202

Denkler K (2010) Surgical complications associated with fasciectomy for Dupuytren's disease: a 20-year review of the English literature. eplasty 10 pmid = 20204055. http://eplasty.com/index.php?option=com_content&view=article&id=413&catid=15&Itemid=116. Accessed Jan 2011

Elliot D (1988) The early history of contracture of the palmar fascia. Part 1: The origin of the disease: the curse of the MacCrimmons: the hand of benediction: Cline's contracture. J Hand Surg Br 13(3):246–253

Foucher G, Medina J, Navarro R (2003) Percutaneous needle aponeurotomy: complications and results. J Hand Surg Br 28(5):427–431

Lermusiaux JL (1997) How should Dupuytren's disease be managed in 1997? Rev Rhum Engl Ed 64:775–776

Tubiana R (1961) Evaluation chiffrée de la déformation dans la maladie de Dupuytren. Mem Acad Chir 87:887–888

Van Rijssen AL, Gerbrandy FSJ, Ter Linden H, Klip H, Werker PMN (2006) A comparison of the direct outcomes of percutaneous needle fasciotomy and limited fasciectomy for Dupuytren's disease: a 6-week follow-up study. J Hand Surg Am 31A:717–725

Dynamic External Fixation in the Treatment of Dupuytren's Contracture

38

George A. Lawson and Anthony A. Smith

Contents

38.1	Introduction	297
38.2	**Treatment of Flexion Contracture at the PIP Joint**	298
38.2.1	Surgical Anatomy Involved in PIP Flexion Contracture	298
38.2.2	Checkrein Ligament Release	298
38.2.3	Techniques in PIP Flexion Contracture Release	298
38.3	**Soft Tissue Shortening in Dupuytren's**	299
38.4	**Soft Tissue Distraction for PIP Joint Flexion Contractures**	299
38.4.1	Historical Background, Distraction Osteogenesis	299
38.4.2	Biologic Basis of Distraction	300
38.4.3	Dynamic External Fixators	300
38.5	**Digit Widget™ as a Dynamic External Fixator in Treatment of Dupuytren's**	301
38.5.1	Digit Widget™ Installation and Treatment	301
38.5.2	Clinical Experience with Digit Widget™	301
38.6	**Discussion**	303
38.7	**Conclusions**	303
	References	303

G.A. Lawson (✉) • A.A. Smith
Department of Surgery, Division of Plastic and Reconstructive Surgery, Mayo Clinic Arizona, 5777 East Mayo Boulevard, Phoenix, AZ 85054, USA
e-mail: lawson.george@mayo.edu; smith.anthony@mayo.edu

38.1 Introduction

The management of Dupuytren's disease is particularly difficult when there is significant flexion contracture of the proximal interphalangeal (PIP) joint. Historically, surgeons have attempted palmar and digital fasciotomy or fasciectomy to treat the Dupuytren's. Review of these efforts has documented disappointing results (Rodrigo et al. 1976; Bryan and Ghorbal 1988).

It was not until HK Watson described the "checkrein" ligament release that the operative management of these proximal interphalangeal joints changed significantly (Watson et al. 1979).

The addition of checkrein ligament release to the commonly employed digital fasciectomy is accepted by many surgeons, but checkrein release still dose not address two critical problems found with long-term PIP joint Dupuytren's contractures: (1) Shortening of the neurovascular digital bundles in recurrent cases, (2) Contraction of the soft tissue envelope.

Correction of the soft tissue deficiency by distraction through external fixators has been shown to be a viable option in the treatment of PIP flexion contracture (Messina and Messina 1991, 1993). The Digit Widget™ (Hand Biomechanics Lab Inc, Sacramento, CA) uses dynamic external boney fixation as a means to correct the soft tissue flexion contracture. Additional surgical treatment of the Dupuytren's contracture after soft tissue lengthening may be necessary to achieve a long-lasting result.

C. Eaton et al. (eds.), *Dupuytren's Disease and Related Hyperproliferative Disorders*,
DOI 10.1007/978-3-642-22597-7_38, © Springer-Verlag Berlin Heidelberg 2012

38.2 Treatment of Flexion Contracture at the PIP Joint

When the MCP joint is significantly involved with Dupuytren's contracture, a single stage operative release will often lead to satisfactory function. Unfortunately, disease at the PIP joint is not so easily treated. Few reports in the literature focus on this difficult joint contracture, and controversy still exists over the most appropriate surgical treatment for severe disease. Precise excision of diseased fascia and gentle manipulation can often correct less severe PIP deformities. Persistent or more severe contractures require a logical and systematic evaluation of the causative forces and altered anatomy of the hand (Crowley and Tonkin 1999). This includes evaluation for the need of checkrein ligament release or capsuloligamentous release.

38.2.1 Surgical Anatomy Involved in PIP Flexion Contracture

The PIP joint is a hinge joint, which is stabilized by the geometric configuration of its articular surface, as well as the by the collateral ligaments and the volar plate. It is supported superficially by the thin retinacular ligament of Landsmeer. The more robust deeper layer consists of the collateral ligaments which originate from the proximal phalanx and insert on the volar plate and middle phalanx (Shin and Amadio 2005). Both sides of the volar plate have a bifurcated ligamentous expansion which extends to the volar proximal phalanx. These anchoring structures are known as the "checkrein" ligaments. In the MCP joint, the volar plate contracts with flexion and re-expands with extension. The volar plate anatomy of the PIP joint behaves differently, as it slides proximally and distally with flexion and extension and does not change in configuration. Therefore, any adhesion or limiting force on the PIP volar plate or checkrein ligaments may cause limitations in full extension of this joint (Shin and Amadio 2005).

38.2.2 Checkrein Ligament Release

HK Watson first described the checkrein ligament release for Dupuytren's (Watson et al. 1979). He describes these entities as two thick ligamentous structures that emanate from the volar plate on each side and insert onto the volar sides of the proximal phalangeal periosteum. He surmised that in order to relieve the PIP contracture without violating the joint space, complete relief of the tethering forces of the volar plate was necessary. His 9 year retrospective review included 52 Dupuytren's contractures among the 115 total cases. His operative strategy included exposing the checkrein ligaments through a palmar approach and releasing them at the proximal edge of the volar plate. Following checkrein release, 110 of the 115 joints achieved full extension intraoperatively. Of those remaining, two required collateral ligament release and three required a second checkrein release during the postoperative period (Watson et al. 1979).

38.2.3 Techniques in PIP Flexion Contracture Release

Although many surgeons consider checkrein ligamentous release as the gold standard in operative therapy for difficult PIP flexion contractures, there is certainly no consensus. Commonly, treatment involves a systematic review of the involved Dupuytren's cords, followed by examination of the PIP flexor apparatus, and an additional assessment of the PIP extensor apparatus (Smith 2002). In those patients who do not acquire full extension after cord release, gentle passive manipulation of the PIP into extension with MCP flexion can be undertaken. The idea is to rupture minor periarticular adhesions involved in the contracture. If the flexion deformity persists, the volar plate and checkrein ligaments (capsuloligamentous structures) are assessed and released if thickened. Failure to achieve full extension at this point may be related to shortened accessory collateral ligaments or shortening of the actual tendon sheath, both of which can be released as well (Smith 2002).

Several studies have importantly compared outcomes using these different techniques for the treatment of Dupuytren's contracture involving the proximal interphalangeal joint. Weinzweig et al. retrospectively compared fasciectomy alone with capsuloligamentous release plus fasciectomy for severe PIP Dupuytren's contractures greater than 60° (Weinzweig et al. 1996). Adequate PIP extension was obtained intraoperatively after fasciectomy alone in a subset of 27 PIP joints. In 15 other PIP joints affected by Dupuytren's, persistent contracture of the PIP joint following fasciectomy necessitated further intervention which involved release of the capsuloligamentous structures (including the checkrein ligaments and sometimes the collateral and accessory collateral ligaments). In both of these groups, there was a significant decrease in PIP flexion contracture following surgical intervention. However, they found no difference in the percentage of contracture correction in the capsulotomy group compared with the noncapsulotomy group. In both cases, the degree of correction maintained at surgery was not maintained postoperatively in follow-up.

Beyermann et al. prospectively followed 43 patients with severely contracted PIP joints who underwent fasciectomy combined with postoperative rehabilitation (Beyermann et al 2004). Eleven of these patients were found to have inadequate release of their flexion contracture (greater than 20° residual flexion) at 6 months. Each of these 11 patients underwent an additional capsuloligamentous release. This additional release resulted in correction of their residual flexion contractures in every case.

Ultimately, a true balance between flexion and extension is necessary to truly correct a difficult flexion deformity in the proximal interphalangeal joint. One must be cognizant of the opposing extensor forces and realize that the extensor apparatus may be incompetent when treating a flexion contracture. After treatment and once the PIP joint can be passively extended, the central slip tenodesis test plays an important role in the complete workup and treatment of PIP Dupuytren's contractures. By flexing the wrist and MCP, the PIP should become fully extended. Otherwise, the central slip may be attenuated due to the flexion contracture. Full extension will never be able to take place without competence of the extensor apparatus. Methods to correct this problem in less severe PIP contractures have included treatment by extension splinting/fixation to heal the extensor apparatus (Smith 2002).

38.3 Soft Tissue Shortening in Dupuytren's

The checkrein ligamentous release plays an important role in the treatment of the severely contracted PIP joint from Dupuytren's. But this and other surgical steps do not address the important problem of soft tissue shortening involved with severe Dupuytren's disease. The soft tissue envelope around the joint is normally redundant and flexible. This laxity and compliance allows for full flexion and extension without creating undue tension on the skin and underlying tissues. During the evolution of a flexion joint contracture, this dynamic covering loses its compliance and shortens. Not only is the skin and underlying soft tissue affected, but the neurovascular bundles can become extremely shortened and fibrotic as well. In the case where the digit extends beyond the ability of the vessels to expand, the vessels may spasm and thrombose. Digital ischemia is an unfortunate result of vigorous passive PIP joint extension in the presence of shortened neurovascular bundles.

In the past, Dupuytren's disease was considered to be end stage at the point in which these neurovascular bundles are fibrosed and shortened (Smith 2002). Surgical correction was considered prohibitive, and amputation or digit shortening arthrodesis were considered salvage options. The soft tissue envelope shortening and resultant problems with wound closure necessitates the use of skin grafting and flap coverage. Each of these techniques sacrifices a donor area, and they may not provide a functional or cosmetically appealing result. Thus, a method of correcting the flexion joint contracture while also stimulating the growth and expansion of the palmar soft tissues would be ideal.

38.4 Soft Tissue Distraction for PIP Joint Flexion Contractures

Traditionally, splints have been used as the extensor force to correct soft tissue deficiencies in joint contractures. The problem with serial splinting and casting is that the skin and soft tissues limit the amount of force that can be applied. Undue pressure can cause pain as well as skin and soft tissue breakdown. Alternatively, by delivering this extensor force to the boney skeleton, much more effective torque can be delivered across a joint without jeopardizing the skin and soft tissues.

38.4.1 Historical Background, Distraction Osteogenesis

Distraction osteogenesis has become an accepted technique for bone lengthening. Ilizarov's work popularized this method for use in difficult cases which require a long bone graft to correct shortening (Ilizarov 1990). Gradual distraction after corticotomy results in long bone formation and bone lengthening. Importantly, as the bone lengthens, the soft tissue structures including nerves and vessels also expand around this construct. Without growth and expansion of the soft tissues, boney distraction could not be successful. This basic principle has fueled the evolution of other methods which use dynamic external fixation for conditions with shortened soft tissue – including joint contractures.

Other upper extremity conditions which require soft tissue lengthening have been successfully treated using distraction. Congenital deficiencies of the radius, involving radius aplasia or hypoplasia, result in a shortened forearm and radially deviated hand (Smith 2002). Centralization of the hand at the distal end of the ulna is commonly used to correct this abnormality. One problem with this correction involves a relative deficiency of radial skin and radial soft tissues that must be dealt with at the time of centralization. Smith and Greene have reported their experience with use of a dynamic external fixator for soft tissue distraction in congenitally deficient forearms (Smith and Greene 1995). In five (four radial deficient, one ulnar deficient) limbs, an Orthofix external distractor (EBI Medical Systems, Inc., Parsipanny, NJ) was placed. For the cases of radially deficient limbs, soft tissue distraction was continued until the hand could be passively centralized without radial deviation This was successfully carried out with a 1 mm/day distraction rate for an average of 1.1 cm total distraction. After formal radial centralization, the limbs remained in proper alignment at a mean of 14 months later.

38.4.2 Biologic Basis of Distraction

In vitro and biochemical analysis of soft tissue distraction demonstrates many interesting results. It is the cross-linking of collagen fibers that delivers the innate soft tissue strength and resistance to expansion. Bailey et al. found increased enzymatic activity (metalloproteinases, collagenase, gelatinase, cathespins) during soft tissue distraction, which led to depolymerization and cross-link breakdown of collagen (Bailey et al. 1994). They believed that the increased tension delivered by the mechanical stressor on the fibrous tissue initiated enzymatic degradation of collagen, thus weakening the fibers and increasing new collagen synthesis. Tarlton et al. confirmed these in vitro results with Dupuytren's tissue and demonstrated that there is a clear correlation between the force applied to the tissue and release of matrix metalloproteinases (Tarlton

et al. 1998). The degraded collagen thus loses its strength due to enzymatic breakdown from mechanical stress and not from other sources such as an inflammatory-mediated etiology.

The microvasculature is also affected in Dupuytren's tissue when external mechanical stress is applied. Brandes et al. demonstrated that dynamic external forces likely change the microfilaments, connections to adherins junctions, and other contacts within endothelial cells (Brandes et al. 1996). The contractile component of the endothelial cell cytoskeleton is altered, which likely helps conform to the external forces applied.

38.4.3 Dynamic External Fixators

The use of dynamic skeletal fixation devices to improve flexion contractures of the PIP joint is not a novel technique. The TEC (Continuous Extension Technique) by A. Messina is perhaps the most studied in the literature.

The TEC device was first reported in the literature in 1991, but in 1993, Messina and Messina reported their expanded results over 5 years in the treatment of patients with Dupuytren's disease (Messina and Messina 1991, 1993). They treated some patients using the device only and others using the device as a preoperative preparation, followed by fasciectomy. The latter group demonstrated fewer flexion contracture recurrences. They concluded that this method of dynamic external fixation offered an alternative to finger amputation or plastic surgical correction of skin and tissue loss in those patients with increased risk for ischemia, necrosis, loss of vascularity, and bad function.

Other soft tissue distractors have been reported to correct PIP joint contracture due to Dupuytren's. These devices include the Pipster (Hodgkinson 1994), Multiplaner Distracter (Kasabian et al. 1998), and S Quattro (Beard and Trail 1996; Rajesh et al. 2000) among others.

Since the evolution and acceptance of soft tissue distraction, there have been various protocols and methods of using the dynamic external fixator. Houshian and Chikkamuniyappa attempted to determine the optimum rate, amount of daily distraction, and the optimum duration of use with a dynamic external fixator (Houshian and Chikkamuniyappa 2007). Two groups were compared using a distraction rate of 0.5 mm/day vs. 1.0 mm/day. Although their study was underpowered, they found no statistically significant differences in the two rates of distraction. This follows common protocols of boney lengthening by distraction in orthognathic surgery that uses rates between 0.5 and 1.0 mm/day.

38.5 Digit Widget™ as a Dynamic External Fixator in Treatment of Dupuytren's

The Digit Widget™ (Hand Biomechanics Lab, Sacramento, CA) is one such device that was particularly developed as a dynamic external fixator for severe PIP flexion contractures. This device, introduced by Dr. John Agee in 2001, has been used with favorable results in the treatment of Dupuytren's PIP contracture. The Digit Widget™ performs soft tissue distraction with accompanying growth of the soft tissue envelope and neurovascular tissues. The external force is transmitted as torque directly to the boney skeleton, thus avoiding the problems associated with splinting and casting which may cause undue soft tissue pressure. An additional benefit with treatment is that full flexion of the PIP may take place with the device in place, thereby encouraging therapy and use of the hand during treatment. The overall treatment plan must include any other steps which may be needed to correct the cause of the flexion deformity (Agee 2010).

38.5.1 Digit Widget™ Installation and Treatment

The Digit Widget™ is installed similar to other external fixators with pins anchored into the middle phalanx bone just distal to the contracted PIP joint (Fig. 38.1). The connector device is then assembled to the anchoring pins and attached to a removable hand cuff (Fig. 38.2). Elastic bands create torque and dictate the extensile force transmitted across the joint. The bands and cuff can be removed for PIP flexion therapy and activity.

38.5.2 Clinical Experience with Digit Widget™

In practice, the Digit Widget™ is used as an adjunct to operative flexion contracture release in those patients felt severe enough to warrant invasive treatment. For these

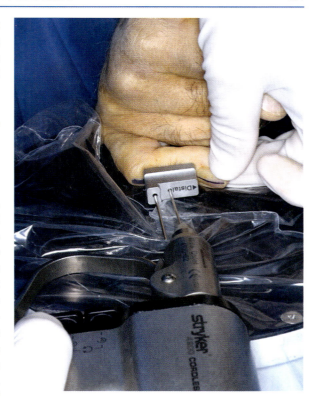

Fig. 38.1 Installation of Digit Widget™: percutaneous pin insertion distal to PIP in dorsal middle phalanx of small finger

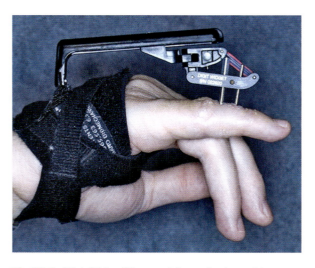

Fig. 38.2 Digit Widget™ external fixator in place with removable hand cuff

cases, the Digit Widget™ can be applied to lengthen the soft tissue envelope and neurovascular structures in preparation for definitive operative treatment of the PIP

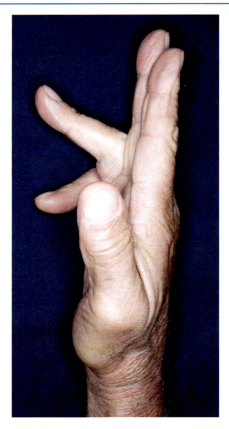

Fig. 38.3 Preoperative view 90° PIP flexion contracture of right small finger due to Dupuytren's before application of Digit Widget™

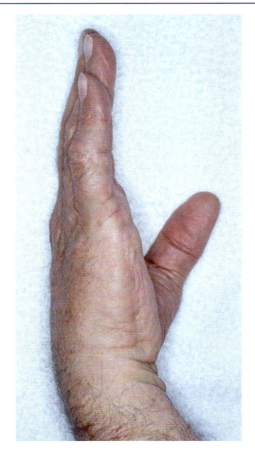

Fig. 38.4 Same patient, 5 months after placement of Digit Widget™. After 6 weeks of soft tissue distraction and hand therapy, the external fixator was removed and the MCP and PIP contractures were surgically released from the right small finger

contracture (often involving exploration of the volar plate and checkrein ligament release) (Figs. 38.3 and 38.4). In some patients, the Digit Widget™ has so completely reversed the contracture that no further intervention has been necessary. This particular strategy may augment operative release of checkrein ligaments in very severe flexion contractures of the PIP joint. Additionally, it seems that the Digit Widget™ may be useful in treating reoperative PIP flexion contractures.

The author's (Smith AA) own experience with the Digit Widget™ has shown promising results. In a series of 30 patients (37 digits), a comparison is made between those who underwent PIP joint checkrein ligament release (CRLR) following fasciectomy versus those who had preoperative placement of the Digit Widget™ (Craft et al. 2011). Of the 20 digits treated with CRLR, a mean of 27.7° of PIP joint extension improvement was observed. But included in this group, 3 of these digits actually developed an increase in flexion contracture, with an average of 16° (2–48°). Comparatively, the average improvement of PIP joint extension in the Digit Widget™ cohort was 54.7°. None of the digits in the Digit Widget™ group experienced worsening contracture, and in fact 3 digits improved to full extension without requiring surgical release. Additionally, the Digit Widget™ group seemed to fare better in those digits with severe PIP joint contractures (61° or greater). Of the 8 CRLR digits with severe preoperative contracture, 1 patient developed worsening contracture of 3° and overall improvement was a mean of 35.3°. In contrast, none of the 10 Digit Widget™-treated joints with severe contractures developed worsening contracture, and mean improvement was 57.3° (Craft et al. 2011).

38.6 Discussion

Dupuytren's disease can be difficult to treat regardless of the location of joint contracture. Proximal interphalangeal joint flexion contractures are particularly problematic. The involvement of fibrous cords, the volar plate, the checkrein ligaments, and incompetent extensor structures make operative treatment difficult. In addition, the soft tissue shortening and accompanying deficiency in neurovascular structures must be addressed as well. Soft tissue distraction using a dynamic external fixator, such as the Digit Widget™, provides an additional tool to combat these difficult PIP contractures. The principles of distraction are sound, and the sparse data on its efficacy in treating the PIP flexion contracture appears promising. Certainly future randomized prospective trials comparing distraction and conventional treatment would be helpful in determining the importance of dynamic external fixation. Ultimately, the treating physician must find the appropriate balance between extension and flexion forces to treat the disease. Dynamic external fixation should be viewed as an important option in the treatment of Dupuytren's disease at the PIP joint.

38.7 Conclusions

- Flexion contractures of the PIP joint in Dupuytren's disease are difficult to treat.
- The surgical treatment of PIP contracture continues to evolve and no consensus exists.
- Soft tissue shortening involved with Dupuytren's contracture presents a significant risk for ischemia and tissue loss after surgical correction.
- Dynamic external fixation is a method of soft tissue distraction that causes the tissues to "grow."
- The Digit Widget™ uses the idea of dynamic external fixation to correct difficult to treat PIP flexion contractures due to Dupuytren's disease.

References

Agee JM (2010) http://www.handbiolab.com/products/digit-widget/. Accessed Sept 2010

Bailey AJ, Tarlton JF, Van Der Stappen J, Sims TJ, Messina A (1994) The continuous elongation technique for severe Dupuytren's disease: a biochemical mechanism. J Hand Surg Br 19(4):522–527

Beard AJ, Trail IA (1996) The "S" Quattro in severe Dupuytren's contracture. J Hand Surg Br 21(6):795–796

Beyermann K, Prommersberger KJ, Jacobs C, Lanz UB (2004) Severe contracture of the proximal interphalangeal joint in Dupuytren's disease: does capsuloligamentous release improve outcome? J Hand Surg Br 29(3):240–243

Brandes G, Reale E, Messina A (1996) Microfilament system in the microvascular endothelium of the palmar fascia affected by mechanical stress applied from outside. Virchows Arch 429(2–3):165–172

Bryan AS, Ghorbal MS (1988) The long-term results of closed palmar fasciotomy in the management of Dupuytren's contracture. J Hand Surg Br 13(3):254–256

Craft RO, Smith AA, Coakley B, Casey WJ, Rebecca AM, Duncan SF (2011) Preliminary soft-tissue distraction vs checkrein ligament release after fasciectomy in the treatment of Dupuytren PIP joint contractures. Plast Reconstr Surg (accepted)

Crowley B, Tonkin MA (1999) The proximal interphalangeal joint in Dupuytren's disease. Hand Clin 15(1):137–147

Hodgkinson P (1994) The use of skeletal traction to correct the flexed PIP joint in Dupuytren's disease. J Hand Surg Br 19(4):534–537

Houshian S, Chikkamuniyappa C (2007) Distraction correction of chronic flexion contractures of PIP joint: comparison between two distraction rates. J Hand Surg Am 32(5):651–656

Ilizarov GA (1990) Clinical application of the tension-stress effect for limb lengthening. Clin Orthop 250:8–26

Kasabian A, McCarthy J, Karp N (1998) Use of a multiplaner distracter for the correction of a proximal interphalangeal joint contracture. Ann Plast Surg 40(4):378–381

Messina A, Messina J (1991) The TEC treatment (continuous extension technique) for severe Dupuytren's contracture of the fingers. Ann Chir Main Memb Super 10:247–250

Messina A, Messina J (1993) The continuous elongation treatment by the TEC device for severe Dupuytren's contracture of the fingers. Plast Reconstr Surg 92(1):84–90

Rajesh KR, Rex C, Mehdi H, Martin C, Fahmy NRM (2000) Severe Dupuytren's contracture of the proximal interphalangeal joint: treatment by two-stage technique. J Hand Surg Br 25(5):442–444

Rodrigo JJ, Niebauer JJ, Brown RL, Doyle JR (1976) Treatment of Dupuytren's contracture: long-term results after fasciotomy and fascial excision. J Bone Joint Surg Am 58(3):380–387

Shin AY, Amadio PC (2005) Stiff finger joints. In: Green DP, Hotchkiss RN, Pederson WC (eds) Green's operative hand surgery, 5th edn. Elsevier, Philadelphia

Smith P (2002) Lister's the hand: diagnosis and indications, 4th edn. Churchill Livingstone, London

Smith AA, Greene TL (1995) Preliminary soft tissue distraction in congenital forearm deficiency. J Hand Surg Am 20A:420–424

Tarlton JF, Meagher P, Brown RA, McGrouther DA, Bailey AJ, Afofke A (1998) Mechanical stress in vitro induces increased expression of MMPs 2 and 9 in excised Dupuytren's disease tissue. J Hand Surg Br 23(3):297–302

Watson HK, Light TR, Johnson TR (1979) Checkrein resection for flexion contracture of the middle joint. J Hand Surg Am 4(1):67–71

Weinzweig N, Culver JE, Fleegler EJ (1996) Severe contractures of the proximal interphalangeal joint in Dupuytren's disease: combined fasciectomy with capsuloligamentous release versus fasciectomy alone. Plast Reconstr Surg 97(3):560–566

Hand Therapy for Dupuytren's Contracture

39

Patricia Davis and Charles Eaton

Contents

39.1	**Introduction**	305
39.2	**Problems Evaluating Therapy for Dupuytren's**	305
39.2.1	Biological Variability	306
39.2.2	Protocol Variability	306
39.2.3	Lack of Evidence	306
39.3	**Preoperative Evaluation**	307
39.4	**Preoperative Therapy**	307
39.5	**Postoperative Management**	307
39.5.1	General Goals	307
39.5.2	The "No-Tension" Program	308
39.5.3	Postoperative Management After Fasciectomy	309
39.5.4	Care After Needle Fasciotomy	312
39.5.5	Care After Enzymatic Fasciotomy	312
39.5.6	Intervention for Complication	313
39.5.7	Home Program	314
39.6	**Summary Points**	314
References		314

P. Davis (✉)
Florida Hand Rehabilitation, 1002 S Old Dixie Hwy #105,
Jupiter, FL 33458, USA
e-mail: alldaviswpb@bellsouth.net

C. Eaton
The Hand Center, Jupiter, FL, USA
e-mail: eaton@bellsouth.net

39.1 Introduction

The unique biology of Dupuytren's disease can make postoperative therapy particularly challenging. Open surgical procedures for Dupuytren's are often followed by prolonged, disproportionate inflammation and fibrosis. Inflammation following surgery for Dupuytren's is easily aggravated by mechanical forces on the soft tissues, and the threshold for this provocation is sometimes only determined in retrospect. More than almost any other situation, therapy following surgery for Dupuytren's contracture tests the therapist's skills of listening, examining, and assessing the effects of every step of therapy. The patient's recovery is not only influenced by individual biology but also by surgical technique, choice of procedure, and timing of therapy. Other comorbid factors include carpal tunnel syndrome, flexor tendinitis, osteoarthritis and postoperative issues of infection, ischemic flaps, local nerve irritation, flare reaction, and reflex sympathetic dystrophy.

39.2 Problems Evaluating Therapy for Dupuytren's

Despite nearly 200 years of collective clinical experience with surgery for Dupuytren's, the exact role of therapy for postoperative Dupuytren's patients remains based on anecdote, experience, and opinion. Three obstacles remain in determining optimum therapy: biological variability, protocol variability, and lack of evidence.

C. Eaton et al. (eds.), *Dupuytren's Disease and Related Hyperproliferative Disorders*,
DOI 10.1007/978-3-642-22697-7_39, © Springer-Verlag Berlin Heidelberg 2012

39.2.1 Biological Variability

The first problem in assessing effectiveness of therapy is the great individual variability in both degree of contracture and biologic aggressiveness. Surgeons attempt to achieve two goals with surgery: correction of deformity and control of disease. The first goal may be elusive, the second, impossible. In mild contractures, the only issue is releasing the deforming force of contracted fascia. More severe contractures may result in secondary anatomic changes of proximal interphalangeal joint capsular contractures, central slip attenuation with boutonniere deformity, sagittal band attenuation with extensor subluxation, intrinsic muscle tightness, and less well-defined changes resulting in stiffness. These issues may be undiagnosed or respond poorly to operative treatment, and their effects strongly influence postoperative recovery. More important is the reality that *even after surgery for Dupuytren's Contracture, the patient still has Dupuytren's Disease*, and their abnormal biology continues through their recovery. By definition, patients with more aggressive Dupuytren's have earlier clinical recurrences. Aggressive or treatment-resistant Dupuytren's is more common in patients with age of onset less than 50, involvement requiring treatment of the small finger, bilateral involvement, thumb or index finger involvement, Garrod's knuckle pads, Ledderhose disease, or more than two fingers involved in one hand (Abe et al. 2004; Bulstrode et al. 2005; Degreef and De Smet 2011). Patients with these risk factors tend to have more inflammation, stiffness, and fibrosis after open surgery for Dupuytren's. All of these considerations influence expectations and make the task of evaluating effectiveness of any one intervention more difficult.

39.2.2 Protocol Variability

The second problem is lack of standardization and individual variation of the surgeons managing patients. In a review of the Dupuytren's management practices of 141 hand surgeons, Au Yong et al. found similar thresholds for recommending surgery with some variation in the type of procedure recommended (e.g., fasciectomy vs. dermofasciectomy). Two-thirds of surgeons surveyed referred all patients for therapy; one-third referred patients as required. Although five out of six surgeons recommended nighttime splinting, there was broad variation in the recommended duration (Au-Yong et al. 2005). This survey was carried out in the United Kingdom, and additional variation would be expected elsewhere in the world. Additional studies of this type are needed, along with greater detail regarding orthotic design and specifics of therapeutic protocols.

39.2.3 Lack of Evidence

The third and largest problem is that there is scant and conflicting evidence in the literature supporting the benefits and risks of hand therapy following surgery for Dupuytren's contracture (Herweijer 2007). This is a significant issue because the soft tissue reactions to surgery, to manipulation, and to immobilization are influenced by the pathologic biology of Dupuytren's and change unpredictably over the months following surgery. At what point does splinting for extension lead to loss of flexion? Given the reactive nature of tissues affected by Dupuytren's, do potential gains from dynamic splinting ever justify the potential risk of reactive inflammation? What is the best way to identify and monitor the threshold of forces used to mobilize soft tissues safely without producing delayed inflammatory reaction? Currently lacking are level 1, evidence-based, randomized controlled studies for physical modalities or exercise protocols following surgery for Dupuytren's contracture (Larson and Jerosch-Herold 2008). Continuous passive motion has been reported to provide no benefit following surgery for Dupuytren's (Sampson et al. 1992). Beyond this, there are few supported recommendations. Postoperative therapeutic orthotic use varies widely among hand surgeons and therapists, and may involve relaxed extension, aggressive extension, tension relieved, or no-tension protocols (Evans et al. 2002; Lubahn 1999; McFarlane 1997; Mackin 1986; Prosser and Conolly 1996; Mullins 1999; Abbott et al. 1987; Jain et al. 1988; Rives et al. 1992; Ebskov et al. 2000; Clare et al. 2004). The "no-tension" regimen described below is the first to correlate the effect of postoperative mechanical stress with the complications of inflammation, sympathetic flare, hypertrophic scar, and functional range of motion (Evans et al. 2002). Currently, a multicenter randomized controlled trial is underway to determine the effectiveness of postoperative orthotic positions and duration of use (Jerosch-Herold

39.3 Preoperative Evaluation

Preoperative evaluation by the therapist is recommended before open surgery for Dupuytren's. The benefits of a single presurgical visit with the therapist include: independent documentation of range of motion; screening for comorbid (e.g., trigger finger, carpal tunnel syndrome) or secondary (e.g., oblique retinacular ligament tightness limiting distal interphalangeal flexion) conditions; reinforcing the surgeon's preoperative discussion regarding the duration of recovery, the need for splinting, and tips for managing with one hand. After a single preoperative consultation with the surgeon, it is common for the patient to discount the possibility of prolonged recovery time and effort described by the surgeon. These patients are then surprised and frustrated if they do have a long recovery. Realistic expectations regarding final outcome can also be discussed, including the likelihood of residual or recurrent contracture following release of proximal interphalangeal joint, the possibility of loss of flexion, and the likelihood of recurrence contractures (Abe et al. 2004; Legge and McFarlane 1980; Misra et al. 2007; Weinzweig et al. 1996).

39.4 Preoperative Therapy

Based on experience with external fixation devices to correct preoperative capsular joint contractures (Bailey et al. 1994; Hodgkinson 1994), preoperative serial casting or static progressive splinting may be helpful in select patients with severe proximal interphalangeal joint flexion contractures. Potential surgical advantages include reduced risk of maceration-related infection, simplifying surgical exposure, shorter rehabilitation, and potentially improving final correction of deformity. The senior demographic of Dupuytren's means that in the USA, Medicare provides insurance and limits the number of covered annual therapy visits. Improperly planned, preoperative therapy might limit the availability of postoperative therapy.

39.5 Postoperative Management

39.5.1 General Goals

There are four groups of goals specific to postoperative care after surgery for Dupuytren's: damage control, maturation guidance, safe intervention, and tissue nutrition.

39.5.1.1 Damage Control
Damage control involves dealing with postoperative problems of infection, ischemic flaps, delayed healing, vasospasm, neuritis/nerve damage, excessive inflammation, hypertrophic scars, surgical scar contracture, and sympathetic dystrophy. Damage control issues require frank and frequent communication with both the surgeon and patient to develop an appropriately individualized plan of care. Previously undiagnosed flexor tendinitis or carpal tunnel syndrome are common problems to surface during the recovery period and may masquerade as postoperative swelling, stiffness, or avoidance of use. Onset of sympathetic dystrophy may do the same. Because these additional diagnoses may require steroid injection, oral medication, or additional testing, and because response is strongly influenced by timing, concerns of this nature should be immediately discussed with and referred to the surgeon.

39.5.1.2 Maturation Guidance
Maturation guidance goals are to encourage uneventful wound healing, reduce swelling, maintain contracture correction, restore finger flexion, and guide collagen remodeling. Specific steps require patient education regarding wound hygiene, retrograde massage, avoidance of tight or elastic circumferential bandages, appropriate splinting, active flexion/extension, and tendon gliding exercises. It is important to remain mindful that after surgery for contracture, the patient still has the abnormal biology of Dupuytren's and is at particular risk for developing tendon adhesions and joint fibrosis during the recovery phase.

39.5.1.3 Safe Intervention
Safe intervention refers to therapy protocol design and execution which does not provoke additional inflammatory reaction. Wound closure, surgical flaps, and grafts may be compromised by stressful exercise. Postoperative tissue loss increases the risk of hypertrophic scar and scar contracture. Anecdotally, inflammation, swelling,

pain, and flap necrosis are much more common when the patient is placed in a full extension splint at the end of the surgical procedure compared to a soft operative bandage. The same applies throughout the entire recovery process.

39.5.1.4 Tissue Nutrition

A helpful concept is to think in terms of tissue nutrition or tissue perfusion instead of range of motion. Tissue nutrition at the capillary level is critically influenced by pressure in the capillary venules and the extravascular tissues. High venous pressure results in edema, tissue protein deposition, and ultimately, impaired arterial inflow. The actual pressures involved are surprisingly low. Normal venous capillary pressure is less than 10 mm of mercury. Muscle interstitial tissue pressures over 15 mm mercury show abnormal physiology (Mubarak and Hargens 1982); sustained tissue pressures over 30 mm of mercury may result in ischemic tissue changes (Gelberman et al. 1981). Repeated exposure to external pressure reduces tolerance to subsequently applied pressure (Reswick and Rogers 1976). Normally, these measurements are obtained with pressure transducers, but what do they actually mean? How do they translate into the real world? A copper penny weighs 2.5 g and has a surface area of about 2.8 cm^2. 15 mm of mercury converts to about 20 g/cm^2, or the pressure beneath a stack of 23 pennies. If an average fingertip pressing down presents a surface area of 1 cm^2, 15 mm of mercury is the pressure generated by a fingertip force of 20 g, or the weight of 8 pennies. *A fingertip pushing with the force of the weight of eight pennies is all the external pressure needed to change tissue perfusion.* Greater forces will trigger inflammatory reaction and ultimately mechanical tissue damage, but detrimental physiologic effects begin at very low sustained pressures and reactive changes to ischemia continue long after the pressure is relieved (Ward 1976).

39.5.2 The "No-Tension" Program

39.5.2.1 Concept

It may seem counterintuitive, but less forceful postoperative therapy for Dupuytren's can yield better final range of motion (Evans et al. 2002). Tension on the soft tissues is a particular problem in the care of patients with Dupuytren's. This is a particular problem

because fingers are usually the most straight at the end of the procedure in the operating room, but during recovery, patients tend to lose this initial correction. *If loss of correction is treated with increasingly aggressive stretching and splinting, the inflammatory response will only make the situation worse in a vicious cycle.* These considerations suggest that a postoperative program which does not involve external wound tension may not only be more comfortable for the patient but results in fewer complications and better final range of motion (Evans et al. 2002).

39.5.2.2 Evidence

Pathologic cellular biology and tissue mechanics of Dupuytren's are reviewed in this textbook (Meinel 2012a; Millesi 2012; Hinz and Gabbiani 2012; Zidel 2012; Phan 2012; Vi et al. 2012; Iqbal et al. 2012) and elsewhere in great detail. Although the relationships are complex, three factors converge to support a no-tension approach: ischemia, edema, and mechanical tension.

Ischemia

The end result of the Dupuytren's biology is ischemic fibrosis and microvascular occlusion from endothelial fibroblast infiltration (Murrell 1992; Kischer and Speer 1984). Conversely, ischemia results in fibroblast proliferation (Hunt et al. 1985), collagen deposition, and the appearance of myofibroblasts (Madden et al. 1975), the key cells in Dupuytren's (Gabbiani and Majno 1972). Some risk factors for Dupuytren's disease – age, diabetes, and smoking tobacco – are also risk factors for microvascular disease (Murrell 1991; Murrell 1992). This is a major issue following surgery for Dupuytren's: tissues which are known to have abnormal tissue perfusion as a baseline are then subjected to ischemic stress during surgery under tourniquet control. Postfasciectomy edema is common in response to the combination of surgical injury and ischemia during surgery. Postfasciectomy edema is greater for at least 4 weeks postoperatively in patients who have had surgery under tourniquet ischemia compared to those operated on without tourniquet (Ward 1976). This *lasting effect of a single episode of ischemia* shows that for Dupuytren's patients, any intervention which provokes even temporary circulatory changes, including tight orthotics, compressive wraps or dynamic splints, may induce a prolonged period of swelling. The threshold for external pressure to provoke circulatory changes is very low, as discussed earlier.

Edema

There is strong anecdotal evidence for a correlation between forceful extension orthotic use, aggressive manual therapy, repetitive strenuous exercise, and prolonged postoperative edema after surgery for Dupuytren's. Tissues respond to mechanical stresses with inflammation and swelling dependent on tissue load, duration, and repetition (Brand 1972; Brand et al. 1999). Local edema produces local ischemia by altering hydrostatic capillary pressure gradients (Hunt et al. 1984; LaVan and Hunt 1990; Knighton et al. 1981). Increasing mechanical forces to compensate for edema-related stiffness compounds the problem in a vicious cycle.

Mechanical Stress

As just noted, mechanical forces exceeding tissue tolerance can result in prolonged swelling and circulatory changes. Compounding this is the finding that tissues affected by Dupuytren's have a lower tolerance to mechanical forces than normal tissues. Laboratory studies have demonstrated that cells from Dupuytren's tissue respond to mechanical stretching forces more than cells from normal fascia (Howard et al. 2003) and that mechanical tension increases both fibroblast proliferation (Curtis and Seehar 1978) and myofibroblast differentiation (Grinnell 1994; Halliday and Tomasek 1995). Myofibroblast activity has been associated with wound site tension (Rudolph et al. 1992), and repetitive mechanical stress has been shown to promote collagen synthesis and deposition (Chvapil and Koopmann 1984). Residual skin tension after fasciotomy increases the likelihood of early disease recurrence (Citron and Hearnden 2003). All of these factors compound each other to make mechanical stresses intolerable in the postoperative Dupuytren's hand.

39.5.3 Postoperative Management After Fasciectomy

As discussed, there is great variation in hand therapy protocols among both surgeons and therapists. Many details of care exist because of training, habit, and availability of supplies rather than any scientific report. The following program is one method, a starting point, based on both published and personal experience, and has proved to be useful for postfasciectomy rehabilitation. Therapy following dermofasciectomy and skin graft is detailed in Ketchum (2012). Some of the following details may be substituted with sensible alternatives, but the no-tension approach should remain the central goal and the patient's comfort and tissue response the guide.

39.5.3.1 Postoperative Care: Weeks One and Two

Dressings and Orthotics

Patients are seen in therapy the day after surgery. Initial wound care is performed with the patient supine to reduce anxiety and in the event of a vasovagal episode. If gauze is adherent, it is saturated with sterile water until it releases easily. Drains are removed if present. Wounds are cleaned with sterile water, and if macerated, allowed to air dry enough to regain normal skin appearance before redressing. Sterile petrolatum or petroleum based antibiotic ointments may be used. Mupirocin ointment is preferred over other antibiotic ointments because of a comparatively lower incidence of allergic contact dermatitis (Sheth and Weitzul 2008). Wounds are redressed with gauze and a lightly applied wrap. Fingers are dressed individually with small sterile gauze squares, 5/8″ tube gauze, and a single layer of lightly applied self-adherent wrap such as Coban™. The hand is fitted with a dorsal extension blocking forearm-based orthotic with the wrist at neutral, metacarpophalangeal joints at 35–45° of flexion, and the interphalangeal joints at comfortable extension (Fig. 39.1). Only the operated digits are included in the orthotic. If the procedure involves the thumb or first web space, the orthotic includes the thumb in comfortable abduction.

Hand Exercise

Patients are seen again in 2 days for wound care and to begin gentle exercise. At this time, wound care is advanced to washing in the sink with mild (fragrance, additive, and alcohol free) soap and tap water, supervised by the therapist, and wounds are dressed as before. Patients are instructed to begin gentle active composite flexion within the confines of the orthotic, avoiding the end ranges of flexion and extension. Because at this point patients begin assuming a more active role in their care, it is important to review the importance of following the program as instructed. If not, patients who are used to being aggressive in work and sports will tend to edit the recommendations, overwork, and overdo. These patients need a firm approach with written instructions and the reminder that "no

Fig. 39.1 Dorsal static protective orthotic and active exercises. This orthotic design is fabricated for the "no-tension" protocol as early as the day after surgery for Dupuytren's contracture and continued for 2–3 weeks. Interphalangeal joints are blocked at comfortable active extension, metacarpophalangeal joints at 35–45°, and the wrist neutral. Only the operated fingers are included. Active range of motion is allowed within the splint with the fingers comfortably strapped in extension in between exercises

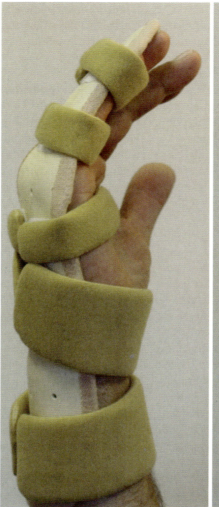
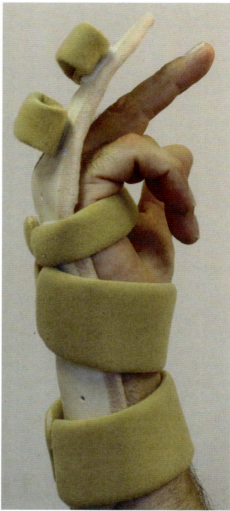

pain, no gain" may be exactly the wrong approach for their optimum outcome. It is helpful to frame the patient's role as paying attention to their body's signals and to explain the nature of delayed inflammatory reaction. *If it increasingly hurts as they do it, they are doing too much; if it aches worse at night or in the morning, they exceeded their tissue threshold hours earlier* ("like a sunburn").

Shoulder Care

Shoulder issues must be anticipated and prevented. The association of Dupuytren's and frozen shoulder (Smith et al. 2001) is reviewed. Instructions are given for ideal shoulder positions for elevation and sleep to avoid impingement as well as shoulder mobilization exercises. During recovery, the upper trapezius and levator scapulae may develop trigger points from disuse and dysfunctional posturing. The therapist must monitor for these, and if symptoms develop, add cervical stretches and myofascial massage to the program.

39.5.3.2 Postoperative Care: Weeks Two and Three
Movement and Exercise

During this phase, flexion/extension exercises are progressively advanced. The therapist begins gentle passive motion of proximal and distal interphalangeal joints using axial traction to prevent cartilage abutment. Aggressive passive mobilization is avoided. If wound healing allows, volar digital orthotics spanning all

39 Hand Therapy for Dupuytren's Contracture

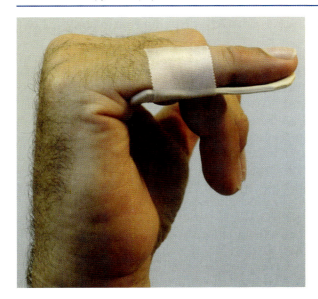

Fig. 39.2 Volar digital orthotics. Two to three weeks after surgery, if wound healing permits, volar orthotics supporting the interphalangeal joints may be used for 10–15 min every 2 h, secured with nonelastic tape. Transparent tape may be used to monitor blanching beneath the tape, which should be avoided

phalanges can be applied four or five times per day with 1-in. tape, applying light extension forces to the PIP joints for up to 15 min (Fig. 39.2). Transparent tape may be used to allow visual confirmation that the underlying skin is not blanched. Functional electrical stimulation (FES) may be used for neuromuscular reeducation and to promote tendon glide. By week three, FES to improve digital extension should be applied for both composite extension and with the MCP joints manually blocked in flexion to transmit forces to the PIP level. Wound care is advanced to lighter dressings, continuing single layer Coban wraps.

Suture Removal

The combination of extensive flap elevation and the biologic effects of Dupuytren's disease delays development of mechanical strength of the healing surgical wounds. *Unless there are signs of suture-related infection, sutures should be left in at least 2 weeks to avoid wound dehiscence.* Suture removal should be *delayed 3 weeks or more if the patient is diabetic, if the flap tips are not stable, or if the wound edges are mobile.* Sutures are removed either when enough time has elapsed and the wounds appear healed or if the wound has dehisced and sutures are no longer providing wound approximation.

Scar Taping

After suture removal, 1″ surgical paper tape is placed longitudinally along incisions and lines of tension where the incision crosses a joint to *stress shield the scar*. Reduction in scar tension is believed to reduce scar inflammation and hypertrophic scar formation (Reiffel 1995; Niessen et al. 1998). Patients are instructed to change the paper tape when they shower. Prior to showering, wounds are massaged with gentle transverse motions. Following shower, the scar and volar tissues are cleaned with isopropyl alcohol to remove residual oil and dried completely before reapplying tape. Silicone gel sheeting is applied to the scar at night instead of tape if the scar is hypersensitive or hypertrophic. The silicone is worn inside the night extension splint. Molded elastomer can be used in combination with a night orthotic for larger palmar areas, but paper tape is less expensive and may be more effective for simple hypertrophic scars than silicone gels or elastomers (Reiffel 1995; Niessen et al. 1998).

Splinting Advancement

During the third week, daytime splinting is discontinued, and the night orthotic is changed to a volar hand-based extension device with straps over the MCP and PIP joints (Fig. 39.3). If there are carpal tunnel symptoms, the night orthotic is made forearm-based with the wrist in slight flexion and ulnar deviation (Burke et al. 1994).

Exercise Advancement

Isolated flexor tendon gliding (Wehbé and Hunter 1985) including hook and full fist are recommended at least five times per day, 15–20 repetitions per exercise. The patient is instructed in intrinsic stretch (MCP extension, PIP and DIP flexion) and oblique retinacular ligament stretch (PIP extension, DIP flexion). Putty and hand grippers are not used, and the patient is warned to avoid strong repetitive composite fisting, which elevates pressures at the A1 pulley (Azar et al. 1983; Evans et al. 1988) and carpal tunnel (Cobb et al. 1994, 1995; Seradge et al. 1995; Siegel et al. 1995), and if overdone, cause flexor tendon inflammation (Evans 2009). The need to avoid aggressive exercise is reinforced.

39.5.3.3 Postoperative Care: Weeks Four to Six

Typically by week four, wounds are epithelialized, edema has improved, and motion has returned. If so,

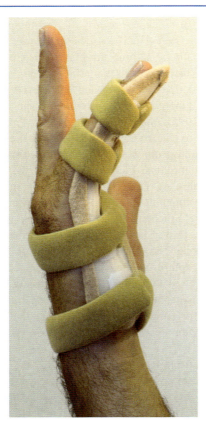

Fig. 39.3 Composite extension splinting. At 3 weeks, a nighttime volar hand-based orthotic may be used to support the hand in the position of maximum comfortable composite extension, continuing daytime intermittent individual digital extension orthotics

therapy can be discontinued or decreased to one or two times per week. Light isometric grip strengthening is begun with a 2-inch dowel. The home exercise program includes these components: intrinsic and ORL stretching, differential flexor gliding, extensor strengthening and MCP/PIP extensor gliding, and wrist extensors and rotator cuff strengthening for return to strenuous activity. Gloves with a palm gel pad are used for sports activities which require grip to increase grip diameter and to shield the palmar skin from shearing forces. Nighttime finger extension orthotics are continued for 3–6 months, with intermittent use of a daytime digital extension orthotic as needed (Rives et al. 1992; Crowley and Tonkin 1999; Misra et al. 2007). Patients benefit from brief periodic visits to the therapist to confirm long-term orthotic use and modify the home program as needed.

39.5.4 Care After Needle Fasciotomy

Patients referred following needle fasciotomy (Lermusiaux and Debeyre 1979; Lermusiaux 2000; Foucher et al. 2003; van Rijssen et al. 2006; Cheng et al. 2008) typically do not require much intervention. Needle fasciotomy patients should avoid strenuous gripping for one full week following their procedure even if they have no discomfort, specifically avoiding golf, racquet sports, fishing, hand tools, yard work, bike/motorcycle riding, carrying bags, and weight training. Needle release patients should be reminded that because the Dupuytren's cords have no sensory innervation, during the first week postrelease, they may not have any pain with grip and will not know that they have overused their hands until it is too late. Overuse risks delayed inflammatory reaction to shearing forces. After 1 week, patients may gradually increase gripping activities. Padded or gel insert padded gloves are recommended for gripping/carrying activities such as racket sports, golf, or gardening. Forceful extension stretching of the hands may provoke the Dupuytren's biology, and these patients should permanently modify their personal pushup and yoga positions by using pushup handles to avoid the forceful extension stress of these activities. Patients with residual contractures after fasciotomy may progressively improve over 4–6 months, particularly if preprocedure composite contractures were over 90°. Residual contractures may gradually improve in response to nighttime splinting with a custom silicone elastomer orthosis (Meinel 2012b). Most of these patients expect to see the therapist for only one or two visits and plan to return to normal activities 1 week postprocedure.

39.5.5 Care After Enzymatic Fasciotomy

The protocol recommended by Auxilium following enzymatic fasciotomy with Xiaflex™ (Hurst et al. 2009) is as follows (Auxilium et al. 2010). Immediately after injection, the hand is wrapped in a soft bulky gauze dressing. The patient is instructed to limit motion and to keep the hand elevated until bedtime. The patient is instructed not to attempt to disrupt the injected cord by self-manipulation. The day after injection, the patient is seen again by the doctor and a manipulation is performed as indicated. Active finger

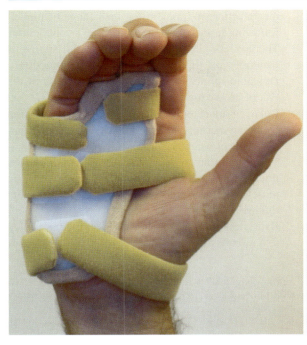 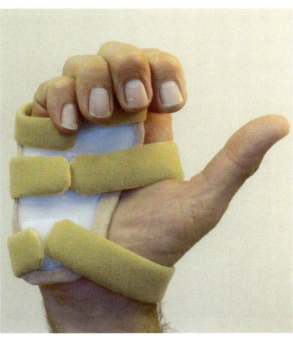

Fig. 39.4 Trigger/intrinsic stretch splint. A volar hand-based splint supporting the metacarpophalangeal joints in neutral extension and allowing interphalangeal joint flexion may be helpful both for trigger-type flexor tendinitis and to allow intrinsic muscle mobilization through active flexion exercises

flexion and extension exercises are recommended several times a day for several months. The patient is fitted with a splint to wear at night for 4 months. The type of splint is not specified by the drug manufacturer, but it would seem reasonable to follow the splint designs outlined previously for the "no-tension" protocol. Beyond this, recommendations outlined above for needle fasciotomy patients should apply. In general, enzymatic fasciotomy produces more initial swelling and bruising than needle release, and may be accompanied by an upper extremity rash, bruising, and tender axillary lymphadenopathy. These effects can be expected to resolve after 1 or 2 weeks. Skin tears are not uncommon and may be monitored until healed.

39.5.6 Intervention for Complication

39.5.6.1 Inflammation and Flare
The therapist should intervene quickly for complications related to worsening inflammation, swelling, suspected infection, or sympathetic flare by referring them back to the surgeon for reassessment and treatment as indicated (Gilron et al. 2006; Koman 2009). Therapy protocols should be tuned to address the specific problem. Sympathetic flare may be due to new or unmasked carpal tunnel syndrome (Figus et al. 2007) and may require carpal tunnel release (Gonzalez and Watson 1991). Diagnosed correctly and treated promptly with steroid injections or surgery, patients with postoperative carpal tunnel syndrome or trigger finger usually resume good progress. Simple postoperative inflammation may respond to changes in exercise patterns, orthotic positions, high-voltage galvanic stimulation, and cold applications. Edema may be treated with Isotoner™ gloves, Coban™ wraps, fluid flushing exercises, and elevation (Villeco 2009). Painful or hypertrophic scars may respond to ultrasound, corticosteroid iontophoresis, paper taping, molded silicone elastomer, desensitization, and massage.

39.5.6.2 Flexor Tendinitis, Intrinsic Tightness, and Joint Stiffness
If steroid injection is not an option, triggering digits may improve by altering forces at the A1 pulley (Evans et al. 1988) with a hand-based MCP extension orthotic (Fig. 39.4) during the day and by limiting repetitive gripping. PIP flexion contractures may respond to serial casting (Fig. 39.5)

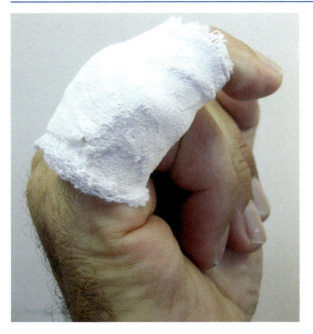

Fig. 39.5 Proximal interphalangeal joint serial casting. Serial casting with plaster to improve proximal interphalangeal joint extension leaves the distal joint free to flex, allowing differential gliding of the profundus and stretching of the oblique retinacular ligament

(Bell-Krotoski 2009) or intermittent use of a palmar digital orthotic held with 1 tape directly over the PIP joint (Fig. 39.2). Poor composite flexion is most often related to intrinsic muscle tightness. If PIP joint flexion or intrinsic tightness is an issue, a volar wrist control with MCPs at 0° can be used for hook grip.

39.5.7 Home Program

A home exercise program is critical to maintaining motion gained in surgery and therapy. Without supervision and reinforcement, most patients will unknowingly drift away from the recommended program, changing their exercise position, repetition, or force once they are discharged from formal therapy. Written exercise programs, discussion in therapy, and quick rechecks after discharge help to ensure compliance with home programs.

39.6 Summary Points

- Ideal management includes preoperative therapy evaluation and early postoperative therapy.
- The "no-tension" protocol reduces risk of inflammatory reaction and maximizes final range of motion following fasciectomy for Dupuytren's contracture.
- Therapy for Dupuytren's must avoid strenuous manipulation, tight orthotics, and wound traction.
- Dynamic splints should be avoided because of the risk of provoking edema and inflammation.
- Delaying suture removal longer than 2 weeks followed by taping incisions for stress shielding reduces complications of wound healing and hypertrophic scars.
- Three common sources of stiffness should be routinely addressed: flexor tendon excursion, intrinsic muscle tightness, and oblique retinacular ligament tightness.
- Extension splinting during sleep is recommended 4–6 months after surgery.

Acknowledgments The authors thank Roslyn Evans, CHT, OTR/L, who was the inspiration and provided the backbone for this chapter.

References

Abbott K, Denney J, Burke FD, McGrouther DA (1987) A review of attitudes to splintage in Dupuytren's contracture. J Hand Surg Br 12(3):326–328

Abe Y, Rokkaku T, Ofuchi S, Tokunaga S, Takahashi K, Moriya H (2004) An objective method to evaluate the risk of recurrence and extension of Dupuytren's disease. J Hand Surg Br 29(5):427–430

Auxilium, Highlights of prescribing information, XIAFLEX™ https://www.xiaflex.com/docs/pi_medguide_combo.pdf. Accessed 13 Sep 2010

Au-Yong IT, Wildin CJ, Dias JJ, Page RE (2005) A review of common practice in Dupuytren's surgery. Tech Hand Up Extrem Surg 9(4):178–187

Azar C, Fleegler E, Culver J (1983) Dynamic anatomy of the flexor pulley system of the fingers and thumb. Second International Meeting for International Federation of Societies for Surgery of the Hand. Boston paper #5.

Bailey AJ, Tarlton JF, Van der Stappen J, Sims TJ, Messina A (1994) The continuous elongation technique for severe Dupuytren's disease. A biochemical mechanism. J Hand Surg Br 19(4):522–527

Bell-Krotoski J (2009) Serial plaster splinting and casting. In: Skirven TM, Fedorczyk J, Osterman AL, Amadio P (eds) Rehabilitation of the hand and upper extremity, 6th edn. Elsevier, New York, chapter 126

Brand PW, National Research Council (U.S.). Committee on Prosthetics Research and Development (1972) Results of work at Public Health Service Hospital, Carville, Louisiana. In: The effect of pressure on soft tissues. National Academy of Sciences, Washington D.C, pp 29–31

Brand PW, Hollister AM, Thompson DE, Brand PW, Hollister AM (1999) Mechanical resistance. In: Clinical mechanics of the hand, 3rd edn. Mosby, St. Louis, pp 184–214

Bulstrode NW, Jemec B, Smith PJ (2005) The complications of Dupuytren's contracture surgery. J Hand Surg Am 30(5):1021–1025

Burke DT, Burke MM, Stewart GW, Cambré A (1994) Splinting for carpal tunnel syndrome: in search of the optimal angle. Arch Phys Med Rehabil 75(11):1241–1244

Cheng HS, Hung LK, Tse WL, Ho PC (2008) Needle aponeurotomy for Dupuytren's contracture. J Orthop Surg (Hong Kong) 16(1):88–90

Chvapil M, Koopmann CF Jr (1984) Scar formation: physiology and pathological states. Otolaryngol Clin North Am 17(2):265–272

Citron ND, Hearnden A (2003) Skin tension in the aetiology of Dupuytren's disease; a prospective trial. J Hand Surg Br 28:528–530

Clare T, Hazari A, Belcher H (2004) Post-operative splinting to maintain full extension of the PIPJ after fasciectomy. Br J Plast Surg 57(2):179–180

Cobb TK, An KN, Cooney WP, Berger RA (1994) Lumbrical muscle incursion into the carpal tunnel during finger flexion. J Hand Surg Br 19(4):434–438

Cobb TK, An KN, Cooney WP (1995) Effect of lumbrical muscle incursion within the carpal tunnel on carpal tunnel pressure: a cadaveric study. J Hand Surg Am 20(2):186–192

Crowley B, Tonkin MA (1999) The proximal interphalangeal joint in Dupuytren's disease. Hand Clin 15:137–147

Curtis AS, Seehar GM (1978) The control of cell division by tension or diffusion. Nature 274(5666):52–53

Degreef I, De Smet L (2011) Risk factors in Dupuytren's diathesis: is recurrence after surgery predictable? Acta Orthop Belg 7:27–32

Ebskov LB, Boeckstyns ME, Sørensen AI, Søe-Nielsen N (2000) Results after surgery for severe Dupuytren's contracture: does a dynamic extension splint influence outcome? Scand J Plast Reconstr Surg Hand Surg 34(2):155–160

Evans RB (2009) Therapists management of carpal tunnel syndrome. In: Skirven TM, Osterman AL, Fedorczyk J, Amadio P (eds) Rehabilitation of the hand and upper extremity, 6th edn. Elsevier, New York, chapter 49

Evans RB, Hunter JM, Burkhalter WE (1988) Conservative management of the trigger finger; a new approach. J Hand Ther 1:59–68

Evans RB, Dell PC, Fiolkowski P (2002) A clinical report of the effect of mechanical stress on functional results after fasciectomy for Dupuytren's contracture. J Hand Ther 15:331–339

Figus A, Iwuagwu FC, Elliot D (2007) Subacute nerve compression after trauma and surgery of the hand. Plast Reconstr Surg 120:705–712

Foucher G, Medina J, Navarro R (2003) Percutaneous needle aponeurotomy: complications and results. J Hand Surg Br 28(5):427–431

Gabbiani G, Majno G (1972) Dupuytren's contracture: fibroblast contraction? An ultrastructural study. Am J Pathol 66(1):131–146

Gelberman R, Garfin S, Hergenroeder P, Mubarak S, Menon J (1981) Compartment syndrome of the forearm: diagnosis and treatment. Clin Orthop 161:252–261

Gilron I, Watson CP, Cahill CM, Moulin DE (2006) Neuropathic pain: a practical guide for the clinician. CMAJ 1(175):265–275

Gonzalez F, Watson HK (1991) Simultaneous carpal tunnel release and Dupuytren's fasciectomy. J Hand Surg Br 16(2):175–178

Grinnell F (1994) Fibroblasts, myofibroblasts, and wound contraction. J Cell Biol 124:401–404

Halliday NL, Tomasek JJ (1995) Mechanical properties of the extracellular matrix influence fibronectin fibril assembly in vitro. Exp Cell Res 217(1):109–117

Herweijer H, Dijkstra PU, Nicolai JP, Van der Sluis CK (2007) Postoperative hand therapy in Dupuytren's disease. Disabil Rehabil. 29(22):1736-41

Hinz B, Gabbiani G (2012) The role of the myofibroblast in Dupuytren's disease: fundamental aspects of contraction and therapeutic perspectives. In: Dupuytren's disease and related hyperproliferative disorders, pp 53–60

Hodgkinson PD (1994) The use of skeletal traction to correct the flexed PIP joint in Dupuytren's disease. A pilot study to assess the use of the Pipster. J Hand Surg Br 19(4):534–537

Howard JC, Varallo VM, Ross DC, Roth JH, Faber KJ, Alman B, Gan BS (2003) Elevated levels of beta-catenin and fibronectin in three-dimensional collagen cultures of Dupuytren's disease cells are regulated by tension in vitro. BMC Musculoskelet Disord 16(4):16

Hunt TK, Knighton DR, Thakral KK, Goodson WH 3rd, Andrews WS (1984) Studies on inflammation and wound healing: angiogenesis and collagen synthesis stimulated in vivo by resident and activated wound macrophages. Surgery 96(1):48–54

Hunt TK, Banda MJ, Silver IA (1985) Cell interactions in post-traumatic fibrosis. CIBA Found Symp 114(1):127–149

Hurst LC, Badalamente MA, Hentz VR, Hotchkiss RN, Kaplan FT, Meals RA, Smith TM, Rodzvilla J, CORD I Study Group (2009) Injectable collagenase clostridium histolyticum for Dupuytren's contracture. N Engl J Med 361(10):968–979

Iqbal SA, Hindocha S, Farhatullah S, Paus R, Bayat A (2012) Dupuytren's disease shows populations of hematopoietic and mesenchymal stem-like cells involving perinodular fat and skin in addition to diseased fascia: implications for pathogenesis and therapy. In: Dupuytren's disease and related hyperproliferative disorders, pp 167–174

Jain AS, Mitchell C, Carus DA (1988) A simple inexpensive postoperative management regime following surgery for Dupuytren's contracture. J Hand Surg Br 13(3):259–261

Jerosch-Herold C, Shepstone L, Chojnowski AJ, Larson D (2008) Splinting after contracture release for Dupuytren's contracture (SCoRD): protocol of a pragmatic, multi-centre, randomized controlled trial. BMC Musculoskelet Disord 30(9):62

Ketchum L (2012) Expanded dermofasciectomies and full-thickness grafts in the treatment of Dupuytren's contracture: a 36-year experience. In: Dupuytren's disease and related hyperproliferative disorders, pp 213–220

Kischer CW, Speer DP (1984) Microvascular changes in Dupuytren's contracture. J Hand Surg Am 9:58–62

Knighton DR, Silver IA, Hunt TK (1981) Regulation of wound-healing angiogenesis-effect of oxygen gradients and inspired oxygen concentration. Surgery 90(2):262–270

Koman AL (2009) Complex Regional Pain Syndrome. In: Skirven TM, Osterman AL, Fedorczyk J, Amadio P (eds) Rehabilitation of the hand and upper extremity, 6th edn. Elsevier, New York, chapter 116

Larson D, Jerosch-Herold C (2008) Clinical effectiveness of postoperative splinting after surgical release of Dupuytren's contracture: a systematic review. BMC Musculoskelet Disord 9:104

LaVan FB, Hunt TK (1990) Oxygen and wound healing. Clin Plast Surg 17(3):463–472

Legge JW, McFarlane RM (1980) Prediction of results of treatment of Dupuytren's disease. J Hand Surg Am 5(6):608–616

Lermusiaux JL (2000) Le traitement médical de la maladie de Dupuytren. Rhumatologi0065 52(4):15–17

Lermusiaux JL, Debeyre N (1979) Le traitement médical de la maladie de Dupuytren. In: De Sèze S, Ryckewaert A, Kahn MF et al (eds) L'actualité rhumatologique. Expansion Scientifique, Paris, pp 338–343

Lubahn JD (1999) Open-palm technique and soft-tissue coverage in Dupuytren's disease. Hand Clin 15(1):127–136

Mackin EJ (1986) Prevention of complications in hand therapy. Hand Clin 2(2):429–447

Madden JW, Carlson EC, Hines J (1975) Presence of modified fibroblasts in ischemic contracture of the intrinsic musculature of the hand. Surg Gynecol Obstet 140(4):509–516

McFarlane R (1997) Dupuytren's disease. J Hand Ther 10(1):8–13

Meinel A (2012a) Palmar fibromatosis or the loss of flexibility of the palmar finger tissue. A new insight into the disease process of Dupuytren's contracture. In: Dupuytren's disease and related hyperproliferative disorders, pp 11–20

Meinel A (2012b) The role of static night splinting after contracture release for Dupuytren's disease. A preliminary recommendation based on clinical cases. In: Dupuytren's disease and related hyperproliferative disorders, pp 333–339

Millesi H (2012) Basic thoughts on Dupuytren's contracture. In: Dupuytren's disease and related hyperproliferative disorders, pp 21–26

Misra A, Jain A, Ghazanfar R, Johnston T, Nanchahal J (2007) Predicting the outcome of surgery for the proximal interphalangeal joint in Dupuytren's disease. J Hand Surg Am 32(2):240–245

Mubarak SJ, Hargens AR (1982) Exertional compartment syndromes. In: Mack RP (ed) Symposium on the foot and leg in running sports. American Academy of Orthopaedic Surgeons, Missouri, pp 141–159

Mullins PA (1999) Postsurgical rehabilitation of Dupuytren's disease. Hand Clin 15(1):167–174

Murrell GA (1991) The role of the fibroblast in Dupuytren's contracture. Hand Clin 7(4):669–680

Murrell GA (1992) An insight into Dupuytren's contracture. Ann R Coll Surg Engl 74(3):156–160, discussion 61

Niessen FB, Spauwen PH, Robinson PH, Fidler V, Kon M (1998) The use of silicone occlusive sheeting (Sil-K) and silicone occlusive gel (Epiderm) in the prevention of hypertrophic scar formation. Plast Reconstr Surg 102(6):1962–1972

Phan HP (2012) Mechanisms of myofibroblast differentiation. In: Dupuytren's disease and related hyperproliferative disorders, pp 61–67

Prosser R, Conolly WB (1996) Complications following surgical treatment for Dupuytren's contracture. J Hand Ther 9(4):344–348

Reiffel RS (1995) Prevention of hypertrophic scars by long-term paper tape application. Plast Reconstr Surg 96(7):1715–1718

Reswick JB, Rogers JE (1976) Experience at Rancho Los Amigos Hospital with devices and techniques to prevent pressure sores. In: Kenedi RM, Cowden JM, Scales JT (eds) Bedsore biomechanics, strathclyde bioengineering seminars. Macmillan Press, London, pp 301–310

Rives K, Gelberman R, Smith B, Carney K (1992) Severe contractures of the proximal interphalangeal joint in Dupuytren's disease: results of a prospective trial of operative correction and dynamic extension splinting. J Hand Surg Am 17(6):1153–1159

Rudolph R, Berg JVD, Ehrlich P (1992) Wound contraction and scar contracture. In: Cohen I, Diegelmann R, Linblad W (eds) Wound healing: biochemical and clinical aspects. WB Saunders, Philadelphia, pp 1296–1314

Sampson SP, Badalamente MA, Hurst LC, Dowd A, Sewell CS, Lehmann-Torres J, Ferraro M, Semon B (1992) The use of a passive motion machine in the postoperative rehabilitation of Dupuytren's disease. J Hand Surg Am 17(2):333–338

Seradge H, Jia YC, Owens W (1995) In vivo measurement of carpal tunnel pressure in the functioning hand. J Hand Surg Am 20A(5):855–859

Sheth VM, Weitzul S (2008) Postoperative topical antimicrobial use. Dermatitis 19(4):181–189

Siegel DB, Kuzma G, Eakins D (1995) Anatomic investigation of the role of the lumbrical muscles in carpal tunnel syndrome. J Hand Surg Am 20(5):860–863

Smith SP, Devaraj VS, Bunker TD (2001) The association between frozen shoulder and Dupuytren's disease. J Shoulder Elbow Surg 10(2):149–151

van Rijssen AL, Gerbrandy FS, Ter Linden H, Klip H, Werker PM (2006) A comparison of the direct outcomes of percutaneous needle fasciotomy and limited fasciectomy for Dupuytren's disease: a 6-week follow-up study. J Hand Surg Am 31(5):717–725

Vi L, Wu Y, Gan BS, O'Gorman DB (2012) Primary Dupuytren's disease cell interactions with the extra-cellular environment: A link to disease progression? In: Dupuytren's disease and related hyperproliferative disorders, pp 151–159

Villeco J (2009) Edema management. In: Skirven TM, Osterman AL, Fedorczyk J, Amadio P (eds) Rehabilitation of the hand and upper extremity, 6th edn. Elsevier, New York, chapter 63

Ward CM (1976) Oedema of the hand after fasciectomy with or without tourniquet. Hand 8(2):179–185

Wehbé MA, Hunter JM (1985) Flexor tendon gliding in the hand. part II. differential gliding. J Hand Surg Am 10:575–579

Weinzweig N, Culver JE, Fleegler EJ (1996) Severe contractures of the proximal interphalangeal joint in Dupuytren's disease: combined fasciectomy with capsuloligamentous release versus fasciectomy alone. Plast Reconstr Surg 97(3):560–566

Zidel P (2012) Dupuytren's contracture versus burn scar contracture. In: Dupuytren's disease and related hyperproliferative disorders, pp 77–83

Severity of Contracture and Self-Reported Disability in Patients with Dupuytren's Contracture Referred for Surgery

40

Christina Jerosch-Herold, Lee Shepstone,
Adrian J. Chojnowski, and Debbie Larson

Contents

40.1	**Introduction**	317
40.2	**Patients and Methods**	318
40.3	**Results**	319
40.4	**Discussion**	320
References		321

40.1 Introduction

Dupuytren's disease (DD) is a fibroproliferative disorder resulting in the formation of nodules and cords in the palmar fascia of hand. These nodules and cords are contractile and often result in one or more fingers becoming flexed into the palm with associated psychosocial and functional deficits for the patient (Pratt and Byrne 2009). It is a common disease with a recent review of prevalence rates reporting a mean of 7% and 14% for women and men respectively at age 45–54 increasing to 23% and 34% over the age of 75 (Hindocha et al. 2009). The standard intervention for DD is surgical excision of the diseased tissue to release the contracted finger (Hurst and Badalamente 1999); however, there is debate regarding whether tissue excision should be minimal to ensure a quick recovery (van Rijssen and Werker 2006) or radical to reduce the risk of recurrence (Hall et al. 1997). The high prevalence of DD together with the impact of surgical treatment on the patient and society warrants a greater understanding of the functional consequences of DD.

The increasing trend in using patient-rated outcome measures is reflected in recently published studies investigating DD. They have included patient-rated activity and participation questionnaires with the Disabilities of the Arm, Shoulder and Hand (DASH) outcome measure (Hudak et al. 1996) being most commonly used (Herweijer et al. 2007; Engstrand et al. 2009; Degreef et al. 2009; Glassey 2001; Skoff 2004; van Rijssen et al. 2006;

C. Jerosch-Herold (✉) • L. Shepstone
Faculty of Health, School of Allied Health Professions,
Institute for Health and Social Science Research, University
of East Anglia,Norwich, UK
e-mail: c.jerosch-herold@uea.ac.uk

A.J. Chojnowski • D. Larson
Department of Orthopaedics, Norfolk and Norwich University
Hospitals NHS Foundation Trust,
Norwich, UK

Reprinted with permission by Elsevier, originally published in the *Journal of Hand Therapy*, Volume 24, Issue 1, pages 6–11 (January 2011).

C. Eaton et al. (eds.), *Dupuytren's Disease and Related Hyperproliferative Disorders*,
DOI 10.1007/978-3-642-22697-7_40, © Springer-Verlag Berlin Heidelberg 2012

Zyluk and Jagielski 2007). The DASH is a region-specific functional outcome measure that has been extensively investigated for validity and reliability with patients with upper limb conditions (Beaton et al. 2001) and has demonstrated acceptable responsiveness with a wide range of hand conditions including patients undergoing Dupuytren's surgery (Gummesson et al. 2003). In an attempt to understand the relationship between DD and function, several studies have examined the correlation between DASH score and either total active range of motion (TAM) or flexion contracture of the affected digits (Zyluk and Jagielski 2007; Herweijer et al. 2007; Engstrand et al. 2009; Degreef et al. 2009).

Herweijer et al. (2007) studied post-operative hand therapy referral patterns in 46 patients with DD. Outcome measures included range of motion and DASH collected pre-operatively and after surgery. Over half of the patients were being operated for recurrent disease and had a mean age of 62 years. They report outcome as total active motion (TAM), calculated as the sum of active metacarpophalangeal (MCP), proximal interphalangeal (PIP) and distal interphalangeal (DIP) joint flexion minus lack of active extension in the same joints. Mean pre-operative TAM was $184°$ ($SD = 49$), and the mean pre-operative DASH score was 12.1 ($SD = 12.9$), indicating a low level of disability.

Three further studies have examined the relationship between range of motion and DASH pre-operatively. Engstrand et al. (2009) assessed 60 patients undergoing surgery. The mean DASH score was 17 points (range 7–28). The degree of flexion contracture was measured by adding MCP, PIP and DIP extension. Sixty patients (81 digits) were included with a mean flexion contracture of $105°$ ($SD = 37$). They reported no significant correlation between DASH and flexion contracture. Degreef et al. (2009) assessed 80 patients before surgery (mean age 60 years). The mean DASH score was 15 points, and mean flexion contracture in the MCP joint was $53°$ and in the PIP joint $60°$. The authors do not report the actual correlation coefficient but state that no significant correlation was found between DASH and flexion contracture.

Zyluk and Jagielski (2007) assessed 74 patients undergoing fasciectomy. Median flexion contracture pre-operatively was $80°$ (range 0–370), and median DASH score was 54 points (range 30–103). They found a weak correlation between total active extension (TAE) and DASH score which was not statistically significant (Spearman correlation $r = 0.26$, $p > 0.05$).

In this chapter, we describe the level of impairment and patient-rated disability in a large cohort of patients undergoing surgery who were enrolled in a multi-centre randomised controlled trial. The aim was to examine the relationship between contracture severity of individual digits as well as the whole hand and self-reported disability.

40.2 Patients and Methods

The pre-operative data in this cohort of 154 patients undergoing surgical release of Dupuytren's contracture were collected as part of a multi-centre, pragmatic, randomised controlled trial of post-operative night splinting (Jerosch-Herold et al. 2008). The trial received multi-centre Ethics Committee approval and Research Governance approval at each of the five participating sites. A total of 16 surgeons at 5 centres in East Anglia were involved in identifying eligible patients. Patients who presented to an operating surgeon with a Dupuytren's contracture affecting one or more digits of the hand and requiring fasciectomy or dermofasciectomy were informed about the study and the trial coordinator notified of their name and address. Two hundred eighteen patients were referred as eligible and invited by mail to take part in the trial. One hundred seventy-two (79%) patients returned written informed consent forms. Eighteen patients were excluded from the trial prior to randomisation for a variety of reasons, including death (1), delayed or cancelled surgery (8), unable to contact (1), already had surgery (6) and not referred to hand therapy/not randomised (1), and one patient withdrew.

A total of 154 patients were thus enrolled into the trial, had surgery and were subsequently randomised. The baseline data for 154 patients are presented here. Assessments of range of motion were taken by two research associates who visited patients in their own homes. This included active range of individual finger joint flexion and extension assessed with a Rolyan (Homecraft, Sutton-in-Ashfield, UK) finger goniometer and following a standardised protocol. Both researchers were not qualified hand therapists but received extensive training in the use of goniometry by a qualified occupational therapist prior to the study including undertaking comparative assessments. For the purpose of this study, flexion contracture (FC) was defined as the summed active extension deficit of DIP, PIP and MCP joints. Total active motion (TAM) was defined as the sum of MCP, PIP and DIP flexion minus

Table 40.1 Demographic characteristics of sample (based on $n = 154$ unless otherwise stated)

Number of patients	154
Mean age (SD/range) in years	67.4 (9.6/36–89)
Ratio of male to female	120 (78%):34 (22%)
Ratio of patients working or seeking work to retired	53 (34.4%):101 (65.6%)
Number of patients being operated on dominant hand	84 (55%)
Number of patients right-handed	133 (86.4%)
Number of patients who had previous surgery for DC	23 (15%)
Operated digit	
Index	7 (4.5%)
Middle	24 (15.6%)
Ring	61 (39.6%)
Small	106 (68.8%)
Ratio of single to multiple fingers (two or more) operated ($n = 153$)[a]	116 (76%):37 (34%)
Mean DASH score (SD/range)	15.87 (14.2/0–62.1)

[a]Missing data for one patient who withdrew

Table 40.2 Mean and standard deviation of flexion contracture (FC), total active flexion (TAF) and total active motion (TAM) by digit measured with goniometry

	FC	PIP joint contracture	MCP joint contracture	TAF	TAM
Index ($n = 154$)	35.5 (20.9)	11.3 (13.9)	21.6 (14.6)	219.5 (20.4)	184 (29.2)
Middle ($n = 153$)[a]	39.1 (22.8)	10.2 (13.8)	27.4 (16.6)	234 (20.3)	194.9 (31.2)
Ring ($n = 153$)[a]	51 (37.2)	17.6 (23.6)	30.4 (19.0)	224.2 (22)	173.3 (42.5)
Small ($n = 152$)[a]	77.8 (43.5)	37.4 (29.5)	32.1 (27.8)	222.2 (20.7)	144.4 (49.4)

FC DIP, PIP and MCP extension loss (full extension = 0), *TAF* DIP, PIP and MCP flexion added, *TAM* TAF minus TAE
[a]Missing values due to one patient with a pre-existing traumatic amputation proximal to the DIP joint of his long and ring fingers and two patients with an amputation of the small finger

extension deficit. Patients were instructed to straighten out each joint as far as they could and the goniometer placed dorsally before reading the degrees of motion to the nearest 2°. Any hyperextension values were set to zero. Patients were sent the Disabilities of the Arm, Shoulder and Hand (DASH) questionnaire by mail to be completed prior to the researchers' visit. The DASH is a standardised, patient-rated, region-specific measure of symptoms and disability (scores 0–100 with higher score indicating greater disability).

Data were entered into an Access database. Statistical analysis was carried out using SAS (SAS v9.1, SAS Institute Inc, Cary, NC, USA). The relationship between the DASH score and range of motion was quantified using Pearson's correlation coefficient and a test of zero correlation carried out.

40.3 Results

Demographic and baseline outcome variables for the cohort are presented in Tables 40.1 and 40.2. The most common presentation was contracture of the MCP and PIP joints of the small finger, followed by the ring finger. The mean flexion contracture for each digit was greatest in the small finger with an ulnar to radial decrease. Total active motion (TAM) was greatest in the radial digits and decreased in a radial to ulnar direction.

The correlation coefficients between self-reported disability (DASH score) and active range of motion measured by goniometry are presented for each digit and the whole hand in Table 40.3. There was a weak, statistically significant correlation between flexion contracture for the whole hand (adding all digits together irrespective of how many or which are affected) and DASH score ($r = 0.264, p < 0.001$). When examining the correlation between flexion contracture and DASH at the single digit level, the strength remained similarly weak in index, middle and ring fingers but became almost absent in the small finger ($r = 0.07, p = 0.41$).

When examining the correlation between DASH score and TAM (a higher TAM indicates greater mobility), a statistically significant weak negative correlation ($r = -0.370, p < 0.0001$) was found for the whole hand. At single digit level, the strength of the correlation decreased from a radial to ulnar direction.

Table 40.3 Pearson correlation coefficients (p-value) between flexion contracture (FC), total active flexion (TAF), total active motion (TAM) and DASH score

	DASH with FC	DASH with TAF	DASH with TAM
Index	0.26 ($p=0.013$)	−0.27 ($p<0.001$)	−0.373 ($p<0.0001$)
Middle	0.28 ($p<0.001$)	−0.14 ($p=0.093$)	−0.291 ($p<0.001$)
Ring	0.21 ($p=0.010$)	−0.24 ($p=0.003$)	−0.308 ($p<0.0001$)
Small	0.07 ($p=0.410$)	−0.24 ($p=0.003$)	−0.161 ($p=0.048$)
Hand (all four digits)	0.264 ($p=0.001$)	−0.26 ($p=0.001$)	−0.370 ($p<0.0001$)

40.4 Discussion

Dupuytren's disease often progresses to a stage where one or more digits in both hands are affected by severe contractures which in turn interfere with everyday activities and result in functional disability (Bayat and McGrouther 2006). Whilst patients with the disease may adapt to these functional limitations initially, eventually, patients seek medical advice with surgery being the only effective intervention for restoring function (Sinha et al. 2002).

In this cohort of patients referred for surgery, the typical presentation was a male patient, aged 60 or over with a contracture of the MCP and PIP of the small and ring fingers. Mean flexion contracture at the PIP joint of the ring and small fingers were 17.6° and 37.4°, respectively, and the mean DASH score was 15 points, indicating low disability. However, the range in the pre-operative demographic and outcome variables also highlights that whilst some patients sought surgical treatment with much milder contracture and self-reported disability, others waited until contractures and functional deficits were severe. The decision to proceed to surgery is often made on a case by case basis (Bayat and McGrouther 2006), and an individual patient's decision to have surgery depends on many factors, such as the appearance of the hand or social embarrassment (shaking hands) and which are not be captured by current outcome measures.

If increasing functional disability is an important factor in patients seeking a surgical opinion, it seems reasonable also to hypothesise that there would be moderate correlation between the severity of the contracture and self-reported disability as assessed by the DASH score. Several other studies have explored this with only one study (Zyluk and Jagielski 2007) finding a weak but statistically significant correlation between pre-operative total active extension and DASH score ($r=0.26$, $p=0.01$), whilst Degreef et al. (2009) and

Engstrand et al. (2009) state that no significant correlations could be found, although the actual coefficients and p-values were not reported in their papers. It is of note that in Zyluk's study, patients also had a much higher median DASH score of 54 points compared to the other studies where mean or median values were ≤17 points including our study. Zyluk and Jagielski (2007), Engstrand et al. (2009) and Degreef et al. (2009) report that they based their correlation coefficients on the affected digits only, whereas in our study, we measured all four fingers irrespective of which was operated on or affected. When taking the summed flexion contracture for all digits, the correlation coefficient is weak and statistically significant ($r=0.264$); however, when examining the correlation at individual digit level, it is surprising that in the small finger, which was the affected digit in 69% of patients and had the worst degree of contracture, any correlation with DASH score is almost absent. One possible explanation is that the intention of the DASH is to determine how well a patient can perform functional activities regardless of how these are carried out, e.g. assistive devices or compensatory strategies are not taken into account. Therefore, the DASH score may underestimate the actual functional impact of DD. Furthermore, it is a region-specific measure and not disease-specific, and difficulties commonly reported by patients with DD like shaking hands, putting on gloves, applying face cream as well as appearance-related concerns are not included in the DASH questionnaire. A further possible explanation of the much weaker correlation between the ulnar digits and the DASH score is that many tasks in the DASH questionnaire rely on tripod grip involving thumb and first two digits only (e.g. writing, turning a key) and that only when the radial digits are affected by contractures is this also reflected in a higher DASH score.

Our study concurs with previously published studies which have shown that the relationship between digital contracture and functional disability appears to be very weak or even absent. This is perhaps not surprising given that range of motion is a measure of body structure, whereas DASH and similar patient-rated questionnaires capture the domains of activity limitation and participation restrictions according to the International Classification of Functioning, Disability and Health (ICF) (WHO 2002). We would argue therefore that measures of impairment such as severity of contracture as well as self-reported disability need to be included in the assessment of outcome of patients undergoing surgical treatment for DD. The question of whether the DASH is the most sensitive and relevant patient-rated outcome measure in this patient group remains unanswered, and further work is needed to compare it to other existing patient-rated outcome measures or to develop a new disease-specific measure.

Acknowledgements The authors are indebted to the patients who participated in the study, the surgeons who assisted in identifying eligible patients and E. Barrett and S. Vaughan for all the data collection.

Funding source: The study was funded by a project grant from Action Medical Research (UK).

References

Bayat A, McGrouther DA (2006) Management of Dupuytren's disease–clear advice for an elusive condition. Ann R Coll Surg Engl 88(1):3–8

Beaton DE, Katz JN, Fossel AH, Wright JG, Tarasuk V, Bombardier C (2001) Measuring the whole or the parts? Validity, reliability, and responsiveness of the disabilities of the arm, shoulder and hand outcome measure in different regions of the upper extremity. J Hand Ther 14(2):128–146

Degreef I, Vererfve P-B, De Smet L (2009) Effect of severity of Dupuytren contracture on disability. Scand J Plast Reconstr Surg Hand Surg 43(1):41–42

Engstrand C, Boren L, Liedberg GM (2009) Evaluation of activity limitation and digital extension in Dupuytren's contracture three months after fasciectomy and hand therapy interventions. J Hand Ther 22(1):21–27

Glassey N (2001) A study of the effect of night extension splintage on post-fasciectomy Dupuytren's patients. Brit J Hand Therapy 6(3):89–94

Gummesson C, Atroshi I, Ekdahl C (2003) The disabilities of the arm, shoulder and hand (DASH) outcome questionnaire: longitudinal construct validity and measuring self-rated health change after surgery. BMC Musculoskelet Disord 4(11):1–6

Hall PN, Fitzgerald A, Sterne GD, Logan AM (1997) Skin replacement in Dupuytren's disease. J Hand Surg Br 22(2): 193–197

Herweijer H, Dijkstra P, Jean-Philippe A, Nicolai A (2007) Postoperative hand therapy in Dupuytren's disease. Disabil Rehabil 29(22):1736–1741

Hindocha S, McGrouther D, Bayat A (2009) Epidemiological evaluation of Dupuytren's disease: incidence and prevalence rates in relation to etiology. Hand 4:256–269

Hudak P, Amadio P, Bombardier C (1996) Development of an upper extremity outcome measure: the DASH (Disabilities of the arm, shoulder, and hand). Am J Ind Med 29:602–608

Hurst L, Badalamente M (1999) Non-operative treatment of Dupuytren's disease. Hand Clin 15(5):97–107

Jerosch-Herold C, Shepstone L, Chojnowski AJ, Larson D (2008) Splinting after contracture release for Dupuytren's contracture (SCoRD): protocol of a pragmatic, multi-centre, randomized controlled trial. BMC Musculoskelet Disord 9(6):1–5

Pratt A, Byrne G (2009) The lived experience of Dupuytren's disease of the hand. J Clin Nurs 18:1793–1802

Sinha R, Cresswell TR, Mason R, Chakrabarti I (2002) Functional benefit of Dupuytren's surgery. J Hand Surg Br 27(4): 378–381

Skoff HD (2004) The surgical treatment of Dupuytren's contracture: a synthesis of techniques. Plast Reconstr Surg 113(2): 540–544

van Rijssen A, Werker P (2006) Percutaneous needle fasciotomy in Dupuytren's disease. J Hand Surg (British and European Volume) 31B:498–501

van Rijssen AL, Gerbrandy FSJ, Ter Linden H, Klip H, Werker PMN (2006) A comparison of the direct outcomes of percutaneous needle fasciotomy and limited fasciectomy for Dupuytren's disease: a 6-week follow-up study. J Hand Surg Am 31(5):717–725

WHO (2002) International classification of functioning, disability and health. World Health Organisation, Geneva

Zyluk A, Jagielski W (2007) The effect of the severity of the Dupuytren's contracture on the function of the hand before and after surgery. J Hand Surg Eur Vol 32E(3):326–329

Night-Time Splinting After Fasciectomy or Dermofasciectomy for Dupuytren's Contracture: A Pragmatic, Multi-centre, Randomised Controlled Trial

41

Christina Jerosch-Herold, Lee Shepstone, Adrian J. Chojnowski, Debbie Larson, Elisabeth Barrett, and Susan P. Vaughan

Contents

41.1	**Background**	323
41.2	**Methods**	324
41.2.1	Patients and Setting	324
41.2.2	Randomisation	324
41.2.3	Interventions	324
41.2.4	Splint Group	324
41.2.5	No Splint Group	325
41.2.6	Outcome Assessment	325
41.2.7	Statistical Approaches	325
41.2.8	Analysis Methods	326
41.3	**Results**	326
41.4	**Discussion**	328
41.5	**Conclusions**	331
41.6	**Bullet Points**	331
References		332

C. Jerosch-Herold • L. Shepstone • E. Barrett • S.P. Vaughan
Faculty of Medicine and Health Sciences,
University of East Anglia,
Norwich, UK

A.J. Chojnowski (✉)
Department of Orthopaedics and Trauma,
Norfolk and Norwich University Hospitals NHS Foundation
Trust, Norwich, UK
e-mail: adrian.chojnowski@nnuh.nhs.uk

D. Larson
Department of Occupational Therapy, Norfolk and Norwich
University Hospitals NHS Foundation Trust,
Norwich, UK

41.1 Background

Dupuytren's disease (DD) is a disabling hand condition that is thought to affect more than two million people in the UK (Townley et al. 2006). Standard surgical treatment includes division of the cords (fasciotomy) or excision (partial or total fasciectomy) (Townley et al. 2006). Long-term recurrence may be reduced by excision of cords/nodules with the overlying skin and full-thickness skin grafting (dermofasciectomy) (Armstrong et al. 2000).

Less invasive percutaneous needle fasciotomy (van Rijssen and Werker 2006) and injectable collagenase ('chemical knife') (Hurst et al. 2009) are alternative outpatient delivered procedures resulting in good short-term contracture release; however fasciotomy is also associated with a much higher recurrence rate compared to limited fasciectomy (van Rijssen et al. 2006).

Surgical excision (fasciectomy) of the diseased cords continues to be a widely used treatment option aimed at correcting the digital contractures and to improve hand function. Rehabilitation post surgery by hand therapists is recommended (Bayat and McGrouther 2006) to control scar formation, prevent secondary complications, and to restore movement and hand function. The use of thermoplastic extension splints worn at night and/or daytime is advocated by many as part of the post-operative rehabilitation (Bayat and McGrouther 2006; Evans et al. 2002). However a systematic review (Larson and Jerosch-Herold 2008) concluded that there is conflicting evidence on the effectiveness of

C. Eaton et al. (eds.), *Dupuytren's Disease and Related Hyperproliferative Disorders*,
DOI 10.1007/978-3-642-22697-7_41, © Springer-Verlag Berlin Heidelberg 2012

post-operative splinting for Dupuytren's disease with both positive and negative results reported.

The paucity of research to date is reflected by the inconsistent use of splinting in clinical practice. A survey of 573 orthopaedic consultants in the UK showed that 33% used splinting most or all of the time (Salim et al. 2006); yet another survey of 141 surgeons found that 84% advocated night splinting (Au-Yong et al. 2005).

Finally, splints may be inconvenient for patients to wear and the materials, therapists' time and skill required to fabricate these custom-made devices are an added expense to health care providers.

The aim of this study was to compare the effect of post-operative static night splinting in addition to hand therapy with hand therapy only on patient reported upper extremity symptoms and disability, composite active digital range of motion, patient satisfaction and recurrence of contracture at 1 year.

41.2 Methods

41.2.1 Patients and Setting

We conducted an open, pragmatic, multi-centre, randomised controlled trial of night-time static splinting worn for 6 months after contracture release to assess the effect on self-reported upper extremity function, active range of movement in all digits and patient satisfaction at 12 months follow-up.

Between October 2007 and January 2009 patients referred with Dupuytren's disease affecting one or more digits of either hand and requiring fasciectomy or dermofasciectomy were invited to participate. Patients had to be over 18 years of age and competent to give fully informed written consent. Patients presenting with contracture of the thumb or first web-space only were excluded.

Identifying eligible patients was conducted in 5 National Health Service (NHS) Hospital Trusts in East Anglia involving a total of 16 operating surgeons. The surgery and all post-operative interventions were delivered within these five secondary care centres. Data collection at baseline and all follow-up assessments for the trial were undertaken in the patients' own homes by two trained research associates.

The protocol was approved by the Cambridgeshire two Research Ethics Committee (REC 07/Q0108/120)

in July 2007 and the Research Governance and Ethics Committee of each participating hospital. All patients gave fully informed written consent.

41.2.2 Randomisation

Patients were randomised after surgical release at their first post-operative appointment by the treating hand therapist (within 2 weeks after surgery and following removal of sutures). Randomisation was stratified by centre (five centres) and by surgical procedure (fasciectomy or dermofasciectomy) in block lengths of four. The allocation sequence was generated and administered independently through a central telephone randomisation service at the Clinical Trials Unit, University of East Anglia. Neither the treating therapists nor the patients were blinded to treatment allocation.

41.2.3 Interventions

The intervention being studied in this trial was static splinting worn at night-time for 6 months after surgical release in addition to usual hand therapy. As this was a pragmatic trial we did not attempt to standardise surgical procedure. Surgeons were allowed to use their preferred surgical techniques tailored to the severity and extent of the contracture. Hand therapy could not be standardised as it is a complex intervention using multiple modalities to treat a wide range of post-operative problems and has to be tailored to the patient's needs. In order to collect data on the range of modalities and treatments used by hand therapists, such as oedema control, exercises or advice, hand therapists were asked to complete a treatment reporting form at each session. This was also used to record post-operative complications and reasons for treatment deviation from protocol.

41.2.4 Splint Group

Patients randomised to the splint group were provided with a custom-made thermoplastic splint fabricated by the treating hand therapist. The splint was designed to accommodate the operated rays of the hand with the metacarpophalangeal joint (MCPJ) and/or proximal interphalangeal joint (PIPJ) held in maximum extension without causing any tension to the wound. After a further 3 weeks when the wound has healed and scar tissue begins to mature, the splint could be remoulded to achieve a greater extension force designed to prevent any loss of extension from surgical scar contracting.

Patients were instructed to wear the splint at night only and were given a splint diary in which they recorded weekly how many nights out of seven they had actually worn the splint and any reasons why the splint was not worn.

41.2.5 No Splint Group

The experimental treatment involved providing usual hand therapy only. However, it was deemed unethical to withhold the application of a splint in patients who developed contractures and which did not respond to hand therapy only. Clinical staff from all five centres were consulted prior to the trial to devise criteria for 'per-protocol' deviations for patients allocated to the no-splint group in the event that they experience a rapid and substantial loss of finger extension. At the first hand therapy visit and following randomisation, active range of movement of MCPJ and PIPJ was measured by the hand therapist with a goniometer and recorded. At the second visit (normally 1 week later) this range of motion was re-measured and if the patient had a net loss of $15°$ or more at the PIPJ and/or a net loss of $20°$ or more at the MCPJ of the operated fingers, they were then given a splint and splint diary. The dates and reasons for these protocol deviations were recorded by the hand therapists and the trial coordinator was notified. Any patients allocated to the no-splint group who were given a splint for any other reasons such as surgeon request were recorded as protocol violations.

41.2.6 Outcome Assessment

The primary outcome measure was self-reported upper extremity function using the 30-item Disabilities of the Arm, Shoulder and Hand (DASH) questionnaire. The DASH is a validated measure of symptoms and physical function for patients with a wide range of musculoskeletal disorders of the upper extremity and has been extensively used in reporting the outcome of surgery for DD before (Zyluk and Jagielski 2007; Herweijer et al. 2007; Engstrand et al. 2009). The questionnaire was mailed to patients for self-completion prior to the research associates' visit at which secondary assessments were taken.

Secondary outcomes were active range of motion of the MCPJ, PIPJ, and distal interphalangeal joint (DIPJ) of operated digits and patient satisfaction. Range of motion was assessed with a Rolyan (Sammons Preston, USA) finger goniometer and following a standardised protocol (Ellis and Bruton 2002). Training was given prior to the trial and both research associates undertook comparative assessments at regular intervals. Individual joint movement of full active flexion and extension was summed for each operated finger and averaged to give a total active extension (TAE) and total active flexion (TAF). Any hyperextension of a joint was recorded but converted to zero for the analysis to prevent underestimation of extension deficit.

Primary and secondary outcomes were assessed prior to surgery, and at 3, 6 and 12 months after surgery. Patient satisfaction was assessed only at 6 and 12 months by asking the patient to rate their satisfaction with the outcome using an 11-point verbal rating scale where 0 indicates complete dissatisfaction and 10 complete satisfaction. The original protocol also indicated recurrence at 1 year as a secondary outcome; however this was abandoned due to the inherent difficulties of distinguishing a true recurrence from a residual scar contracture, the lack of agreed definition of recurrence (Dias and Braybrooke 2006) and the subjectivity in visually inspecting and palpating the hand.

41.2.7 Statistical Approaches

41.2.7.1 Sample Size

Using the DASH as the primary outcome measure, where a difference of 15 points is considered to be a minimal important change (MIC) (Beaton et al. 2001) and using a between-group standard deviation of 22 points (Gummesson et al. 2003) a total of 51 patients would be needed in each group for a power of 90%. Allowing for a 20% loss to follow-up a total of 128 randomised patients was aimed for.

41.2.8 Analysis Methods

Baseline demographic and clinical characteristics were compared between groups using descriptive statistics to assess any potential disparities between groups.

The primary outcome, the DASH score, was found to be very right-skewed and therefore a logarithmic transformation was applied to produce a more symmetric distribution, assumed to be Normal. A general linear model was used to formally analyse the between-group mean difference adjusting for the baseline DASH score, recruiting hospital and type of surgery (the latter two variables were used to stratify randomisation).

Range of motion that is total active flexion (TAF) and total active extension (TAE), both appeared to follow a Normal distribution. These were also analysed using a general linear model with adjustment for baseline TAF or TAE values, recruiting hospital and type of surgery. Similarly, at 6 and 12 months, the patient satisfaction score was analysed using a general linear model with adjustment for recruiting hospital and type of surgery.

A Poisson model was used to analyse number of therapy sessions with adjustment for recruiting hospital and surgery type. Similarly, a Logistic regression model was used to analyse the use of a dynamic splint again with adjustment for recruiting hospital and surgery type.

As appropriate to pragmatic trials an intention-to-treat approach was used as the primary analysis strategy in which all patients were analysed according to their initial group allocation. However, no data imputation was used for missing follow-up data as these were very few.

A secondary per-protocol analysis was conducted comprising those individuals that adhered to the treatment protocol. In the splint group, adherence was defined *a priori* as wearing the splint for at least 50% of nights in the first 3 months after surgery. In the no-splint group the per-protocol analysis included those individuals who did not use a splint or were managed as 'per protocol' and given a splint once their extension loss exceeded the criterion agreed by the trial management group.

For the intention-to-treat analysis the statistician (LS) was subgroup blind.

The trial was registered as an International Standard Randomised Controlled Trial, number ISRCTN57079 614 on http://www.controlled-trials.com. The trial was funded by Action Medical Research Charity, UK.

41.3 Results

Between October 2007 and January 2009, 218 patients were referred as eligible and invited to participate. Forty six patients declined, one patient withdrew and one patient died. A further 16 patients were excluded because either their surgery had been cancelled or postponed ($n = 8$), they were mistakenly referred after surgery ($n = 6$), 1 patient could not be contacted and 1 patient was not referred to hand therapy.

A total of 154 patients were thus enrolled into the trial from December 2007 to January 2009 and randomly allocated to either trial arm (see Fig. 41.1). Follow-up continued until January 2010 and six patients were lost to follow-up (4%). Of the 77 patients allocated to receive a splint, 1 patient refused the splint and was also lost to follow-up. In the no-splint group, 69 of the 77 patients received the allocated intervention of hand therapy only. There were eight protocol violations in the no-splint group: One patient was given a splint by mistake prior to randomisation and seven patients were given a splint immediately at their first hand therapy appointment either due to surgeon request or because the patient already presented with a loss of extension. Thirteen patients allocated to the no-splint group (17%) went on to develop a contracture of the PIPJ which exceeded the agreed threshold and were subsequently given a splint as per protocol.

The baseline demographic and clinical characteristics for the two groups are given in Table 41.1. Both groups were similar with regard to clinical characteristics except for the proportion of patients who had one or more digits operated with a slightly larger proportion of multiple digit involvement in the no-splint group. A fasciectomy was the most common procedure with only 16 patients receiving a dermofasciectomy.

Table 41.2 presents the results of the ITT analysis for primary and secondary outcomes at 3, 6 and 12 month by treatment group and the adjusted mean difference with 95% confidence interval. There were no statistically significant differences at 12 months between the two groups in DASH score (0.66, -2.79 to 4.11, $p = 0.703$), degrees of total active flexion of operated digits (-2.02, -7.89 to 3.85, $p = 0.493$), degrees of total active extension deficit of operated digits (5.11, 2.33 to -12.55, $p = 0.172$). Both groups were satisfied with the outcome at 12 months (mean 8.5 splint group and 8.9, no-splint group) and did not differ significantly (-0.35, -1.04 to 0.34, $p = 0.315$). Similarly, no significant differences were found at 3 or 6 months.

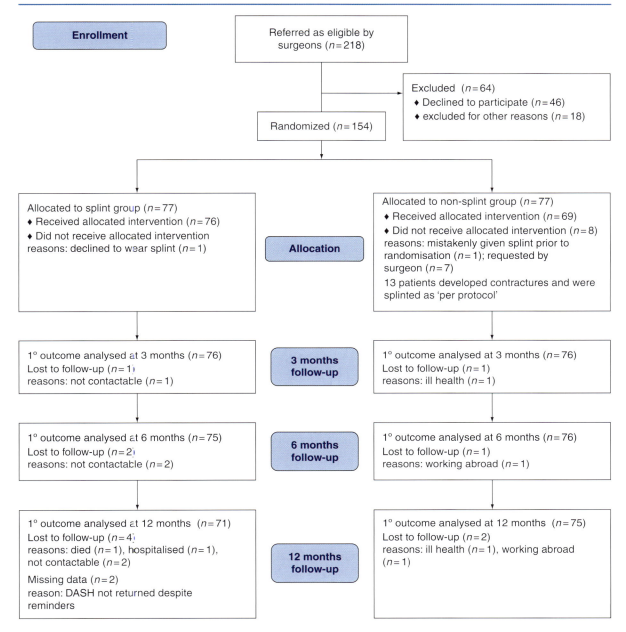

Fig. 41.1 CONSORT flowchart for SCoRD trial

The mean number of therapy sessions was 5.1 (SD 2.5) in the splint group and 5.6 (SD 3.5) in the no-splint group. There were no significant differences in number of therapy sessions between the two groups (adjusted odds ratio: 0.93, 0.81–1.07, $p = 0.305$). The use of subsequent dynamic daytime splints for residual PIPJ contractures was similar for both groups (13 patients in splint group and 14 in no-splint group) and was not statistically significant (adjusted odds ratio: 0.91, 0.35–2.36, $p = 0.839$).

A secondary per-protocol analysis was conducted on all those patients in whom the treatment protocol was adhered to. This included those patients allocated to the splint group and wore the splint for at least 50% of nights in the first 3 months. In those allocated to the no-splint it includes the 13 patients given a splint due

Table 41.1 Baseline demographic and clinical characteristics

		Splint group N = 77	No splint group N = 77
Centre	Cambridge	13 (17%)	13 (17%)
	Ipswich	17 (22%)	18 (23%)
	Norwich	30 (39%)	29 (38%)
	Peterborough	5 (6%)	4 (5%)
	West Suffolk	12 (16%)	13 (17%)
Age	Mean (SD)	67.2 (10.0)	67.5 (9.2)
Sex	Ratio male: female	61:16	59:18
Occupation	Working	24 (31%)	29 (38%)
	Seeking work	1 (1%)	0
	Retired/not working	52 (68%)	48 (62%)
Surgery type	Dermofasciectomy	7 (9%)	9 (12%)
	Fasciectomy	70 (91%)	68 (88%)
Operated digit	Index	5 (7%)	3 (4%)
	Long	7 (9%)	16 (21%)
	Ring	37 (49%)	26 (34%)
	Small	56 (74%)	53 (69%)
No operated rays	1	50 (66%)	60 (78%)
	2	23 (30%)	13 (17%)
	3	3 (4%)	4 (5%)
Previous surgery	Yes	11 (14%)	12 (16%)
	No	66 (86%)	65 (84%)
Woodruff grade	2 (MCP only)	3 (4%)	7 (9%)
	3 (MCP and PIP, single digit)	42 (55%)	45 (58%)
	4 (as 3 multiple digits)	32 (41%)	25 (33%)
Initial DASH score	Mean (SD)	16.4 (15.1)	15.4 (13.2)
Initial TAF	Mean (SD)	223.8 (20.9)	226.2 (15.0)
Initial TAE	Mean (SD)	50.7 (22.2)	51.1 (18.8)

TAF total active flexion of MCPJ, PIPJ and DIPJ of operated digit(s) only; *TAE* total active extension of MCPJ, PIP and DIPJ of operated digit(s) only

to ensuring contracture. Table 41.3 gives the results for the per-protocol analysis for primary and secondary outcomes at 3, 6 and 12 months. No statistically significant differences were found on any of the outcomes and at any time points.

Mean adherence to splint wear in the first 3 months was 74.6% of nights (SD = 29.4%) and only 12 patients did not meet the adherence criterion (splint worn ≥50% of night for first 3 months). Reasons for non-adherence or discontinuing splint wear were documented in the splint diary. The most commonly cited reason (n = 12) was the patient no longer perceiving any benefit from wearing the splint, other reasons were: causing hand stiffness, causing discomfort or pain, sleep disturbance, advised to discontinue by surgeon, ill fitting or causing a rash.

41.4 Discussion

This pragmatic trial has shown that the policy of using routine night-time static splints in addition to usual post-operative hand therapy does not offer any additional benefit in terms of self-reported hand function and disability, active composite range of flexion or extension or patient satisfaction. Both groups improved over the 12-month follow-up period in their DASH score. However any between-group differences were not statistically significant and the 95% confidence intervals included values of 5 points or less which are well below the threshold for a minimal important change in DASH.

As surgery is primarily aimed at releasing contracted tissues and splints designed to maintain this extension,

41 Night-Time Splinting After Fasciectomy or Dermofasciectomy for Dupuytren's Contracture

Table 41.2 Intention-to-treat analysis for primary and secondary outcomes (mean and standard deviation)

		Splint group	No splint group	Adjusted difference 95% C.I.	p-value
3-month	DASH (0–100)	9.6 (12.8)	10.8 (12.5)	−1.48	0.403
		$n=76$	$n=76$	(−5.02 to 2.06)	
	LogDASH	1.74 (1.17)	1.87 (1.18)	−0.16	0.372
		$n=76$	$n=76$	(−0.50 to 0.19)	
	TAF (degrees)	213.0 (26.5)	217.6 (22.5)	−3.49	0.326
		$n=75$	$n=76$	(10.57 to −3.59)	
	TAE (degrees)	−32.9 (19.6)	−30.9 (20.7)	3.30	0.209
		$n=75$	$n=76$	(1.93 to −8.53)	
6-month	DASH	7.9 (11.4)	7.1 (10.7)	0.20	0.890
		$n=75$	$n=76$	(−2.72 to 3.12)	
	LogDASH	1.47 (1.21)	1.38 (1.21)	0.07	0.704
		$n=75$	$n=76$	(−0.29 to 0.43)	
	TAF	220.6 (25.2)	225.8 (21.6)	−4.16	0.199
		$n=74$	$n=76$	(−10.6 to 2.29)	
	TAE	−31.0 (23.3)	−28.4 (21.1)	4.52	0.142
		$n=74$	$n=76$	(−1.61 to 10.65)	
	Patient satisfaction (0–10)	8.7 (1.89)	9.0 (1.23)	−0.28	0.286
		$n=75$	$n=76$	(−0.81 to 0.24)	
12-month	DASH	7.0 (14.6)	6.0 (9.2)	0.66	0.703
		$n=71$	$n=75$	(−2.79 to 4.11)	
	LogDASH	1.24 (1.21)	1.23 (1.20)	−0.02	0.914
		$n=71$	$n=75$	(−0.38 to 0.34)	
	TAF	223.8 (25.7)	227.3 (19.5)	−2.02	0.493
		$n=72$	$n=75$	(−7.89 to 3.85)	
	TAE	−32.9 (27.4)	−29.6 (23.3)	5.11	0.172
		$n=72$	$n=75$	(−2.33 to 12.55)	
	Patient Satisfaction	8.5 (2.33)	8.9 (1.79)	−0.35	0.315
		$n=73$	$n=75$	(−1.04 to 0.34)	

Table 41.3 Per-protocol analysis for primary and secondary outcomes at all time points

		Splint group	No splint group	Adjusted difference 95% C.I.	p-value
		$n=65$	$n=68$		
3-month	DASH (0–100)	9.8 (13.5)	10.7 (13.0)	−2.19 (−6.15 to 1.77)	0.270
	LogDASH	1.72 (1.20)	1.84 (1.20)	−0.20 (−0.58 to 0.18)	0.302
	TAF (degrees)	211.9 (26.5)	218.7 (21.5)	−4.51 (−12.2 to 3.2)	0.245
	TAE (degrees)	33.0 (19.4)	31.1 (21.0)	3.49 (−2.06 to 9.04)	0.210
		$n=64$	$n=68$		
6-month	DASH	8.4 (12.1)	7.4 (11.0)	−0.13 (−3.35 to 3.09)	0.936
	LogDASH	1.51 (1.24)	1.38 (1.24)	0.05 (−0.34 to 0.44)	0.793
	TAF	220.4 (23.0)	226.5 (21.7)	−3.92 (−10.59 to 2.75)	0.242
	TAE	30.9 (23.5)	29.0 (21.9)	4.38 (−2.23 to 10.99)	0.188
	Patient satisfaction (0–10)	8.65 (2.00)	9.00 (1.23)	−0.34 (−0.92 to 0.24)	0.254
		$n=62$[a]	$n=67$		
12-month	DASH	7.4 (15.5)	6.1 (9.6)	0.44 (−3.41 to 4.29)	0.821
	LogDASH	1.27 (1.22)	1.20 (1.23)	0.02 (−0.37 to 0.41)	0.919
	TAF	223.4 (23.4)	228.0 (19.3)	−1.87 (−7.78 to 4.04)	0.527
	TAE	32.6 (27.7)	30.1 (24.4)	5.12 (−3.01 to 13.3)	0.211
	Patient satisfaction	8.68 (2.17)	8.85 (1.84)	−0.18 (−0.90 to 0.54)	0.622

[a]For DASH and log DASH splint group $n=61$

total extension deficit is an important clinical measure of change and a more proximate outcome. However, the ITT analysis found no statistically significant differences between the two groups on either active extension or flexion.

A potential weakness of the trial is that the primary outcome measure was patient reported and participants could not be blinded. Secondary outcomes were collected by the research associates who were also not blinded, although they were independent of the clinical staff delivering the interventions. The lack of blinding could introduce a bias but this bias is more likely to be in favour of splinting (i.e. those patients with an active intervention more likely to report favourable results). The fact that the trial did not find evidence in support of splinting would mitigate against the possible assessment bias from the patients' or researchers' expectations to have a better outcome from splinting.

Our trial exceeded the required sample size for 90% power, had a very high follow-up rate (96%) and even in the secondary per-protocol analysis the sample size still exceeds 51 in each group; therefore the possibility of a Type II error remains low, and yet the confidence intervals exclude the minimally important difference for the DASH.

There are several possible explanations for our results. The primary outcome measure is a well-validated outcome measure for upper limb function and disability. However, DASH is a region-specific upper extremity measure and not disease-specific. It may therefore lack sensitivity to change in patients with Dupuytren's contracture. A clinically important change of 15 points as a criterion is a large effect size especially when considering that the baseline mean score prior to surgery was only 16 points, thus indicating minimal disability. Range of movement of digital joints could be argued as a more proximate and objective indicator of contracture severity, yet the differences between groups were also non-significant with small and narrow confidence intervals, confirming that a splint does not offer any additional benefit in terms of active extension or flexion of affected digits.

A second possible reason for a lack of difference could be dilution bias especially through non-adherence in the splint group. Patients were asked to complete a weekly splint diary; however overall mean adherence with splint wear was high and only 12 patients in the

splint group were deemed as non-adherent (15.6%) at 3 months. The results of the per-protocol analysis which includes only those who met the adherence criterion of splint wear for ≥50% differences were still non-significant for all primary and secondary outcomes, indicating that even when the splint is worn or adhered to a lack of effect is still evident. One weakness is that these adherence rates relied on patient completed diaries. Whilst the diaries were collected by research associates (not the treating therapists or surgeon) and therefore encouraged patients to be honest, independent verification of actual splint wear was not possible.

A third plausible reason for the lack of effect could be that the amount of tension provided through a static night splint is not sufficient to remodel scar tissue. In a study investigating full time casting in patients with an orthopaedic injury improvement in PIP, flexion contracture was related to the total time that the cast was worn with greater extension achieved the longer the cast was worn (Flowers and LaStayo 1994). However, it is unknown if the same principle applies to an intermittent application of force, such as the use of a night splint only in post-operative Dupuytren's disease.

The use of composite joint motion, that is adding MCPJ, PIPJ and DIPJ range, is a potential limitation; however separate analysis by joint means multiple hypotheses tests and increases the risk of a Type I error. It is also widely acknowledged that correction of PIPJ contractures presents a greater challenge than in patients with MCPJ involvement only. The trial was not adequately powered for subgroup analyses, and hence, results of such secondary analyses need to be interpreted with caution. We did conduct one such subgroup analysis based on those patients who had surgery involving the PIPJ of the little finger ($n = 109$, 71% of total sample). No statistically significant differences were found between the groups on DASH or PIPJ flexion or extension. These results concur with the primary analysis.

Our trial was pragmatic and its broad inclusion criteria, the fact that it was a multi-centre trial across 5 hospitals and involved 16 surgeons and around 26 therapists mean that generalisability is good. The baseline clinical and demographic characteristics of the whole cohort of 154 patients is typical of this patient group and although we were unable to collect data on non-consenting patients the fact that 73% of those invited consented further supports the external validity of this trial. Furthermore we have no evidence of selection bias in the method by which surgeons screened patients for eligibility.

The interventions used in this pragmatic trial were consistent with current practice within the five trusts and we used practical criteria based on clinical reasoning to agree protocol deviations, although the exact thresholds for net loss of extension and therefore when to apply a splint were arbitrary and could be reconsidered.

Our results are generalisable to patients managed surgically by fasciectomy or dermofasciectomy; however caution is needed in extrapolating these findings to other surgical or less invasive procedures where the role of post-operative hand therapy including splinting remains largely unknown.

41.5   Conclusions

Contrary to the widespread belief in the value of post-op night splinting for up to 6 months after fasciectomy or dermofasciectomy, we found no evidence of its short- or long-term effect. The policy of splinting all patients referred for hand therapy immediately after fasciectomy or dermofasciectomy needs to be reconsidered. This phase III trial provides evidence of a lack of effect of splinting when adhered to for at least 50% of nights in the first 3 months compared to hand therapy and splinting only when contractures occur. Patients receiving post-operative hand therapy by a specialised occupational therapist or physiotherapist had at least as good an outcome as those given an additional night splint. Only a small proportion (17%) of patients allocated to hand therapy went on to develop contractures of the PIPJ which exceeded the agreed threshold and needed a splint. Given the added expense of therapists' time, thermoplastic materials and the potential inconvenience to patients having to wear a device the policy of routine addition of night-time splinting after fasciectomy or dermofasciectomy should no longer be advocated but only where a loss of extension has occurred, particularly if the loss is rapid and early in the post-operative period.

41.6   Bullet Points

- Randomized controlled study of night splinting after Dupuytren's contracture release surgery.
- Outcome measures – DASH, patient satisfaction and measured range of motion.
- Intention to treat analysis showed no difference between groups at 3, 6, 9 or 12 months follow-up.
- This study does not support the routine use of a night splint after Dupuytren's contracture release surgery.

Editorial Statements

Competing Interests   The authors declare that they have no competing interests.

Authors' Contributions   CJH, LS, AJC and DL all contributed to the trial concept and design, interpretation of data and drafting of the manuscript. LS undertook the statistical analysis. EB and SV conducted all data collection. CJH, LS, AJC and DL obtained funding. All authors revised the manuscript for important intellectual content and have read and approved the final version.

Acknowledgements   Action Medical Research Charity funded the trial costs including all consumables and research associate salaries (AP1074). CJH and LS were funded by the Faculty of Health, University of East Anglia. The National Institute for Health Research (NIHR) funded CJH through a Career Development Fellowship from January 2009. The study received support by NIHR through the Comprehensive Local Research Network.

The SCoRD Trial Group included:

Investigators: C Jerosch-Herold, L Shepstone, A Chojnowski, D Larson.
Surgeons and sites: P Chapman, A Chojnowski, A Logan, M Meyer, A Patel (Norwich); G Cormack, J Hopkinson-Woolley, I Grant (Cambridge); M Wood (Bury St Edmunds); J Jones, A White, A Doran (Peterborough); P Crossman, C Roberts, M Shanahan (Ipswich). *Lead Hand Therapists and sites:* D Larson (Norwich), M Hayden (Cambridge); Laura Smith (Bury St Edmunds); Jill Frusher (Peterborough), J Dinley (Ipswich). *Trial research staff:* E Barrett, S Vaughan. *Independent Trial Steering Committee members:* DGI Scott, S Spooner. *Local PPIRes members:* C Handford, V Hawes, C Williams.

Previous Publication   This chapter has been published first in BMC Musculoskeletal Disorders 2011, 12:136 doi:10.1186/1471-2474-12-136. It is re-printed in a slightly modified form and with permission by the authors.

References

Armstrong JR, Hurren JS, Logan AM (2000) Dermofasciectomy in the management of Dupuytren's disease. J Bone Joint Surg Br 82(1):90–94

Au-Yong ITH, Wildin CJ, Dias JJ, Page RE (2005) A review of common practice in Dupuytren surgery. Tech Hand Up Extrem Surg 9(4):178–187

Bayat A, McGrouther DA (2006) Management of Dupuytren's disease-clear advice for an elusive condition. Ann R Coll Surg Engl 88(1):3–8

Beaton D, Davis A, Hudak P, McConnell S (2001) The DASH (Disabilities of the Arm, Shoulder and Hand) outcome measure: what do we know about it now? Br J Hand Ther 6(4):109–118

Dias JJ, Braybrooke J (2006) Dupuytren's contracture: an audit of the outcomes of surgery. J Hand Surg Br 31(5):514–521

Ellis B, Bruton A (2002) A study to compare the reliability of composite finger flexion with goniometry for measurement of range of motion in the hand. Clin Rehabil 16(5):562–570

Engstrand C, Boren L, Liedberg GM (2009) Evaluation of activity limitation and digital extension in Dupuytren's contracture three months after fasciectomy and hand therapy interventions. J Hand Ther 22(1):21–26

Evans RB, Dell PC, Fiolkowski P (2002) A clinical report of the effect of mechanical stress on functional results after fasciectomy for Dupuytren's contracture. J Hand Ther 15(4):331–339

Flowers KR, LaStayo P (1994) Effect of total end-range time on improving passive range of motion. J Hand Ther 7(3):150–157

Gummesson C, Atroshi I, Ekdahl C (2003) The Disabilities of the Arm, Shoulder and Hand (DASH) outcome questionnaire: longitudinal construct validity and measuring self-rated health change after surgery. BMC Musculoskelet Disord 4:11

Herweijer H, Dijkstra PU, Nicolai J-P, Van der Slius CK (2007) Postoperative hand therapy in Dupuytren's disease. Disabil Rehabil 29(22):1736–1741

Hurst LC, Badalamente MA, Hentz VR, Hotchkiss RN, Kaplan FTD, Meals RA, Smith TM, Rodzvilla J, Group CIS (2009) Injectable collagenase clostridium histolyticum for Dupuytren's contracture. N Engl J Med 361(10):968–979

Larson D, Jerosch-Herold C (2008) Clinical effectiveness of post-operative splinting after surgical release of Dupuytren's contracture: a systematic review. BMC Musculoskelet Disord 9:104

Salim J, Walker AP, Sau I, Sharara KH (2006) Dupuytren's contracture: postoperative management survey in United Kingdom. EFNAOT proceedings. J Bone Joint Surg Br 88-B(Suppl 1):35

Townley WA, Baker R, Sheppard N, Grobbelaar AO (2006) Dupuytren's contracture unfolded. BMJ 332(7538):397–400

van Rijssen AL, Werker P (2006) Percutaneous needle fasciotomy in Dupuytren's disease. J Hand Surg Eur Vol 31B:498–501

van Rijssen AL, Gerbrandy FSJ, Ter Linden H, Klip H, Werker PMN (2006) A comparison of the direct outcomes of percutaneous needle fasciotomy and limited fasciectomy for Dupuytren's disease: a 6-week follow-up study. J Hand Surg [Am] 31(5):717–725

Zyluk A, Jagielski W (2007) The effect of the severity of the Dupuytren's contracture on the function of the hand before and after surgery. J Hand Surg Eur Vol 32E(3):326–329

The Role of Static Night Splinting After Contracture Release for Dupuytren's Disease: A Preliminary Recommendation Based on Clinical Cases

42

Albrecht Meinel

Contents

42.1	Introduction	333
42.2	**Static Night Splinting in the Treatment of Dupuytren's Disease**	333
42.2.1	Pathogenesis and the Effect of Splinting	333
42.2.2	The Splint Application	334
42.2.3	The Finger Splint with an Existing Extension Deficit	336
42.2.4	The Unusual Case	337
42.3	**Discussion**	338
42.4	**Conclusions**	339
References		339

A. Meinel
Dupuytren-Ambulanz, Kardinal-Döpfner-Platz 1,
97070 Würzburg, Germany
e-mail: meinel@dupuytren-ambulanz.de

42.1 Introduction

The recommendation of night splinting of the surgically treated Dupuytren finger is as old as the literature on the disease itself. The wine importer who was treated with open fasciotomy by Dupuytren on June 12, 1831, afterwards wore a night splint "for another month and an excellent result was achieved" (Elliot 1988). A hand or finger splint has remained an integral part of the treatment of Dupuytren's disease to this day in many surgical schools. Yet there has long been insufficient evidence of the actual efficacy of splinting. With the increasing popularity of the percutaneous needle fasciotomy, finger splinting as a part of the treatment of Dupuytren's disease has experienced somewhat of a renaissance. My own experience with finger splinting secondary to percutaneous needle fasciotomy has been entirely positive. Static night splinting appears to enhance the efficacy and sustainability of this surgical treatment. These observations and other effects of splinting are presented and critically examined in case studies taken from my own practice.

42.2 Static Night Splinting in the Treatment of Dupuytren's Disease

42.2.1 Pathogenesis and the Effect of Splinting

As is discussed in this book (Meinel 2012), the Dupuytren finger contracture is not the result of tissue contraction but of a loss of mobility in the compressed and folded soft tissue lying above the flexed fingers. The connective tissue conglomerate of newly formed

C. Eaton et al. (eds.), *Dupuytren's Disease and Related Hyperproliferative Disorders*,
DOI 10.1007/978-3-642-22697-7_42, © Springer-Verlag Berlin Heidelberg 2012

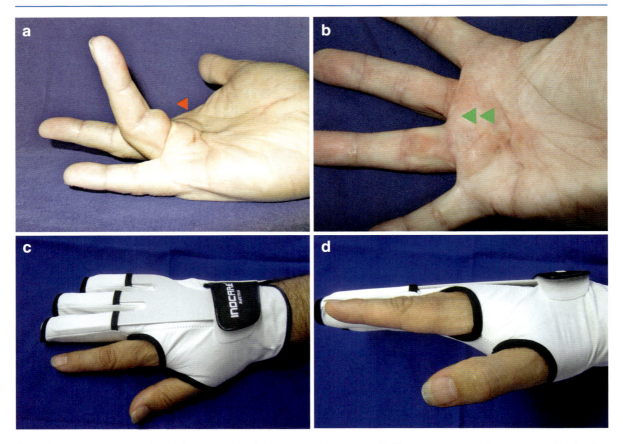

Fig. 42.1 Percutaneous needle fasciotomy and static night splinting. (**a**) and (**b**) Dupuytren finger before and immediately after PNF; Tubiana II to Tubiana 0. (**c**) and (**d**) the FixxGlove splint system viewed from above and from the side

and preexisting tissue in palmar fibromatosis can no longer be expanded. As a result, it prevents extension of the affected fingers. The Dupuytren finger contracture represents an extension block in the finger as a result of tissue changes. The histogenesis and morphogenesis of the tissue mix occurring in fibromatosis is decisively influenced by stresses that act on the tissue via the mobile fingers. This produces the typical clinical picture with cords and bent fingers.

Percutaneous needle fasciotomy fragments the Dupuytren tissue, allowing it to be distracted. The fingers can again be extended. This minimally invasive procedure converts the process back to an earlier stage of the disease. In the most favorable case, Tubiana stage 0 is achieved (Fig. 42.1a, b). In percutaneous needle fasciotomy (PNF), the tissue remains in situ, and during sleep, the hand rests in flexion. There is a risk that this posture will bring the distracted tissue back into apposition, where scarring could join it together again. Such a process would recreate an extension deficit.

Therefore, it is recommended to immobilize the finger in extension to keep the fragmented Dupuytren tissue apart during the postoperative scarring phase (Fig. 42.1c, d). In the early stage of the disease characterized by nodule development and prior to loss of extension in the finger, the extension splint removes the skin anchoring fibers from their flexion position, counteracting the immobilizing effect of the proliferative tissue and thus avoiding permanent flexion of the finger.

42.2.2 The Splint Application

42.2.2.1 The Standard Splint in the Treatment of Dupuytren's Disease

Night splinting was prescribed for a period of up to 6 months or even longer. As strict long-term compliance is crucial to success, it was important to find a splint model that offered maximum comfort. With this in mind, the FixxGlove splint system was developed

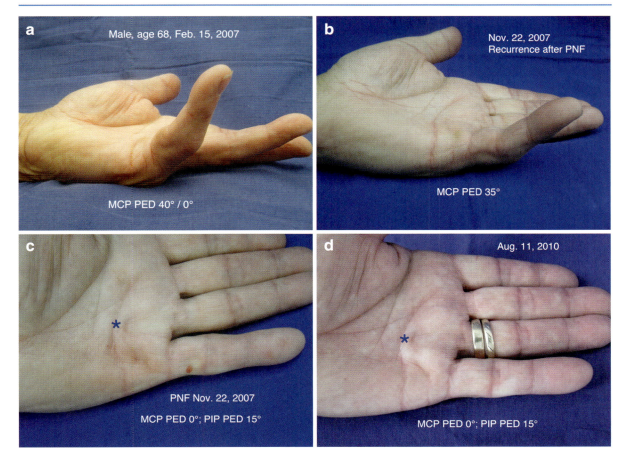

Fig. 42.2 A long-term observation. Extension deficits in the little finger. (**a**) Findings before first percutaneous needle fasciotomy; (**b**) recurrent extension deficits before second PNF; (**c**) findings immediately after second fasciotomy; (**d**) nearly 3 years later. No splinting before second fasciotomy; long-term night splinting after second fasciotomy: *Dupuytren nodule with skin dimple in the same size and shape over nearly 3 years

from a golf glove in cooperation with Inocare International (Heiligkreuzsteinach, Germany, www.inocare.de). The system consists of a three-fingered glove splint with an aluminum insert on the extensor side that holds the fingers in extension (Fig. 42.1c, d). The glove is limited to the three typical Dupuytren fingers, which reflects an intentional compromise. These three fingers form a functional unit due to their muscular connections, and they are most often affected by fibromatosis. The thumb and forefinger can also be involved. Yet because this occurs far less often, it was felt that it was more important to preserve their freedom of movement for the pinch grip by excluding them from the splint complex. This standard splint is thus suitable for treating the most common manifestations of the disease in the little, ring, and middle fingers. Yet its glove form and the freedom of movement it allows for the pinch grip make it very comfortable to wear, which is crucial to promoting patient compliance.

42.2.2.2 A Long-Term Observation

In this example of Dupuytren's disease, a man who was 68 years old at the onset of treatment was observed over a three-year period. The results demonstrate that long-term night splinting can indeed enhance the sustainability of the correction achieved by percutaneous needle fasciotomy. Figure 42.2a shows the findings prior to the first percutaneous needle fasciotomy in February 2007. The passive extension deficit (PED) of 40° in the metacarpophalangeal joint was successfully reduced to 0°. The patient did not wear a splint and presented again 9 months later with a recurrent flexion deformity in the metacarpophalangeal joint of the little finger. A nodule and fold indicative of progressive disease had also

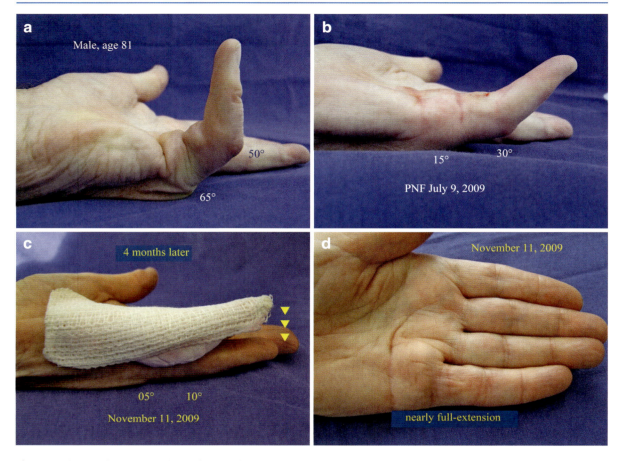

Fig. 42.3 Observations when splinting fingers with extension deficits. (**a**) Before PNF; (**b**) immediately after PNF; (**c, d**) 4 months after PNF. The postoperative extension deficits have almost completely disappeared with splinting with a silicone bed

developed over the ring finger. At the patient's request, the PNF was repeated in November 2007. The procedure succeeded in completely eliminating the extension deficit of the metacarpophalangeal joint. However, it was not possible to achieve any significant reduction of the extension deficit of 15° in the proximal interphalangeal joint (Fig. 42.2c). A glove splint was prescribed after the second fasciotomy. The patient returned in August 2010 because he was now unable to extend the little finger of the other hand. He reported that function in the left little finger, which had last been treated nearly 3 years previously, continued to be very good. Objective findings were identical to postoperative findings after the second fasciotomy in November 2007: PED was 0° in the MCP joint and 15° in the PIP joint. The nodule and fold formation over the ring finger was also identical to the findings in November 2007. The patient reported having worn the glove splint every night for over 6 months. After that, he wore the splint every second or third night during the last 2 years. He decided on his own to do this because he felt good doing so, and it gave him a sense of security. Wearing the splint over a period of years like this had been neither prescribed nor recommended. It did not lead to any sort of impairment of finger mobility.

42.2.3 The Finger Splint with an Existing Extension Deficit

In this 81-year-old man, PNF significantly reduced the extension deficits in the metacarpophalangeal and proximal interphalangeal joints of the left little finger. As was expected, an extension deficit of 30° remained in the proximal interphalangeal joint in particular (Fig. 42.3b). With extension impairments of 20° or

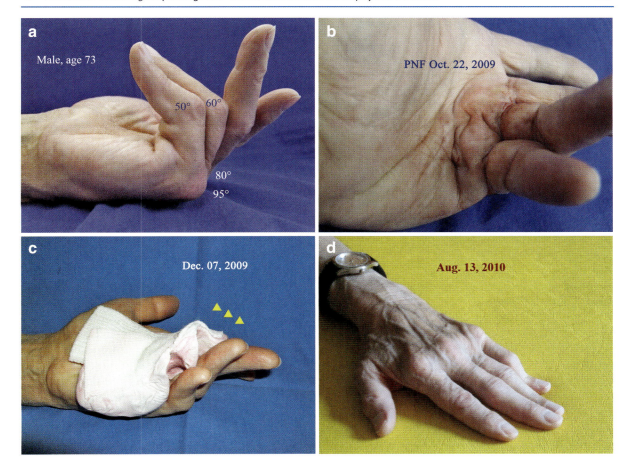

Fig. 42.4 The unusual case. (**a**) Initial findings: D5 and D4 Tubiana IV; (**b**) immediately after PNF; (**c**) reduced extension deficits 6 weeks after PNF. Splinting with silicone bed; (**d**) table test 10 months after PNF with rigorous adherence to regime of night splinting. Only one PNF procedure at the beginning of the treatment

more in one or more fingers, the glove can no longer be worn without problems. The aluminum splint itself can be bent to fit. However, with some contractures, it may be difficult or impossible to put the glove on and to wear it. In such cases, manufacturing a custom splint with a form-fitted silicone bed for the finger has proven effective (Fig. 42.3c). Thermoplastic bandage material stabilizes and supports the splint. The silicone bed splint is fixed in place either with an adhesive elastic gauze bandage or with Velcro strips. The patient presented again 4 months later. Amazingly, the extension impairment in the little finger had nearly completely disappeared. The subcutaneous indurations had also become fewer and softer (Fig. 42.3c, d). A second fasciotomy was no longer indicated. The splint therapy could now be continued with a glove splint.

42.2.4 The Unusual Case

The 73-year-old man did not desire surgical treatment as he had had bad experience with it in the right hand. Because of the narrowed approach, needle fasciotomy could initially be performed only over the metacarpophalangeal joints. It led to a slight improvement in range of motion (Fig. 42.4b). An initial silicone bed splint was applied 8 days postoperatively once the skin permitted splinting. The follow-up examination 6 weeks later showed that the extension deficits were significantly reduced as evidenced by the increased extension in the fingers on the splint bed (Fig. 42.4c). Two further adjustments to the splint were subsequently made. These led to further reductions in the extension deficits. This unexpected clinical course obviated the need for the planned repeat fasciotomy.

The middle and ring fingers now have nearly their full range of motion. The impairment in the proximal interphalangeal joint of the little finger was attributable to articular causes and did not bother the patient (Fig. 42.4d). The hyperextended distal phalanx of the little finger in the table test could be actively flexed. The last picture shows nearly the entire hand in contact with the table. This picture was sent by the patient who was very pleased with the clinical course. I had never imagined that such a Dupuytren hand could be treatable in four short outpatient sessions (one percutaneous needle fasciotomy, three splint fittings). In a comparable case, a similar result has been successfully maintained for over 3 years. Both these patients have rigorously adhered to the regime of night splinting.

42.3 Discussion

Searching the literature for results after needle fasciotomy with and without finger splinting has not been very fruitful. The work group around P.M.N. Werker in Groningen, Netherlands, has employed percutaneous needle fasciotomy for years with very good results. However, the treated fingers were not splinted. At the symposium in Miami, van Rijssen reported on the initial long-term results from Groningen (van Rijssen et al. 2010). In this study, the rate of recurrence following percutaneous needle fasciotomy was 85%. This was frightfully high compared with 23.8% following limited fasciectomy. The recurrences following percutaneous needle fasciotomy were also significantly earlier than those following limited fasciectomy. There were no available studies on finger splinting after percutaneous needle fasciotomy.

Can adequate splinting improve the results of percutaneous needle fasciotomy? I am not yet able to provide convincing numbers on the efficacy of splinting after percutaneous needle fasciotomy. However, I can present case studies that suggest that appropriate splinting can indeed influence the flexion deformity in the fingers. It apparently does this in several possible ways. First, finger splinting delays or prevents a recurrent flexion deformity in the finger. Second, splinting leads to partial or complete resolution of an existing extension impairment. Third, the splint also prevents the Dupuytren nodule from progressing to a finger contracture. Ball and Nanchahal reported observations of this nature (Ball and Nanchahal 2002). They examined the effect of long-term static night splinting as a "nonsurgical treatment for Dupuytren's disease." Six patients in various stages of the disease who did not undergo surgery were included in a pilot study. The authors found that the static night splint could halt progression of the clinical picture. They also observed improvements in the initial range of motion. Such phenomena among my own patients continue to be a source of fascination.

The prophylactic effect of the finger splint in preventing a flexion deformity following percutaneous needle fasciotomy is attributable to its maintaining the gap in the Dupuytren tissue created by surgery. The effect of the splint in preventing a flexion deformity in the previously untreated hand can be seen in how it withdraws the skin anchoring fibers from the flexion position. The improvement in an existing flexion deformity under splinting is best understood in light of the altered biomechanical stresses acting on the Dupuytren tissue. It is not yet known whether the silicone finger bed may also have an effect. Silicone is a suitable material for the finger bed for several reasons. Silicone can be easily and precisely molded to fit the finger. It offers maximum comfort, and it has proven effective in the treatment of scarring. The question of whether silicone can enhance the effect of the splint warrants further study. This is an interesting field of inquiry for clinical research. The suspicion that simple long-term night splinting can prevent a Dupuytren nodule from developing into a finger deformity is based on initial observations and is still somewhat speculative. Yet in light of the socioeconomic significance of this widespread disorder, it is an option that may have a significant impact.

Finally, there is a historical dimension that Wylock alluded to in his book on the life and times of Dupuytren published in 2010. Wylock describes the open fasciotomy performed by Dupuytren on the wine importer M. L. on June 12, 1831, as a milestone in the history of the treatment of Dupuytren's disease. Wylock operated on a similarly diseased hand with all the means of modern medicine. Today's medicine with anesthesia, a bloodless surgical field, asepsis, and skin transplantation doubtlessly ensures far more comfort and safety. Yet the actual treatment of Dupuytren's disease itself has hardly progressed in 180 years. The hand shown in Fig. 42.4 corresponds to Dupuytren's case of 1831 and to Wylock's case of 2010. It is amazing to consider the alteration of the clinical course that can be achieved with minimalistic means. Yet this also shows that new treatment options are not always as new as they might seem. Fasciotomy and night splinting were successfully applied by Dupuytren himself.

42.4 Conclusions

Splinting of the Dupuytren finger, whether trapped in flexion or still mobile, whether postsurgical or still untreated, opens up fascinating therapeutic options that deserve greater attention in both clinical practice and research. Yet the case studies presented here justify the use of the splint as a low-risk, low-cost treatment concept. The splint with a silicone bed appears to be particularly important in the management of Dupuytren's disease.

Disclosure The author developed the concept of the FixxGlove night splint and receives royalties from the sales of the FixxGlove night splint.

References

Ball C, Nanchahal J (2002) The use of splinting as a non-surgical treatment for Dupuytren's disease: a pilot study. Br J Hand Ther 7(3):76–78

Elliot DE (1988) The early history of contracture of the palmar fascia. J Hand Surg 13B:246–253

Meinel A (2012) Palmar fibromatosis or the loss of flexibility of the palmar finger tissue. A new insight into the disease process of Dupuytren contracture. In: Dupuytren's disease and related hyperproliferative disorders, pp 11–20

Van Rijssen A, Ter Linden H, Werker PMN (2010) 5-year results of first-ever randomised clinical trial on treatment in Dupuytren's disease: percutaneous needle fasciotomy versus limited fasciectomy. Presented at: International Symposium on Dupuytren's Disease, Miami FL, May 22–23, 2010

Wylock P (2010) The life and times of Guillaume Dupuytren, 1777–1835. University Press, Brussels

Part VII

Additional and New Treatment Options

Editor: M. Heinrich Seegenschmiedt

Injectable Collagenase (*Clostridium histolyticum*) for Dupuytren's Contracture: Results of the CORD I Study

43

Marie A. Badalamente

Contents

43.1	Introduction	343
43.2	Methods	344
43.3	Results	345
43.4	Discussion	345
43.5	Conclusions	346
References		346

43.1 Introduction

Dupuytren's contracture is a progressive disorder of pathologic collagen deposition characterized by nodules and cords in the palm and fingers. These pathologic changes cause pitting of the overlying skin and flexion contractures of the fingers (Hueston and Tubiana 1974; McFarlane 1974; Brickley-Parsons et al. 1981; Murrell and Hueston 1990).

Myofibroblasts are the important pathologic cells in development of Dupuytren's disease (Gabbiani and Majno 1972). Myofibroblasts mediate increased collagen production, particularly type-III collagen in the early stages of the disease (Brickley-Parsons et al. 1981; Murrell and Hueston 1990; Murrell et al. 1991). In the early stages of the disease process, nodules form within the palm (Hueston and Tubiana 1974). As the condition progresses, collagen cords cause fingers to progressively flex at the metacarpophalangeal (MP) and proximal interphalangeal (PIP) joints, resulting in a fixed-flexion deformity of the fingers and an extension deficit (Hueston and Tubiana 1974; McFarlane 1974; Rayan 2007).

The global prevalence of Dupuytren's contracture among Caucasians is estimated at 3–6% (Early 1962; Yost et al. 1955). Certain patient groups have been identified in which the incidence of Dupuytren's contracture is substantially higher than others. The incidence is reported as higher in men compared to women (Early 1962). A strong association exists between onset of Dupuytren's contracture and age. Most patients are older than 50 years at presentation (Loos et al. 2007). Among patients with diabetes, the incidence of Dupuytren's disease has been estimated at 10.5% (Del Rosso et al. 2006), although other reports suggest the incidence may be

M.A. Badalamente
Department of Orthopaedics, State University of New York at Stony Brook, Stony Brook, NY, USA
e-mail: mbadalamente@nctes.cc.sunysb.edu

C. Eaton et al. (eds.), *Dupuytren's Disease and Related Hyperproliferative Disorders*,
DOI 10.1007/978-3-642-22697-7_43, © Springer-Verlag Berlin Heidelberg 2012

much higher (Balci et al. 1999). In patients with thyroid disease, the incidence for Dupuytren's disease has been reported to be 8.8% (Cakir et al. 2003).

At present, surgical fasciectomy is most often the technique of treatment choice (Rayan 2007; Tubiana et al. 2000; Van Rijssen et al. 2006). Minimal invasive percutaneous needle fasciotomy is also used as a treatment option (Van Rijssen et al. 2006; Eaton 2012). Since most patients with Dupuytren's disease are elderly or may have other significant comorbidities, they may not represent ideal candidates for invasive procedures. In addition, neurovascular injury, hematoma, and infection can occur during or following surgery, and in patients with severe contractures digital nerve damage is a risk. Reflex sympathetic dystrophy and complex regional pain syndrome can also develop after surgery. Recurrence of Dupuytren's contracture after surgery is a risk. An average of 30% of patients experience a recurrence during the first and second postoperative years, then an additional 15% experience a recurrence during the third to fifth years, 10% between the fifth and tenth years, and <10% after 10 years (Tubiana et al. 2000).

Preclinical, Phase 2 and single center Phase 3, FDA-regulated, open label and randomized, double-blind, placebo-controlled clinical trials have indicated that injectable collagenase (*Clostridium histolyticum*) had merit as a nonsurgical treatment option for Dupuytren's contracture (Badalamente and Hurst 1996, 2000, 2007; Badalamente et al. 2002; Hurst and Badalamente 1999; Starkweather et al. 1996). The herein presented Phase 3 FDA-regulated, multicenter, randomized, double-blind, placebo-controlled clinical trial (Hurst et al. 2009) was undertaken to confirm the results of the prior pilot and phase 2 studies in a larger patient population. This trial was termed the *C*ollagenase *O*ption for *R*eduction of *D*upuytren's –the CORD I – study.

43.2 Methods

Three hundred six patients with Dupuytren's disease were analyzed for efficacy. The patients were enrolled at 16 participating centers across the USA. There were 245 (80%) males and 61 (20%) females, mean age 62.7 years. Patients were in good health, were ≥18 years old, had MP contractures between 20° and 100° or PIP contractures between 20° and 80°, and had an inability to simultaneously place the affected finger and palm flat on a table. Female patients were required to be postmenopausal or practicing contraception. Exclusion criteria included nursing or pregnancy, bleeding disorder, recent stroke, previous treatment of the primary joint (first joint injected) within 90 days of study start, collagenase treatment or treatment with any investigational drug within 30 days of study start, use of a tetracycline derivative within 14 days of study start, anticoagulant within 7 days of study start, allergy to collagenase, and chronic muscular, neurologic, or neuromuscular disorder affecting the hands. The study was reviewed and approved by human subjects review boards at each participating institution. All patients provided written informed consent.

Before initiating treatment, study investigators identified a primary joint (first joint) for treatment in each patient. Secondary and tertiary joints were also identified for potential subsequent injections, maximum three injections. Primary joints were stratified by type (two MP: one PIP) and by severity of joint contracture (MP ≤50° or >50°, PIP ≤40° or >40°) and then randomized 2:1 to injectable Clostridial collagenase or placebo. Clostridial collagenase (0.58 mg per injection) was reconstituted in sterile diluent and injected directly into affected cords, 0.25 ml (MP joints) or 0.20 ml (PIP joints). Placebo (10 mM Tris per 60 mM sucrose reconstituted in diluent) was administered similarly. If needed, all joints were manipulated up to three times using a standardized procedure (finger extension) the day after injection to attempt cord rupture. Patients were given a splint to wear nightly for up to 4 months. Follow-up visits occurred 1, 7, and 30 days post injection.

A treatment cycle comprised injection, manipulation, and 30-day follow-up. Each affected cord contracting the joint could undergo a maximum of three treatment cycles, and each patient could receive a maximum of three injections during the double-blind phase. If the primary joint met the primary endpoint in fewer than three injections, a secondary joint could be treated. If the primary and secondary joints met primary endpoint in fewer than three injections, a tertiary joint could be treated. The primary efficacy endpoint was reduction in contracture to zero to 5° of normal extension (0°), 30 days after the last injection. The primary efficacy endpoint and clinical improvement were analyzed using the Cochran-Mantel-Haenszel test, controlling for joint type and baseline contracture severity. Percent reduction in contracture and change from baseline in arc of motion were analyzed using an ANCOVA with a factor for treatment group, and

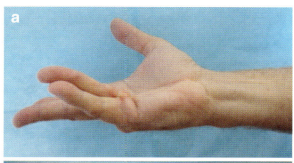
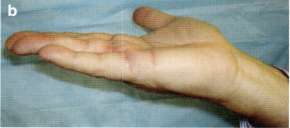

Fig. 43.1 (a) A 59-year-old male patient with contractures of the right hand little and ring finger MP joints, prior to collagenase injection. Natatory cords were present to these finger contractures. The "Y" point of the natatory cords was injected. (b) The same patient as in (a), 30 days after a collagenase injection. A reduction to 0° of both finger contractures was achieved

baseline contracture severity, and joint type as covariates. The log rank test was used to analyze times to meet the primary endpoint between treatment groups. Analyses were also conducted separately by joint type.

43.3 Results

More joints treated with collagenase than placebo (64.0% vs. 6.8%, $p<0.001$) achieved a reduction in contracture to 0–5° of full extension 30 days after the last injection (the primary endpoint) (Fig. 43.1a, b).

Two of seven joints in the placebo group to achieve reduction of contracture of 0–5° were erroneously treated with collagenase during their second injection, potentially contributing to the response rate observed in the placebo group. More than half of the collagenase-treated joints that did not meet primary endpoint did not receive the maximum allowable number of collagenase injections (three per cord) most commonly because investigators could not palpate a cord or patients were satisfied with the result. Median time to meet primary endpoint for collagenase-treated joints was 56 days. Mean change in contracture from baseline to 30 days after last injection was 50.2–12.2° for collagenase-treated and 49.1–45.7° for placebo-treated joints ($p<0.001$). The mean change in range of motion from baseline to 30 days after the last injection was an increase from 43.9° to 80.7° in the collagenase-treated joints (mean 36.7°) and from 45.3° to 49.5° in the placebo-injected joints ($p<0.001$).

Additionally, of those patients who received collagenase injections, 84.7% achieved a ≥50% reduction in contracture vs. 11.7% for those who received placebo.

The percentage of joints that achieved the primary endpoint of 0–5° of normal extension 30 days after the last injection by joint type was: MP joints, 76.7% collagenase vs 7.2% placebo ($p<0.001$), PIP joints, 40% collagenase vs. 5.9% placebo ($p<0.001$).

In reviewing the response to collagenase treatment by baseline contracture severity and by joint type, the following results were noted: if an MP joint contracture was ≤50° at baseline, 88.9% reached the primary endpoint of 0–5° normal extension; if an MP joint contracture was ≥50° at baseline, 57.7% reached the primary endpoint of 0–5° normal extension; if a PIP joint was ≤40° at baseline, 80.9% reached the primary endpoint of 0–5° normal extension; and finally, if a PIP joint was ≥40° at baseline, 22.4% reached the primary endpoint of 0–5° normal extension.

Patients who received collagenase injections had injection/finger manipulation-related adverse events. The most common of these events were edema, contusion, injection site pain, injection site hemorrhage, and transient regional lymph node swelling/pain. All of these events resolved without intervention in a median of 10 days. There were no adverse systemic immune events, no adverse events involving nerves or vessels. Three serious adverse events were deemed related to collagenase treatment: one case of complex regional pain syndrome and two tendon ruptures which required surgical correction.

43.4 Discussion

In this study, injectable collagenase (*Clostridium histolyticum*) was significantly superior to placebo in reducing contractures and improving range of motion in affected joints and was generally well tolerated. This novel nonsurgical injection is a treatment option in patients with Dupuytren's disease. The primary endpoint of this randomized, placebo-controlled, double-blind, multicenter clinical trial was reduction of contracture to within 0–5° full extension in the primary joint 30 days after the last injection. This endpoint was rigorous. Overall, 64% of primary joints – 77% of MP joints and 40% of PIP joints – treated with collagenase met this rigorous endpoint with significant gains in range of finger motion. The results further indicate that if a joint had a less severe contracture, defined in this clinical trial as ≤50° for MP joints and ≤40° for PIP joints, it was more likely to respond to collagenase injection treatment. This may indicate that an earlier intervention, before the contracture severity is high, if possible, may be an effective approach to treatment.

We found that collagenase injections had associated mild to moderate adverse events related to the injection itself and/or the manipulation in extension on the following day for cord rupture. These included bruising, pain, and swelling which resolved without intervention in a median of 10 days. Collagenase injections in this study caused no injuries to nerves or vessels nor did it negatively affect flexion or grip.

In summary, this study showed the efficacy and safety of injectable collagenase as an alternative to surgery. Collagenase injection as a nonsurgical treatment for Dupuytren's disease was approved by the US Food and Drug Administration in February 2010 as Xiaflex. Follow-up studies of patients who participated in the CORD I clinical trial are now ongoing to assess recurrence and disease extension rates. Results of a study at 2 years in Cord I patients indicate a recurrence rate of 19.6% (Auxilium Pharmaceuticals Public Announcement, June 2010). CORD I recurrence was defined as return of contracture in the treated finger of greater than or equal to 20 degrees, which was the minimum criterion for study entry. There was a positive opinion in December 2010 from the European Medicines Agency's (EMA) Committee for Medicinal Products for Human Use (CHMP) recommending European Union (EU) approval for XIAPEX® (collagenase clostridium histolyticum) as treatment for Dupuytren's contracture.

43.5 Conclusions

- Collagenase (Xiaflex) injection is a safe and effective method for the treatment of Dupuytren's contracture.
- Two-year recurrence data from the CORD I clinical trials indicate a relatively low recurrence rate of 19.3%.

Acknowledgments The author wishes to acknowledge the substantial contributions of the CORD I investigators as follows: *Edward Akelman, MD*, Brown University School of Medicine, Providence, RI, *Brian Bear, MD*, Rockford Orthopedic Associates, Rockford, Il, *Mark R. Belsky, MD*, Tufts University School of Medicine, Boston, MA, *Philip Blazar, MD*, Harvard University School of Medicine, Boston, MA, *Eric N. Britton, MD*, Hand Surgery Associates, Denver, CO, *Bronier Costas, MD*, Hand and Upper Extremity Center of Georgia, Altanta, GA, *Joel L. Frazier, MD*, Health Research Institute, Oklahoma City, OK, *Vincent R. Hentz, MD*, Stanford University School of Medicine and University Medical Center, Palo Alto, CA, *Robert N. Hotchkiss, MD*, Hospital for Special Surgery, New York, NY, *Lawrence C. Hurst MD*, Department of Orthopaedics, SUNY, Stony Brook, NY, *F. Thomas D. Kaplan, MD*, Indiana Hand Center, Indianapolis, IN, *John Lubahn, MD*, Hand, Microsurgery and Reconstructive Orthoapedics, Erie, PA, *Roy A. Meals, MD*, University of California at Los Angeles, CA, *Scott McPherson, MD*, Tria Orthopaedic Center, Minneapolis, MN, *Theodore M. Smith, PhD*, Biometrics, Auxilium Pharmaceuticals, Malvern, PA, *Clayton A. Peimer, MD*, Marquette University Hospital, Marquette, MI, *Douglas Roeshot, MD*, University Orthopedics Center, State College, PA

Disclosure The author has received research support for the CORD I trial and consulting fees from Auxilium Pharmaceuticals, Inc. The author holds partial royalty rights from Biospecific Technologies Corp.

References

Badalamente MA, Hurst LC (1996) Enzyme injection as a nonoperative treatment for Dupuytren's disease. Drug Deliv 3:35–40

Badalamente MA, Hurst LC (2000) Enzyme injection as nonsurgical treatment of Dupuytren's disease. J Hand Surg [Am] 25:629–636

Badalamente MA, Hurst LC (2007) Efficacy and safety of injectable mixed collagenase subtypes in the treatment of Dupuytren's contracture. J Hand Surg [Am] 32:767–774

Badalamente MA, Hurst LC, Hentz VR (2002) Collagen as a clinical target: nonoperative treatment of Dupuytren's disease. J Hand Surg [Am] 27:788–798

Balci N, Balci MK, Tuzuner S (1999) Shoulder adhesive capsulitis and shoulder range of motion in type II diabetes mellitus: association with diabetic complications. J Diabetes Complications 13:135–140

Brickley-Parsons D, Glimcher MJ, Smith RJ, Albin R, Adams JP (1981) Biochemical changes in the collagen of the palmar fascia in patients with Dupuytren's disease. J Bone Joint Surg Am 63:787–797

Cakir M, Samanci N, Balci N, Balci MK (2003) Musculoskeletal manifestations in patients with thyroid disease. Clin Endocrinol (Oxf) 59:162–167

Del Rosso A, Cerinic MM, De Giorgio F, Minari C, Rotella CM, Seghier G (2006) Rheumatological manifestations in diabetes mellitus. Curr Diabetes Rev 2:455–466

Early PF (1962) Population studies in Dupuytren's contracture. J Bone Joint Surg Am 44B:602–613

Eaton Ch (2012) A technique of needle aponeurotomy for Dupuytren's contracture. In: Dupuytren's disease and related hyperproliferative disorders, pp 267–279

Gabbiani G, Majno G (1972) Dupuytren's contracture. A fibroblast contraction? An ultrastructural study. Am J Pathol 66: 131–146

Hueston JT, Tubiana R (1974) Dupuytren's disease. Churchill Livingstone, Edinburgh

Hurst LC, Badalamente MA (1999) Nonoperative treatment of Dupuytren's disease. Hand Clin 15:97–107

Hurst LC, Badalamente MA, Hentz VR, Hotchkiss RN, Kaplan TD, Meals RA, Smith TN, Rodzvilla J (2009) Injectable collagenase clostridium histolyticum for Dupuytren's contracture. New Engl J Med 361:968–979

Loos B, Puschkin V, Horch RE (2007) 50 Years experience with Dupuytren's contracture in the Erlangen university hospital– a retrospective analysis of 2919 operated hands from 1956 to 2006. BMC Musculoskelet Disord 8:60

McFarlane RM (1974) Pattern of the diseased fascia in the fingers in Dupuytren's contracture. Plast Reconst Surg 54:31–36

Murrell GAC, Hueston JT (1990) Aetiology of Dupuytren's contracture. Aust NZ J Surg 60:247–252

Murrell GAC, Francis MJO, Bromley L (1991) The collagen changes of Dupuytren's contracture. J Hand Surg [Br] 16:263–266

Rayan GM (2007) Dupuytren's disease: anatomy, pathology, presentation, and treatment. J Bone Joint Surg [Am] 89: 189–198

Spring M, Fleck H, Cohen BD (1970) Dupuytren's contracture. Warning of diabetes? N Y State J Med 70:1037–1041

Starkweather KD, Lattuga S, Hurst LC et al (1996) Collagenase in the treatment of Dupuytren's disease: an in vitro study. J Hand Surg [Am] 21:490–495

Tubiana R, Leclercq C, Hurst LC, Badalamente MA, Mackin EJ (2000) Dupuytren's disease. Martin Dunitz Ltd, London

Van Rijssen AL, Gerbrandy FS, TerLinden H, Klip H, Werker PM (2006) A comparison of the direct outcomes of percutaneous needle fasciotomy and limited fasciectomy for Dupuytren's disease: a 6 week follow-up. J Hand Surg [Am] 31:717–725

Yost J, Winters T, Fett HC Sr (1955) Dupuytren's contracture; a statistical study. Am J Surg 90:568–571

44

Long-Term Outcome of Radiotherapy for Early Stage Dupuytren's Disease: A Phase III Clinical Study

Michael Heinrich Seegenschmiedt,
Ludwig Keilholz, Mark Wielpütz, Christine Schubert,
and Fabian Fehlauer

Contents

44.1	**Introduction**	349
44.2	**Patients, Materials, and Methods**	353
44.2.1	Patient Characteristics	353
44.2.2	Site Characteristics	353
44.2.3	Disease Predisposition	353
44.2.4	Pretreatment	353
44.2.5	Stage of Disease	353
44.2.6	Objective Signs	354
44.2.7	Subjective Symptoms	354
44.2.8	Radiotherapy	354
44.2.9	Randomization	354
44.2.10	Evaluation and Statistics	355
44.3	**Results**	358
44.3.1	Treatment Compliance	358
44.3.2	Treatment Toxicity	358
44.3.3	Primary Study Endpoints	358
44.3.4	Secondary Study Endpoints	358

44.3.5	Overall Relapse/Progression	359
44.3.6	Prognostic Parameters	359
44.4	**Discussion**	359
44.4.1	Rationale of Radiotherapy	360
44.4.2	Clinical Results of Radiotherapy	361
44.4.3	Prognostic Factors	363
44.4.4	Potential Side Effects of Radiotherapy	363
44.4.5	Radiotherapy and Surgery	364
44.5	**Conclusions**	364
References		369

M.H. Seegenschmiedt (✉)
Strahlenzentrum Hamburg
Strahlentherapie & Radioonkologie, Hamburg, Germany

Klinik für Strahlentherapie und Radioonkologie,
Alfried Krupp Krankenhaus, Essen, Germany
e-mail: mhs@szhh.info

L. Keilholz
Klinik für Strahlentherapie,
Klinikum Bayreuth, Bayreuth, Germany

M. Wielpütz • C. Schubert
Klinik für Strahlentherapie und Radioonkologie,
Alfried Krupp Krankenhaus, Essen, Germany

F. Fehlauer
Strahlenzentrum Hamburg
Strahlentherapie & Radioonkologie, Hamburg, Germany
e-mail: fehlauer@szhh.info

44.1 Introduction

Dupuytren's disease (DD) is *a proliferative disorder* of the connective tissue involving the palmar fascia of the hand. In its early stage, *subcutaneous nodules* appear, which may be fixed to the overlying skin. Later, *tough cords* develop and become predominant in what is called Dupuytren's contracture. With further progression, the cords reach the periosteum of the hand bones and lead to advanced DD which is characterized by the contraction of the palm and the medial phalangeal (MP) and proximal interphalangeal (PIP) joints. This creates the typical *flexion deformity* of the palm and an increasing *extension deficit* of the involved fingers. The clinical staging of DD according to Tubiana et al. (1966) is based on this functional loss of the finger movement (Görlich 1981; McFarlane et al. 1990; Millesi 1981; Moorhead 1956; Schink 1978) (Table 44.1).

DD was initially described by Felix Platter (1614) and Sir Astley Cooper (1822) but is named after the French Guillaume Dupuytren (Dupuytren 1832, 1834). Its prevalence is 1–3% in Central Europe (McFarlane et al. 1990;

C. Eaton et al. (eds.), *Dupuytren's Disease and Related Hyperproliferative Disorders*,
DOI 10.1007/978-3-642-22697-7_44, © Springer-Verlag Berlin Heidelberg 2012

Table 44.1 Classification of Dupuytren's disease (DD) according to Tubiana et al. (1966)

Stage	Clinical symptoms	Extent of extension deficit
Stage N	Nodules, cords, skin retraction and fixation, etc.	None, i.e., no flexion deformity
Stage N/I	As stage N plus deformity of fingers	1–10°[a]
Stage I	As stage N plus flexion deformity of fingers	11–45°
Stage II	As stage N plus flexion deformity of fingers	46–90°
Stage III	As stage N plus flexion deformity of fingers	91–135°
Stage IV	As stage N plus flexion deformity of fingers	>135°

[a]Stage N modified from Keilholz et al. (1996)

Viljanto 1973) but varies widely worldwide (Strickland et al. 1990). Caucasians are believed to be mostly affected (Early 1962; Brenner et al. 1994). Very high prevalence is noted in regions of Ireland, Scotland, and France (Rafter et al. 1980; Brouet 1986) but more recently also in other European countries like Belgium (Degreef and de Smet 2010) and Bosnia (Zerajic and Finsen 2012). DD starts usually in the fourth decade and peaks in the fifth to sixth decade with a male to female ratio of 3:1 (Yost et al 1955). Two-thirds of the patients may develop a bilateral affliction (McFarlane et al. 1990; Hueston 1987). A family background is more pronounced among female than male patients (Early 1962; Ling 1963; McFarlane et al. 1990).

Etiology and pathogenesis are still poorly understood: In the past, DD has been often associated with certain risk factors including alcohol or nicotine abuse, diabetes, and epilepsy (Brenner et al. 1994) but results are still contradictory, and more recently occupation is also being considered as a potential influence of DD onset (Al-Qattan 2006; Descatha 2012).

The clinical course and the typical pathological features of DD are divided in (a) a *proliferative phase* (increased fibroblasts, nodule formation), (b) an *involutional phase* (increased myofibroblasts in diseased fiber bundles) which leads to contracture, and (c) a *residual phase* (collagenous fibers dominate in the connective tissues) (Luck 1959; Tomasek et al. 1987; Mohr and Wessinghage 1994). The different cellular composition especially regarding the low cellularity of proliferating fibroblasts and myofibroblasts in normal tendons and scar tissue and the high cellularity of nodules and cords of the palmar fascia in Dupuytren's disease is shown in Fig. 44.1. This underlines the important role of proliferating fibroblasts and myofibroblasts in the initial disease progression and final transformation into scarring tissue with functional deficit (Dave et al. 2001; Moyer et al. 2002).

Unlike aggressive fibromatosis (desmoids), DD never exhibits an invasion of voluntary muscles (Allen

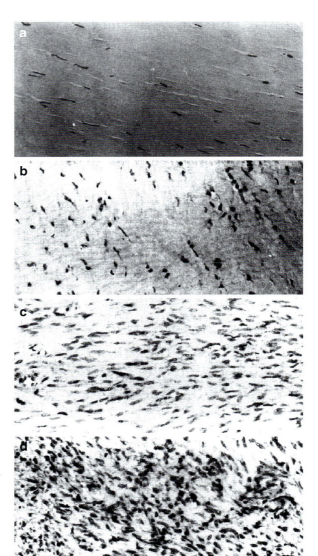

Fig. 44.1 Histopathogenesis of Dupuytren's disease and related tissues. (a) Typical tendon tissue with low cellularity. (b) Typical scar tissue with low cellularity. (c) Typical Dupuytren's cord tissue with increased cellularity. (d) Typical Dupuytren's nodular tissue with increased cellularity

1977). DD may progress slowly, sometimes stabilizes for years, but only rarely regresses spontaneously. Without any therapy, DD progresses in about 30–50% within 5 years leading to functional deficiencies and requiring surgical correction (Millesi 1981). Thus, any successful early treatment strategy requires at least 5 years follow-up (FU) for long-term evaluation.

Several noninvasive treatment options have been suggested for prophylaxis of DD progression, but so far no specific drugs (including steroids, allopurinol, DMSO, NSAIDs, enzymes, vitamin E) have been able to prevent the disease progression in the early DD stages (Falter et al. 1991). Injection of corticosteroids did not provide effective long-term results (Ketchum and Donahue 2000). Recently, in more advanced DD stages the injection of collagenase has been examined and found to provide effective release of contracted tissue especially for PIP joints; long-term data over several years are not yet available (Badalamente and Hurst 2012). In addition, minimal invasive surgical techniques like needle fasciotomy have been developed in France and implemented to provide effective release in contracted fingers (Badois et al. 1993). Both minimal invasive techniques provide quick recovery and alleviate repetitive application but with short or uncertain recurrence periods, respectively. Furthermore, both techniques show limited results for PIP joints. Surgery, including fasciotomy and local excision, partial or total fasciectomy, is reserved for advanced *DD stages*, when flexion deformity and function-limiting extension deficits are more prominent and disturb the daily activities. The principal aim is not to cure but to restore normal hand function (Murrell and Francis 1994). Unfortunately, all surgical results are impaired by complication rates in the range of 15–20% and high relapse or progression rates of 30–50% despite successful surgical removal of diseased areas (McFarlane et al. 1990; Falter et al. 1991; Murrell and Francis 1994; Geldmacher 1994; Au-Yong et al. 2005; Loos et al. 2007; Denkler 2010; Becker and Davis 2010). Additional postoperative splinting seems to offer no benefit (Jerosch-Herold et al. 2012). Nevertheless, repeated surgical procedures are required throughout the lifetime (Millesi 1981; Hueston 1987). Moreover, unilateral affliction can develop into bilateral affliction, and additional Ledderhose's disease (LD) may affect previously uninvolved feet.

The *radiobiological potential* of ionizing radiation is clearly limited to the early DD stages, as long as the proliferating fibroblasts exist as predominant radiosensitive target. In addition, the excessively expressed growth factors – platelet-derived growth factor (= PDGF) and tumor growth factor beta (= TGFβ) – can be influenced and downregulated, as they are responsible for the disturbed growth regulation of the fibroblastic system with rapid increase and ongoing stimulation of the myofibroblast proliferation and an aberrant collagen production. Thus, the highly activated monocyte-macrophage system in DD can be regarded as another important radiosensitive target, which is responsible for and initiates the extensive myofibroblast proliferation, at least in the early stages of DD, i.e., during the periods when nodules and cords are developing, but not in the phase of tissue scarring (Lubahn et al. 1984; Terek et al. 1995; Tomasek and Rayan 1995; Rayan et al. 1996; Rubin et al. 1999; Kampinga et al. 2004), Fig. 44.2a, b.

Several uncontrolled clinical studies – mostly from Europe and Germany – support the concept of prophylactic RT (Kaplan 1949; Finney 1955; Wasserburger 1956; Dewing 1965; Braun-Falco et al. 1976; Lukacs et al. 1978; Vogt and Hochschau 1980; Hesselkamp et al. 1981; Haase 1982; Köhler 1984; Herbst and Regler 1986; Keilholz et al. 1996, 1997). Long-term analysis has revealed a decreasing response rate with increasing follow-up and increasing stage of DD, but so far RT has not been accepted as a "standard treatment," (Order and Donaldson 1990; Suit and Spiro 1999) although recently some countries have changed their policies regarding the use of RT for early stage DD. For example, the National Institute for Health and Clinical Excellence (NICE) has issued full guidance to the NHS in England, Wales, Scotland, and Northern Ireland on radiation therapy for early Dupuytren's disease (NICE 2010). Nevertheless, the professional awareness for the use of RT and practical skills among radiation therapists and the interdisciplinary cooperation have still to grow in the future (Leer et al. 2007). More important, however, is the fact that treating early stage DD by RT has been increasingly recognized as a means to postpone or even avoid surgery (Dupuytren Society 2011) but is still far from being a generally accepted treatment option.

Although several RT dose concepts have been successfully applied in the past, RT has never been tested in a prospective clinical study against a control group. The first 1-year interim results of our group's prospectively controlled randomized clinical trial were presented (Seegenschmiedt 2001) was designed to establish a dose-response relationship and to optimize the radiotherapeutic treatment management.

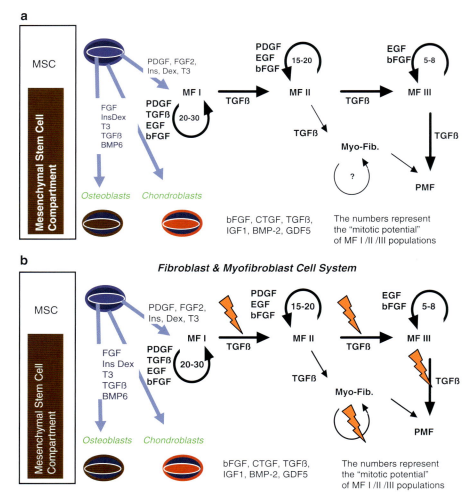

Fig. 44.2 (**a**) Pathomechanism of hyperproliferation in the soft tissue. Fibroblasts like osteoblasts and chondroblasts derive from the unique Mesenchymal Stem Cell Compartment (*MSC*). The proliferation and differentiation of the Fibroblast Cell System (*FCS*) is regulated by multiple growth factors and cytokines including the Platelet-Derived Growth Factor (*PDGF*), the basic Fibroblast Growth Factor (*bFGF*), the Epidermal Growth Factor (*EGF*), and the Tissue Growth Factor β (*TGF β*). The PDGF, bFGF, and EGF all act as mitogenetic stimulus for the myofibroblast generations *MF I-*, *MF II-*, and *MF-III-*Fibroblasts derived from the precursor compartment MSC; while PDGF is only weakly mitogenetic for MF-III-Fibroblasts, *TGFβ* induces a rapid mitosis and differentiation of the MF-I-Fibroblasts and their further differentiation into MF-II- and MF-III-Fibroblasts. Simultaneously, *TGFβ* has a leading role for the induction of myofibroblasts and the activation of the collagen synthesis. As seen in the graphic, *TGFβ* supports the shortcut from the proliferative MF II-Fibroblasts to the postmytotic myofibroblasts (*PMF*) via myofibroblasts (*MF*) in an unknown quantity. (**b**) Radiogenic targets to affect the soft tissue hyperproliferation in DD. Ionizing radiation (*RT*) interacts with all generations of myofibroblasts (*MF I, MF II and MF III*) through the Tissue Growth Factor ß (*TGFβ*) leading to a termination of the proliferation and increased transfer into the inactive and postmitotic myofibrocyte population (*PMF*)

44.2 Patients, Materials, and Methods

44.2.1 Patient Characteristics

From January 1997 to December 2009, 624 patients with clinically evident and progressive early stage DD were referred to our clinic for RT or further counseling by orthopedists, surgeons, and family physicians. As of January 2011, a total of 489 patients (198 females; 291 males) had reached a minimum follow-up (FU) of at least 5 years and therefore have been included in our study and were analyzed. The overall mean age was 61.6 ± 10 (median 61, range 29–81) years. Females were older (mean 63.2 ± 9) than males (60.6 ± 11 years). After clinical examination, extensive counseling about the different treatment options including a "wait and see" strategy, 83 patients decided not to receive prophylactic RT for personal or other reasons and served as control group without RT in long-term follow-up. The other 406 patients, who decided to undergo RT were randomized between two different RT concepts: 199 patients received 21 Gy (7×3 Gy) ("low-dose RT") total dose, while 207 patients received 30 Gy (10×3 Gy) ("high-dose RT") total dose. All patients completed the prescribed RT protocol and all FU evaluations at 3 and 12 months and at last FU after RT in December 2010.

44.2.2 Site Characteristics

A total of 258 (53%) patients presented with unilateral DD, while 230 (47%) had bilateral DD, which resulted in a total of 718 hands (sites) included in this study. A positive family record in the first generation (parents and siblings) was found in 142 (28.5%) patients for DD, in 66 (13.5%) patients for LD, and in 21 (4%) patients for other DD-related conditions such as Garrod's disease (GD) and frozen shoulder syndrome. The time period from first recognition of typical DD symptoms until presentation at our clinic and onset of treatment was 24 ± 12 (range: 62–163) months.

44.2.3 Disease Predisposition

By using a structured questionnaire (Appendix) and careful interview, the following predisposing factors for DD were identified in the patients' record: A *positive family history* was found in 165 (34%) patients (92 of 198 (46%) females, 73 of 291 (25%) males); *Morbus Ledderhose* of the plantar fascia was found in 92 (19%) patients (51 females; 41 males); *Garrod's disease (knuckle pads)* was observed in 13 (3%) patients (7 females; 6 males); a *history of keloids/hypertrophic scar* after trauma or surgery was reported by 19 (4%) patients (11 females; 8 males); a *trauma* of the upper extremity and hand was documented in 39 (8%) patients (14 females; 25 males); *diabetes mellitus* was actually present in 36 (7%) patients (16 females; 20 males); an *epileptic disorder* was reported by 10 (2%) patients (3 females; 7 males); *liver disease/cirrhosis* in 28 (6%) was known in 28 (6%) patients (9 females; 19 males); the regular use of *nicotine* was stated by 22% patients (43 females; 65 males); regular *alcohol consumption* was reported by 62 (13%) patients (24 females; 38 males); combined use of regular alcohol and nicotine intake was stated by 47 (10%) of all patients, but these later figures regarding alcohol have to be taken with some uncertainty.

44.2.4 Pretreatment

One hundred and thirty-two (27%) patients underwent one or more of the following treatments prior to the use of RT: surgical procedures including local excisions and partial fasciectomy in 65 (13%) patients, topical use of steroids (injections) in 36 (7%), systemic NSAID in 28 (6%), vitamin E in 45 (9%) or other drugs in 14 (3%) patients, and other unspecified therapeutic measures in 16 (3%) patients.

44.2.5 Stage of Disease

Staging was conducted according to Tubiana et al. (1966), which is based on the measurable total flexion deformity of palm and involved MP/PIP/DIP finger joints (Table 44.1). As *stage I* comprises a very large range of function loss (1–45°) allowing no differentiation between initial and later changes, an *intermediate stage N/I* was defined for angle deficits of 1–10° (Keilholz et al. 1996, 1997). According to this modified classification, stage N occurred in 470 (65.5%) sites, stage N/I in 124 (17%), stage I in 106 (15%), and stage II in 18 (2.5%) sites. According to the patient's record, all involved sites had experienced progressive symptoms at least within the last 6–12 months before RT.

44.2.6 Objective Signs

The dimensions and consistency of nodules, cords, skin changes, and finger mobility were assessed by clinical inspection, palpation, and measurements with a linear ruler. All findings were drawn onto the skin and photographed or photocopied (Herbst and Regler 1986; Keilholz et al. 1996). An example is given in Fig. 44.3.

A total of 2,849 nodules were diagnosed in almost all patients and sites, i.e., 712 (99%) hands exposed a mean number of 4 nodules and a mean size of 1.1 cm in diameter for the respective largest nodule. In addition, 866 cords were diagnosed in 360 (50%) hands with a mean number of 2.4 and a mean length of 2.0 cm. Typical skin retractions or pits were found in 251 (31%) sites. An extension of the DD from the palmar region into the fingers (digital involvement) was found in 233 (32%) hands; an objective angle deficit was measured in 248 (34.5%) hands. The overall mean angle deficit of the most involved digit was 17.3°.

44.2.7 Subjective Symptoms

The following subjective symptoms were reported prior to the onset of RT: Patients complained about *pressure* in the palm in 75 (10%) sites, *tension* in the palm or in the fingers in 140 (19.5%) sites, *pain sensation* in 29 (4%) sites, and *burning or itching sensations* in 45 (6%) sites. Regarding hand dysfunction in daily life, 152 (21%) sites were affected, and 89 (12%) sites were affected for special functions during profession (e.g., musician, crafts work, etc.) or sports activities. Patients scored their symptoms on a 10-scale linear analogue scale (LAS). Overall, the symptom score for all patients at the time of first presentation and before onset of any treatment was 3.1 ± 1.7.

44.2.8 Radiotherapy

Local RT was applied depending on the individual grade and extent of DD. It was common policy in our clinic to treat the whole afflicted area of the palm including all palpable and visible nodes and cords with sufficient distal and proximal (1–2 cm) and lateral margins (1 cm) (Fig. 44.4). An orthovoltage unit[1] was used with 120 kV X-rays (20 mAs/2 mm Al filter) and two cones of 6 × 8 cm and 10 × 12 cm with a source to skin distance (SSD) of 40 cm. All uninvolved areas of the palm and digits were individually shielded using 3-mm-thick lead rubber plates (Fig. 44.5). In addition, all other recommended radiation protection measures (appropriate beam direction, patient positioning, use of lead apron, etc.) were applied to minimize radiation exposure to the patient.

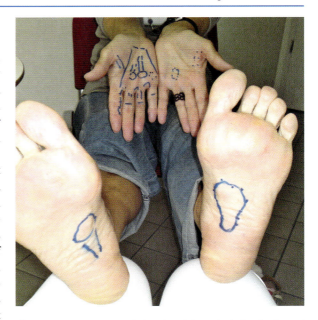

Fig. 44.3 A 49-year old female with typical distribution of nodes and cords in the right hand and two large nodes in both feet (combined Dupuytren and Ledderhose's disease). Stage N Dupuytren's disease in the right-hand palm plus early signs in the left-hand palm; stage I Ledderhose's disease in the right and stage II Ledderhose's in the left foot sole

44.2.9 Randomization

After full informed consent about the typical disease progression and all possible treatment options including RT, patients could decide between observation only and radiotherapy:

(a) *Eighty-three patients* (166 hands) decided to be observed and were regarded as "control group" (group A).

Those who decided to be treated were randomized to receive one of the following two RT schedules:

(b) *One hundred and ninety-nine patients* (293 hands) received 7 fractions of 3 Gy every other day (total dose: 21 Gy) in *one RT series* (total treatment time: 15 days or 2 weeks) (group B).

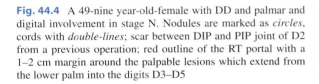
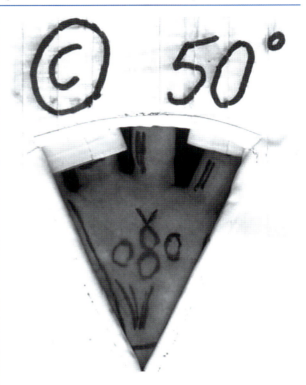

Fig. 44.4 A 49-nine year-old-female with DD and palmar and digital involvement in stage N. Nodules are marked as *circles*, cords with *double-lines*; scar between DIP and PIP joint of D2 from a previous operation; red outline of the RT portal with a 1–2 cm margin around the palpable lesions which extend from the lower palm into the digits D3–D5

Fig. 44.5 Individual shielding of uninvolved areas by 3-mm-thick lead rubber plate

44.2.10 Evaluation and Statistics

(c) *Two hundred and seven patients* (404 hands) received a total of 10 fractions of 3 Gy (total dose: 30 Gy) in 2 *series* of each 5×3 Gy in 1 week separated by 10–12 weeks (total treatment time: 12–16 weeks) (group C).

Most of the relevant patient and site characteristics were equally distributed between control and RT and between both RT groups (Tables 44.2 and 44.3). Minor differences were only observed between males and females; recurrent disease and DD stage II–IV disease was slightly more frequent in the control group (each 9%) as compared to the RT groups. All other differences were not statistically significant between the three groups.

All patients in this study completed at least 5 years follow-up (FU). Mean FU was 102 months and median FU 104 months. The clinical evaluation (treatment side effect and efficacy) was performed at 3 and 12 months and at last follow-up (FU) after RT. Final evaluation was in December 2010. Acute and chronic radiogenic toxicity was scored according to the Common Toxicity Criteria (CTC) (Trotti et al. 2000, 2003) and the Late Effects Normal Tissue (LENT) criteria (Pavy et al. 1995; Rubin et al. 1995; Seegenschmiedt 1998), each with 4 grades of severity. The *primary endpoints* of the study were *objective clinical signs of progression* and *necessity of surgery* or *salvage surgery*. Secondary endpoints were treatment of side effects and specific objective disease parameters (number and size of nodules, cords, flexion deformity of the palm, extension deficit of fingers) and subjective criteria (symptoms and function) and patient's subjective satisfaction using the 10-scale LAS.

The statistical analysis was performed with the software program SPSS (Chicago, IL). For categorical

Table 44.2 Patient characteristics

	A: control	B: RT 21 Gy	C: RT 30 Gy	All
Patients	83	199	207	489
– Females	34 (41%)	83 (42%)	81 (39%)	198 (40%)
– Males	49 (59%)	116 (58%)	126 (61%)	291 (60%)
Age (years) @ 1st Exam				
– Mean	61.3+11	62.1+13	62.6+9	61.6+10
– Median	61	63	62	62
– Range	29–74	34–79	33–81	29–81
Affected hands	122 (73%)	293 (74%)	303 (73%)	718 (73%)
# Hands (# pts × 2)	166	398	414	978
– Uninvolved	44 (27%)	105 (26%)	109 (26%)	258 (26%)
– Unilateral	44	105	109	258
– Bilateral	39	94	97	230
Positive family record (first degree)				
– Dupuytren's disease	27 (31%)	56 (28%)	59 (28.5%)	142 (28.5%)
– Ledderhose's disease	13 (16%)	27 (13.5%)	26 (12.5%)	66 (13.5%)
– Others (GD, FS etc.)	3 (3%)	8 (4%)	10 (5%)	21 (4%)
Comorbidity				
– Ledderhose's disease	17 (20.5%)	38 (19%)	37 (18%)	92 (19%)
– Garrod's disease (GD)	3 (4%)	6 (3%)	4 (2%)	13 (3%)
– Peyronie's disease (M)	3 (6%)	5 (4%)	4 (3%)	12 (3%)
– Frozen shoulder (FS)	6 (7%)	9 (4.5%)	8 (4%)	23 (5%)
– Keloid/Hypertr. Scar	4 (5%)	8 (4%)	7 (3%)	19 (4%)
– Any "Hand Trauma"	9 (11%)	14 (7%)	16 (8%)	39 (8%)
– Diabetes mellitus	7 (8%)	14 (7%)	15 (7%)	36 (7%)
– Any liver disease	5 (6%)	11 (5.5%)	12 (6%)	28 (6%)
– Epileptic disorder	2 (2%)	4 (2%)	4 (1.5%)	10 (2%)
Risk factors				
– Nicotine abuse (NA)	18 (22%)	46 (23%)	44 (21%)	108 (22%)
– Alcohol abuse (AA)	13 (16%)	26 (13%)	23 (11%)	62 (13%)
– Combined NA+AA	10 (12%)	19 (10%)	18 (9%)	47 (10%)
First symptoms (months) before RT				
– Mean	26±12	23±11	24±13	24±12
– Median	22	21	21	21
– Range	6–240	12–264	9–248	6–264
Follow-up (months)				
– Minimum	60	61	62	61
– Mean	102±18	103±19	102±21	102±20
– Median	104	105	104	104
– Range	60–160	61–162	62–163	62–163

DD Dupuytren's disease, *LD* Ledderhose's disease, *GD* Garrod's disease (knuckle pads), *FS* frozen shoulder, *NA* nicotine abuse, *AA* alcohol abuse

None of the above parameters were statistically significantly different between the treatment groups ($p < 0.05$)

44 Long-Term Outcome of Radiotherapy for Early Stage Dupuytren's Disease: A Phase III Clinical Study

Table 44.3 Treatment site characteristics

	A: control	B: RT 21 Gy	C: RT 30 Gy	All
Patients (Table 44.1)	83	199	207	489
Overall # hands	166	398	414	978
Affected hands	122 (73%)	293 (74%)	303 (73%)	718 (73%)
– Uninvolved	44 (27%)	105 (26%)	109 (27%)	258 (27%)
– Right hand (RH)	(23)	(54)	(52)	129
– Left hand (LH)	(21)	(51)	(57)	129
– Bilateral (RH+LH)	39 (47%)	94 (47%)	97 (47%)	230 (47%)
– Primary disease	113 (91%)	290 (99%)	299 (99%)	702 (98%)
– Recurrent (post Sx)	9 (9%)	3 (1%)	4 (1%)	16 (2%)
Nodes				
– Present (yes)	120 (98%)	291 (99%)	301 (99%)	712 (99%)
– Mean #	4.0 ± 2.3	4.1 ± 2.4	3.8 ± 2.0	4.0 ± 2.4
– Mean size (cm²)	1.0 ± 0.8	1.1 ± 0.9	1.2 ± 0.8	1.1 ± 0.9
Cords				
– Present (yes)	59 (48%)	146 (50%)	155 (51%)	360 (50%)
– Mean #	2.1 ± 1.3	2.4 ± 1.5	2.4 ± 1.5	2.4 ± 1.5
– Mean length (cm)	1.8 ± 1.2	2.1 ± 1.3	1.9 ± 1.1	2.0 ± 1.2
Pits				
– Present (yes)	46 (38%)	102 (35%)	103 (34%)	251 (35%)
Classification				
– Stage N	76 (62%)	195 (67%)	199 (66%)	470 (65,5%)
– Stage N/I	21 (21%)	50 (17%)	53 (17%)	124 (17%)
– Stage I	16 (16%)	43 (14,5%)	47 (16%)	106 (15%)
– Stage II–IV*	9 (9%)	5 (2%)	4 (1%)	18 (2.5%)
Clinical symptoms				
Digital involvement	41 (34%)	92 (31%)	100 (33%)	233 (32%)
Extension deficit	46 (38%)	98 (33%)	104 (34%)	248 (34.5%)
Mean deficit (°)*	26.6 ± 14.3	19.2 ± 6.9	15.0 ± 5.9	17.3 ± 9.1
– Pressure	14 (11.5%)	30 (10%)	31 (10%)	75 (10%)
– Tension	23 (19%)	56 (19%)	61 (20%)	140 (19.5%)
– Pain	6 (5%)	11 (4%)	12 (4%)	29 (4%)
– Itching & Other S.	8 (6.5%)	16 (5.5%)	21 (7%)	45 (6%)
Symptom score	3.3 ± 1.8	3.1 ± 1.6	3.0 ± 1.5	3.1 ± 1.7
Functional impairment				
– Any dysfunction	29 (24%)	62 (23%)	61 (20%)	152 (21%)
– Special functions (sports, hobbies)	18 (15%)	36 (12%)	35 (11.5%)	89 (12%)

DD Dupuytren's disease, *LD* Ledderhose's disease, *GD* Garrod's disease (knuckle pads), *FS* frozen shoulder, *NA* nicotine abuse, *AA* alcohol abuse, *n.a* not available

*$p < 0.05$

variable numbers and percentage values and for continuous variable median, mean and range values were calculated. Statistical testing for independence of categorical and continuous variables between different groups, time points, and study endpoints included the Student-t, the Cochran-Mantel-Haenszel, and the Wilcoxon test. Univariate and multivariate analyses were performed using the logistic regression analysis. P-values lower than 0.05 were defined as statistical significant for two-sided tests.

44.3 Results

44.3.1 Treatment Compliance

A total of 2 (1%) patients in group B (21 Gy total dose) received only 15 Gy, and 7 (3%) patients in group C (30 Gy total dose) did not receive the second RT series after completion of the first series (15 Gy) for various reasons. All patients were followed and evaluated according to the "intention-to-treat" concept in their specific treatment groups.

44.3.2 Treatment Toxicity

Acute toxicity within 6 weeks after RT was observed in 166 of 596 (28%) irradiated sites, in 151 (25%) cases presenting as redness or dryness of the skin (CTC grade 1), and in only 16 (2%) cases as an extensive erythema, moist desquamation, or with pronounced local swelling (CTC 2°). Most of these reactions were limited to the RT portal. Acute toxicity occurred more often and intensively after 7 fractions of 3 Gy (group B) than after each of the two RT series with each 5 fractions of 3 Gy (group C) (93/293 = 32% versus 74/303 = 24%, $p = 0.046$).

Chronic side effects at last FU occurred in 83 (14%) sites, either as *dryness*, *increased desquamation*, or *mild skin atrophy* accompanied by *slight subcutaneous fibrosis* which required occasionally to daily use moist ointments (LENT grade 1); in a few sites, alteration of heat and pain sensation occurred. In addition, the incidence of late effects was higher in the 21 Gy group (48 of 293 = 16%) as compared to the 30 Gy group (35 of 303 = 11.5%) ($p = 0.088$, n.s.), with a statistical trend in favor of the 30 Gy group.

44.3.3 Primary Study Endpoints

At last FU, an overall *DD stage progression* was observed in 176 of 718 (24.5%) sites. The differences in the DD stage progression between the control group with 63 of 122 hands progressing (52%) and the 21 Gy group with 64 of 293 hands (22%) ($p < 0.001$) and the 30 Gy group with 49 of 303 (16%) progressing ($p < 0.001$) were highly significant; however, the difference between the two RT groups showed only a statistical trend ($p = 0.077$). When *all clinical signs of progression* were included in the analysis, the progression rate of the control group was 76 of 122 (62%) versus 71 of 293 (24%) in the 21 Gy group and 59 of 303 (19.5%) in the 30 Gy group ($p < 0.001$); again, the difference between the RT groups was not statistically significant but with a statistical trend in favor of the 30 Gy group ($p = 0.106$). Similarly, when considering the number of sites which required surgery due to ongoing progression of the disease, the differences between the control group (37 of 122 = 30%) and the 21 Gy group (35 of 293 = 12%) and the 30 Gy group (25 of 303 = 8%) were highly statistically significant ($p < 0.001$), while the differences between the RT groups were not significant ($p = 0.134$).

44.3.4 Secondary Study Endpoints

Similar, several other details in treatment outcome showed a clear advantage of the two RT groups (21 and 30 Gy) versus the control group:

(a) The mean *number of nodes per site* increased in the control group (plus 1.2–5.2 nodes), while it was reduced in the 21 Gy (−0.4 to 3.7 nodes) and 30 Gy group (−0.6 to 3.6 nodes) (both p < 0.001).

(b) The mean *number of cords per site* increased in the control group (plus 1.1–3.2 cords), while it was reduced in the 21 Gy (− 0.4 to 2.0 cords) and 30 Gy group (−0.3 to 2.1 cords) (both $p < 0.001$).

(c) The *digital involvement* at last FU increased in the control group in 37 of 122 (30%) sites as compared to the 21 Gy group with 16 of 293 (5.5%) and the 30 Gy group with 9 of 303 (3%) (both $p < 0.001$).

(d) The *extension deficit* at last FU increased in the control group in 43 of 122 (35%) sites as compared to the 21 Gy group with 21 of 293 (7%) and the 30 Gy group with 13 of 303 (4%) (both $p < 0.001$).

(e) The *mean angle of the extension deficit* at last FU increased in the control group by an average of 13.2° as compared to 2.2° (21 Gy group) and 0.9° (30 Gy group) (both $p < 0.05$).

(f) The *mean symptom score* at last FU increased in the control group by an average of 1.4–4.7 points as compared to a reduction of 0.5 points to 2.6 points in the 21 Gy group and of 0.7 points to 2.3 points in the 30 Gy group (both $p < 0.05$). Symptom relief occurred in 4 of 51 (8%) affected sites in the control group as compared to 24 of 113 (21%) in the 21 Gy group and 32 of 125 (26%) in the 30 Gy group (both $p < 0.001$).

(g) The *overall satisfaction with the disease status* at last FU was 12 of 122 (10%) in the control group and 141 of 293 (48%) in the 21 Gy group and 155 of 303 (51%) in the 30 Gy group (both $p < 0.001$).

44.3.5 Overall Relapse/Progression

At last FU 63 of 122 sites in the control group revealed disease progression in the "potential RT portal," i.e., within an initially suggested RT area. In contrast, progression or relapse within an irradiated area was only present in 28 of 293 (9.5%) sites of the 21 Gy groups and in 22 of 303 (7%) sites of the 30 Gy group (both $p < 0.001$). However, additional progression outside the irradiated area occurred in 63 of 293 (21.5%) hands of the 21 Gy group and in 51 of 303 (17%) hands of the 30 Gy group. This indicates, that sometimes RT portals may have been chosen too small, or ongoing trigger mechanisms have initiated further disease in untreated areas as compared to treated areas. Salvage treatments included surgery (as mentioned above) and salvage RT in 24 of 122 (20%) of the control group and in 16 of 293 (5.5%) hands in the 21 Gy group and in 18 of 303 (6%) hands in the 30 Gy group (both $p < 0.001$).

44.3.6 Prognostic Parameters

Differences in treatment outcome were analyzed for the two endpoints "progression of disease" and "surgery required" at last FU. As already shown, the use of RT treatment with either 21 Gy or 30 Gy was far superior to avoid disease progression than with observation only, while the differences between the two RT groups were not significant but revealed a statistical trend in favor of the 30 Gy group over the 21 Gy group with regard to DD stage progression ($p = 0.077$) and overall signs of progression ($p = 0.106$).

Several *patient-related parameters* were analyzed: With regard to *gender*, 68 of 198 (34%) females and 108 of 291 (37%) males experienced progression (n.s.); with regard to *age*, 85 of 263 (32%) patients older than 60 years had progression as compared to 91 of 225 (40%) patients younger than 60 years. Regarding the *use of nicotine*, 49 of 108 (45%) smokers experienced progression as compared to 129 of 381 (33%) non-smokers ($p = 0.028$); regarding the *use of alcohol*, 29 of 62 (47%) patients with regular alcohol intake experienced progression as compared to 147 of 427 (34%) abstinent patients ($p = 0.028$).

Patients with a longer *symptom duration* prior to RT had a higher rate of progression than those with a shorter interval. Using a cutoff value of 24 months, 98 of 231 (42%) with longer duration of symptoms developed progression as compared to 78 of 258 (30%) with shorter duration.

The *DD stage prior to RT* was the most important prognostic factor for treatment outcome independent from the treatment group. Forty-seven of 470 (10%) sites with stage N, 51 of 124 (41%) sites with stage N/I, 62 of 106 (58%) sites with stage I, and 16 of 18 (89%) sites with stages II, III, and IV progressed in long-term FU. In summary, patients with a higher DD stage developed higher progression rates ($p < 0.0001$) (Table 44.4).

The relevant prognostic parameters from the univariate analysis were also used for the final multivariate analysis using a logistic regression process. Table 44.5 summarizes the result: Only symptom duration >24 months, advanced stage of disease (N versus N/I and more), digital involvement, and the use of RT were statistically significant parameters; use of smoking showed a statistical trend. In addition, the difference between the two dose groups showed a statistical trend in favor of the 30 Gy group.

44.4 Discussion

This clinical study is the first to document the long-term outcome of untreated DD versus DD treated with RT applied in two different dose levels. The distribution

Table 44.4 Stage of DD prior to RT and DD stage progression at last FU

	A: control	B: RT 21 Gy	C: RT 30 Gy	All
Progression	$n = 122$	$n = 293$	$N = 303$	$N = 718$
DD stage				
Stage N	26 of 76 (34%)	14 of 195 (7%)	7 of 199 (3.5%)	47 of 470 (10%)
Stage N/I	14 of 21 (67%)	21 of 50 (42%)	16 of 53 (30%)	51 of 124 (41%)
Stage I	14 of 16 (87.5%)	25 of 43 (58%)	23 of 47 (49%)	62 of 106 (58%)
Stage II–IV	9 of 9 (100%)	4 of 5 (80%)	3 of 4 (75%)	16 of 18 (89%)
DD stage progression	63 of 122 (52%)	64 of 293 (22%)	49 of 303 (16%)	176 of 718 (24,5%)

Statistical analysis with 8 degrees of freedom: $p < 0.0001$

Table 44.5 Prognostic parameters for disease progression in multivariate analysis

Parameter	Partition (favorable first)	*p*-value	Odds ratio
Patient			
Gender	Female vs. male	= 0.26, n.s.	1.29
Age	≥60 vs. <60 years	= 0.18, n.s.	1.43
Smoking	Non-smoking vs. smoking	= 0.08	1.58
Alcohol	Non-alcohol vs. alcohol	= 0.12, n.s.	1.36
Disease			
Symptom duration	<24 vs. ≥24 months	= 0.007	1.86
Stage of disease	Stage N vs. N/I–IV	<0.001	3.41
Extension deficit	0–5° vs. >6° to >90°	<0.001	2.67
Digital involvement	No involvement vs. involvement	<0.01	1.78
Treatment			
RT vs. No RT	RT (21 & 30) vs. control	<0.0001	6.32
RT dose	RT 21 vs. 30 Gy	=0.08	1.61

of all relevant data regarding the patient and site-specific characteristics enable a direct comparison of outcomes. Thus, it is necessary to understand the basic rationale for the use of ionizing radiation in the early stages of DD, as only the early stages of DD seem to be most responsive to the use of ionizing radiation.

44.4.1 Rationale of Radiotherapy

Early stages of DD are characterized by *proliferation of fibrous tissue* in the form of nodules or cords; they have several features in common with benign neoplastic fibromatosis (McFarlane et al. 1990; Luck 1959). The evolution of DD acts similar to the *wound healing* through contraction and maturation of fibrous tissue (Rodemann and Bamberg 1995; Mutsaers et al. 1997). The fibro-fatty tissue between the skin and palmar aponeurosis is regarded as primary site of disease onset. The abnormal fibrous tissue develops around ligamentous cords that have a predominantly longitudinal orientation and follow the tension lines

of the palm. *Pathological forces* and *mechanical stress* play an important role in the pathogenesis and development of DD (Flint 1990a). From a radiobiological view, the *proliferation process* is the most important component of DD. It is driven by *immature fibroblast and myofibroblasts* (Gabbiani et al. 1971; Rudolph and Vande Berg 1991), which produce the extracellular matrix consisting of fibronectin, laminin, collagen type IV, and tenascin (Berndt et al. 1994). Myofibroblast phenotypes and growth factor gene synthesis are present in active proliferating nodules of DD (Berndt et al. 1994). Similar to the wound healing process in DD, increased *growth factor* levels are found including the messenger-RNA for interleukin-1, basic fibroblast growth factor (bFGF), transforming growth factor beta (TGF-beta), platelet-derived growth factor (PDGF) (Terek et al. 1995; Tomasek and Rayan 1995; Kampinga et al. 2004), epidermal growth factor (EGF), and connective tissue growth factor (CTGF) which stimulate the fibroblast proliferation (Baird et al. 1993; Brenner et al. 1996; Igarashi et al. 1996).

It has been suggested that in DD, local ischemia is induced by microvessel narrowing, which produce free radicals and damage the surrounding stroma and stimulate perivascular fibroblast proliferation; repeated pericyte damage, fibroblast proliferation, and collagen deposition further enhance microvessel ischemia, thereby self-propagating the pathogenetic process (Gabbiani et al. 1971; Kischer and Speer 1986; Murrell et al. 1989, 1990). However, so far there is not a clear concept of what really initiates the pathological proliferation in DD: a *traumatic process*, i.e., rupture of fascial fibers (Skoog 1948; Flint 1990b; Rodemann and Bamberg 1995) or an *inflammatory process* with adhesions between ligamentous structures (Andrew et al. 1991; McGrouther 1982). In the latter situation, additional radiosensitive targets are available.

In summary, the pathogenesis of DD provides a good rationale for using ionizing radiation in early DD stages: (a) *Proliferating fibroblasts and myofibroblasts* are radiosensitive target cells; (b) the radiogenic induction of free radicals damages fibroblasts, impairs their proliferative activity, and thereby may reduce cell density (Murrell and Francis 1994); (c) RT interferes with the over-expressed growth factors, especially PDGF and TGF beta (Terek et al. 1995; Tomasek and Rayan 1995; Rayan et al. 1996; Kampinga et al. 2004); (d) *activated monocytes and macrophages* are very radiosensitive target cells which interact with the inflammatory and reparative processes and the onset and extent of myofibroblast proliferation (Rubin et al. 1999). In the past, similar pathogenetic pathways and radiosensitive target cells have been identified for the prophylactic effects of intravascular RT to inhibit arterial restenosis (Crocker 1999; Tripuraneni et al. 1999) or for use of external beam RT to avoid relapses after resection of keloids (Suit and Spiro 1999) or pterygium of the eye (Smitt and Donaldson 1999) or to influence progression Morbus Ledderhose (Seegenschmiedt & Attassi, 2003) and in Peyronie's disease (Incrocci et al. 2008). Moreover, in the radiotherapy community the awareness and skills about the use of RT for benign conditions has clearly increased over the past decade (Leer et al. 2007).

44.4.2 Clinical Results of Radiotherapy

Besides our present study, the efficacy of local RT to impact on the early stages of DD has been shown in many clinical trials since the early 1950s of the last century (Finney 1955; Wasserburger 1956; Lukacs et al. 1978; Vogt and Hochschau 1980; Hesselkamp et al. 1981; Haase 1982; Köhler 1984; Herbst and Regler 1986; Keilholz et al. 1996, 1997) (Table 44.6). However, the first clinical studies were limited by short FU: Lukacs et al. (1978) observed "no disease progression" in 36 sites at 1 year. Hesselkamp et al. (1981) reached "improved or stable conditions" for over 2 years in 93% of 46 sites. Vogt and Hochschau (1980) found 94% of 109 irradiated sites "stable" or "improved" after more than 3 years. Köhler (1984) reported 82% of 33 sites "improved or stable," and 6 "progressed" after 3 years. Herbst and Regler (1986) observed all 45 sites "stable or improved" after a median of 1.5 years.

It was the group in Erlangen (Germany) which reported the first 5-year results which could be compared with the reported outcome in published surgical series: Keilholz et al. (1996, 1997) found 72% of 142 sites with "regression of nodules and cords" at last FU; of 57 sites with a minimum FU of 5 years, only 5 (9%) sites progressed outside and 8 (14%) inside the RT portal; thus the overall local control was 77%. Adamietz et al. (2001) conducted an extended analysis of the same study population, but with a longer median FU of 10 years, and confirmed the results from the pilot study. They also identified a DD stage-dependent response pattern, with better outcome in early DD stages as compared to more advanced DD stages: In stage N 84% and stage N/I 67% of cases remained stable, while 65% of stage I and 83% in stage II had progressive nodules and cords. In case of DD progression, no complications occurred after a further RT series or after salvage surgery. Recently, Betz et al. (2010) increased the median FU of the same study population to 13 years and confirmed the stage-dependent outcome which corresponds well with the stage-dependent outcome in our own study.

Ten years ago, our pilot study (Seegenschmiedt et al. 2001) was the first to analyze the impact of different RT dose regimens on treatment outcome. In the actual update of this study, the long-term analysis, not only a DD stage-dependent response pattern can be confirmed but also a superiority of RT versus observation only. All together, our clinical data demonstrate and confirm that the observed progression rate in early DD stages is much lower after irradiation than the expected 50% progression rate within 5 years for untreated patients or for patients who have to undergo

Table 44.6 Clinical results of radiotherapy for Dupuytren's contracture (literature review)

Study (year)	Patients (sites) (Stage)	(N)	RT concept Fractioning	RT dose	Follow-up N (%)	Clinical outcome [N (%)] "Regression"	"No change"	"Progression"
Finney (1955)	43	NA	1–3 × RT Ra-Moulage	1–3.000 r	FU: NA 25 (58%) sites	15/25 (60%) "Good functional result"		
Wasserburger (1956)	213	NA	1–3 × RT Ra-Moulage	1–3.000 r	"Long–term" 146 (69%) pts	"Long-term cure" stage I: 62 of 69 (90%); Stage II: 26 of 46 (57%); stage III: 10 of 31 (32%)		
Lukacs et al. (1978)	106	(I: 140) (II: 18)	RT day 1+2 4 series á 2 mos	4 Gy SD 32 Gy TD	FU: NA 36 (23%) sites	I: 26 of 32 (81%) II: 3 of 4 (75%)	I: 6 of 32 (19%)	None
Vogt and Hochschau (1980)	(I: 98) (II: 4) (III: 7)	(154)	RT day 1+2 5 series á 2 mos	4 Gy SD 32 Gy TD	FU>3 years 109 (63%) pts	I: 21 of 98 (21%) II: 1 of 4 (25%) III: --	I: 73 of 98 (74%) II: 2 of 4 (50%) III: 6 of 7 (86%)	I: 4 of 98 (4%) II: 1 of 4 (25%) III: 1 of 5 (20%)
Hesselkamp et al. (1981)	46	(65)	RT day 1+2 5 series á 3 mos	4 Gy SD 40 Gy TD	FU 1–9 years 46 (53%) pts	Total: 24 (52%)	Total: 19 (41%)	Total: 3 (7%);
Köhler (1984)	31	(38)	RT 3–5×/week 1 series	2 Gy SD 20 Gy TD	FU 1–3 years 33 (87%) sites	Total: 7 (21%)	Total: 20 (61%)	Total: 6 (18%)
Herbst et al. 1986	33	(46)	RT 5×/week 2 series á 1–3 mos	3 Gy SD <42 Gy TD	FU>1,5 years 46 (100%) sites	None	Total: 45 (98%)	Total: 1 (2%)
Keilholz et al. (1997)	96 pts 142 hands	(N: 82) (N/I: 17) (I: 30) (II: 13)	RT 5×/week 6 weeks break 2 series á 2 mos	3 Gy SD 30 Gy TD	FU 1–12 years; median: 6 years	10(7%) improved @ 3 months,, 130 (92%) stable, 2 (1%) progressed Stages N: 99%, N/I: 88%, I: 77%, II–IV: 54% progression-free 13 (23%) progression inside (8 cases) or outside (5 cases) of RT field.		
Adamietz et al. (2001)	99 pts 176 hands	(N: 81) (N/I: 15) (I: 65) (II: 15)	Same RT concept	3 Gy SD 30 Gy TD	FU 7–18 years; median: 10 years	Stages N: 84%, N/I: 67%, I: 35%, II–IV: 17% remain progression-free		
Betz et al. (2010)	135 pts 208 hands	(N: 115) (N/I: 33) (I: 50) (II: 10)	Same RT concept	3 Gy SD 30 Gy TD	FU 2–25 years; median: 13 years	20 (10%) improved, 123 (59%) remained stable, 65 (31%) progressed Stages N 87%, N/I: 70%, I: 38%, II–IV: 14% progression-free		
Seegenschmiedt et al. (2001)	2 arms			3 Gy SD		Subjective/Objective	Subjective/ Objective	Subjective/Objective
	A: 63	(95)	RT 5×/week (×2)	30 Gy TD	FU>1 year all (100%) pts	55 (56%) symptoms	35 (37%) symptoms	7 (7%) symptoms
	B: 66	(103)	RT 3×/week	21 Gy TD		55 (53%) symptoms	39 (38%) symptoms	9 (9%) symptoms

surgery in advanced DD stages (Millesi 1981). In the more advanced DD stages, stage I to stage IV, however, RT appears not to be as effective, which corresponds well with a relatively presence of proliferating fibroblast and myofibroblasts in these DD stages.

Moreover, our actual clinical study has been conducted in a controlled prospective design which overcomes the previous criticism of using only a retrospective analysis. Thus, our study is the first clear proof of a "therapeutic window" for RT in the early stage of DD. Although the differences between the two RT groups were not yet statistically significant, there is a statistical trend in favor of the higher RT dose of 30 Gy applied in a protracted regimen over 3 months as compared to the lower dose of 21 Gy applied over 2 weeks. With higher numbers for patients and sites, this difference in efficacy and probably less acute side-effects may become statistically significant. Nevertheless, multicenter clinical data are required to confirm these monocentric results.

44.4.3 Prognostic Factors

Köhler (1984) suggested a total dose of at least 20 Gy (10×2 Gy) to avoid DD progression, but his regimen was less successful than most other studies using higher total RT doses, such as 32–40 Gy (4 Gy single dose) (Vogt and Hochschau 1980; Hesselkamp et al. 1981). In the first clinical studies, single doses of 1,000r (corresponding to 10 Gy) every 3–6 months up to a total dose of 3,000r (30 Gy) had been successfully applied (Finney 1955; Finck 1955; Wasserburger 1956). The three clinical studies from Erlangen obtained good long-term outcome using 30 Gy total dose in two RT series of each 5×3 Gy. Our study confirms that a total dose of 30 Gy seems to be more effective than a lower dose of 21 Gy despite using the same single doses (3 Gy). Both dose- and time-dependent effects can be responsible for observed differences in long-term outcome. It is interesting to note that the 21 Gy group developed more acute side effects than the 30 Gy group, while the chronic side effects were similar in both groups.

Using an appropriate RT technique seems to be another important factor for treatment outcome: While some groups have recommended the "whole palm irradiation" (Köhler 1984; Hesselkamp et al. 1981), which is far more than we would recommend, others includ-

ing ourselves have treated the diseased areas only but with sufficient safety margin (Vogt and Hochschau 1980; Keilholz et al. 1996, 1997). We usually apply an individual shielding of all uninvolved parts of the palm similar to the procedures proposed by Keilholz et al. (1996, 1997); however, this may allow DD progression outside the RT portal if the longitudinal and lateral extension of the disease have been underestimated. Thus, large safety margins of at least 1–2 cm around all visible and palpable lesions should avoid this problem. We do not apply total palm irradiation to avoid unnecessary side effects. We believe that out-field DD progression occurs not very often is then to a second RT series, as long as no major overlap with the primary RT portals exist; in contrast, in-field progression may require surgery. With regard to RT technique, there appears to be no difference between orthovoltage photons (120–150 kV) or linac electrons (3–6 MeV) as long as all nodes and cords are sufficiently covered; this may require a penetration depth of 5–15 mm down to the periosteum of the hand bones. The use of 120 kV/20mAs orthovoltage RT with a half-value layer of 33 mm is sufficient to reach this depth (Kaplan 1949; Finney 1955; Finck 1955; Dewing 1965). Historic RT studies have implemented the radium grip cylinder or radium molds (Wasserburger 1956; Dewing 1965). Nowadays, careful dosimetry and RT dose prescription according to the ICRU 50/62 and diligent RT application to all involved areas of DD are important requirements to achieve a favorable long-term outcome in DD and avoid possible relapses and unnecessary side effects.

44.4.4 Potential Side Effects of Radiotherapy

Ionizing radiation of 30 Gy induced only mild early or late radiogenic toxicity including minor effects like dryness of the skin; major fibrosis has been observed only in few patients, especially in previously operated sites. Simple skin care using moisture and greasy ointments is used to deal with these minor radiogenic sequelae. Late adverse side effects of grade 2 and more have never occurred in long-term FU. Our observations have been confirmed by others in long-term FU (Adamietz et al. 2001; Betz et al. 2010; Heyd et al. 2010). So single neoplasm was similar to the Erlangen study with long-term outcome

(Betz 2010) doses used for DD and LD are associated with a theoretical risk for induction of soft tissue sarcoma or skin cancer in the RT portals estimated to be in the range of 0.5–1% after latency periods of 8–30 years (Jansen et al. 2005; Trott and Kamprad 2006; Seegenschmiedt 2008), but only children and younger adults up to the age of 30 years may have an increased risk. Thus, critical indication after individual risk and benefit assessment and careful RT technique is required for this age group. However, at the present time, no single case of cancer induction has ever been reported after the use of RT for treatment of LD, DD, keloids, hypertrophic scars, or other benign hyperproliferative disorders.

44.4.5 Radiotherapy and Surgery

Among most hand surgeons, prophylactic RT is not only poorly known but also criticized for various reasons, e.g., long-term inefficacy (Finck 1955), surgery complications after application of RT (Falter et al. 1991; Weinzierl et al. 1993), or observed side effects (Falter et al. 1991). Although we doubt the latter observations as they lack controlled published data, we agree that advanced DD stage II–IV may not benefit from RT due to the loss of appropriate target cells, the actively proliferating fibroblast (Wasserburger 1956; Vogt and Hochschau 1980). In our study, DD stage I to stage IV were insufficiently treated with RT; even in DD stage N/I, only 58% in the 21 Gy group and 70% in the 30 Gy group were controlled in long-term FU without progression, which is still much better than the 33% in the control group. However, the best long-term results were achieved in DD stage N with over 90% of the irradiated sites remaining in a stable or even slightly improved condition. From this analysis, our advice is to transfer patients with advanced stages I–IV and/or recurrent lesions primarily to the hand surgeons. Close cooperation with hand surgeons is always important, as prophylactic RT should not impair possible good surgical results. In our study all those sites, which required hand surgery due to DD progression after prophylactic RT in long-term FU, were operated without surgical complications or enhanced perioperative morbidity.

In summary, the rationale for prophylactic RT applies to the early DD stage N and stage N/I with a maximum extension deficit of 10° because in this stage the clinical symptoms and functional deficits are still limited, and radiosensitive target cells and target mechanisms are still active. Otherwise, in the more advanced DD stages I to IV, more than 50% of patients will progress and suffer functional loss; at least 30% will require hand surgery within the next 5 years. It will be of great interest for the medical community if there might be a further role for RT in case of an early relapse after surgery, as this relapse may be driven by renewed fibroblast and myofibroblast proliferation. However, this question can only be answered in a prospective clinical study and in close cooperation with the hand surgeons.

44.5 Conclusions

The use of RT in early stage DD is superior to observation only. In long-term FU, the stage N and to some extent also stage N/I patients and sites clearly benefit from the prophylactic irradiation.

Both tested RT regimens (21 and 30 Gy) have been well accepted and tolerated by the patients. Acute toxicity was slightly enhanced in the low-dose group (21 Gy) compared with the medium-dose group (30 Gy), probably due to the time factor of a higher total dose within one RT series. Response to RT or avoidance of DD progression or surgery was slightly better in the 30 Gy group as compared to the 21 Gy group (statistical trend).

Important prognostic factors in univariate analysis were gender, age, alcohol and nicotine consumption, time interval of first symptoms to first treatment, DD stage, and DD stage-dependent parameters such as involvement of fingers and amount of extension deficit. The most important independent prognostic factor in multivariate analysis was DD stage and use of RT as compared to observation only.

Additional potential for RT may be relevant for those patients who develop a rapid progression or early relapse after surgery assuming that myofibroblasts and proliferating fibroblasts are also active in these situations; further prospective clinical trials and prognostic testing are required.

Appendix A

Morbus Dupuytren - Documentation		

Date of 1st Contact   ⌞ ⌟D⌞ ⌟M⌞ ⌟Y

Name .... **Birth Date** ⌞ ⌟D⌞ ⌟M⌞ ⌟Y

General Data :   ⌞ ⌟ **Right Handed**   ⌞ ⌟ **Left Handed**

Dupuytren in Family History?   ⌞ ⌟No; ⌞ ⌟ Yes, who? ....

Related Diseases Existing?   ⌞ ⌟M. Peyronie   ⌞ ⌟M. Ledderhose

....   ⌞ ⌟Knuckle Pads   ⌞ ⌟Keloid

Other Diseases Existing?   ⌞ ⌟Diabetes mellitus   ⌞ ⌟Epilepsy

Alcohol Intake ⌞ ⌟No ⌞ ⌟Yes   ⌞ ⌟Liver Disease, which: ....

Smoking   ⌞ ⌟No ⌞ ⌟Yes   ⌞ ⌟Artheriosclerosis, where: ....

Trauma involving Hands?   ⌞ ⌟which : ....

Professional / Leisure Hand Activities   ⌞ ⌟Rough Activities   ⌞ ⌟Fine Activities

Which Professional / Leisure Activity?   ....

1st Clinical Symptoms recognized since ....…....….... (months/years)

Clinical Symptoms Which?		Right Hand when?		Left Hand when?
Itching and Burning?	⌞ ⌟N	⌞ ⌟Y	⌞ ⌟N	⌞ ⌟Y
Tension Feeling?	⌞ ⌟N	⌞ ⌟Y	⌞ ⌟N	⌞ ⌟Y
Pressure Feeling?	⌞ ⌟N	⌞ ⌟Y	⌞ ⌟N	⌞ ⌟Y
Pain at Rest?	⌞ ⌟N	⌞ ⌟Y	⌞ ⌟N	⌞ ⌟Y
Pain during Motion?	⌞ ⌟N	⌞ ⌟Y	⌞ ⌟N	⌞ ⌟Y
Skin Retraction? / when?	⌞ ⌟N	⌞ ⌟Y /	⌞ ⌟N	⌞ ⌟Y /
Palpable Nodules? / when?	⌞ ⌟N	⌞ ⌟Y /	⌞ ⌟N	⌞ ⌟Y /
Palpable Cords? / when?	⌞ ⌟N	⌞ ⌟Y /	⌞ ⌟N	⌞ ⌟Y /
Flexion Deformity? / when?	⌞ ⌟N	⌞ ⌟Y /	⌞ ⌟N	⌞ ⌟Y /
Other Symptoms? / which?	⌞ ⌟N	⌞ ⌟Y /	⌞ ⌟N	⌞ ⌟Y /

Free Text (Disease Development)

Have clinical symptoms increased within the past period? ⌊ ⌋ No; ⌊ ⌋ Yes,

within ⌊ ⌋ the past 4 weeks: .... ⌊ ⌋ the past 3 months: .....…..........................

⌊ ⌋ the past 12 months: ..…..…........ ⌊ ⌋ the past ⌊ ⌋ years : ....

Intercurrent stabilisation? ⌊ ⌋ no; ⌊ ⌋ yes, ……………………...............…….......…...............

Which physicians did you consult ?

⌊ ⌋ General Practitioner ⌊ ⌋ Specialist/Name : ....

Which treatment(s) has (have) been performed for the involved hand(s)?

Therapy :	Right Hand	Left Hand
Medication		
Steroids		
Allopurinol		
Antirheumatics/Antiphlogistics		
Vitamines		
Enzymes		
Tissue softening agents		
Others:		
Surgical Procedures (Date, Sx Type)		
Radiotherapy: (Date, RT Dose)		
Local Injections Date, Drug		
Lokal Ointments		
Other Therapies		

44 Long-Term Outcome of Radiotherapy for Early Stage Dupuytren's Disease: A Phase III Clinical Study

Basic Findings   **Date** ⌊ ⌋D⌊ ⌋M⌊ ⌋Y   **(prior to RT Start)**

Findings	Right Hand					Left Hand				
Digits	D 1	D 2	D 3	D 4	D 5	D 5	D 4	D 3	D 2	D 1
Skin Fixation (F)										
Skin Retraction (R)										
Nodules (N) [largest size [cm]										
Cords (C) [largest size [cm]										
Flexion Deformity [angle in degree "°"] – DIP joints < °	-------	-------	-------	-------	-------	-------	-------	-------	-------	-------
– PIP joints < °	-------	-------	-------	-------	-------	-------	-------	-------	-------	-------
– MP joints < °	------	------	------	------	------	------	------	------	------	------
Total Deficit : < °										
Hyperextension (H)										
Ankylosis (A)										
Other Findings: e.g. Surgical Scars etc.										
Symptom Score (LAS - scale 0–10)										
Disease Stage										

Abbreviations: finding at the palm (palmar) = **P**; findings at the fingers (digital) = **D**; combined = **PD**
Notes:

RT indication for ⌊ ⌋**Right Hand / D** .... ⌊ ⌋**Left Hand** ....

Obtain photo or photocopy of drawn findings and the planned RT treatment portal !

Date, Signature (Physician): ....

Follow-Up Findings   Date └   ┘D└   ┘M└   ┘Y   **(at** .... **months after RT)**

Findings	Right Hand					Left Hand				
Digits	**D 1**	**D 2**	**D 3**	**D 4**	**D 5**	**D 5**	**D 4**	**D 3**	**D 2**	**D 1**
Skin Fixation (F)										
Skin Retraction (R)										
Nodules (N) [largest size [cm]										
Cords (C) [largest size [cm]										
Flexion Deformity [angle in degree "°"] – DIP joints < °	-------	-------	-------	-------	-------	-------	-------	-------	-------	-------
– PIP joints < °	-------	-------	-------	-------	-------	-------	-------	-------	-------	-------
– MP joints < °	------	------	------	------	------	------	------	------	------	------
Total Deficit : < °										
Hyperextension (H)										
Ankylosis (A)										
Other Findings: e.g. Surgical Scars etc.										
Symptom Score (LAS-scale 0–10)										
Disease Stage										

Abbreviations: finding at the palm (palmar) = **P**; findings at the fingers (digital) = **D**; combined = **PD**
Change after RT: Improved (↑)"+++ 100% / ++ > 50% / + > 25%"; Stable"="; Worsened (↓)"– / – / –";

Notes:

Clinical Status: └   ┘ **Progression**   └   ┘ **Progression**
└   ┘ **Stable Disease**   └   ┘ **Stable Disease**
└   ┘ **Remission (%) :** ....   └   ┘ **Remission (%):** ....

Date, Signature (Physician): ....

References

Adamietz B, Keilholz L, Grünert J, Sauer R (2001) Radiotherapy of early stage Dupuytren disease. Long-term results after a median follow-up period of 10 years. Strahlenther Onkol 177(11):604–610, in German

Allen PW (1977) The fibromatoses: a clinicpathologic classification based on 140 cases. Am J Surg Pathol 1:255–270

Al-Qattan MM (2006) Factors in the pathogenesis of Dupuytren's contracture. J Hand Surg [Am] 31(9):1527–1534

Andrew JG, Andrew SM, Ash A, Turner B (1991) An investigation into the role of inflammatory cells in Dupuytren's disease. J Hand Surg [Br] 16:267–271

Au-Yong IT, Wildin CJ, Dias JJ, Page RE (2005) A review of common practice in Dupuytren's surgery. Tech Hand Up Extrem Surg 9:178–187

Badalamente MA, Hurst LC (2012) Injectable collagenase (clostridium histolyticum) for Dupuytren's contracture: results of the CORD I study. In: Dupuytren's disease and related hyperproliferative disorders, pp 343–347

Badois FJ, Lermusiaux JL, Masse C, Kuntz D (1993) Traitement non chirurgical de la maladie de Dupuytren par aponévrotomie à l'aiguille. Rev Rhum 60:808–813

Baird KS, Crossan JF, Ralston SH (1993) Abnormal growth factor and cytokine expression in Dupuytren's contracture. J Clin Pathol 46:425–428

Becker GW, Davis TR (2010) The outcome of surgical treatments for primary Dupuytren's disease – a systematic review. J Hand Surg Eur Vol 35(8):623–626

Berndt A, Kosmehl H, Katenkamp D, Tauchmann V (1994) Appearance of the myofibroblast phenotype in Dupuytren's disease is associated with a fibronectin, laminin, collagen type I and tenascin extracellular matrix. Pathobiology 62:55–58

Betz N, Ott OJ, Adamietz B, Sauer R, Fietkau R, Keilholz L (2010) Radiotherapy in early-stage Dupuytren's contracture. Long-term results after 13 years. Strahlenther Onkol 186(2):82–90

Braun-Falco O, Lukacs S, Goldschmidt H (1976) Dermatologic radiotherapy, 1st edn. Springer, Berlin/Heidelberg/New York

Brenner P, Mailänder P, Berger A (1994) Epidemiology of Dupuytren's disease. In: Berger A, Delbrück A, Brenner P, Hinzmann R (eds) Dupuytren's disease – Patho-biochemistry and clinical management. Springer, Berlin/Heidelberg, pp 244–254

Brenner P, Sachse C, Reichert B, Berger A (1996) Expression of monoclonal antibodies in nodules and band stage in Dupuytren's disease. Handchir Mikrochir Plast Chir 28:322–327

Brouet JP (1986) Etude de 1000 dossiers de maladie de Dupuytren. In: Tubiana R, Hueston JT (eds) La maladie de Dupuytren. Expansion Scientifique Française, Paris, pp 98–105

Cooper AP (1822) On dislocation of the fingers and toes - dislocation from contracture of the tendons. A treatise on dislocations and fractures of the joints. Longman and Co.:524–525

Crocker I (1999) Radiation therapy to prevent coronary artery restenosis. Semin Radiat Oncol 9:134–143

Dave SA, Banducci DR, Graham WP 3rd et al (2001) Differences in alpha smooth muscle actin expression between fibroblasts derived from Dupuytren's nodules or cords. Exp Mol Pathol 71:147–155

Degreef I, de Smet L (2010) A high prevalence of Dupuytren's disease in Flanders. Acta Orthop Belg 76(3):316–320

Denkler K (2010) Surgical complications associated with fasciectomy for Dupuytren's disease: a 20-year review of the English literature. EPlasty 10:e15

Descatha A (2012) Dupuytren's disease and occupation. In: Dupuytren's disease and related hyperproliferative disorders, pp 45–49

Dewing SB (1965) Disorders of function and overgrowth. In: Dewing SB (ed) Radiotherapy of benign disease. Thomas, Springfield, pp 78–171

Dupuytren G (1832) Leçons orales de clinique chirurgicale, faites à l'Hôtel-Dieu de Paris. Bd. I. Germer Baillière, Paris

Dupuytren G (1834) Permanent retraction of the fingers, produced by an affection of the palmar fascia. Lancet 2:222–225

Dupuytren Society (2011) Listing of clinics offering radiotherapy for Dupuytren's disease. http://www.dupuytren-online.info/radiotherapy_clinics.html. Accessed Jan 2011

Early PF (1962) Population studies in Dupuytren's contracture. J Bone Joint Surg Br 44:602–613

Falter E, Herndl E, Muhlbauer W (1991) Dupuytren's contracture. When operate? Conservative preliminary treatment? Fortschr Med 109:223–226

Finck KW (1955) Zur Frage der Dupuytrenschen Fingerkontaktur und ihrer Behandlung mit Radium. Strahlentherapie 97:608–612

Finney R (1955) Dupuytren's contracture. Br J Radiol 28:610–613

Flint M (1990a) Connective tissue biology. In: McFarlane RM, McGrouther DA, Flint M (eds) Dupuytren's disease. Biology and treatment, vol 5, The hand and upper limb series. Churchill Livingstone, Edinburgh, pp 13–24

Flint M (1990b) The genesis of the palmar lesion. In: McFarlane RM, McGrouther DA, Flint M (eds) Dupuytren's disease. Biology and treatment, vol 5, The hand and upper limb series. Churchill Livingstone, Edinburgh, pp 136–154

Gabbiani G, Ryan GB, Majno G (1971) Presence of modified fibroblasts in granulation tissue and their possible role in wound contraction. Experimentia 27:549–550

Geldmacher J (1994) Limited fasciectomy. In: Berger A, Delbrück A, Brenner P, Hinzmann R (eds) Dupuytren's disease. Springer, Berlin/Heidelberg, pp 257–263

Görlich W (1981) Die Dupuytrensche Kontraktur. Chir Praxis 28:91–98

Haase W (1982) Strahlentherapie hypertrophischer Prozesse des Bindegewebes. Therapiewoche 32:4856–4864

Herbst M, Regler G (1986) Dupuytrensche Kontraktur. Radiotherapie der Frühstadien. Strahlentherapie 161:143–147

Heyd R et al. "Strahlentherapie bei frühen Stadien des Morbus Ledderhose" Strahlentherapie und Onkologie 186 (2010) p 24–29

Hesselkamp J, Schulmeyer M, Wiskemann A (1981) Röntgentherapie der Dupuytrenschen Kontraktur im Stadium I. Therapiewoche 31:6337–6338

Hueston JT (1987) Dupuytren's contracture and occupation. J Hand Surg [Am] 12:657–658

Igarashi A, Nashiro K, Kikuchi K, Sato S, Ihn H, Fujimoto M, Grotendorst GR, Takehara K (1996) Connective tissue growth factor gene expression in tissue sections from localized scleroderma, keloid, and other fibrotic skin disorders. J Invest Dermatol 106:729–733

Incrocci L, Hop WC, Seegenschmiedt MH (2008) Radiotherapy for Peyronie's disease: a European survey. Acta Oncol 47:1110–1112

Jansen JT, Broerse JJ, Zoetelief J, Klein C, Seegenschmiedt HM (2005) Estimation of the carcinogenic risk of radiotherapy of benign diseases from shoulder to heel. Radiother Oncol 76(3):270–277

Jerosch-Herold C, Shepstone L, Chojnowski AJ, Larson D (2012) Night-time splinting after fasciectomy or dermofasciectomy for Dupuytren's Contracture: a pragmatic, multicentre, randomized controlled trial. In: Dupuytren's disease and related hyperproliferative disorders, pp 323–332

Kampinga HH, van Waarde-Verhagen MA, van Assen-Bolt AJ et al (2004) Reconstitution of active telomerase in primary human foreskin fibroblasts: effects on proliferative characteristics and response to ionizing radiation. Int J Radiat Biol 80:377–388

Kaplan II (1949) Clinical radiation therapy, 2nd edn. Hoeber, New York

Keilholz L, Seegenschmiedt MH, Sauer R (1996) Radiotherapy for prevention of disease progression in early-stage Dupuytren's contracture: initial and long-term results. Int J Radiat Oncol Biol Phys 36:891–897

Keilholz L, Seegenschmiedt MH, Born AD, Sauer R (1997) Radiotherapy in the early stages of Dupuytren's disease: indication, technique, long-term results. Strahlenther Onkol 173:27–35

Ketchum LD, Donahue TK (2000) The injection of nodules of Dupuytren's disease with triamcinolone acetonide. J Hand Surg 25:1157–1162

Kischer CW, Speer DW (1986) Microvascular changes in Dupuytren's contracture. J Hand Surg 9A:58–62

Köhler AH (1984) Die Strahlentherapie der Dupuytrenschen Kontraktur. Radiobiol Radiother 25:851–853

Leer JW, van Houtte P, Seegenschmiedt MH (2007) Radiotherapy of non-malignant disorders: where do we stand? Radiother Oncol 83:175–177

Ling RSM (1963) The genetic factor in Dupuytren's disease. J Bone Joint Surg Br 45:709–718

Loos B, Puschkin V, Horch RE (2007) 50 years experience with Dupuytren's contracture in the Erlangen University Hospital - a retrospective analysis of 2919 operated hands from 1956–2006. BMC Musculoskelet Disord 8:60–69

Lubahn JO, Lister GD, Wolfe T (1984) Fasciectomy of Dupuytren's disease, comparison between the open-palm technique and wound closure. J Hand Surg 9A:53–58

Luck JV (1959) Dupuytren's contracture. J Bone Joint Surg [Am] 41:635–664

Lukacs S, Braun Falco O, Goldschmidt H (1978) Radiotherapy of benign dermatoses: indications, practice, and results. J Dermatol Surg Oncol 4:620–625

McFarlane RM, McGrouther DA, Flint MH (1990) Dupuytren's disease. Biology and treatment, vol 5, The hand and upper limb series. Churchill Livingstone, Edinburgh

McGrouther DA (1982) The microanatomy of Dupuytren's contracture. Hand 13:215–236

Millesi H (1981) Dupuytren-Kontraktur. In: Nigst H, Buck-Gramcko D, Millesi H (eds) Handchirurgie, Band I. Thieme, Stuttgart/New York, pp 1500–1557

Mohr W, Wessinghage D (1994) Morphology of Dupuytren's disease. In: Berger A, Dellbrück A, Brenner P, Hinzmann R (eds) Dupuytren's disease. Springer, Berlin/Heidelberg, pp 3–15

Moorhead JJ (1956) Dupuytren's contracture. Review of the disputed etiology 1831–1956. NY J Med 56:3686–3703

Moyer KE, Banducci DR, Graham WP 3rd et al (2002) Dupuytren's disease: physiologic changes in nodule and cord fibroblasts through aging in vitro. Plast Reconstr Surg 110:187–193

Murrell GAC, Francis MJO (1994) Oxygen free radicals and Dupuytren's disease. In: Berger A, Delbrück A, Brenner P, Hinzmann R (eds) Dupuytren's disease. Springer, Berlin/Heidelberg, pp 227–234

Murrell GAC, Francis MJO, Howlett CR (1989) Dupuytren's contracture. Fine structure in relation to aetiology. J Bone Joint Surg Br 71:367–372

Murrell GAC, Francis MJO, Bromley L (1990) Modulation of fibroblast proliferation by oxygen free radicals. Biochem J 165:659–665

Mutsaers SE, Bishop JE, McGrouther G, Laurent GJ (1997) Mechanisms of tissue repair: from wound healing to fibrosis. Int J Biochem Cell Biol 29:5–17

National Institute for Health and Clinical Excellence (NICE) (2010) Radiation therapy for early Dupuytren's disease: guidance. http://guidance.nice.org.uk/IPG368. Accessed Jan 2011

Order SE, Donaldson SS (1990) Radiation therapy of benign diseases – A clinical guide. Springer, Berlin/Heidelberg/New York

Pavy JJ, Denekamp J, Letschert J, Littbrand B, Mornex F, Bernier J, Gonzales-Gonzales D, Horiot JC, Bolla M, Bartelink H (1995) EORTC Late Effects Working Group. Late Effects toxicity scoring: the SOMA scale. Int J Radiat Oncol Biol Phys 31(5):1043–1047

Platter F (1614) Observationum un Hominis Affectibus. Libri tres. Basel, L. König: 140–146

Rafter D, Kenny R, Gilmore M, Walsh CH (1980) Dupuytren's contracture – a survey of a hospital population. Ir Med J 73:227–228

Rayan GM, Parizi M, Tomasek JJ (1996) Pharmacological regulation of Dupuytren's fibroblast contraction in vitro. J Hand Surg [Am] 21:1065–1070

Rodemann HP, Bamberg M (1995) Cellular basis of radiation induced fibrosis. Radiother Oncol 35:83–90

Rubin P, Constine LS, Fajardo LF, Phillips TL, Wasserman TH (1995) RTOG Late Effects Working Group. Overview. Late Effects of Normal Tissues (LENT) scoring system. Int J Radiat Oncol Biol Phys 31(5):1041–1042

Rubin P, Soni A, Williams JP (1999) The molecular and cellular biologic basis for radiation treatment of benign proliferative diseases. Semin Radiat Oncol 9:203–214

Rudolph R, Vande Berg J (1991) The myofibroblast in Dupuytren's contracture. Hand Clin 7:683–692

Schink W (1978) Die Dupuytrensche Kontraktur. Med Klin 73:1371–1379

Seegenschmiedt MH (1998) Interdisciplinary documentation of treatment side effects in oncology. Present status and perspectives. Strahlenther Onkol 174(Suppl 3):25–29

Seegenschmiedt MH, Attassi M (2003) Strahlentherapie beim Morbus Ledderhose – Indikation, und klinische Ergebnisse. Strahlenther Onkol 179:847–853

Seegenschmiedt MH, Olschewski T, Guntrum F (2001) Optimierung der Radiotherapie beim Morbus Dupuytren: erste Ergebnisse einer kontrollierten Studie. Strahlenther Onkol 177:74–81

Seegenschmiedt MH (2008) Morbus Dupuytren/Morbus Ledderhose (Chapter 9) In Seegenschmiedt MH, Makoski H-B, Trott KR, Brady L (Eds) Radiotherapy for Non-Malignant Disorders, ISBN 978-3-540-62550-6. Springer (Berlin, New York, 2008) pp 161 – 191

Skoog T (1948) Dupuytren's contraction with special reference to aetiology and improved surgical treatment, its occurence in epileptics. Acta Chir Scand 96(Suppl):139

Smitt MC, Donaldson SS (1999) Radiation therapy for benign disease of the orbit. Semin Radiat Oncol 9:179–189

Strickland JW, Idler RS, Creighton JC (1990) Dupuytren's disease. Indiana Med 83:408–409

Suit H, Spiro I (1999) Radiation treatment of benign mesenchymal disease. Semin Radiat Oncol 9:171–178

Terek RM, Jiranek WA, Goldberg MJ, Wolfe HJ, Alman BA (1995) The expression of platelet-derived growth-factor gene in Dupuytren contracture. J Bone Joint Surg Am 77:1–9

Tomasek J, Rayan GM (1995) Correlation of alpha-smooth muscle actin expression and contraction in Dupuytren's disease fibroblasts. J Hand Surg [Am] 20:450–455

Tomasek JJ, Schultz RJ, Haaksma CJ (1987) Extracellular matrix-cytoskeletal connections at the surface of the specialized contractile fibroblast (myofibroblast) in Dupuytren disease. J Bone Joint Surg Am 68:1400–1407

Tripuraneni P, Giap H, Jani S (1999) Endovascular brachytherapy for peripheral vascular disease. Semin Radiat Oncol 9:190–202

Trott KR, Kamprad F (2006) Estimation of cancer risk from radiotherapy of benign diseases. Strahlenth Onkol 182:431–436

Trotti A, Byhardt R, Stetz J, Gwede C, Corn B, Fu K, Gunderson L, McCormick B, Morrisintegral M, Rich T, Shipley W, Curran W (2000) Common toxicity criteria: version 2.0. an improved reference for grading the acute effects of cancer treatment: impact on radiotherapy. Int J Radiat Oncol Biol Phys 47(1):13–47

Trotti A, Colevas AD, Setser A, Rusch V, Jaques D, Budach V, Langer C, Murphy B, Cumberlin R, Coleman CN, Rubin P (2003) CTCAE v3.0: development of a comprehensive grading system for the adverse effects of cancer treatment. Semin Radiat Oncol 13(3):176–181

Tubiana R, Michon J, Thomine JM (1966) Evaluation chiffree des deformations dans la maladie de Dupuytren. In: Maladie du Dupuytren, monographies du G.E.M. Expansion Scientifique Francaise, Paris

Viljanto JA (1973) Dupuytren's contracture: A review. Semin Arthritis Rheum 3A:155–176

Vogt HJ, Hochschau L (1980) Behandlung der Dupuytrenschen Kontraktur. Münch Med Wschr 122:125–130

Wasserburger K (1956) Therapie der Dupuytrenschen Kontraktur. Strahlenther 100:546–560

Weinzierl G, Flügel M, Geldmacher J (1993) Fehlen der Effektivität der alternativ nicht-chirurgischen Behandlungsverfahren beim Morbus Dupuytren. Chirurg 64:492–494

Yost J, Winter T, Fett H (1955) Dupuytren's contracture. A statistical study. Am J Surg 90:568–571

Zerajic D, Finsen V (2012) The epidemiology of Dupuytren's disease in Bosnia. In: Dupuytren's disease and related hyperproliferative disorders, pp 123–127

Outcomes of Using Bioengineered Skin Substitute (Apligraf®) for Wound Coverage in Dupuytren's Surgery

45

E. Anne Ouellette, Melissa Diamond, and Anna-Lena Makowski

Contents

45.1	Introduction	373
45.2	Materials and Methods	374
45.3	Results	375
45.4	Discussion	376
45.5	Conclusions	377
References		377

E.A. Ouellette (✉)
Physicians for The Hand, Miami, FL, USA
e-mail: eouellette@thehandplace.com

M. Diamond
Department of Pediatrics, Jackson Memorial Hospital,
Miami, FL, USA
e-mail: mbdiamond@med.miami.edu

A.-L. Makowski
The Hand Place, LLC, Miami, FL, USA
e-mail: amakowski@thehandplace.com

45.1 Introduction

Dupuytren's disease is a thickening of the palmar aponeurosis which consists of diseased collagen and contractile elements leading to a contraction of the involved digits. This condition was originally described by Baron Guillaume Dupuytren in 1831, and he developed an open surgical technique for releasing the contracture by fasciotomy, or division of the cords (Dupuytren 1834). Recurrence of Dupuytren's contracture is inherently difficult to ascertain as recurrence may be confused with disease progression. Recurrence is defined as disease within the area already operated on (Gordon 1957; Tonkin et al. 1984; Adam 1992; Honner et al. 1971) with nodules reappearing anywhere in the ray previously operated on (Moermans 1996). Scar and joint contracture or intrinsic tendon imbalance may be confused with recurrence (Tonkin et al. 1984). Progression is regarded as disease affecting an area not previously operated on (Gordon 1957). Incidence of recurrence or progression of the disease has been documented as high as 40–50% at 5 years post-surgery (Gordon 1957). The diseased collagen in the aponeurosis can be difficult to detect at the time of surgery, and remaining diseased collagen is the source of recurrence of the Dupuytren's contracture (Högemann et al. 2009). Total aponeurectomy has a recurrence rate of 10% in contrast to limited fasciectomy with a recurrence rate of up to 66% (Högemann et al. 2009; De Maglio et al. 1996; McGrouther 1999; Norotte et al. 1988; Tubiana and Leclercq 1985; Hakstian 1966; Tonkin et al. 1984; Foucher et al. 1992; Adam and Loynes 1992; Cools an Verstreken 1994; Hueston 1963; Makela et al. 1991). Recurrence of the Dupuytren's contracture is also

C. Eaton et al. (eds.), *Dupuytren's Disease and Related Hyperproliferative Disorders*,
DOI 10.1007/978-3-642-22697-7_45, © Springer-Verlag Berlin Heidelberg 2012

stimulated by tension in the palmar fascia (Citron and Hearnden 2003). Application of a skin graft or leaving the wounds open after surgery allows for wound coverage without adding tension by suturing the skin. The usual time for wound closure with the open technique is 2–3 weeks. Final range of motion depends on the severity of the contracture at the time of surgery.

Removing the skin over a fasciectomy was noted to be associated with a decrease in recurrence of the contractures (Hueston 1969, 1984). The presence of myofibroblasts in the skin has been associated with the areas of contractions or nodules in Dupuytren's disease (McMann et al. 1993; VandeBerg et al. 1982). As a result of these findings, removing the skin as part of treatment for Dupuytren's contracture was suggested (McMann et al. 1993; VandeBerg et al. 1982; Hueston 1984, 1985; Ullah et al. 2009). Use of the aggressive technique dermofasciectomy and skin autografts as primary treatment in Dupuytren's surgery remains controversial as predicting recurrence is difficult (Villani et al. 2008) Dermofasciectomy reduces the recurrence values to around 10% (Armstrong et al. 2000; Hall et al. 1997; Ketchum and Hixson 1987). This is particularly true for the diffuse type of Dupuytren's disease that involves the skin and does not produce well-defined cords (Armstrong et al. 2000). Aggressive Dupuytren's disease with a history of recurrence was successfully treated with dermofasciectomy in 20 of 23 hands according to an 8-year follow-up study recently performed by Villani (Villani et al. 2008). Resurfacing the fasciectomy in a smaller area combined with other closure techniques has proven to be an effective "firebreak" in stopping the progression or recurrence of the contractures (Hueston 1984, 1985; Gonzales 1971). A recent study using the smaller "firebreak" skin graft technique and comparing it to Z-plasties after fasciectomy showed no difference in the recurrence rate (12%) between the two groups at 3 years' follow-up (Ullah et al. 2009).

Many patients are not prepared to undergo a total palmar fasciectomy or dermofasciectomy and opt for smaller incisions with the understanding that they may have to redo the surgery at a later time in case of recurrence of the contractures. To improve protection against recurrence but delaying or avoiding the need for dermofasciectomy with its need for donor sites for skin grafts, the use of tissue-engineered bilayered skin graft in conjunction with limited fasciectomy was evaluated. By using this technique, the benefit of the "firebreak" graft is utilized.

Bioengineered skin graft was developed for use in skin coverage of ulcers such as diabetic foot and venous leg ulcers that are not healing after 3–4 weeks with conventional therapies (DeCarbo 2009). It has been shown safe and effective in providing skin coverage. In a meta-analysis of the effectiveness for complete wound closure in diabetic foot ulcers, 42.89% (199/464) of patients with bioengineered skin grafts healed completely compared to 29.57% (123/416) of the patients receiving conventional treatment (Teng et al. 2010).

In our practice we have experience using bioengineered skin graft for treatment of epidermolysis bullosa in six hands. After release of palmar joint contractures and removal of pseudo-membranes from cocooned hand, the bioengineered skin graft was applied. The graft took in all cases; wounds were healed by 6 weeks, and all patient regained functional use of their hands.

Based on our experience with the use of bioengineered skin graft on EB cases, we started using this graft for wound coverage after the McCash incision in our Dupuytren cases. Using the skin graft, allow for a wait-and-see approach, starting with a less aggressive fasciectomy, apply the skin graft, and if there is recurrence, treatment can continue with a more aggressive fasciectomy or dermofasciectomy. Furthermore, using bioengineered skin avoid donor site morbidity from obtaining an autologous skin graft. Observation of our patients receiving the bioengineered skin graft indicated decrease of recurrence rate, increase in range of motion, and overall patient satisfaction after using the bioengineered skin graft. A retrospective review of previous Dupuytren patients was conducted to evaluate these observations.

45.2 Materials and Methods

A chart review of 137 patients (153 hands) that were undergoing surgery to release Dupuytren's contracture between 1999 and 2007 was conducted. The limited fasciectomy technique developed by McCash (McCash 1964) was applied and involved transverse incisions over the diseased area (Fig. 45.1).

These incisions were used to identify and protect the neurovascular bundles to each digit and for the removal of the diseased fascia. Based on the 137 charts reviewed, 36 patients had the wounds covered with the bioengineered skin graft cut in pieces to cover the

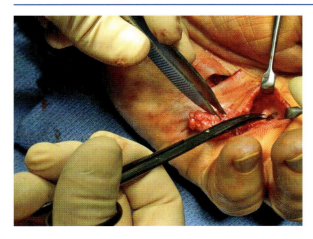

Fig. 45.1 Transverse McCash incision for removal of the diseased fascia

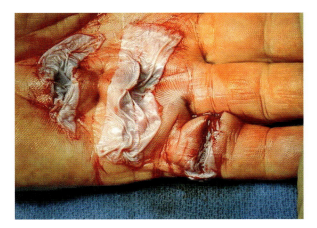

Fig. 45.2 The incisions are covered with tissue-engineered skin graft

incision. The grafts were sewn into place with 6-0 sutures (Fig. 45.2).

The graft was covered with non-adhering dressing which was soaked in ophthalmic antibiotic drops. A second gauze layer was applied and soaked with saline. A typical hand bundle dressing is applied. One week after surgery, the dressing was removed in hand therapy, leaving the non-adhering dressing in place. The wounds were again treated with ophthalmic antibiotic drops and redressed with dry gauze. The ophthalmic drops were added twice per day at the time of dressing changes. The bioengineered skin graft dried out after 7–10 days. Soap and water washes were started and continued until wounds were clean.

All 36 patients who had the McCash incisions followed by application of bioengineered skin substitute during this time period were contacted for follow-up evaluation. Eleven patients (17 rays) (31%) agreed to participate in the follow-up study and filled out an Upper Extremity Disabilities of the Arm, Shoulder, and Hand (DASH) questionnaire collecting information on pain level, range of motion, and activities of daily living. The patients also submitted pictures of their palmar scar. Descriptive statistics was used to present DASH scores.

45.3 Results

Ten of 11 patients with the bioengineered skin substitute applied to their surgical wounds submitted completed DASH questionnaires. One patient omitted five responses on the DASH questionnaire, and a score could not be calculated. Average follow-up time was 6 years (range 2.5–11 years). Average DASH score for this group was 8. Dash score distribution was $n=8$ (DASH 0–10), $n=1$ (11–20), $n=0$ (21–30), $n=1$ (31–40), $n=0$ (41–100) (Fig. 45.3). The highest score with an average of 2.2 was given to question 30, which states "I feel less capable, less confident or less useful because of my arm, shoulder or hand problem." The activities given the highest scores were opening a tight or new jar (average 1.6) and recreational activities in taking force or impact through arm shoulder or hand (average 1.6).

Five of the ten patients responded to the work module portion of the DASH with an average score of 5. DASH score distribution was $n=3$ (DASH 0–10), $n=2$ (11–20). The most common complaint was mild difficulty (a score of 2) in doing work as well as would have been liked.

Four of the ten patients responded to the sports/performing arts module of the DASH with an average of 23. At this point, the sample size has dropped dramatically from the original 10 which would alter the impact of the numbers. One patient gave a score of 4 or 5 (moderate or severe difficulty) to every question. This is the same patient that had an overall DASH score of 40, showing that there was difficulty from the surgery. The other three patients that responded to this portion mostly noted mild difficulty (score of 2) with playing the musical instrument or sport.

Range of motion, ROM, before surgery and at the time of wound closure (average 4 weeks; range 21–35 days) was available for the affected finger in seven patients receiving the bioengineered skin graft. In the skin graft group, the average percentage improvement in ROM was 29% (range: 0% increase in ROM to 70%

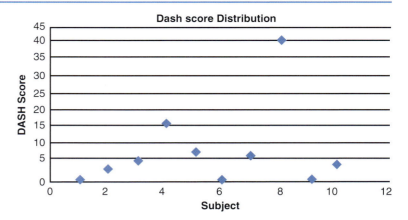

Fig. 45.3 Dash score from ten patients at long-term follow-up

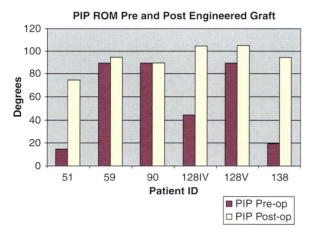

Fig. 45.4 Range of motion for proximal interphalangeal joints before and after Dupuytren's surgery using bioengineered skin graft

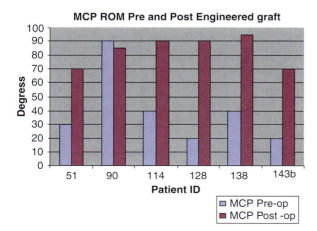

Fig. 45.5 Range of motion for metacarpophalangeal joints before and after Dupuytren's surgery using bioengineered skin graft

increase in ROM, 0=90° pre- and post-surgery) for the PIP joint and 47% (range: 5% decrease in ROM to 75% increase in ROM) for the MCP joint. Actual pre- and post-surgery values are presented in Figs. 45.4 and 45.5.

Wounds covered with bioengineered skin substitute ($n=11$) took an average of 40 days to heal. The scars healed well for all patients (Fig. 45.6).

45.4 Discussion

The patients in our small long-term follow-up study all had good outcomes and high patient satisfaction after application of bioengineered skin graft to the McCash incisions. In this small group there was no recurrence of contracture, but we are unable to draw a meaningful conclusion of recurrence since this is was not a randomized controlled prospective study. Range of motion improvement of 29% in the PIP joint and 47% in the MCP joint after surgery using the tissue engineered skin graft was noted, but we are unable to draw any conclusions regarding if application of bioengineered skin graft improves range of motion as compared to uncovered McCash incisions in this limited study.

Obvious advantages of using allograft material to cover the wounds in the McCash incisions or after complete dermofasciectomy are no donor side morbidity and the creation of epithelial coverage and a biologic barrier, preventing microbial penetration and fluid loss. It is possible that the engineered skin graft works like a firebreak much like resurfacing fasciectomy described in the literature (Hueston 1984, 1985; Gonzales 1971; Ullah et al. 2009). Certainly, applying wound coverage without tension removes this trigger

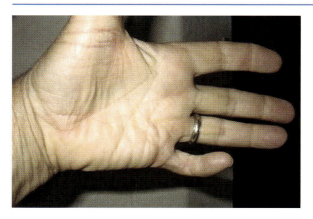

Fig. 45.6 Patient 5 years after surgery using bioengineered skin graft to cover the McCash incisions

for recurrence of the contractures. Using the bilayered skin substitute (Apligraf®) has the added benefit of bringing in live fibroblasts and keratinocytes to the wound, producing biological factors such as growth factors, natural antibiotics, and proteoglycans important for wound healing. The bilayered skin graft also serves as a matrix for new skin (cell migration) and neovascularization.

A potential mechanism of action for why Apligraf could be preventing recurrence of the Dupuytren contractures may be the presence of relaxin, a peptide in the insulin growth factor family, present in the human skin and linked to tissue homeostasis by reducing the fibroblasts' production of collagen and stimulating an increase in collagenase production (Unemori and Amento 1990; Unemori et al. 1993). Postoperative incisional scarring, maintenance of connective tissue in the extracellular matrix, and controlling collagen turnover are linked to the involvement of relaxin (Cooney et al. 2009). The basal lamina keratinocytes in human skin has receptors for relaxin. It is unknown at this time if keratinocytes of the Apligraf have relaxin receptors as well. Further investigation of the potential role of relaxin and general mechanism of action of bilayered skin graft application after fasciectomy in Dupuytren's disease should be evaluated.

Future research using a randomized prospective controlled study comparing patients with bioengineered skin graft covering the McCash incision to patients with open McCash incision left to heal by secondary intent should be conducted. Range of motion measurements should be done pre- and post-surgery and follow-up should be 5 years.

45.5 Conclusions

- Bilayered skin graft provides barrier protection after McCash incision.
- Bilayered skin graft readily available; no donor site morbidity.
- Initial clinical data are promising; retrospective data, compromised by limited number of cases.
- Controlled clinical trials necessary to confirm the preliminary data.

References

Adam RF, Loynes RD (1992) Prognosis in Dupuytren's disease. J Hand Surg [Am] 17:312–317

Armstrong JR, Hurren JS, Logan M (2000) Dermofasciectomy in the management of Dupuytren's disease. J Bone Joint Surg [Br] 82:90–94

Citron N, Hearnden A (2003) Skin tension in the aetiology of Dupuytren's disease; a prospective trial. J Hand Surg [Br] 6:528–530

Cools H, Verstreken J (1994) The open palm technique in the treatment of Dupuytren's disease. Acta Orthop Belg 60: 413–420

Cooney T, Schober J, Lubahn J, Konieczko E (2009) Relaxin's involvement in extracellular matrix homeostasis: Two diverse lines of evidence. Ann N Y Acad Sci 1160:329–335

De Maglio A, Timo R, Feliziani G (1996) Recidive ed estensioni nel morbio di Dupuytren trattato con apineurectomia selettiva. Revisioni clinica di 124 casi. Chir Organi Mov 86:43–48

DeCarbo WT (2009) Bilayered bioengineered skin substitute to augment wound healing. Foot Ankle Spec 2:303–305

Dupuytren G (1834) Permanent retraction of the fingers, produced by an affection of the palmer fascia. Lancet ii:222–225

Foucher G, Cornill C, Lenoble E (1992) Open palm technique for Dupuytren's disease: a five year follow-up. Ann Chir Main Memb Super 11:362–366

Gonzales R (1971) Open fasciectomy and Wolfe grafts for Dupuytren's contracture. In: Hueston JT (ed) Transactions of the fifth international congress of plastic and reconstructive surgery. Butterworth, London

Gordon S (1957) Dupuytren's contracture: recurrence and extension following surgical treatment. Br J Plast Surg 9:286–288

Hakstian RW (1966) Long term results of extensive fasciectomy. Br J Plast Surg 19:140–149

Hall PN, Fitzgerald GD, Sterne GD, Logan AM (1997) Skin replacement in Dupuytren's disease. J Hand Surg [Br] 22(2):193–197

Högemann A, Wolfhard U, Kendoff D, Board TN, Olivier LC (2009) Results of total aponeurectomy for Dupuytren's contracture in 61 patients: a retrospective clinical study. Arch Orthop Trauma Surg 129:195–201

Honner R, Lamb DW, James JIP (1971) Dupuytren's contracture, long term result after fasciectomy. J Bone Joint Surg 53B:240–246

Hueston JT (1963) Recurrent Dupuytren's contracture. Plast Reconstr Surg 31:66–69

Hueston JT (1969) The control of recurrent Dupuytren's contracture by skin replacement. Br J Plast Surg 22(2):152–156

Hueston JT (1984) "Firebreak" grafts in Dupuytren's disease. Aust N Z J Surg 54:277

Hueston JT (1985) The role of the skin in Dupuytren's disease. Ann R Coll Surg Engl 67:372

Ketchum L, Hixson F (1987) Dermofasciectomy and full thickness grafts in the treatment of Dupuytren's contracture. J Hand Surg [Am] 12(5):659–664

Makela EA, Jaroma H, Harju A, Anttila S, Vainio J (1991) Dupuytren's contracture: the long term results after day surgery. J Hand Surg [Br] 16:272–274

McCash CR (1964) The open palm technique in Dupuytren's contracture. Br J Plast Surg 17:271–280

McGrouther DA (1999) Dupuytren's contracture. In: Green DP, Hotchkiss RN, Pederson WC (eds) Green's operative hand surgery. Churchill Livingstone, London

McMann BG, Logan A, Warn A, Warn RM (1993) The presence of myofibroblasts in the dermis of patients with Dupuytren's contracture. J Hand Surgery [Br] 18:656–661

Moermans JP (1996) Long-term results after segmental aponeurectomy for Dupuytren's disease. J Hand Surg [Br] 21(6):797–800

Norotte G, Apoil A, Travers V (1988) Résultat à plus de dix ans de maladie de Dupuytren. A propos de cinquante-huit observations. Ann Chir Main 7:277–281

Teng YJ, Li YP, Wang JW, Yang KH, Zhang YC, Wang YJ, Tian JH, Ma B, Wang JM, Yan X (2010) Bioengineered skin in diabetic foot ulcers. Diabetes Obes Metab 12:307–315

Tonkin MA, Burke FD, Varian JPW (1984) Dupuytren's contracture: a comparative study of fasciectomy and dermofasciectomy in one hundred patients. J Hand Surg [Br] 9: 156–162

Tubiana R, Leclercq C (1985) Recurrent Dupuytren's disease. In: Hueston JT, Tubiana R (eds) Dupuytren's disease, 2nd edn. Churchill Livingstone, Edinburgh

Ullah AS, Dias JJ, Bhowal B (2009) Does a "firebreak" full-thickness skin graft prevent recurrence after surgery for Dupuytren's contracture? A prospective, randomized trial. J Bone Joint Surg [Br] 91:374–378

Unemori E, Amento E (1990) Relaxin modulates synthesis and secretion of procollagenase and collagen by human dermal fibroblasts. Biol Chem 265:10681–10685

Unemori E, Beck S, Lee W (1993) Human relaxin decreases collagen accumulation in vivo in two rodent models of fibrosis. J Invest Dermatol 101:280–285

VandeBerg JS, Rudolph R, Gelberman R, Woodward MR (1982) Ultrastructural relationship of skin to nodule and cord in Dupuytren's contracture. Plast Reconstr Surg 69(5): 835–844

Villani F, Choughri H, Pelissier P (2008) Intérêt de la greffe de peau dans la prévention des récidives de la maladie de Dupuytren. Chir Main 28(6):349–351

Highly Dosed Tamoxifen in Therapy-Resisting Dupuytren's Disease

46

Ilse Degreef, Sabine Tejpar, and Luc De Smet

Contents

46.1	**Introduction**	379
46.2	**Tamoxifen: Concept**	379
46.3	**Trial Design**	380
46.3.1	Standards for Clinical Trials in Dupuytren's Surgical Outcome	380
46.3.2	Tamoxifen Trial	381
46.4	**Preliminary Results of Tamoxifen in High-Risk Dupuytren's Disease**	381
46.5	**Discussion**	384
46.5.1	Tamoxifen in Clinical Practice	384
46.5.2	Overall Evidence	385
46.6	**Conclusions**	385
References		385

I. Degreef (✉) • L. De Smet
Department of Orthopaedic Surgery,
Leuven University Hospitals, Pellenberg, Belgium
e-mail: ilse.degreef@uzleuven.be

S. Tejpar
Department of Gastroenterology,
Leuven University Hospitals, Leuven, Belgium

46.1 Introduction

Since Dupuytren's disease is a progressive fibroproliferative disease, the various surgical techniques can only correct contractures. Recurrence or expansion of the disease remains a major unpredictable problem. Indeed, recurrence rates, ranging from 0% to 71%, have been mentioned (Roush and Stern 2000).

Several authors have tried to estimate the risk for recurrence and/or extension. A risk evaluation method has been suggested by Abe et al. It is based on clinical signs, namely, bilateral involvement, little finger surgery, early onset, plantar fibrosis, and knuckle pads and radial side involvement; these variables were significantly correlated with recurrence. Certainly in "high-risk" patients, future treatments would ideally aim for disease control, which implies ceasing this excessive fibroproliferative process.

46.2 Tamoxifen: Concept

Active fibroblasts (myofibroblasts) have been shown to be a major component of the involved tissue in Dupuytren's disease. These cells are able to contract and probably contribute to the eventual finger contracture as seen in this condition. Different in vitro studies on myofibroblast cultures in collagen lattices have been run to examine the influence of several agents on the contractile properties of these cells. Transforming growth factors (TGF) beta-1 and beta-2 play an important role in the progressive fibrosis of

---

C. Eaton et al. (eds.), *Dupuytren's Disease and Related Hyperproliferative Disorders*,
DOI 10.1007/978-3-642-22697-7_46, © Springer-Verlag Berlin Heidelberg 2012

Dupuytren's disease, and their downregulation may be useful in the treatment (Tse et al. 2004). In one study, the effect of tamoxifen (a synthetic non-steroidal anti-estrogen known to modulate the production of TGF beta) on fibroblast function and TGF (beta2) downregulation in palmar fascia affected by Dupuytren's disease was clearly demonstrated on cultures in vitro: the contraction rate of collagen lattices, populated with fibroblasts obtained from Dupuytren-affected fascia, and TGF (beta1) expression decreased under the influence of tamoxifen (Kuhn et al. 2002). Tamoxifen has been applied in vivo in aggressive fibrotic diseases, for example, idiopathic retroperitoneal fibrosis and recurrent desmoid tumors. Although the primary clinical application of this drug is breast cancer in female patients, it has also been used in males with breast cancer, gynaecomastia, prostate cancer, and acromegaly and is well tolerated (Novoa et al. 2002). In these pathologies, treatment strategies include low-dose tamoxifen (30 mg orally per day) and high-dose tamoxifen (60–120 mg orally per day).

46.3 Trial Design

Although the literature on Dupuytren's disease and surgical treatment methods are abundant and increasing every day, there is almost no standardization on trial design and outcome evaluation. Therefore, it is impossible to compare surgical techniques as Davis recently stated (Becker and Davis 2010). Specific reports on particular surgical techniques all show reasonably good outcome, but as we have seen in our retrospective report on self-reported recurrence, not one technique guarantees indefinite success (Degreef et al. 2009). What's more, differences in outcome appear to depend on fibrosis diathesis more than anything else. In some patients, fast postoperative recurrence can be feared and is fairly predictable if a risk profile is made. At this moment, this risk profile is only possible by using clinical parameters. No clear genetic or histological findings are reliable to help in this patient evaluation (Degreef et al. 2009). Therefore, we have designed a standardized clinical research method to conduct comparable clinical outcome studies with a high efficiency in evaluating a difference.

46.3.1 Standards for Clinical Trials in Dupuytren's Surgical Outcome

46.3.1.1 High-Risk Patients

As fibrosis diathesis is the most important factor determining outcome and recurrence in surgical procedures for Dupuytren's contractures, it should always be taken into account. However, only a minority of patients are high-risk patients for Dupuytren's disease. Most studies, however, have no criteria on diathesis for patient recruitment, and therefore, any conclusions on outcome may be compromised. What's more, if real differences in treatment outcome need to be compared, high numbers of patients need to be included. However, in low-risk patients, minimal surgery will almost guarantee high satisfaction rates. Taking all these remarks into account, restricting patient recruitment to a high-risk group increases the efficiency of research, lowering the required inclusion numbers for an acceptable power of the study. It is also ethical: no need for "experimenting" in patients wherein minimal treatment will already provide good outcome.

We use the score of Abe, since we have confirmed its efficacy in our own work (Degreef and De Smet 2011) and it is easy to use (Abe et al. 2004). We added a positive family history, although it may statistically not make a difference in the end score, since patients with a high fibrosis diathesis appear to almost always have a positive anamnesis with relatives with Dupuytren's disease.

46.3.1.2 Clinical Outcome

In prospective studies, outcome needs to be standardized to make true comparison possible, not only in the study but also in the literature (Becker and Davis 2010). Although many scores have been suggested, we have shown earlier that the DASH score on disability is not reliable in Dupuytren's disease (Degreef et al. 2009). This does not mean the contractures are not disabling, but the score is not influenced by the specific impairment of Dupuytren's disease. One of the reasons is that the disease is painless and that finger flexion remains intact (at least before surgery). The most reliable outcome parameter is an independent, measurable one that can easily be documented. Therefore, we now use standardized photos with a maximal extension of the fingers in a lateral view and measure the outcome with digital photography (Smith et al. 2009). Because the patient's opinion is of course the most important parameters in Dupuytren's treatment, we use a visual 10-graded analogue score for satisfaction. These parameters do not yet include the description of nodules or an extension of the disease, nor does it define "recurrence." These items need to be addressed in the future because we firmly believe that the tamoxifen trial is an important step toward "disease control." To evaluate the effect in early stages, before contractures become obvious, we need to have an independent and well-documenting technique for these issues. Perhaps the methods of Seegenschmiedt in his evaluations of radiotherapy in early Dupuytren's disease may be a first step in this direction (Seegenschmiedt et al. 2001).

46.3.1.3 Study Design – CONSORT Method

The consolidated standards of reporting clinical trials (CONSORT) is a reliable method to design, conduct, and report randomized trials and has proven its efficiency in hand surgery as well (Moher et al. 2001; Sauerland and Davis 2004; Plint et al. 2006). We therefore use these standards in current and future study design, and this will enhance comparisons to other trials if conducted in a similar fashion.

46.3.2 Tamoxifen Trial

We have conducted a prospective randomized double-blind study on the possible adjuvant effect of tamoxifen on segmental fasciectomy in patients with Dupuytren's disease who show a high risk for recurrence (Abe grade 4 or more, Fig. 46.1). Double blinding was provided to optimize the value of the suggested trial (the randomization process, the physicians and patients as to therapy and to ongoing results).

$D = a + b + c + d + e + f$

D is the diathesis score

a	bilateral hand involvement	(with = 1, without = 0)
b	little finger surgery	(with = 1, without = 0)
c	early onset of disease	(with = 1, without = 0)
d	plantar fibrosis	(with = 2, without = 0)
e	knuckle pads	(with = 2, without = 0)
f	radial side involvement	(with = 2, without = 0)
$D > 4$	high risk of recurrence and extension	
$D < 4$	little risk of recurrence and extension	

Fig. 46.1 Risk score as introduced by Abe et al.

The protocol was made up according to the CONSORT standards. A total of 30 patients were enrolled with double-blinded randomization: 15 patients with tamoxifen and 15 patients with placebo (Fig. 46.2).

Since we have shown earlier that segmental fasciectomy had no reported disadvantages of higher disease recurrence, we used this surgical technique as a standard in the trial setting. We looked at the effect of adding highly dosed neo-adjuvant tamoxifen. Based on the experience in desmoid tumors, we administered 80 mg tamoxifen daily, starting 6 weeks before and continuing 12 weeks after surgery (since the most important part of scar tissue is formed within these 3 months). Standardized parameters were digital photography of the extension lack in the most affected ray and a visual analogue score for satisfaction. Complications were noted as were possible side effects of the medication. Contraindications were malignancy, pre-menopausal women, history of thrombosis, and known allergy, and these patients were excluded from the study. Rehabilitation was standardized with nighttime extension splinting for 8 weeks and daytime splinting on an on/off basis for the first 4 weeks. Follow-up was scheduled at 6 weeks, 3 months, 6 months, 1 year, and 2 years. The data was gathered and analyzed blindly. The data monitor helped with blinded analysis of the data after 3 months of follow-up after the last inclusion, to evaluate preliminary results.

46.4 Preliminary Results of Tamoxifen in High-Risk Dupuytren's Disease

The period of recruitment was 14 months between January 2008 and March 2009. Follow-up is now over 2 years. The clinical follow-up is continued in a double-blinded fashion, and outcome was blindly evaluated with the help of two data monitors. Here, preliminary outcome is reported at 3 months after surgery with a further 1-year follow-up.

Illustrated in Tables 46.1 and 46.2, the groups were very similar with a mean age of 64 and 62 years. In group 1, there were four female patients and one in group 2. All patients had a high risk score of Abe, higher than 4. The mean Abe score was 6 in both groups. Both groups have a similar preoperative finger extension lack. Group 2 had a slightly worse extension lack, mostly in the PIP joints, which was statistically insignificant.

Fig. 46.2 Participant flow. The flow diagram illustrates the participant flow from assessment of the eligibility, through the randomization, and toward the exact numbers that are analyzed in the end

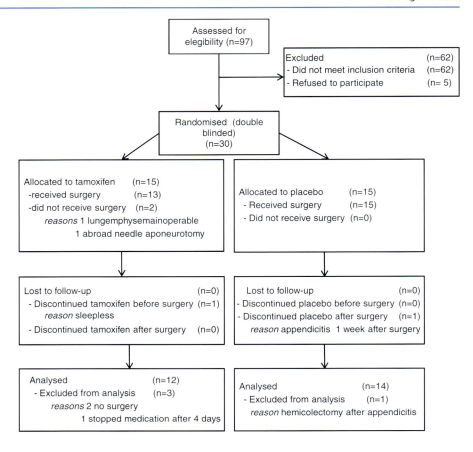

Table 46.1 Group 1 with the placebo: goniometric results 3 months after surgery

Nr	Ray	Abe	Gain% PIP	Total short pre	Total short post	Total gain	% Gain
1	5	8	−50	42	34	8	19
2	5	7	40	100	49	51	51
3	5	7	23	128	62	66	52
6	5	5	11	114	80	34	30
8	5	7	48	58	30	28	48
9	4	5	86	90	10	80	89
10	5	7	55	126	35	91	72
13	5	7	0	45	17	28	62
14	5	5	47	122	38	84	69
16	5	5	56	135	32	103	76
17	5	7	69	32	10	22	69
19	5	5	100	29	0	29	100
21	3	5	100	30	25	5	17
22	4	5	100	40	0	40	100
	Mean	6	49	78	30	48	61
	SD		43.0	42.0	22.9	31.7	26.8

Nr number, *ray* operated finger included in the measurements, *pre* preoperative measurements, *post* postoperative measurements, *MCP* metacarpophalangeal joint, *PIP* proximal interphalangeal joint, *SD* standard deviation

Table 46.2 Group 2 with the tamoxifen: goniometric results 3 months after surgery

Nr	Ray	Abe	Gain% PIP	Total short pre	Total short post	Total gain	% Gain
4	4	5	100	34	0	34	100
5	5	5	100	125	0	125	100
7	4	5	100	110	0	110	100
12	5	5	72	60	20	40	67
15	4	7	100	149	0	149	100
18	5	7	34	51	25	38	75
20	2	6	100	48	0	48	100
25	5	7	61	120	35	85	71
26	5	6	100	78	0	78	100
27	5	5	100	54	0	54	100
29	5	7	100	112	0	112	100
30	5	5	100	157	0	157	100
	Mean	6	89	92	7	86	93
	SD		21.7	42.3	12.5	44.1	13.2

Nr number, *ray* operated finger included in the measurements, *pre* preoperative measurements, *post* postoperative measurements, *MCP* metacarpophalangeal joint, *PIP* proximal interphalangeal joint, *SD* standard deviation

During surgery, a full finger extension was achieved in all patients, except in one of group 2. A PIP contracture was not fully corrected during surgery, even after releasing the check rain ligaments. The achieved correction remained unchanged after surgery, even after 3 months.

In group 1, there was one dropout due to appendicitis. In group 2, we had one dropout due to known lung emphysema; one patient had sleepless nights and one patient was lost for follow-up after having second thoughts about surgery

Goniometric outcome was statistically different between both groups, student *t* test $p=0.001$ (Tables 46.1 and 46.2). A relative gain as calculated by the Tubiana index of 61% (39–100, SD 26.8) was seen in group 1, compared to 93% (67–100, SD 13.2) in group 2 (Fig. 46.3). It was 49% in the PIP joints (−50–100, SD 43.0) in group 1 and 89% (34–100, SD 21.7) in group 2, also significantly different ($p=0.007$).

The VAS for satisfaction also was significantly different between both groups ($p=0.02$) (Fig. 46.4). Preoperative VAS score in group 1 was 7.6 (SD 1.4) and did not improve significantly ($p=0.3$) after the operation, with an 8.2 score (SD 2.0). Although preoperative visual analogue scores for satisfaction were somewhat worse (7.1, SD 2.1) in group 2, they significantly ($p=0.0006$) improved to a 9.7 score (SD 0.9), demonstrating a high patient satisfaction with the technique.

There were no serious complications, and all possible side effects occurred in the placebo group (group 1).

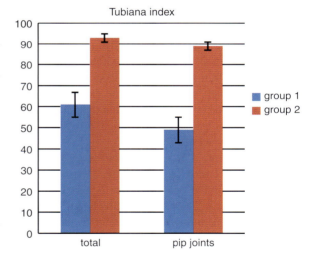

Fig. 46.3 Comparison of the Tubiana relative correction coefficient in both groups 3 months after surgery

In the placebo group, a transient carpal tunnel syndrome was seen in three patients (two males), and during the blinded trial, it was suspected that this might be enhanced by the use of the active component, which is an anti-estrogen, and carpal tunnel syndrome is seen mostly in female patients. In the two male patients, the symptoms ceased 4 months after surgery, and the female patients underwent a successful decompression of the carpal tunnel after 6 months. Although two male patients complained of impotence, 1 transient and 1 continuing after 1 year, they both appeared to have taken the

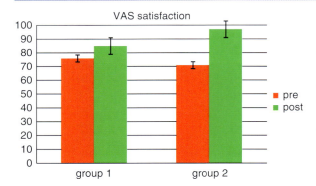

Fig. 46.4 Patient satisfaction. Illustration of the significant difference ($p=0.0006$) in postoperatively improved visual analogue scale for satisfaction in the tamoxifen patients (group 2) but not in the pacebo group ($p=0.3$) (group 1). Results 3 months after surgery

placebo. A male patient mentioned severe weight gain; again he belonged to group 1. A severe enteritis in a female patient with a hospital stay for 5 days, 4 weeks after the operation, also occurred in group 1.

All wounds healed uneventfully, except in one patient of group 2 with the tamoxifen, with a slow wound granulation process for 3 weeks. The patient had physiotherapy, and although the extension of his finger was full, he could only bend the finger passively. A flexor adhesiolysis was performed 3 months after surgery and was successful.

In one patient, a recurrent contracture was seen 3 months after tamoxifen stop. After this, the extension lack appeared to stabilize in the 1-year follow-up. Although it occurred only once, this event does not rule out a possible rebound effect when the medication is ceased abruptly.

46.5 Discussion

The results in this study show a significant improvement in outcome of segmental fasciectomy in Dupuytren's disease in patients with a high risk for recurrence and high diathesis. Also, the satisfaction appears to be high and complications low with the neo-adjuvant use of highly dosed tamoxifen. No side effects were noted, and the study seems to stress the psychological aspect of impotence. The one wound problem that was seen cannot lead to any conclusions, but monitoring of later use of this medication does need to confirm the safety of highly dosed tamoxifen, considering the wound healing process. The patient with a possible rebound effect also drew some attention. Although this recurrent extension lack stabilized after 3 months, he did lose some of the correction. Although this only happened in one patient, future monitoring may reveal the real risk of this possible complication. In patients with severe forms of Dupuytren's disease, it may therefore be necessary to either continue the medication for longer periods (possibly in lower dosages), if not indefinitely as is often done in desmoids patients, or at least not to stop the medication too abruptly.

Naturally, the study needs more follow-up to evaluate long-term outcome, and therefore, the monitoring will continue and a later report will be completed in term.

Strengths of the study are its double blinding, the CONSORT standards that were strictly followed, its strict randomization, the single surgeon and single technique, and the similar populations with a high risk for bad outcomes, which increases the possible effect of the medication. Weaknesses are the limited patient groups and the relatively high dropout in the active group. However, differences are indisputably statistically significant, although future studies are needed to confirm these findings and further assess potential risks.

46.5.1 Tamoxifen in Clinical Practice

Although the use of tamoxifen may not be indicated in all patients with Dupuytren's disease, this study does bring enough evidence to certainly consider the use in patients with severe recurrent forms and a high family occurrence, in which case patients may even already have a negative personal experience of surgery, due to bad outcome and rapid recurrences. Here, neo-adjuvant tamoxifen may help in the fight against a disease which will never cure but can only be pushed into a state of remission after surgery for the finger contractures. Since patients with Dupuytren's disease almost always present to the surgeon when contractures have already been established, the necessity for a surgical intervention will never disappear. However, with the new approach of identifying risk patients and considering tamoxifen, disease recurrence and high-risk re-operations may be prevented in a significant amount of patients in the near future. This may avoid the amputations that were sometimes needed after revision surgery and severe recurrent disease. Patients with severe Dupuytren's disease, need a lifetime monitoring for timely intervention and, if necessary, considering the (periodical) use of tamoxifen if it flares. This disease control protocol is somewhat comparable with the treatment practice of patients with rheumatoid arthritis.

On the other hand, the use of tamoxifen may also be considered in other wound healing problems as keloid formation in patients known with this problem or in families with systematic keloid formation. There are even families known with an associated keloid occurrence and Dupuytren's disease, which suggests a possible common pathway and/or genetic background. There might even be a place for tamoxifen use in posttraumatic keloid formation as is known in burns.

46.5.2 Overall Evidence

The use of tamoxifen is mostly known in breast cancer due to its anti-estrogen effect. In this pathology, a long-term experience with the drug has confirmed its safety as well as its efficacy in this pathology. Due to its fibroblast-repressing effect, the use in desmoids tumors is also common. However, due to the rarity of this tumor, no large series have been studied and some controversy about its effectiveness does exist (Bauernhofer et al. 1996; Hansmann et al. 2004). In retroperitoneal fibrosis, there are some studies confirming the possible positive effect on outcome (Bourouma et al. 1997; Ergun et al. 2005). In vitro studies of Dupuytren's myofibroblasts in the lab have confirmed a positive effect of tamoxifen on the cellular differentiation and contractility (Kuhn et al. 2002). Our study appears to confirm a positive effect on the outcome in Dupuytren's disease. This may be due to the suppression effect on the specific myofibroblasts in this disease. Also a generalized antifibrotic effect of the tamoxifen may have a positive effect on the result, since the wound healing process on itself is a fibroblastic proliferating and contracting event. This may also add to the wound healing problem seen in the one patient, and therefore careful monitoring in future use is obligatory.

Most naturally, future randomized, placebo-controlled clinical trials in larger numbers of patients are necessary before advocating for the use of a drug with known side effects relating to estrogen, which may concern male patients even more than female patients.

46.6 Conclusions

- Neo-adjuvant highly dosed tamoxifen may improve the surgical outcome of segmental fasciectomy in Dupuytren's disease.
- Improved finger extension with 32% and high patient satisfaction.
- No reported serious side effects within this relatively short period of time.
- In high-risk patients, highly dosed tamoxifen should be considered.
- In therapy-resisting patients, tamoxifen may never be discontinued.

References

Abe Y, Rokkaku T, Ofuchi S, Tokunaga S, Takahashi K, Mariya H (2004) An objective method to evaluate the risk of recurrence and extension of Dupuytren's disease. J Hand Surg Br 29:427–430

Bauernhofer T, Stoger H, Schmid M, Smola M, Gurtl-Lackner B, Hofler G, Ranner G, Reisinger E, Samonigg H (1996) Sequential treatment of recurrent mesenteric desmoid tumor. Cancer 77:1061–1065

Becker GW, Davis TR (2010) The outcome of surgical treatments for primary Dupuytren's disease - a systematic review. J Hand Surg Eur Vol 35(8):623–626

Bourouma R, Chevet D, Michel F et al (1997) Treatment of idiopathic retroperitoneal fibrosis with Tamoxifen. Nephrol Dial Transplant 12:2407–2410

Degreef I, De Smet L, Sciot R, Cassiman JJ, Tejpar S (2009) Beta-catenin overexpression in Dupuytren's disease is unrelated to disease recurrence. Clin Orthop Relat Res 467:838–845

Degreef I, De Smet L (2011) Risk factors in Dupuytren's diathesis: is reurrence after surgery predictable? Acta Orthop Belg 77:37–32

Ergun I, Keven K, Canbakan B, Ekmekci Y, Erbay B (2005) Tamoxifen in the treatment of idiopathic retroperitoneal fibrosis. Int Urol Nephrol 37:341–343

Hansmann A, Adolph C, Vogel T, Unger A, Moeslein G (2004) High-dose tamoxifen and sulindac as first-line treatment for desmoid tumors. Cancer 100:612–620

Kuhn MA, Wang X, Payne WG, Ko F, Robson MC (2002) Tamoxifen decreases fibroblast function and downregulates TGF beta2 in Dupuytren's affected palmar fascia. J Surg Res 103:146–152

Moher D, Schulz KF, Altman D, CONSORT Group (Consolidated Standards of Reporting Trials) (2001) The CONSORT statement: revised recommendations for improving the quality of reports of parallel-group randomized trials. JAMA 285:1987–1991

Novoa FJ, Boronat M, Carillo A, Tapia M, Diaz-Cremades J, Chirino R (2002) Effects of tamoxifen on lipid profile and coagulation parameters in male patients with pubertal gynecomastia. Horm Res 57:187–191

Plint AC, Moher D, Morrison A, Schulz K, Altman DG, Hill C, Gaboury I (2006) Does the CONSORT checklist improve the quality of reports of randomised controlled trials? A systematic review. Med J Aust 185:263–267

Roush TF, Stern PJ (2000) Results following surgery for recurrent Dupuytren's disease. J Hand Surg Am 25:291–296

Sauerland S, Davis TR (2004) The Consolidated Standards of Reporting Trials (CONSORT): better presentation of surgical trials in the Journal of Hand Surgery. J Hand Surg Br 29(6):621–624

Seegenschmiedt MH, Olschewski T, Guntrum F (2001) Radiotherapy optimization in early-stage Dupuytren's contracture: first results of a randomized clinical study. Int J Radiat Oncol Biol Phys 49(3):785–798

Smith RP, Dias JJ, Ullah A, Bhowal B (2009) Visual and computer software-aided estimates of Dupuytren's contractures: correlation with clinical goniometric measurements. Ann R Coll Surg Engl 91(4):296–300

Tse R, Howard J, Wu Y, Gan BS (2004) Enhanced Dupuytren's disease fibroblast populated collagen lattice contraction is independent of endogenous active TGF-beta2. BMC Musculoskelet Disord 5:41

Screening of Prodrugs on Cells Grown from Dupuytren's Disease Patients

47

Davor Jurisic

Contents

47.1   **Introduction** 387

47.2   **Materials and Methods** 388
47.2.1 Samples and Cell Cultures 388
47.2.2 Proliferation Assays and Compounds 388
47.2.3 Immunofluorescence 388

47.3   **Results** 389

47.4   **Discussion and Conclusion** 390

References 391

Abbreviations

DD	Dupuytren's disease
D	Cells grown from the affected palmar fascia tissue samples
ND	Cells grown from patient-matched non-diseased fascia
K	Control cells
5-FU	5-Fluorouracil
DMEM	Dulbecco's modified Eagle's medium
PBS	Phosphate-buffered saline
FBS	Fetal bovine serum
α-SMA	α-Smooth muscle actin

47.1 Introduction

Dupuytren's disease (DD) is a fibroproliferative disorder which is treated in the advanced stages by means of surgery. Due to the fact that surgical excision of the affected fascia does not completely cure the disease nor solve problems of recurrence, nonsurgical treatments are being investigated – among them, drugs with antiproliferative action. Thus, the therapeutic potential of new cytostatic drugs was evaluated for DD treatment and/or for reduction of postoperative recurrence rates. The N-sulphonylpyrimidine derivative, amidino-substituted benzimidazo[1,2-a]quinoline, and amidino dihydrothienothienyl[2,3-c]quinolone hydrochloride – known to affect proliferation processes, as shown in our previous studies on several tumor cell lines

D. Jurisic
Department for Plastic and Reconstructive Surgery,
University Hospital Center Rijeka,
Brace Fucak 5a, 51000 Rijeka, Croatia
e-mail: davor_jurisic@inet.hr

C. Eaton et al. (eds.), *Dupuytren's Disease and Related Hyperproliferative Disorders*,
DOI 10.1007/978-3-642-22697-7_47, © Springer-Verlag Berlin Heidelberg 2012

(Zinic et al. 2003; Hranjec et al. 2007; Jarak et al. 2006), and to show antiproliferative activity in vivo (Pavlak et al. 2005) – were tested for their antiproliferative activity on primary fibroblasts/myofibroblasts cell cultures derived from the palmar fascia of patients affected by DD.

47.2 Materials and Methods

47.2.1 Samples and Cell Cultures

Surgical samples were collected from eight male patients (mean age 60.5 years, six primary and two recurrent cases of DD) undergoing regular surgical procedures for Dupuytren's contracture. For that purpose, the affected palmar fascia tissue samples localized in the palmodigital area (D), along with patient-matched nondiseased fascia tissue as a biopsy from a macroscopically unaffected area at the edge of primary incision (ND), were collected. Control samples (K) were obtained from six patients undergoing carpal tunnel decompressions. The cells were grown according to standard cell-growth procedures.

47.2.2 Proliferation Assays and Compounds

The panel cell lines were inoculated into a series of standard 96-well microtiter plates on day 0 at 2,000 cells per well. Test agents and control agent 5-fluorouracil (5-FU, compound **1**) (PLIVA, Croatia) which was used for comparison with antiproliferative effects of tested compounds as suggested by several authors (Bulstrode et al. 2005; Jemec et al. 2000), N-sulphonylpyrimidine derivative (compound **2**), amidino-substituted benzimidazo[1,2-a]quinoline (compound **3**), and amidino dihydrothienothienyl[2,3-c] quinolone hydrochloride (compound **4**) were then added in five ten-fold dilutions (1×10^{-8} M–1×10^{-4} M) and further incubated for 3, 6, and 14 days. For the MTT assay, cells were inoculated onto a series of standard 96-well microtiter plates on day 0 at 5,000 cells per well. Test agents were then added in five ten-fold dilutions (1×10^{-8}–1×10^{-4} M) and incubated for further 3, 6, and 13 days. Working dilutions were freshly prepared on the day of testing in the growth medium. The solvent (DMSO) was also tested for eventual inhibitory activity by adjusting its concentration to be the same as in the working concentrations (DMSO concentration never exceeded 0.1%). After incubation, the cell growth rate was evaluated by performing the MTT assay: experimentally determined absorbance values were transformed into a cell percentage growth (PG) using the formulas proposed by NIH and described previously (Gazivoda et al. 2005). This method directly relies on control cells behaving normally at the day of assay because it compares the growth of treated cells with the growth of untreated cells in control wells on the same plate – the results are therefore a percentile difference from the calculated expected value. The IC50 values for each compound were calculated from dose–response curves using linear regression analysis by fitting the mean test concentrations that give PG values above and below the reference value. If, however, all of the tested concentrations produce PGs exceeding the respective reference level of effect (e.g., PG value of 50) for a given cell line, the highest tested concentration is assigned as the default value (in the screening data report that default value is preceded by a ">" sign). Each test point was performed in quadruplicate in three individual experiments. The results were statistically analyzed (ANOVA, Tukey's post hoc test at $p < 0.05$). Finally, the effects of the tested substances were evaluated by plotting the mean percentage growth for each cell type in comparison to control on dose–response graphs.

47.2.3 Immunofluorescence

D, ND, and K cells were seeded on 8-well glass chamber slides (Nunc, USA) in 10% Dulbecco's modified Eagle's medium (DMEM) at 2×105 cells/well and incubated for 1 day at 37°C in a humid atmosphere with 5% CO_2. After 24 h of incubation, the cells were treated with compounds **1–4** at their IC50 concentrations (50% inhibitory concentration is the compound concentration required to inhibit cell proliferation by 50%).

After the 24-h and 48-h treatments, the cells were washed in the phosphate-buffered saline (PBS) and fixed in formaldehyde (Kemika, Croatia). After washing with PBS, the blocking buffer (Dako, USA) was added, and cells were incubated for further 20 min at room temperature. Primary FITC-conjugated antibody against α-SMA (Monoclonal Anti-Actin,

Fig. 47.1 Dose–response graphs obtained by MTT assay. Cells' percentage of growth was plotted as a function of compound concentration and compared across different compounds, cell types, and days. When compared to D and ND cells, the growth of K cells was less inhibited by compound **4** in days 3, 6, and 13

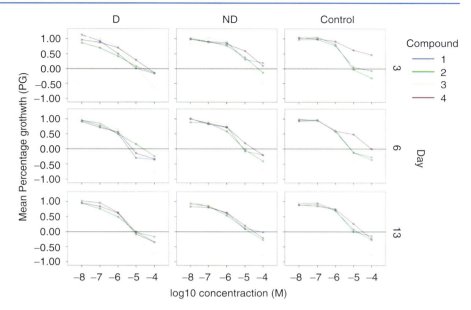

α-Smooth Muscle–FITC antibody produced in mouse; Sigma) at concentration 1:250 was allowed to bind in the dark overnight at 4°C in a humid atmosphere. The cells were washed with PBS and mounted in glycerol medium (Glycergel Dako, SAD). The prepared samples were analyzed under UV illumination at ×100 magnification using Olympus BX51 microscope and Olympus DP50 camera. The total number of cells per field and the number of positively staining cells (α-SMA positive cells – green fluorescence) were counted, and a percentage of myofibroblasts was derived for each treated or untreated cell line

47.3 Results

Upon successful establishment of stable D, ND, and K cell cultures, a series of proliferative assays were performed in order to test the activity of tested compounds on the growth of Dupuytren's fibroblasts/myofibroblasts (Fig. 47.1). These experiments were aimed at determining the IC50 values for compounds (Table 47.1) as well as to find the compound(s) that will exhibit differential antiproliferative effects either between fibroblasts obtained from Dupuytren's disease patients (D and ND) and control fibroblasts (K) or, alternatively, between D and ND cells. As 5-FU (compound **1**) was extensively studied for its effect on the

Table 47.1 IC$_{50}$ values

Compound	Treatment/days	IC$_{50}$ D	ND	K
1	3	1.1	7.0	4.4
	6	1.0	3.6	2.5
	14	2.9	3.0	3.8
2	3	0.7	7.2	4.4
	6	1.1	2.3	2.0
	14	1.0	1.8	3.9
3	3	4.1	7.7	5.2
	6	2.7	4.5	2.1
	14	2.4	3.4	2.3
4	3	5.5	27.5	81.2
	6	1.8	4.7	8.7
	14	2.5	3.8	5.7

IC$_{50}$ values presented in μM concentrations for each tested compound and each cell line (D, ND, and K), determined after the 3-, 6-, and 14-day treatments. LC$_{50}$ values were >100 μM for compounds **1**, **2**, and **4** and ~75 μM for compound **3**. (IC$_{50}$: 50% inhibitory concentration, or compound concentration required to inhibit cell proliferation by 50%; LC$_{50}$: the concentration that reduces the initial cell number by 50%)

growth of Dupuytren's fibroblasts (Bulstrode et al. 2005; Jemec et al. 2000), it was used as a control substance. The expression levels of α-SMA were additionally monitored by immunofluorescence, and results showed higher α-SMA expression in D cells in

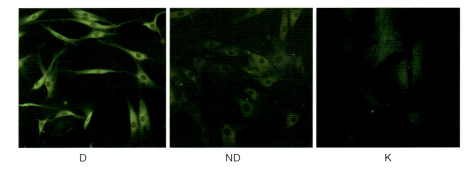

Fig. 47.2 Representative pictures of immunofluorescence staining for α-smooth muscle actin in cultured cells. Representative pictures of immunofluorescence staining for α-smooth muscle actin in cultured cells grown from affected (*D*) and nondiseased (*ND*) palmar fascia and control fibroblasts (*K*). The green fluorescence observed under UV illumination (*green intracellular filaments*) is indicative for α-smooth muscle actin expression and is clearly visible in D cells

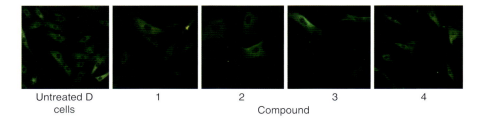

Fig. 47.3 Immunofluorescence of untreated D cells and those treated with the tested compounds (compounds **1**, **2**, and **4** at 5×10^{-6} M, compound **3** at 1×10^{-7} M). The *green* fluorescence is in direct correlation with α-SMA expression. Results of immunofluorescence analysis of untreated D cells and those treated with the tested compounds (compounds **1**, **2**, and **4** at 5×10^{-6} M, compound **3** at 1×10^{-7} M) revealed morphological changes of cells and antiproliferative effects (enlarged cells in treatment with compounds **1**, **2**, and **3** that point to cell cycle arrest and lower number of cells in all treatments, varying 3–8% only after 24-h treatment)

comparison to ND cells, while no α-SMA expression has been detected in control cells K.

Among all tested compounds, substance **4** has been identified as potential target for future investigations on selective treatment of cells affected by Dupuytren's contracture due to its differential effect on the growth of D cells (Fig. 47.2). Indeed, statistical analysis ($p<0.05$) revealed that this compound selectively inhibited the growth of D cells in comparison with ND cells while showing low cytotoxicity on control cells (K) at all tested time points. Especially, low cytotoxicity (approximately ten times lower in comparison to other tested compounds) was observed for compound **4** at prolonged incubation time of cells (Table 47.1) (Fig. 47.3).

47.4 Discussion and Conclusion

Drugs with antiproliferative action may be valuable in DD treatment. Assuming that proliferation of cultured fibroblasts is a key process preceding myofibroblast differentiation, which is highly important for arising of symptoms in DD (Fig. 47.2), we tested the antiproliferative activities of the newly synthesized compounds **2**, **3**, and **4** on cells from DD patients cultured as monolayers. Such approach is a basic approach to drug selection for further preclinical evaluation (Prekupec et al. 2005). 5-FU has been used as experimental control due to previously reported good antiproliferative activity in vitro for this compound (Bulstrode et al. 2005; Jemec et al. 2000). There were no significant growth rate differences between the cultured cell lines treated with 5-FU. However, IC50 values after 3 days of in vitro culturing pointed to a differential antiproliferative effect of 5-FU on D cells in comparison to ND cells.

The strongest antiproliferative effect was observed for amidino-substituted benzimidazo[1,2-a]quinoline (compound **3**), but it was nonspecific. This compound showed to be the most cytotoxic among the tested compounds. This compound binds ct-DNA in vitro and causes DNA damage, and additionally acts as a catalytic inhibitor of topoisomerase II (Hranjec et al. 2007).

It, thus, seems likely that compound **3** induces fibroblast/myofibroblast apoptosis due to DNA damage in a dose-related manner, possibly due to its intercalative properties. The most interesting among all the tested compounds was the amidino dihydrothienothienyl[2,3-c]quinolone hydrochloride (compound **4**), belonging to a class of compounds that specifically inhibit mammalian topoisomerase activity; bind ct-DNA, causing DNA damage (Jarak et al. 2006); and interfere with tubulin polymerization (Xia et al. 2001). Compound **4** exerted a differential activity on the growth of D cells. The antiproliferative activity of compound **4** on Dupuytren's fibroblasts/myofibroblasts is probably linked both to intercalation into DNA and to its ability to inhibit cytoskeletal changes leading to the differentiation process of myofibroblasts (Jarak et al. 2006). These molecular mechanisms probably induce both cell apoptosis and prevent the acquisition of myofibroblast phenotype. Due to its high specificity observed for D cells, this compound could be interesting for selective treatment of Dupuytren's cells at early disease stages characterized by high proliferation rates of cells as well as for early postoperative application related to the wound-healing process, especially due to its low toxicity on all tested cell cultures. Low cytotoxicity of compound **4** has been documented in previous in vitro studies as well (Jarak et al. 2006).

Out of the four tested substances, compound **4** appeared to be a best choice for further preclinical studies and optimization as it acted in a highly specific manner on cells derived from diseased fascia of DD patients and exhibited a low cytotoxic effect.

Acknowledgments   This report was financially supported by the Croatian Ministry of Science, Education and Sport grant "Molecular characteristic of myofibroblasts derived from Dupuytren's contracture" (098-0982464-2393) and the National Employment and Development Agency grant "Development of a drug intended for treating Dupuytren's disease patients" (14 V09809).

References

Bulstrode NW, Mudera V, McGrouther DA, Grobbelaar AO, Cambrey AD (2005) 5-fluorouracil selectively inhibits collagen synthesis. Plast Reconstr Surg 116:209–221

Gazivoda T, Plevnik M, Plavec J, Kraljevic S, Kralj M, Pavelic K, Balzarini J, De Clercq E, Mintas M, Raic-Malic S (2005) The novel pyrimidine and purine derivatives of L-ascorbic acid: synthesis, one- and two-dimensional H-1 and C-13 NMR study, cytostatic and antiviral evaluation. Bioorg Med Chem 13:131–139

Hranjec M, Kralj M, Piantanida I, Sedic M, Suman L, Pavelic K, Karminski-Zamola G (2007) Novel cyano- and amidino-substituted derivatives of styryl-2-benzimidazoles and benzimidazo[1,2-a]quinolines. Synthesis, photochemical synthesis, DNA binding and antitumor evaluation. J Med Chem 50:5696–5711

Jarak I, Kralj M, Piantanida I, Suman L, Zinic M, Pavelic K, Karminski-Zamola G (2006) Novel cyano- and amidino-substituted derivatives of thieno[2,3-b]- and thieno[3,2-b]thiophene-2-carboxanilides and thieno[3′,2′: 4,5]thieno- and thieno[2′,3′: 4,5]thieno [2,3-c]quinolones: synthesis, photochemical synthesis, DNA binding, and antitumor evaluation. Bioorg Med Chem 14:2859–2868

Jemec B, Linge C, Grobbelaar AO, Smith PJ, Sanders R, McGrouther DA (2000) The effect of 5-fluorouracil on Dupuytren fibroblast proliferation and differentiation. Chir Main 19:15–22

Pavlak M, Stojković R, Radacić-Aumiler M, Kasnar-Samprec J, Jercić J, Vlahović K, Zinić B, Radacić M (2005) Antitumor activity of novel N-sulfonylpyrimidine derivatives on the growth of anaplastic mammary carcinoma in vivo. J Cancer Res Clin Oncol 131(12):829–836

Prekupec S, Makuc D, Plavec J, Kraljevic S, Kralj M, Pavelic K, Andrei G, Snoeck R, Balzarini J, De Clercq E, Raic-Malic S, Mintas M (2005) Antiviral and cytostatic evaluation of the novel 6-acyclic chain substituted thymine derivatives. Antivir Chem Chemother 16:327–338

Xia Y, Yang ZY, Hour MJ, Kuo SC, Xia P, Bastow KF, Nakanishi Y, Nampoothiri P, Hackl T, Hamel E, Lee KH (2001) Antitumor agents. Part 204: synthesis and biological evaluation of substituted 2-aryl quinazolinones. Bioorg Med Chem Lett 11: 1193–1196

Zinic B, Krizmanic I, Glavas-Obrovac L, Karner I, Zinic M (2003) Synthesis and antitumor activity of N-sulfonyl derivatives of nucleobases and sulfonamido nucleoside derivatives. Nucleosides Nucleotides Nucleic Acids 22: 1623–1625

Relaxin: An Emerging Therapy for Fibroproliferative Disorders

48

Chrishan S. Samuel

Contents

48.1	**Introduction**	393
48.2	**Pathophysiology of Dupuytren's Disease**	394
48.3	**Relaxin**	394
48.4	**Antifibrotic Effects of H2 Relaxin That Are Relevant to Dupytren's Disease**	395
48.4.1	Relaxin Abrogates Profibrotic Cytokine-Induced Matrix Secretion and Deposition	395
48.4.2	Relaxin Promotes Matrix-Metalloproteinase-Induced Collagen Degradation	396
48.4.3	Relaxin Abrogates Myofibroblast Differentiation	397
48.4.4	Relaxin Interferes with TGF-β1 Signal Transduction and Activity	397
48.5	**Other Actions of H2 Relaxin That Are Relevant to Dupuytren's Disease**	397
48.6	**Translational Issues from Experimental Studies to Human Pathology**	398
48.7	**Conclusion**	398
References		398

C.S. Samuel
Department of Biochemistry and Molecular Biology,
Howard Florey Institute, The University of Melbourne,
Melbourne, Australia
e-mail: chrishan.samuel@florey.edu.au

The Department of Pharmacology,
Monash University, Melbourne, Australia
e-mail: chrishan.samuel@monash.edu

48.1 Introduction

While surgical resection of diseased tissue from patients with Dupuytren's disease (DD) remains the most successful (and in some cases the only) form of treatment, it does not always fully eliminate contracture of the fingers or the inevitability of recurrence and has therefore had variable success rates. Indeed, approximately 2–60% (with a mean rate of 33%) of patients with DD are subject to recurrence, which can vary depending on the type of surgery conducted and time of assessment performed postoperatively (Loos et al. 2007; Rayan 2007), and therefore need additional (new) surgery. Furthermore, as the effectiveness of surgery can be influenced by several factors, including the age and condition of patients, the type and location of the injury presented, the amount of tension on the wound, the condition of the underlying soft tissue, and the level of contamination of the affected tissue, the utility of novel nonsurgical forms of treatment and their potential ability to enhance surgical intervention requires further investigation.

Given that DD is a connective tissue disorder characterized as nodular palmar fibromatosis, a commonly held belief is that agents that can alter connective tissue turnover and remodeling can ameliorate and even reverse the scar formation and resultant contracture that accompanies the disease. This chapter will summarize the growing body of evidence that suggests that the naturally occurring hormone, relaxin, is a potential antifibrotic therapy for developing and established scarring that is associated with fibroproliferative disorders such as DD.

C. Eaton et al. (eds.), *Dupuytren's Disease and Related Hyperproliferative Disorders*,
DOI 10.1007/978-3-642-22697-7_48, © Springer-Verlag Berlin Heidelberg 2012

48.2 Pathophysiology of Dupuytren's Disease

Although the etiology of DD remains poorly understood, the palmar nodule that is involved in contracture is thought to be formed by fibroblast proliferation and myofibroblast-mediated collagen deposition (MacCallum and Hueston 1962; Gabbiani and Manjo 1972); leading to uncontrolled proliferation and thickening of the palmar fascia (Revis 2010) in addition to "collagen shrinkage" (Wong and Rogers 2010). The thickened fascia, in turn, becomes more susceptible to hypoxia and hemorrhaging of microvessels, which contributes to disease progression (Tubiana 1999). The origin of the myofibroblast in DD still remains unknown, but as in other granulating wounds that contract, myofibroblast differentiation is thought to occur in the perivascular zone (Wong and Rogers 2010) and becomes the main offending cell that contributes to the pathophysiology of the disease.

An array of tissue factors have now been shown to influence myofibroblast activity at various stages of contracture and disease pathology (reviewed in Cordova et al. 2005). These include prostaglandins, plasminogen-activating enzymes and thrombin, fibronectin, angiotensin II, serotonin, interlukin-1α and -1β (Wong and Rogers 2010), granulocyte–macrophage colony-stimulating factor, and interferon-γ, in addition to a number of growth factors such as transforming growth factor (TGF)-α, -β1, and -β2; platelet derived growth factor (PDGF); and epidermal growth factor (EGF). TGF-β1 is upregulated in DD (Zhang et al. 2008) and is the primary stimulator of myofibroblast activity (Badalamente et al. 1996).

The extracellular matrix (ECM) of the Dupuytren's contracture mainly consists of collagens, fibronectin, and proteoglycans, where upregulation of TGF-β1-stimulated collagen and fibronectin (Ignotz and Massagué 1986), including "immature" collagen subtypes (such as type III collagen), and various glycosaminogylcans are typically found. Collagen cross-linking is also apparent. However, collagen shortening and contraction of collagen fibers are not thought to contribute to contracture of the palmar fascia (Brickley-Parsons et al. 1981). Myofibroblasts are the key cells involved in synthesizing collagen and other matrix proteins associated with DD, as they not only contain myofibrils but also have intercellular connections to each other which permit the generation of synchronized contractile forces (Revis 2010); and

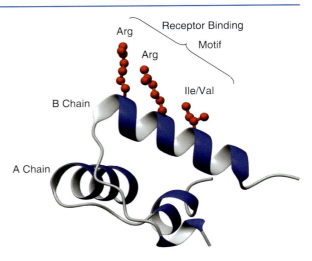

Fig. 48.1 Schematic representation of the structure of H2 relaxin. Representation of the structure of H2 relaxin with its constituent A and B chains, linked by inter- and intramolecular (A-chain) disulfide bonds. The conserved residues incorporating the relaxin binding motif (Arg-X-X-X-Arg-X-X-Ile/Val) on the B-chain are also shown (kindly provided by Dr Johan Rosengren, Institute for Molecular Biology, University of Queensland, Brisbane, Australia)

have been identified throughout the palmar fascia. Therefore, agents that can abrogate the influence of factors that promote myofibroblast differentiation and/or contractility, while enhancing those that inhibit myofibroblast activity (Pittet et al. 1994), offer a novel therapeutic approach to potentially combating the pathology of DD.

48.3 Relaxin

Relaxin is a small (6 kDa) dimeric peptide hormone that is structurally related to the insulin family of peptides (Fig. 48.1) and has a diverse range of biological actions with significant therapeutic and clinical implications (reviewed in Sherwood 2004; Bathgate et al. 2006a; Dschietzig et al. 2006; Samuel et al. 2006, 2007a, b; Bani et al. 2009; Bennett 2009; Conrad 2010). Discovered over 80 years ago (Hisaw 1926), relaxin is primarily produced in the ovary (corpus luteum) of pregnant women (O'Byrne et al. 1978; Weiss et al. 1978) and has long been regarded as a hormone of pregnancy, based on its numerous actions that help facilitate gestation, childbirth, and lactation. Many of these functions are centered around its ability to regulate collagen turnover, specifically through a reduction in collagen synthesis and promotion of matrix-metalloproteinase (MMP)-induced collagen degradation. Based on these actions, more recent studies (reviewed in Sherwood 2004; Bathgate et al. 2006a; Dschietzig et al. 2006; Samuel et al. 2006, 2007a, b; Bani et al. 2009; Bennett 2009; Conrad 2010) have demonstrated that relaxin is also a potent regulator of aberrant matrix turnover in several nonreproductive organs of various mammalian species, including the skin, heart, lung, liver, and kidneys, where it has emerged as an antifibrotic and anti-inflammatory agent that plays important roles in the regulation of vasodilation, angiogenesis, wound healing, and organ protection.

To date, three relaxin genes have been identified in humans which are termed *RLN1*, *RLN2*, and *RLN3* and which encode the peptides, H1 relaxin, H2 relaxin, and H3 relaxin, respectively (Sherwood 2004; Bathgate et al. 2006a). The H2 relaxin protein is the major stored and circulating form of relaxin and will be the form of relaxin mainly discussed in this chapter. On the other hand, a functional role for the H1 peptide is yet to be elucidated (Bathgate et al. 2006a), while the most recently discovered H3 relaxin peptide (Bathgate et al. 2002) is predominantly expressed in the brain and is thought to be a neuropeptide involved in regulating arousal, feeding, learning, and memory (van der Westhuizen et al. 2008). Many of the actions of H2 relaxin are mediated via a leucine-rich-repeat (LGR)-containing G-protein-coupled receptor, originally discovered as LGR7 (Hsu et al. 2002), and recently renamed relaxin family peptide receptor 1 (RXFP1), which is part of a subgroup (type C) of LGRs that include receptors for follicle-stimulating hormone, luteinizing hormone, and thyroid-stimulating hormone (Bathgate et al. 2006b).

48.4 Antifibrotic Effects of H2 Relaxin That Are Relevant to Dupytren's Disease

The production of highly purified recombinant and synthetic forms of H2 relaxin has been a major advance in relaxin biology, providing the opportunity to determine its therapeutic relevance. Recombinant H2 relaxin is biologically active in animals and has therefore been evaluated in several in vitro and in vivo systems for its ability to modify connective tissue. Several studies have demonstrated that relaxin is able to inhibit fibrogenesis and the aberrant collagen overexpression that is associated with organ fibrosis. It is important to note that while several of these actions of relaxin are consistently identified in multiple tissues, some of its actions are organ-specific or vary between organs, suggesting that relaxin inhibits fibrosis through common and specific mechanisms:

48.4.1 Relaxin Abrogates Profibrotic Cytokine-Induced Matrix Secretion and Deposition

Over the past two decades, a number of studies have clearly demonstrated the antifibrotic potential of H2 relaxin in several human/rat (myo)fibroblast cultures in vitro (Table 48.1) and experimental models of injury/disease in vivo (reviewed in Samuel et al. 2007a, b). H2 relaxin has been shown to dose-dependently downregulate TGF-β1-stimulated collagen and/or fibronectin synthesis and secretion from human dermal (Unemori and Amento 1990), pulmonary (Unemori et al. 1996), and renal (Heeg et al. 2005) fibroblasts in vitro, while decreasing TGF-β1 expression itself when administered to experimental models of chronic renal disease (Garber et al. 2001) and myocardial infarction (Samuel et al. 2011) in vivo. Likewise, H2 relaxin abrogated the aberrant collagen synthesis and deposition that was stimulated by interleukin-1β in human dermal fibroblasts (Unemori and Amento 1990) and by angiotensin II in neonatal rat atrial and ventricular fibroblasts (Samuel et al. 2004a), while also being able to ameliorate collagen production (either alone or in combination with interferon-γ) from scleroderma patient-derived dermal fibroblasts (Unemori et al. 1992). In all cases, H2 relaxin decreased the newly formed collagen secretion in the presence of collagen overexpression that was induced by these profibrotic factors, while markedly inhibiting collagen deposition into the cell layers of these stimulated cells. Importantly though, H2 relaxin did not demonstrate any effects on basal collagen/fibronectin expression, highlighting its safety as a potential therapeutic.

In keeping with these findings, a number of in vivo studies have demonstrated that H2 relaxin is a potent antifibrotic with rapid occurring efficacy under experimental conditions. A continuous 1–4 week infusion of H2 relaxin, in the form of subcutaneously implanted

Table 48.1 Fibroblast culture models that have been used to evaluate the matrix remodeling effects of H2 relaxin in vitro

| Species | Fibroblast source | Stimulus used | Effect of H2 relaxin: | | | |
			Myofibroblast differentiation	Matrix production	MMP activity	TIMP activity
Human	Skin[a-c]	TGF-β1, IL-1β	↓	↑	↑	↓
	Lung[d]	TGF-β1	↓	↓	↑	↓
	Kidney[e]	TGF-β1	↓	↓	↑	
	Lower uterus[f]				↑	↓
	Pelvic tissues[g]				↑	–
Rat	Liver[h,i]	TGF-β1	↓	↓	–[h]/↑[i]	↓[h]/↑[i]
	Kidney Cortex[j,k]	TGF-β1 (Ang II)	↓	↓	↑	
	Cardiac atria, ventricles[l]	TGF-β1, Ang II	↓	↓	↑	↓
	Pulmonary artery[m]	TGF-β1		↓		

"–" denotes no change detected
[a]Unemori and Amento (1990); [b]Unemori et al. (1992); [c]Samuel et al. (2005); [d]Unemori et al. (1996); [e]Heeg et al. (2005); [f]Palejwala et al. (2001); [g]Chen et al. (2005); [h]Williams et al. (2001); [i]Bennett et al. (2003); [j]Masterson et al. (2004); [k]Mookerjee et al. (2009); [l]Samuel et al. (2004); [m]Tozzi et al. (2005)

osmotic minipumps, consistently prevents and/or reverses the extracellular matrix (primarily collagen and/or fibronectin) production and accumulation (fibrosis) that results from tissue injury and aberrant wound healing, from a diverse array of pathologies (reviewed in Samuel et al. 2007a, b). Inclusive of this, H2 relaxin significantly reduced collagen accumulation in two rodent models of fibrotic-implant-induced dermal scarring over a 2-week treatment period (Unemori et al. 1993), where it both lowered collagen deposition within the affected regions and loosened the densely packed arrays of collagen fibers to those that were less abundant and randomly orientated. Interestingly, H2 relaxin abrogated both cardiac and renal fibrosis in spontaneously hypertensive rats (Lekgabe et al. 2005), suggesting that the hormone may simultaneously ameliorate similar pathologies in multiple organs. Furthermore, in most cases, the effects of H2 relaxin were demonstrated to be rapid and effective when its administration resulted in circulating levels of ~30–50 ng/mL – the physiological range of serum relaxin that has been measured in pregnant rodents and in women undergoing multiple pregnancies, but higher than that measured in women undergoing single pregnancies (which reach a maximum of 1–2 ng/mL) (Sherwood 2004; Bathgate et al. 2006a). Most importantly, control groups in several studies have shown that H2 relaxin does not affect basal matrix content in unaffected tissues, further highlighting its safety as a potential therapeutic. With these encouraging findings in mind, it should be noted that the ability

of H2 relaxin to prevent and/or reverse fibrosis progression diminishes when applied to more established stages of age-related (Samuel et al. 2003, 2005) and injury-related (Hewitson et al. 2010) fibrosis at the experimental level, where it fully abrogates aberrant collagen overexpression at early phases of disease progression, but only reduces collagen levels by 25–75% at more established stages, depending on the affected organ studied and timing of assessment. At the clinical level, relaxin administration to scleroderma patients with moderate symptoms (over 24 weeks) reduced skin thickening and improved their renal function, but could not sustain these beneficial actions when applied to patients with severe/end-stage disease symptoms (Erikson and Unemori 2001), indicating that its optimal therapeutic efficiency is demonstrated when applied to the early onset of disease progression.

48.4.2 Relaxin Promotes Matrix-Metalloproteinase-Induced Collagen Degradation

In addition to preventing aberrant collagen synthesis and secretion, H2 relaxin promotes matrix (collagen, fibronectin, and/or elastin) degradation via a number of matrix metalloproteinases (MMPs). These can include MMP-1 [collagenase-1] (Unemori and Amento 1990; Unemori et al. 1996; Qin et al. 1997), MMP-2 [gelatinase A] (Samuel et al. 2004; Heeg et al. 2005; Lekgabe et al. 2005), MMP-3 [stromelysin-1] (Qin et al. 1997), MMP-9 [gelatinase B] (Qin et al. 1997), MMP-12 [elastase] (Chen et al. 2005), and MMP-13 [collagenase-3] (Samuel et al. 2008). However, while H2 relaxin only prevents collagen production in the presence of profibrotic stimuli, it can increase MMP levels and inhibit the expression and activity of the tissue inhibitors of metalloproteinases (TIMPs) (Unemori and Amento 1990; Williams et al. 2001; Samuel et al. 2008), or at least alter the balance between MMPs and TIMP to favor a net increase in collagenase/gelatinase activity, in the presence or absence of profibrogenic stimuli (Table 48.1). It should be noted that the type of MMPs and TIMPs affected by H2 relaxin is dependent upon the species and particular organ studied, with MMP-1 being the major collagenase that is promoted by H2 relaxin in human organs (Unemori and Amento 1990; Unemori et al. 1996; Qin et al. 1997). At the in vivo level though, the H2-relaxin-mediated promotion of collagenase activity appears secondary to its ability to abrogate aberrant collagen production (Hewitson et al. 2010).

48.4.3 Relaxin Abrogates Myofibroblast Differentiation

While limited studies have demonstrated that H2 relaxin can inhibit profibrotic factor–stimulated fibroblast proliferation (Samuel et al. 2004), several investigations have revealed that the hormone consistently abrogates myofibroblast differentiation (Table 48.1) and is emerging as both an endogenous (Samuel et al. 2005) and exogenous inhibitor of myofibroblast activity, which is of direct relevance to DD. H2 relaxin downregulated α-SMA expression in a dose-dependent manner when applied to cortical myofibroblasts derived from the obstructed kidneys of rats (Masterson et al. 2004) and ameliorated TGF-β1-stimulated α-SMA expression from rat hepatic stellate cells (Bennett et al. 2003), rat cardiac myofibroblasts (Samuel et al. 2004), and human renal myofibroblasts (Heeg et al. 2005). Furthermore, H2 relaxin decreased α-SMA levels in the left ventricle of spontaneously hypertensive rats (Lekgabe et al. 2005) and in the skin of aging relaxin-deficient mice (Samuel et al. 2005) in vivo, suggesting that its inhibitory effects on myofibroblast differentiation are species- and organ-independent and are consistent with its ability to abrogate matrix production.

48.4.4 Relaxin Interferes with TGF-β1 Signal Transduction and Activity

Given the consistent ability of H2 relaxin to antagonize the effects of TGF-β1 in cell culture and animal models of injury/disease, more recent attention has focused on the level at which the hormone interferes with TGF-β1 signal transduction. TGF-β1 activity is driven to a large extent by the regulatory Smad family of proteins, where the phosphorylation of Smad2 and Smad3, the formation of (Smad2/Smad3) complexes with Smad4, and the translocation of these (Smad2/Smad3/Smad4) complexes from the cytosol to the nucleus are required to promote this process. Studies using TGF-β1-stimulated human renal myofibroblasts (Heeg et al. 2005) were able to demonstrate that H2 relaxin specifically inhibited the phosphorylation and translocation of Smad2 to the nucleus and interfered with the complexing of Smad2 to Smad3 (without having any direct effects on Smad3 or Smad4) to disrupt TGF-β1 activity and its influence on myofibroblast differentiation, collagen/fibronectin production, and MMP activity. A follow-up study was able to extend these findings by demonstrating that H2 relaxin signals through RXFP1 and the nitric oxide pathway to interfere with Smad2 phosphorylation and TGF-β1-mediated myofibroblast differentiation and collagen production (Mookerjee et al. 2009). These findings are of significance, given that Smads play an important role in the regulation of collagen accumulation. However, as cross-talk among a variety of pathways is necessary for the maximal regulation of collagen expression (Schnaper et al. 2003), H2 relaxin, like many other ligands for G-protein-coupled receptors, is likely capable of activating multiple signal transduction pathways, which warrants further investigation. A better understanding of these pathways will identify novel therapeutic targets that can optimize the antifibrotic potential of H2 relaxin.

48.5 Other Actions of H2 Relaxin That Are Relevant to Dupuytren's Disease

In addition to its well-documented antifibrotic actions, H2 relaxin has been shown to promote vasodilation in the kidney, heart, uterus, placenta, mammary gland, and liver of pregnant and nonpregnant mammals (reviewed in Sherwood 2004; Bathgate et al. 2006a; Dschietzig et al. 2006; Samuel et al. 2006, 2007a; Bani et al. 2009; Conrad 2010). In rat aortic and mesenteric arteries, the vasodilatory effects of H2 relaxin were mediated in part through attenuation of endothelin-1 and angiotensin-II-induced vasoconstriction (Dschietzig et al. 2003), while as a consequence of these actions in the kidney, H2 relaxin increased effective renal plasma flow and glomerular filtration rate, attenuated the renal circulatory response to angiotensin II, and reduced plasma osmolality regardless of gender. Based on these promising findings, H2 relaxin is currently being evaluated in clinical trials for its vasodilatory benefits in acute heart failure patients (Teerlink et al. 2009).

It is also known that vasodilatory hormones often demonstrate angiogenic properties: H2 relaxin has been shown to stimulate blood vessel growth in the endometrial lining of the uterus and expression of the angiogenic cytokine vascular endothelial growth factor (VEGF) in human endometrial cells (Unemori et al. 1999) and experimental models of heart disease (Formigli et al. 2007). Relaxin has also been shown to stimulate new blood vessel formation, particularly at ischemic wound sites, and induce various isoforms of VEGF and basic fibroblast growth factor (bFGF) in cells, collected from wound sites of experimental models in vivo (Unemori et al. 2000; Formigli et al. 2007). Since the administration of exogenous VEGF can reduce fibrosis and stabilize organ function (Kang et al. 2001), an H2-relaxin-mediated promotion of angiogenesis (and vasodilation) may be beneficial to scarring.

48.6 Translational Issues from Experimental Studies to Human Pathology

While the pleiotropic nature of H2 relaxin as a potential therapeutic has primarily been demonstrated in animal studies, a number of caveats to translating these findings to human therapeutics exist. Most of our understanding of relaxin biology comes from studies in rodents, and significant differences in relaxin physiology can exist between species. As with other peptide therapeutics, another challenge to developing relaxin as a therapy is the requirement for continuous administration (by microinfusion pumps) due to its relatively short half-life (of 5–10 min). Nevertheless, H2 relaxin has been evaluated in several clinical trials to date

(reviewed in Samuel et al. 2007a; van der Westhuizen et al. 2008), has demonstrated efficacy in treating moderate forms of dermal scarring/thickening in scleroderma patients (Erikson and Unemori 2001), and has demonstrated an excellent safety profile, suggesting that it may have a promise as a therapy for fibroproliferative disorders. These trials have highlighted specific biological activities of the hormone in patients with varying pathologies, while future trials are aimed at validating its significance in human pathology.

48.7 Conclusion

- The ability of H2 relaxin to inhibit TGF-β1 signal transduction and hence, TGF-β1-stimulated myofibroblast differentiation and myofibroblast-mediated matrix (collagen/fibronectin) production highlights its potential therapeutic significance for fibroproliferative disorders including DD.
- The fact that H2 relaxin only inhibits TGF-β1-stimulated fibrosis without affecting basal matrix turnover suggests that it may represent a better therapeutic alternative to TGF-β blockers (which nullify both negative and positive effects of TGF-β1).
- Further clinical evaluation of H2 relaxin is required to validate its significance in human pathology.
- Further clinical trials using the potential of H2 relaxin in hyperproliferative disorders are waranted.

Acknowledgments Chrishan S. Samuel is supported by a National Heart Foundation of Australia (NHFA) and National Health and Medical Research Council (NHMRC) of Australia R.D. Wright Fellowship.

References

Badalamente MA, Sampson SP, Hurst LC, Dowd A, Miyasaka K (1996) The role of transforming growth factor beta in Dupuytren's disease. J Hand Surg Am 21:210–215

Bani D, Yue SK, Bigazzi M (2009) Clinical profile of relaxin, a possible new drug for human use. Curr Drug Saf 16:915–928

Bathgate RAD, Samuel CS, Burazin TCD, Layfield S, Claasz AA, Reytomas IGT, Dawson NF, Zhao C, Bond C, Summers RJ, Parry LJ, Wade JD, Tregear GW (2002) Human relaxin gene 3 (H3) and the equivalent mouse relaxin (M3) gene. J Biol Chem 277:1148–1157

Bathgate RAD, Hsueh AJ, Sherwood OD (2006a) Physiology and molecular biology of the relaxin peptide family. In:

Knobil E, Neill JD (eds) Physiology of reproduction, 3rd edn. Elsevier, New York

Bathgate RAD, Ivell R, Sanborn BM, Sherwood OD, Summers RJ (2006b) International Union of Pharmacology LVII: recommendations for the nomenclature of receptors for relaxin family peptides. Pharmacol Rev 58:7–31

Bennett RG (2009) Relaxin and its role in the development and treatment of fibrosis. Transl Res 154:1–6

Bennett RG, Kharbanda KK, Tuma DJ (2003) Inhibition of markers of hepatic stellate cell activation by the hormone relaxin. Biochem Pharmacol 66:867–874

Brickley-Parsons D, Glimcher MJ, Smith RJ, Albin R, Adams JP (1981) Biochemical changes in the collagen of the palmar fascia in patients with Dupuytren's disease. J Bone Joint Surg Am 63:787–797

Chen B, Wen Y, Yu X, Polan ML (2005) Elastin metabolism in pelvic tissues: is it modulated by reproductive hormones? Am J Obstet Gynecol 192:1605–1613

Conrad KP (2010) Unveiling the vasodilatory actions and mechanisms of relaxin. Hypertension 56:2–9

Cordova A, Tripoli M, Corradino B, Napoli P, Moschella F (2005) Dupuytren's contracture: an update of biomolecular aspects and therapeutic perspectives. J Hand Surg Br 30:557–562

Dschietzig T, Bartsch C, Richter C, Laule M, Baumann G, Stangl K (2003) Relaxin, a pregnancy hormone, is a functional endothelin-1 antagonist: attenuation of endothelin-1-mediated vasoconstriction by stimulation of endothelin type-B receptor expression via ERK-1/2 and nuclear factor-kappaB. Circ Res 92:32–40

Dschietzig T, Bartsch C, Baumann G, Stangl K (2006) Relaxin-a pleiotropic hormone and its emerging role for experimental and clinical therapeutics. Pharmacol Ther 112:38–56

Erikson MS, Unemori EN (2001) Relaxin clinical trials in systemic sclerosis. In: Tregear GW, Ivell R, Bathgate RA, Wade JD (eds) Relaxin 2000: proceeding of the third international conference on relaxin and related peptides. Kluwer Academic Publishers, Amsterdam

Formigli L, Perna AM, Meacci E, Cinci L, Margheri M, Nistri S, Tani A, Silvertown J, Orlandini G, Porciani C, Zecchi-Orlandini S, Medin J, Bani D (2007) Paracrine effects of transplanted myoblasts and relaxin on post-infarction heart remodelling. J Cell Mol Med 11:1087–1100

Gabbiani G, Manjo G (1972) Dupuyten's contracture: fibroblast contracture? An ultrastructural study. Am J Path 66:131–146

Garber SL, Mirochnik Y, Brecklin CS, Unemori EN, Singh AK, Slobodskoy L, Grove BH, Arruda JAL, Dunea G (2001) Relaxin decreases renal interstitial fibrosis and slows progression of renal disease. Kidney Int 59:876–882

Heeg M, Koziolek MJ, Vasko R, Schaefer L, Sharma K, Muller GA, Strutz F (2005) The antifibrotic effects of relaxin in human renal fibroblasts are mediated in part by inhibition of the Smad2 pathway. Kidney Int 68:96–109

Hewitson TD, Ho WY, Samuel CS (2010) Antifibrotic properties of relaxin: in vivo mechanism of action in experimental renal tubulointerstitial fibrosis. Endocrinology 151:4938–4948

Hisaw F (1926) Experimental relaxation of the pubic ligament of the guinea pig. Proc Soc Exp Biol Med 23:661–663

Hsu SY, Nakabayashi K, Nishi S, Kumagai J, Kudo M, Sherwood OD, Hsueh AJ (2002) Activation of orphan receptors by the hormone relaxin. Science 295:671–674

Ignotz RA, Massagué J (1986) Transforming growth factor-beta stimulates the expression of fibronectin and collagen and

their incorporation into the extracellular matrix. J Biol Chem 261:4337–4345

Kang DH, Hughes J, Mazzali M, Schreiner GF, Johnson RJ (2001) Impaired angiogenesis in the remnant kidney model: II. Vascular endothelial growth factor administration reduces renal fibrosis and stabilizes renal function. J Am Soc Nephrol 12:1448–1457

Lekgabe ED, Kiriazis H, Zhao C, Xu Q, Moore XL, Su Y, Bathgate RA, Du XJ, Samuel CS (2005) Relaxin reverses cardiac and renal fibrosis in spontaneously hypertensive rats. Hypertension 46:412–418

Loos B, Puschkin V, Horch RE (2007) 50 years experience with Dupuytren's contracture in the Erlangen University Hospital-a retrospective analysis of 2919 operated hands from 1956 to 2006. BMC Musculoskelet Disord 8:60

MacCallum P, Hueston JT (1962) The pathology of Dupuytren's contracture. ANZ J Surg 1:241–253

Masterson R, Hewitson TD, Kelynack K, Martic M, Parry L, Bathgate R, Darby I, Becker G (2004) Relaxin down-regulates renal fibroblast function and promotes matrix remodelling in vitro. Nephrol Dial Transplant 19:544–552

Mookerjee I, Hewitson TD, Halls ML, Summers RJ, Mathai ML, Bathgate RA, Tregear GW, Samuel CS (2009) Relaxin inhibits renal myofibroblast differentiation via RXFP1, the nitric oxide pathway, and Smad2. FASEB J 23:1219–1229

O'Byrne EM, Flitcraft JF, Sawyer WK, Hochman J, Weiss G, Steinetz BG (1978) Relaxin bioactivity and immunoactivity in human corpora lutea. Endocrinology 102:1641–1644

Palejwala S, Stein DE, Weiss G, Monia BP, Tortoriello D, Goldsmith LT (2001) Relaxin positively regulates matrix metalloproteinase expression in human lower uterine segment fibroblasts using a tyrosine kinase signaling pathway. Endocrinology 142:3405–3413

Pittet B, Rubbia-Brandt L, Desmoulière A, Sappino AP, Roggero P, Guerret S (1994) Effect of gamma-interferon on the clinical and biologic evolution of hypertrophic scars and Dupuytren's disease: an open pilot study. Plast Reconstr Surg 93: 1224–1235

Qin X, Garibay-Tupas J, Chua PK, Cachola L, Bryant-Greenwood GD (1997) An autocrine/paracrine role of human decidual relaxin. I. Interstitial collagenase (matrix metalloproteinase-1) and tissue plasminogen activator. Biol Reprod 56:800–811

Rayan GM (2007) Dupuytren disease: anatomy, pathology, presentation, and treatment. J Bone Joint Surg Am 89:189–198

Revis DR Jr (2010) Dupuytren contracture. eMedicine specialties > plastic surgery > hand. http://emedicine.medscape.com/article/329414-overview. Updated 10 Feb 2010

Samuel CS, Zhao C, Bathgate RA, Bond CP, Burton MD, Parry LJ, Summers RJ, Tang ML, Amento EP, Tregear GW (2003) Relaxin deficiency in mice is associated with an age-related progression of pulmonary fibrosis. FASEB J 17:121–123

Samuel CS, Unemori EN, Mookerjee I, Bathgate RAD, Layfield SL, Mak J, Tregear GW, Du X-J (2004) Relaxin modulates cardiac fibroblast proliferation, differentiation, and collagen production and reverses cardiac fibrosis in vivo. Endocrinology 145:4125–4133

Samuel CS, Zhao C, Yang Q, Wang H, Tian H, Tregear GW, Amento EP (2005) The relaxin gene knockout mouse: a model of progressive scleroderma. J Invest Dermatol 125:692–699

Samuel CS, Du X-J, Bathgate RAD, Summers RJ (2006) 'Relaxin' the stiffened heart and arteries: the therapeutic potential for relaxin in the treatment of cardiovascular disease. Pharmacol Ther 112:529–552

Samuel CS, Hewitson TD, Unemori EN, Tang MLK (2007a) Drugs of the future: the hormone relaxin. Cell Mol Life Sci 64:1539–1557

Samuel CS, Lekgabe ED, Mookerjee I (2007b) The effects of relaxin on extracellular matrix remodeling in health and fibrotic disease. In: Agoulnik AI (ed) Relaxin and related peptides. Landes Bioscience/Springer, Austin/New York

Samuel CS, Hewitson TD, Zhang Y, Kelly DJ (2008) Relaxin ameliorates fibrosis in experimental diabetic cardiomyopathy. Endocrinology 149:3286–3293

Samuel CS, Cendrawan S, Gao XM, Ming Z, Zhao C, Kiriazis H, Xu Q, Tregear GW, Bathgate RAD, Du XJ (2011) Relaxin remodels fibrotic healing following myocardial infarction. Lab Invest 91:675–690

Schnaper HW, Hayashida T, Hubchak SC, Poncelet AC (2003) TGF-beta signal transduction and mesangial cell fibrogenesis. Am J Physiol Renal Physiol 284:F243–F252

Sherwood OD (2004) Relaxin's physiological roles and other diverse actions. Endocr Rev 25:205–234

Teerlink JR, Metra M, Felker GM, Ponikowski P, Voors AA, Weatherley BD, Marmor A, Katz A, Grzybowski J, Unemori E, Teichman SL, Cotter G (2009) Relaxin for the treatment of patients with acute heart failure (Pre-RELAX-AHF): a multicentre, randomised, placebo-controlled, parallel-group, dose-finding phase IIb study. Lancet 373:1429–1439

Tozzi CA, Poiani GJ, McHugh NA, Shakarjian MP, Grove BH, Samuel CS, Unemori EN, Riley DJ (2005) Recombinant human relaxin reduces hypoxic pulmonary hypertension in the rat. Pulm Pharmacol Ther 18:346–353

Tubiana R (1999) Dupuytren's disease of the radical side of the hand. Hand Clin 15:149–159

Unemori EN, Amento EP (1990) Relaxin modulates synthesis and secretion of procollagenase and collagen by human dermal fibroblasts. J Biol Chem 265:10681–10685

Unemori EN, Bauer EA, Amento EP (1992) Relaxin alone and in conjunction with interferon-gamma decreases collagen synthesis by cultured human scleroderma fibroblasts. J Invest Dermatol 99:337–342

Unemori EN, Beck LS, Lee WP, Xu Y, Siegel M, Keller G, Liggitt HD, Bauer EA, Amento EP (1993) Human relaxin decreases collagen accumulation in vivo in two rodent models of fibrosis. J Invest Dermatol 101:280–285

Unemori EN, Pickford LB, Salles AL, Piercy CE, Grove BH, Erikson ME, Amento EP (1996) Relaxin induces an extra-cellular matrix-degrading phenotype in human lung fibroblasts in vitro and inhibits lung fibrosis in a murine model in vivo. J Clin Invest 98:2739–2745

Unemori EN, Erikson ME, Rocco SE, Sutherland KM, Parsell DA, Mak J, Grove BH (1999) Relaxin stimulates expression of vascular endothelial growth factor in normal human endometrial cells in vitro and is associated with menometror-rhagia in women. Hum Reprod 14:800–806

Unemori EN, Lewis M, Constant J, Arnold G, Grove BH, Normand J, Deshpande U, Salles A, Pickford LB, Erikson ME, Hunt TK, Huang X (2000) Relaxin induces vascular endothelial growth factor expression and angiogenesis selectively at wound sites. Wound Repair Regen 8:361–370

van der Westhuizen ET, Halls ML, Samuel CS, Bathgate RAD, Unemori EN, Sutton SW, Summers RJ (2008) Relaxin family peptide receptors – from orphans to therapeutic targets. Drug Discov Today 13:640–651

Weiss G, O'Byrne EM, Hochman J, Steinetz BG, Goldsmith L, Flitcraft JG (1978) Distribution of relaxin in women during pregnancy. Obstet Gynecol 52:569–570

Williams EJ, Benyon RC, Trim N, Hadwin R, Grove BH, Arthur MJ, Unemori EN, Iredale JP (2001) Relaxin inhibits effective collagen deposition by cultured hepatic stellate cells and decreases rat liver fibrosis in vivo. Gut 49:577–583

Wong WW, Rogers FR (2010) Hand, Dupuytren disease. eMedicine specialties > plastic surgery > hand. http://emedicine.medscape.com/article/1285422-overview. Updated 30 Jul 2010

Zhang AY, Fong KD, Pham H, Nacamuli RP, Longaker MT, Chang J (2008) Gene expression analysis of Dupuytren's disease: the role of TGF-beta2. J Hand Surg Eur Vol 33:783–790

Cryotherapy and Other Therapeutical Options for Plantar Fibromatosis

49

Terry L. Spilken

Contents

49.1	**Introduction**	401
49.2	**Inheritance, Prevalence, and Histology**	402
49.3	**Symptoms and Diagnosis**	402
49.4	**Classification Schemes**	404
49.5	**Risk Factors and Related Diseases**	404
49.6	**Early Stage Treatment**	404
49.7	**Surgical Treatment Options**	405
49.8	**Cryosurgery**	405
49.8.1	The Cryosurgery Technique	405
49.8.2	A Cryosurgery Example	406
49.9	**Results**	407
References		407

T.L. Spilken
Foot Care of Livingston, Livingston, NJ, USA
e-mail: tlee10@aol.com

49.1 Introduction

Plantar fibromatosis is a condition that affects the plantar aponeurosis. This condition is also sometimes called Ledderhose disease, Morbus Ledderhose, or, wrongly, plantar aponeurosis. The condition was named after Georg Ledderhose, a German surgeon, who first described it in 1897 (Ledderhose 1897).

Ledderhose disease is a non-malignant thickening of the deep connective tissue, the fascia, in the arch of the foot (Fig. 49.1). It is a fibrotic tissue disorder. There is presence of excessive collagen or fibrotic tissue. It is important to emphasize that this is non-cancerous. Some researchers even label fibromatosis as a wound healing disorder.

The origin of plantar fibromatosis is unknown. In his original paper in 1897, Georg Ledderhose suspected trauma causing the nodules: when a foot is fixed in a cast for a longer period of time, proliferation might start, and when the cast is removed and the foot is used again, the middle part of the plantar aponeurosis can be subject to one or several micro-cracks or tears which then develop into hypertrophic scarring. Yet Ledderhose realized that patients might develop this disease with seemingly healthy feet, without wearing a prior cast. Today, despite various theories, the cause for some people contracting this disease still cannot be definitively known. As Ledderhose suspected, the disorder may be an aggressive healing response to small tears in the plantar fascia. Basically, the fascia is over repairing itself after an injury. Tears in the fascia may occur from thickening and tightening caused by plantar fasciitis. Fibroblasts in the aponeurosis produce collagen,

C. Eaton et al. (eds.), *Dupuytren's Disease and Related Hyperproliferative Disorders*,
DOI 10.1007/978-3-642-22697-7_49, © Springer-Verlag Berlin Heidelberg 2012

Fig. 49.1 Typical location of plantar fibromatosis

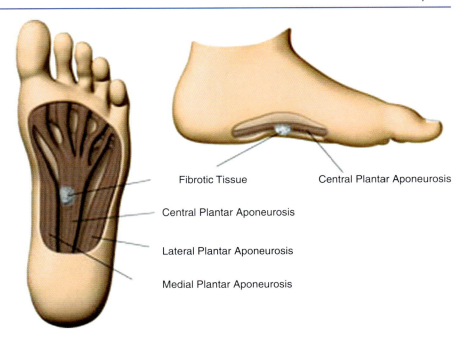

fibronectin, and glycosaminoglycans responsible for plantar fibromatosis formation.

49.2 Inheritance, Prevalence, and Histology

As stated above, the root cause of plantar fibromatosis formation is not yet understood. It is believed to be an inherited disease. There are typically variable occurrences in the same family. The necessary genes for this condition to develop may remain dormant in the family for over several generations. It also may be present in multiple individuals in the same generation.

Plantar fibromatosis is most commonly seen in the middle aged and elderly, but it can affect all ages (Fleischmajer et al. 1973; Rao and Luthra 1988). It affects men more frequently than women, although some groups report equal distribution (Sammarco and Mangone 2000; de Bree et al. 2004). Possibly, the relation depends on age as known for Dupuytren's disease (Ross 1999). A parent or close relative may also have Ledderhose disease. It is typically seen bilaterally and progresses slowly but not indefinitely. It is most common in Caucasians of Northern European descent. The condition rarely affects Asians, at least little is known about prevalence in Asia.

Histologically, we see dense fibrocellular tissue (de Palma et al. 1999). Mature collagen and fibrocytes in various stages of maturation are seen. There are no prominent atypical features or abnormal activity. The epidermis and superficial dermal tissue are normal. The neoformation grows upward and downward replacing the normal adipose tissue. There is a proliferation of uniform but well-differentiated spindled cells, mainly composed of myofibroblasts. This proliferation involves many cellular foci surrounded by scar-like connective tracts. The fibrocytic component is dense with the cells packed very closely.

49.3 Symptoms and Diagnosis

One form of Ledderhose disease is superficial fibromatosis. It is most common in children and young adults. It might be due to myofibroblast proliferation more than fibroblast overgrowth. Superficial fibromatosis, as a condition, is very uncommon. The cells are round or oat-shaped, and the stoma is chondroid. The hamartomatous form is associated with proteus syndrome. Proteus syndrome is also known as Wiedemann's syndrome. There is skin overgrowth, atypical bone development with tumors covering half of the body. It is commonly referred to as neurofibromatosis, the elephant man. This is a very rare condition. Only aggressive infantile fibromatosis has an invasive course. It grows rapidly and infiltrates the subcutaneous tissue, aponeurosis, and muscles. It is still not considered

49 Cryotherapy and Other Therapeutical Options for Plantar Fibromatosis

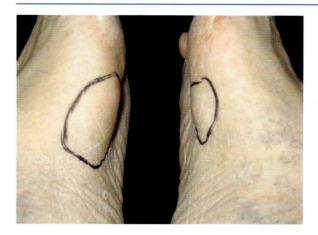

Fig. 49.2 Ledderhose nodules in the arch of the foot

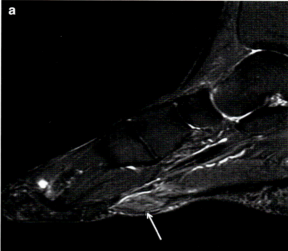

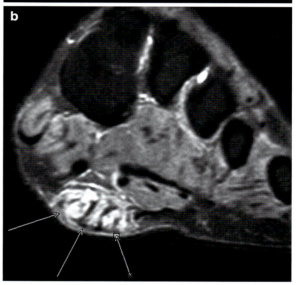

Fig. 49.3 Magnetic resonance image (MRI) of plantar fibromatosis. Plantar fibromatosis of a female patient, 41 years old. The arrows are indicating the fibromatosis. (Courtesy Prof. MH Seegenschmiedt, Strahlenzentrum Hamburg, Germany)

metastatic. This form is the only form that can spontaneously regress, although it also can persist.

There are many conditions that can be included in the differential diagnosis. They include scar, keloids, fasciitis, neurofibroma, achromic neuroid nevus, malignant melanoma, serous tendinous cyst, mucoid cyst, calcinosis, osteoma, calcaneal spur, and gout.

Symptoms include nodules that form in the medial and central portions of the plantar fascia. These are firm nodular masses (Fig. 49.2). They are typically slow growing. The cords in the fascia band can thicken. This can lead to stiffening of the toes with plantar contracture in 25% of the patients. Walking becomes painful for the patient. These nodules may lie dormant, or they may begin rapid and unexpected growth. It is most commonly seen on the medial border. The nodule itself is usually painless, and there is no tenderness on palpation. The pain occurs when the patient ambulates and has contact with the ground. Thus, standing or walking can elicit symptoms. There is repetitive pressure occurring with standing and walking that impinges on the healthy tissue. The overlying skin remains freely movable. If contracture will occur, it will be in the later stages.

Some research indicates that plantar fibromatosis occurs in both feet 25% of the time. Other research indicates that plantar fibromas are typically bilateral (Sammarco and Mangone 2000). The disease may infiltrate the dermis and the adipose tissue. Very rarely is the flexor tendon sheath involved. Except for superficial fibromatosis, this condition is not known to resolve on its own. They often increase in size and density over time, eventually stopping.

Sonographic techniques are versatile and often sufficient to determine the extent of the nodule (Bedi and Davidson 2001). Magnetic resonance imaging (MRI) provides better resolution but is still somewhat poorly defined (Fig. 49.3). There is a low signal in both T1- and T2-weighted images. There is an infiltrative mass in the aponeurosis next to the plantar muscles showing its margins. Heterogeneity is seen in the signal intensity. The MRI shows the extent of the lesion. It shows the degree of deep invasion. It does not reveal the tissue composition. One should be aware that the fibrosarcoma will show the same MRI readings.

49.4 Classification Schemes

The Enneking Classification system for plantar fibromatosis is the same as tumors:

Stage I: Latent stage: tumors are usually static or inactive and asymptomatic.

Stage II: Active stage: tumors are actively growing and cause clinical symptoms.

Stage III: Local aggressive growth stage: tumors are locally aggressive, histologically immature, and show progressive growth.

A different classification scheme is proposed by Sammarco and Mangone (2000). Here the focus is on disease extension:

Grade 1: FOCAL disease isolated to a small area on the medial and/or central aspect of the fascia, NO adherence to the skin, NO deep extension to the flexor sheath.

Grade 2: MULTIFOCAL disease, with or without proximal or distal extension, NO adherence to the skin, NO deep extension to the flexor sheath.

Grade 3: MULTIFOCAL disease, with or without proximal or distal extension, EITHER adherence to the skin OR deep extension to the flexor sheath.

Grade 4: MULTIFOCAL disease, with or without proximal or distal extension, adherence to the skin AND deep extension to the flexor sheath.

49.5 Risk Factors and Related Diseases

Dupuytren's disease has a lot in common with Ledderhose disease. Dupuytren's disease affects the hands causing bent hands and fingers. The histological and ultrastructural features of both diseases are identical (de Palma et al. 1999), and we might therefore assume that both have common etiologies and pathogenesis. About 28% of people with plantar fibromatosis also have Dupuytren's disease (Sammarco and Mangone 2000). Two to twenty percent of people with Dupuytren's disease will develop Ledderhose disease.

Risk factors for development of plantar fibromatosis include a family history. There is a significantly higher incidence in males. Patients with these conditions have an increased risk factor: Dupuytren's disease, Peyronie's disease, epilepsy, other seizure disorders, diabetes mellitus, chronic liver disease, and hypothyroidism.

There is also a possible link with patients taking certain medications. These include beta adrenergic blocking agents (beta blocker) used for high blood pressure. There could also be a link with anti-seizure medicine such as phenytoin (Dilantin). Certain supplements such as glucosamine and chondroitin as well as large doses of vitamin C can also influence the development of plantar fibromatosis. There is a suspected but unproven link with alcoholism, smoking, liver disease, thyroid problems, and stressful work.

49.6 Early Stage Treatment

The medical treatments for plantar fibromatosis almost always fail. The occasional success is probably due to spontaneous involution of the plantar fibroma, and that typically only occurs in the superficial fibromatosis form. The most success with treatment is found in the very early stages of the condition. The medical treatments in the early stages with a single small nodule include (Lee et al. 1993; Wheeless and van der Bauwhede 2010):

1. Avoid direct pressure.
2. Soft inner soles or custom orthotics.
3. Protective padding with dispersion.
4. Corticosteroid injections.
5. Clobetasol ointment – a corticosteroid used for eczema and psoriasis.
6. Methotrexate – an antimetabolite and antifolate used for cancer and autoimmune diseases.
7. Stretching.
8. Physical therapy.

Recently, Transdermal Verapamil 15% gel has been used as a conservative treatment. It is applied to the skin above the nodules twice a day. This medication is a calcium channel blocker. Fibroblasts need calcium to produce collagen. The theory is that this medication will decrease the production and release of collagen and fibronectin from the fibroblast. The medication is supposed to increase the activity of collagenase that will help breakdown excess collagen. Research is being done to determine the efficacy of this treatment. Anecdotal evidence and patients' comments in the Dupuytren/Ledderhose forum so far are fairly negative (Dupuytren Society website 2010).

Other conservative treatments include radiation therapy (Seegenschmiedt and Attassi 2003; Seegenschmiedt et al. 2012a). Radiation therapy is increasingly applied for Dupuytren patients (Seegenschmiedt 2008; Seegenschmiedt et al. 2012b) and may become a successful standard treatment for plantar fibromatosis. Some have tried administering gadolinium which is used as a contrast agent for an MRI. Other treatments include skin grafts, shock wave therapy (ESWT), injections of collagenase, and, last not least, cryosurgery.

49.7 Surgical Treatment Options

Surgical treatments for plantar fibromatosis have traditionally two approaches. The first is to excise the plantar fibroma in toto. The surgeon must avoid the tendons, nerves, and muscles which are located close to each other. Damaging them could result in unpleasant side effects. Portions of the diseased tissue may accidentally be left in the foot and start to re-grow. This procedure of removing only the plantar fibroma has a very high recurrence rate of 85% (Durr et al. 1999; Sammarco and Mangone 2000). The leading cause of recurrence is probably inadequate removal of the nodule. The surgeon would need to take at least 1.5 cm of normal fascial tissue when removing the mass.

The other procedure is a radical plantar fasciectomy. This is currently the most common surgical treatment. It requires complete removal of the plantar fascia. There is a long recovery time and can lead to walking and other podiatric problems. The surgeon needs to make a Z- or S-shaped incision that will allow complete exposure to the entire plantar fascia. A drain is needed to reduce the risk of hematoma formation and flap necrosis. The patient must be non-weight bearing in a Jones compression dressing for at least 21 days. Accommodative orthoses are needed after the surgical correction.

Biopsies performed reveal that the diseased area is not encapsulated. The clinical margins are hard to define on biopsy. What is seen is predominantly cellular. The biopsy is frequently misdiagnosed as fibrosarcoma.

49.8 Cryosurgery

49.8.1 The Cryosurgery Technique

Cryosurgery is a minimally invasive procedure that can be performed in an office setting (Allen et al. 2007). It involves a small dose of local anesthesia. The procedure can be performed in a short amount of time with no sutures required. There is minimal post-operative discomfort. Cryosurgery does not require use of a surgical shoe, and the patient can bath within 24 h.

Hippocrates recognized the use of freezing for injuries. I.S. Cooper developed one of the first cryosurgical devices in 1962 which continued to be improved (Amoils 1967; Garamy 1968). J.W. Lloyd was the first to use cryoanalgesia in 1976 for pain management (Barnard 1980). Today, cryoanalgesia is used by dermatology, plastic surgery, gynecology, pain management, and other allopathic physicians (Cavazos et al. 2009). A. Trescott perfected the use of cryoanalgesia for the management of pain and indicated its use for the foot and ankle in 2003. That same year, the FDA approved cryoanalgesia for peripheral nerves of the foot. The mechanism of action has cryoneurolysis providing long-term pain relief when pain has been shown to be caused by sensory nerves. The application of cold ($-70°C$) to tissues creates a conduction block, similar to the effect of local anesthetics. Long-term pain relief from nerve freezing occurs because ice crystals create vascular damage to the vaso nervorum, which produces severe endoneural edema. Cryoanalgesia disrupts the nerve structure and creates Wallerian degeneration, but leaves the myelin sheath, perineurium, and epineurium intact. Cryoneurolysis is far superior to other methods of peripheral nerve destruction because it is NOT followed by neuritis or neuralgia. The treatment blocks the pain perception of the sensory nerve endings and has NO EFFECT on motor function.

The principle of cryosurgery has nitrous oxide forced under the pressure of 600–800 psig between the inner and outer tubes of the cryoprobe. The gas is released through a small opening into a chamber at the tip of the probe. The gas expands and results in a rapid drop in temperature called the Joule-Thompson effect. An ice ball forms at the uninsulated end of the probe. The ice ball can range from 3.5 to 10 mm. The temperature reaches $-70°C$, and no gas escapes from the cryoprobe.

Cryosurgery is referred to as cryoneurolysis or cryogenic neuroablation. Nerve cells are destroyed by the freezing process. Cold causes destruction of the axon with breakdown of the myelin sheath and Wallerian degeneration. The breakdown of the axon is more complete with repeated freezes and thawing. The epineurium and perineurium are preserved, permitting ordered axonal regeneration, preventing the formation of amputation or stump neuromas. Cellular necrosis causes the release of tissue proteins, facilitating a

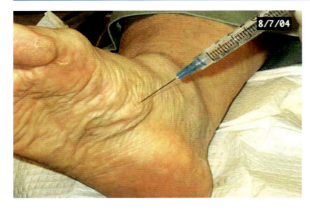

Fig. 49.4 Administration of local anesthesia

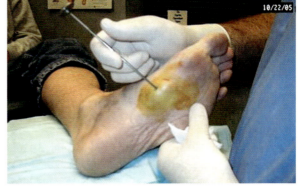

Fig. 49.5 Trochar inserted and needling of a plantar fibroma

Fig. 49.6 Plantar fibroma with probe inserted and freeze cycles performed

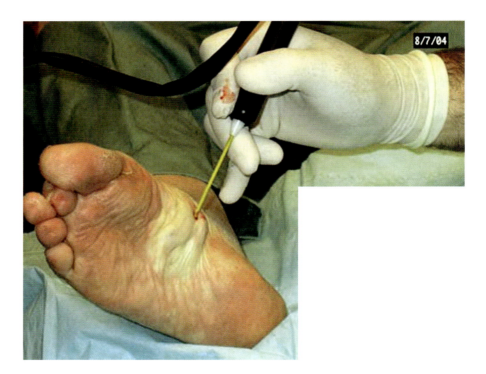

change in protein antigenic properties. An autoimmune response explains the prolonged analgesic relief.

49.8.2 A Cryosurgery Example

The procedure starts by administering local anesthesia; 0.5% marcaine with epinephrine 1:200,000 is recommended (Fig. 49.4).

A trochar is then inserted into the plantar fibroma, and a needling type technique is employed to create channels into the nodule (Fig. 49.5).

Next the probe is inserted, and several freeze cycles are performed (Fig. 49.6). Each freeze is accompanied by a defrost cycle.

An anti-inflammatory is then injected into the site. Celestone Soluspan is a very effective agent. The area is cleaned with Betadine and an antibiotic ointment applied. A dry sterile compression dressing is then applied and kept in place for 24 h.

49.9 Results

We have been performing cryosurgery for plantar fibromatosis for 4 years. We follow up with our patients to determine the success of the procedure. Success is measured by a decrease in the size and mass of the lesion but more importantly, the absence of pain. It takes up to 2 months for the full effectiveness of this procedure. If pain is still present after this time, then we recommend another cryosurgical procedure. The procedure can be performed many times without any negative consequences. We have treated 27 patients. Twenty-one were considered successful, with no more pain or discomfort from the lesions. That translates to 78%, which is comparable to data reported elsewhere (Caporusso et al. 2002; Goldstein 2005). Most patients who did not have complete success with the first procedure responded to one additional procedure to accomplish a successful outcome. Only two required a third procedure. A minimum of 2 months is needed between subsequent procedures. There is no long-term analysis of the success of cryosurgery for plantar fibromatosis available because it is too new of a modality.

We conclude that for plantar fibromatosis, cryosurgery is an excellent alternative to traditional surgical intervention. It is minimally invasive, and there is less post-operative healing with fewer risks of complication. Cryosurgery provides excellent pain relief with minimal recovery time. There is also a high patient satisfaction rate. The procedure can be repeated several times.

References

Allen BH, Fallat LM, Schwartz SM (2007) Cryosurgery: an innovative technique for the treatment of plantar fasciitis. J Foot Ankle Surg 46:75–79

Amoils SP (1967) The Joules Thompson cryoprobe. Arch Opthalmol 78:201–207

Barnard D (1980) The effects of extreme cold on sensory nerves. Ann R Coll Surg Engl 62:180–187

Bedi DG, Davidson DM (2001) Plantar fibromatosis: most common sonographic appearance and variations. J Clin Ultrasound 29:499–505

Caporusso EF, Fallet LM, Savoy-Moore R (2002) Cryogenic neuroablation for the treatment of lower extremity neuromas. J Foot Ankle Surg 41:286–290

Cavazos GJ, Khan KH, D'Antoni AV, Harkless LB, Lopez D (2009) Cryosurgery for the treatment of heel pain. Foot Ankle Int 30:500–505

De Bree E, Zoetmulder FAN, Keus RB, Peterse HL, van Coevorden F (2004) Incidence and treatment of recurrent plantar fibromatosis by surgery and postoperative radiotherapy. Am J Surg 187:33–38

de Palma L, Santucci A, Di Giulio A, Carloni S (1999) Plantar fibromatosis; an immunohistochemical and ultrastructural study. Foot Ankle Int 20:253–257

Dupuytren Society website (2010) Specifically on transdermal verapamil: http://www.dupuytren-online.info/dupuytren_anecdotal.html and http://www.dupuytren-online.info/Forum_English/board/other-therapies/verapamil-2_49.html. Accessed 6 Nov 2010

Durr HR, Krodel A, Truillier H, Lienemann A, Refior HJ (1999) Fibromatosis of the plantar fascia: diagnosis and indications for surgical treatment. Foot Ankle Int 20:13–17

Fleischmajer R, Nedwich A, Reeves JRT (1973) Juvenile fibromatoses. Arch Dermatol 107:574–579

Garamy G (1968) Engineering aspects of cryosurgery. In: Rand RW, Rinfret A, von Leden H (eds) Cryosurgery. Charles C. Thomas, Springfield

Goldstein SH (2005) Frozen in time. Podiatry management. 1–5

http://www.wheelessonline.com/ortho/ledderhose_disease_plantar_fibromatosis. Accessed 6 Nov 2010

Ledderhose G (1897) Zur Pathologie der Aponeurose des Fusses und der Hand. Langenbecks Arch Klin Chir 55:694–712

Lee TH, Wapner KL, Hecht PJ (1993) Current concepts review: plantar fibromatosis. J Bone Joint Surg [Br] 75:1080–1084

Rao GS, Luthra PK (1988) Dupuytren's disease of the foot in children: a report of three cases. Br J Plast Surg 41:313–315

Ross D (1999) Epidemiology of Dupuytren's disease. In: Tubiana R, Rayan G (eds) Dupuytren's disease. Hand Clin 15

Sammarco GJ, Mangone PG (2000) Classification and treatment of plantar fibromatosis. Foot Ankle Int 21:563–569

Seegenschmiedt MH (2008) Morbus Dupuytren/Morbus Ledderhose. In: Seegenschmiedt MH, Makoski HB, Trott KR, Brady L (eds) Radiotherapy for non-malignant disorders. Springer, Berlin/New York, pp 161–192

Seegenschmiedt MH, Attassi M (2003) Strahlentherapie beim Morbus Ledderhose – Indikation und Ergebnisse. Strahlenther Onkol 179(12):847–853

Seegenschmiedt MH, Wielpütz M, Hanslian E, Fehlauer F (2012a) Long-term outcome of radiotherapy for primary and recurrent Ledderhose disease. In: Dupuytren's disease and related hyperproliferative disorders, pp 409–427

Seegenschmiedt MH, Keilholz L, Wielpütz M, Schubert Ch, Fehlauer F (2012b) Long-term outcome of radiotherapy for early stage Dupuytren's disease: a phase III clinical study. In: Dupuytren's disease and related hyperproliferative disorders, pp 349–371

Wheeless CR, van der Bauwhede J (2010) Ledderhose disease: plantar fibromatosis. In: Wheeless' textbook of orthopaedics online

Long-Term Outcome of Radiotherapy for Primary and Recurrent Ledderhose Disease

50

Michael Heinrich Seegenschmiedt, Mark Wielpütz, Etienne Hanslian, and Fabian Fehlauer

Contents

50.1	**Introduction**	409
50.2	**Patients and Methods**	411
50.2.1	Study Design and Evaluation Criteria	411
50.2.2	Patients' Characteristics	413
50.2.3	Patients' Symptoms and Classification of Disease	413
50.2.4	Radiation Therapy	413
50.2.5	Documentation	416
50.2.6	Statistics	416
50.3	**Results**	416
50.3.1	Primary Study Endpoints	416
50.3.2	Secondary Study Endpoints: Nodules and Cords	417
50.3.3	Secondary Study Endpoints: Symptoms	417
50.3.4	Treatment Side Effects	417
50.3.5	Comparison with Control Group	419
50.3.6	Uni- and Multivariant Analysis	419

50.4	**Discussion**	419
50.4.1	Comparison with Other RT Studies	419
50.4.2	Radiobiologic Targets and Mechanisms	420
50.4.3	Potential Side Effects of Radiotherapy	421
50.4.4	Surgery Alone	421
50.4.5	Surgery Plus Postoperative Radiotherapy	421
50.5	**Conclusions**	423
Appendix A		423
References		426

M.H. Seegenschmiedt (✉)
Strahlenzentrum Hamburg,
Strahlentherapie & Radioonkologie, Hamburg, Germany

Klinik für Strahlentherapie und Radioonkologie,
Alfried Krupp Krankenhaus, Essen, Germany
e-mail: mhs@szhh.info

M. Wielpütz • E. Hanslian
Klinik für Strahlentherapie und Radioonkologie,
Alfried Krupp Krankenhaus, Essen, Germany

F. Fehlauer
Strahlenzentrum Hamburg,
Strahlentherapie & Radioonkologie, Hamburg, Germany
e-mail: fehlauer@szhh.info

50.1 Introduction

Plantar fibromatosis/Ledderhose disease (LD) is a hyperproliferative non-malignant disorder of unknown cause with low incidence rate of 1–2 cases per 100,000 hospital admissions (Ledderhose 1897; Pickren et al. 1951; Seegenschmiedt 2007). The disease is named after the German surgeon *Georg Ledderhose* (Fig. 50.1).

The concomitant palmar fibromatosis (so-called Dupuytren's disease, DD) occurs in up to 35% of all Ledderhose patients, while knuckle pads (Garrod's disease) or penile fibromatosis (Peyronie's disease) occurs in only up to 5% of patients affected by DD/LD (Allen et al. 1955; Aviles et al. 1971). For unknown reasons, LD has a much higher incidence among Caucasians as compared to the African or Asian populations (Delgadillo and Arenson 1985). Males are up to two times more often affected than females (Allen et al. 1955). Various etiologic and risk factors have been discussed, including genetic factors, long-term nicotine and alcohol abuse, concomitant disorders like diabetes mellitus (Seegenschmiedt 2007), and/or long-term use of antiepileptic medication such as phenobarbiturate (Strzelczyk et al. 2008), but the major cause for disease onset and continuation remains unclear. The

C. Eaton et al. (eds.), *Dupuytren's Disease and Related Hyperproliferative Disorders*,
DOI 10.1007/978-3-642-22697-7_50, © Springer-Verlag Berlin Heidelberg 2012

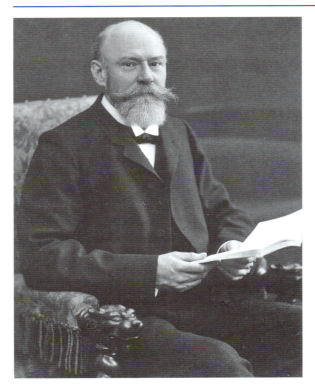

Fig. 50.1 The German surgeon Georg Ledderhose (1855–1925) (Reprinted with permission by Stadtarchiv Munich, Germany)

Table 50.1 International classification of Ledderhose disease (IC-LD)

Grade	Short description	Explanation
1	Unifocal disease	One nodule/cord or one well-circumscribed region involved without adherence to skin or extension to the flexor sheath (plantar fascia)
2	Multifocal disease	Several nodules/cords or several regions involved without adherence to the skin or extension to the flexor sheath (plantar fascia)
3	Multifocal disease, deep extension into ONE direction	Several nodules/cords or several regions involved; deep extension to EITHER skin (= 3A) OR flexor sheath (plantar fascia) (= 3B)
4[a]	Multifocal disease, deep extension into TWO directions	Several nodules/cords or several regions involved; deep extension to skin (3A) AND flexor sheath (plantar fascia) (3B), i.e., stage 3C
Suffix R	Recurrent disease	Any status or stage progression after previous surgical therapy
Other suffices	Specific disease, parameters	Nodules (N), cords (C), pain symptoms (P), other symptoms (S), walking disorder (W)

[a]Stages 3 and 4 can be combined and specified into three categories A, B, C

typical symptoms of LD usually start one decade earlier than in DD, namely, in the third to fourth decade (Classen and Hurst 1992; Seegenschmiedt 2007). Also children, adolescents, and young adults can be affected by LD (Fetsch et al. 2005; Godette et al. 1997; Rao and Luthra 1988). Often LD starts unilaterally, but bilateral disease is common in later stages and observed in long-term follow-up (Classen and Hurst 1992).

Typical signs of LD are "bumps" attached to the plantar fascia or "bunions" on the ball of the foot which may be palpable for smaller nodules and visible for large size nodules. Typical subjective complaints expressed by patients are "tension, pressure, and/or burning sensations" of parts or the whole foot sole causing discomfort while standing and alteration of gait while walking (Seegenschmiedt and Attassi 2003; Seegenschmiedt 2007). In most cases, single (= unifocal disease) or multiple nodules or cords (= multifocal disease) are localized on the central and medial part of the plantar fascia (Aviles et al. 1971; Beckmann et al. 2004; Cavolo and Sherwood 1982); however, other distributions are possible with involvement of the forefoot or the lateral part of the plantar fascia.

The typical onset of LD is characterized by a rapid growth of one or more nodules over a few weeks to months, followed by stationary or very slow progressive disease phases over many years (Classen and Hurst 1992). In early stages, the overlying skin is not attached to the nodules and the fibroblastic hyperplasia is embedded within the tissue of the plantar fascia, but in later stages, the nodules and cords may extend to the subcutaneous tissue layer or the deeper structures of the flexor tendon sheath (Kashuk and Pasternack 1981); however, in contrast to the aggressive type of fibromatosis, in LD, the plantar muscles or bones are rarely infiltrated (Johnston et al. 1992; Seegenschmiedt 2007). Moreover, "contracture of toes" occurs less often than it has been observed for fingers in DD (Beckmann et al. 2004). Recently, a classification system of LD has been proposed with four different stages, unifocal disease (stage 1), multifocal disease (stage 2), with extension to the superficial (stage 3) and deep foot structural stage (stage 4) (Sammarco and Mangone 2000). For practical reasons, some modifications of this staging system were applied in our study (Table 50.1).

Histopathology of the fibrous tissue helps to differentiate between different phases of LD. Immunochemical histological studies found type III/I collagen ratio to correspond with progression of DD (Herovici 1961). The amount of type III collagen as percentage of the total collagen corresponds with disease progression: clinical stage 1 has >35% type III collagen, clinical stage 2 range between 20% and 35%, and clinical stage 3 has <20% type III collagen (Lam et al. 2010). In our clinical study, histological confirmation was only achieved for pre-operated cases. The following clinical phases have been described in agreement with the staging that Luck (1959) proposed for Dupuytren's disease:

- *First LD phase*: The initial LD stage is characterized by proliferating fibroblasts, which are responsible for the formation of nodules of high cellularity, which later transform into the cords which are of moderate cellularity.
- *Second LD phase*: During this second so-called involutional stage, the existing proliferating fibroblasts differentiate into the mitotic and postmitotic myofibroblasts which slowly initiate the contraction process forming cords and fibrotic scars (low cellularity).
- *Third LD phase*: The final and so-called residual stage is histologically dominated mostly by existing collagenous fibers with a low cellularity similar to scars.

Due to the low incidence and actual lack of cure so far, no standard treatment has been established. Thus, at the present time, most family physicians, general practitioners, and orthopedists will recommend surgery as the primary treatment step, but the few published studies indicate high relapse rates ranging from 8% to 73% (Allen et al. 1955; Alusio et al. 1996; Aviles et al. 1971; Beckmann et al. 2004; Dürr et al. 1999; Haedicke and Sturim 1989; Mirabell et al. 1990; Pickren et al. 1951; Wapner et al. 1995; Wu 1994), depending upon the LD stage and applied surgical techniques. The situation for recurrent LD is even worse and requires more and more aggressive surgery (Landers et al. 1993). Due to the high relapse rate, some authors have suggested to use the radical total plantar fasciectomy as primary surgical procedure (Parnitzke et al. 1991). For the surgical treatment, it is possible to differentiate between local, segmental, or wide excision procedures (LE, SE, WE) with a small safety margin of 2–3 cm, and subtotal or total radical fasciectomy with a larger safety margin and with or without skin grafting for far advanced or recurrent lesions (LD stages 3 and 4). The other available treatment options are noninvasive and include the prescription of orthotic devices; physical therapy; local steroid injections; systemic medication like vitamin E; and other supportive measures like weight reduction, reduction of special foot's strain, and avoidance of nicotine and alcohol abuse (Pentland and Anderson 1985; Beckmann et al. 2004).

Radiotherapy (RT) as primary treatment of early LD stages – similar to its already known application for early DD stages – has been first successfully implemented by our group at Alfried Krupp Hospital in Essen in 2003 (Seegenschmiedt and Attassi 2003) and independently confirmed by another German group in Offenbach (Heyd et al. 2010). This chapter is an update and long-term analysis of our ongoing clinical study with a much higher number of patients and treated sites (feet) and much more extended long-term follow-up to obtain better basic back ground data of this disorder and clinical information concerning the efficacy of RT either as a primary treatment or as a salvage treatment after surgery.

50.2 Patients and Methods

50.2.1 Study Design and Evaluation Criteria

This prospective cohort study comprises all consecutive patients presented to our institution between January 1997 and December 2009 (13 years). Patients' characteristics (gender, age, involved sites, risk factors, disease record, etc.) and details of affected feet were assessed with standardized documentation. All patients were examined and counseled about different treatment options including: (1) "wait and see" strategy without treatment, (2) possible medication, e.g., vitamin E, (3) local radiotherapy, and (4) possible surgical methods. Patients who did not qualify for or consented to RT (due to disease-related or personal reasons) were continuously followed and served as control group ("control"). All other patients (sites) were submitted to a prospective RT protocol with predefined RT technique and annual follow-up. Primary study endpoints were: (a) *prevention of disease progression* and (b) *avoidance of surgical intervention*. Secondary study endpoints were: (c) *objective effects on morphological signs* (number and size of nodules and cords, LD stage), and (d) *subjective effects on functional and symptomatic aspects* such as pain (P; no, slight, moderate, severe pain), walking ability (W; no limitations, >1 km, <1 km, walking disability with/without orthotics), and (e) overall *satisfaction with disease status* (10-point linear analogue scale: "0" = "completely satisfied status" up to "10" "completely

Table 50.2 CTC and LENT scale for skin and subcutaneous tissue

CTC grade 0	Grade 1 "minor"	Grade 2 "moderate"	Grade 3 "severe"	Grade 4 "life-threatening"
None	Faint erythema or dry desquamation	Moderate to brisk erythema or a patchy moist desquamation, mostly confined to skin folds and creases; moderate edema	Confluent moist desquamation $\geq$1.5 cm diameter and not confined to skin folds; pitting edema	Skin necrosis or ulceration of full thickness dermis; may include bleeding not induced by minor trauma or abrasion

Table 50.3 Patient characteristics

	All n (%)	RT group	Control	Statistics
Patients (%)	158 (100%)	91 (58%)	67 (42%)	
– Females	77 (49%)	44 (48%)	33 (49%)	ns
– Males	81 (51%) (+)	47 (52%)	34 (51%)	ns
– Adolescents <18 years	(+) 3	(+) 2	(+) 1	–
Age (years)				
– Mean	49	48	51	ns
– Median	52	51	53	ns
– Range	9–81	9–79	21–81	ns
Sites (pats × 2)	316	182	134	
– Unilateral	68	46	22	*
– Bilateral	77	45	32	ns
– Overall feet	316	182	134	
Affected feet (Table 50.4)	222 (70%)	136 (61%)	86 (39%)	ns
Positive family record (first degree)				
– Dupuytren's disease	36 (23%)	21 (23%)	15 (22%)	ns
– Ledderhose disease	12 (8%)	9 (10%)	3 (4%)	ns
– Other (e.g., Garrod's disease)	6 (3%)	3 (3%)	3 (4%)	ns
Comorbidity				
– Dupuytren's disease	72 (46%)	46 (51%)	26 (39%)	ns
– Garrod's disease	9 (6%)	6 (7%)	3 (4%)	ns
– Peyronie's disease	5 (3%)	3 (3%)	2 (3%)	ns
– Frozen shoulder	15 (9%)	9 (9%)	6 (9%)	ns
– Keloid/hypertrophic scar	12 (8%)	8 (9%)	4 (6%)	ns
– Any "foot trauma"	14 (9%)	9 (10%)	5 (7%)	ns
– Diabetes mellitus	12 (8%)	7 (8%)	5 (7%)	ns
– Liver disease	9 (6%)	6 (7%)	3 (4%)	ns
– Epileptic disorder	3 (2%)	2 (2%)	1 (1,5%)	ns
Risk factors				
– Nicotine abuse (NA)	41 (26%)	24 (26%)	17 (25%)	ns
– Alcohol abuse (AA)	25 (16%)	14 (15%)	11 (16%)	ns
– Combined NA+AA	19 (12%)	9 (10%)	10 (15%)	ns
Time of first symptoms (months) before RT				
– Mean	29	30	27	ns
– Median	18	20	16	ns
– Range	6–264	12–264	6–84	ns
Follow-up (months)				
– Mean	68	68	66	ns
– Median	61	62	60	ns
– Range	24–160	24–160	24–156	ns

DD Dupuytren's disease, *LD* Ledderhose disease, *GD* Garrod's disease (knuckle pads), *NA* nicotine abuse, *AA* alcohol abuse, *ns* not statistically significant
*Statistically significant with $p < 0.05$

unsatisfied status") before RT and at last follow-up (FU). Acute side effects were analyzed according to NCI's Common Toxicity Criteria (CTC; up to 90 days after RT) and chronic side effects according to Late Effects Normal Tissue (LENT; more than 90 days after RT) classification, which provides five grades of severity (0=none; 1=mild; 2=moderate; 3=severe; 4=life-threatening) (Trotti et al. 2000; Mornex et al. 1997) (Table 50.2).

50.2.2 Patients' Characteristics

From January 1997 to December 2009, 158 consecutive patients (91 males, 67 females) were referred to our clinic because of obvious and/or symptomatic LD. Their mean age was 49 (median 52, range 9–81) years. For most disease aspects, no gender difference was found. Concomitant DD was noted in 36 (23%) patients, 9 (6%) had additional Garrod's disease, 12 (8%) hypertrophic scars or keloids, and 12 (8%) diabetes mellitus. Fourteen (9%) patients reported a former "foot injury or trauma". Forty-one (26%) patients stated long-term smoking and 25 (16%) regular alcohol intake. Patient data (including genetic and other possible risk factors) are summarized in Table 50.3 (Patient Characteristics) and site-specific data in Table 50.4 (Site Characteristics).

After careful physical examination (all conducted by the first author), 222 (75%) feet (i.e., sites) were found to be affected by one or more typical signs of LD (84 bilateral, 35 right and 33 left foot), while 74 (25%) feet were unaffected. Additional ultrasound and magnetic resonance imaging was used to confirm palpated and suspected disease if necessary and to assess the depth of the lesion (Fig. 50.2).

After initial assessment, patients were counseled about all possible treatment options including a "wait and see strategy," conservative options like stretching, orthotics, nonsteroidal drugs, local cortisone-injections and physiotherapy, radiotherapy, and surgical options. The final decision was left at the discretion of the individual patient. From the initial 158 patients, 91 (61.5%) patients (47 males and 44 females) representing 136 (46%) affected feet decided to undergo RT and signed the informed consent; the remaining 67 (38.5%) patients representing 134 feet did not undergo RT and served as control group ("control"), either due to less advanced LD (wait & see approach) or because other treatment options were considered as more promising.

50.2.3 Patients' Symptoms and Classification of Disease

Prior to the first visit at our clinic, most patients had counseling by family practitioners, orthopedists, or specialized foot surgeons or had performed Internet research themselves. They presented with symptomatic progressive LD for at least 6–12 months; the mean time from first observation of any sign of LD up to the first presentation at our institution was 29 (median 18, range 6–264) months. All 91 treated patients (or 136 feet) had developed an increasing size or number of nodules (N), cords (C), or other specific symptoms, i.e., 88 (97%) patients had progressive LD symptoms (S) in 118 (87%) feet including pain symptoms (P), numbness (N), and/or any other discomfort (O); 86 (95%) patients representing 114 (84%) feet had walking difficulties (W) due to pain or used orthotics in at least one affected foot. Most patients had received nonsurgical treatments like local massage, special insoles, steroid injections into growing nodules and cords, or systemic non-steroidal anti-inflammatory drugs (NSAID) due to local pain. Thirty-five (26%) feet had recurrent progressive LD after surgical procedures and 8 (6%) feet had received prior RT. The site characteristics of the RT and control group prior to RT onset are summarized in Table 50.4 (Treatment Site Characteristics).

50.2.4 Radiation Therapy

RT was applied to almost all feet (133, 98%) by means of 125–150 kV photons/20 mA and 4-mm Aluminum filter for beam correction (until 06/2000: Philips 250, Hamburg, Germany; since 07/2000 Gulmay Medical, Bristol, UK). The RT tubes (6×8 and 10×15 cm^2) were directly positioned onto the lesions with a focus-to-skin-distance of 40 cm. The RT portal encompassed all visible and palpable lesions and disease detected by means of ultrasonic or magnetic resonance imaging with a 2 cm safety margin. Uninvolved areas were shielded with 3-mm thick lead rubber plates (Figs. 50.3–50.5). Two adolescents (9 and 15 years, 3 affected feet) obtained RT with 6 MeV electron beam and en-face portals with plantar to dorsal beam direction and additional 10-mm skin bolus due to a more complex target volume and better radioprotection for normal tissue; shielding was achieved by means of

Table 50.4 Site characteristics

	All n (%)	RT group	Control	Statistics
Patients/Table 50.3	158	91	67	ns
Overall # feet	316	182	134	
Affected # feet = N	222	136	86	
Unilateral involvement	68 (31%)	46 (34%)	22 (26%)	*
– Right foot (RF)	(35)	(24)	(11)	
– Left foot (LF)	(33)	(22)	(11)	
Bilateral (RF+LF)	77	45 (66%)	32	*
Uninvolved	94 (30%)	46 (25%)	48 (36%)	ns
– Primary disease	170 (77%)	101 (74%)	69 (80%)	ns
– Recurrent (post Tx)	52 (23%)	35 (26%)	17 (20%)	ns
1 surgical procedure	(38)	(30)	(8)	
≥2 surgical procedures	(14)	(12)	(2)	
Nodes #/size				
– Present (yes/no)	218 (98%)	136 (100%)	82 (95%)	ns
– Mean #	2.3	2.2	2.5	ns
– Mean size (cm^2)	13±7	14±7	12±8	ns
– Range (cm^2)	1.0–36	1.5–30	1.0–36	ns
Cords #/size				
– Present (yes/no)	162 (73%)	102 (75%)	60 (70%)	ns
– Mean #	1.4	1.6	1.3	ns
– Mean length (cm)	2.0±1.2	2.0±1.2	1.5±1.1	ns
– Range (min–max)	0.5–5.0	0.5–4.5	0.5–5.0	ns
LD classification				
– Stage 1/unifocal	72 (32%)	46 (34%)	26 (30%)	ns
– Stage 2/multifocal	92 (41%)	60 (44%)	32 (37%)	ns
– Stage 3/deep fixation	58 (26%)	30 (22%)	28 (33%)	ns
Symptoms				
Any symptom	168 (76%)	104 (76%)	64 (74%)	ns
– Pressure	157 (71%)	100 (72%)	57 (66%)	ns
– Tension	98 (44%)	62 (45%)	36 (42%)	ns
– Pain @ walking	132 (59%)	86 (62%)	46 (53%)	ns
– Pain @ rest/stand	71 (32%)	47 (34%)	24 (28%)	ns
– Other: itching, numbness	34 (15%)	22 (16%)	12 (14%)	ns
Symptom score	6.3	6.4	6.1	ns
Function status				
– Any dysfunction	109 (49%)	69 (51%)	40 (47%)	ns
– Walking disorder	75 (34%)	49 (36%)	26 (30%)	ns
– Obvious limp	33 (15%)	23 (17%)	10 (12%)	ns
– Use of insoles	71 (32%)	41 (30%)	30 (35%)	ns
– Other dysfunction(s) (sports)	48 (22%)	29 (21%)	19 (22%)	ns

*statistically $p < 0.05$
DD Dupuytren's disease, *LD* Ledderhose disease, *GD* Garrod's disease (knuckle pads), *NA* nicotine abuse, *AA* alcohol abuse, *ns* not statistically significant

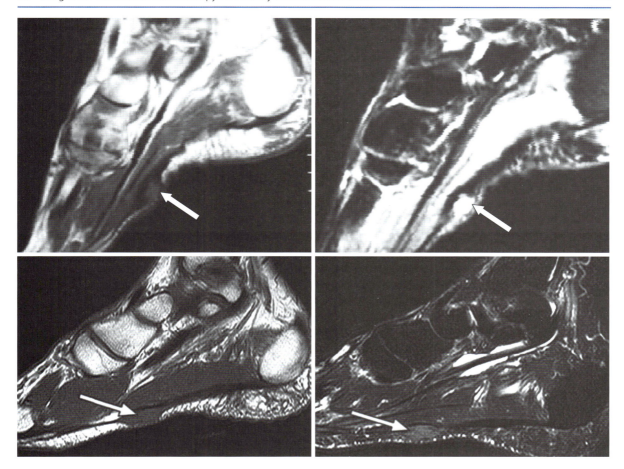

Fig. 50.2 Magnetic resonance imaging of Ledderhose disease. Typical magnetic resonance imaging (MRI) findings without (*left*) and with contrast media (*right*)

10-mm lead blocks inserted into the electron tube mounting of the linear accelerator (Mevatron™ or Primus™, Siemens, Erlangen, Germany).

The RT reference dose for all lesions was prescribed at mean lesion depth, i.e., for most lesions at 1 cm depth; for superficial lesions, the reference depth was assumed at the skin surface, while for lesions of >2 cm depth and >5 cm diameter, the depth was additionally measured by ultrasonic or magnetic resonance imaging and individually adjusted. All RT sessions were performed either with the patient standing, knee bended 90°, and the affected foot positioned onto the treatment table or with patient in prone position. Details of RT planning and treatment setup are shown in Figs. 50.3–50.5. The RT protocol prescribed two RT series consisting of 5 weekly fractions of 3 Gy or five fractions within 1 week (7 days), repeated after 12 (range 10–15) weeks with the same scheme up to 30 Gy total dose; three patients (5 feet) received only one RT series.

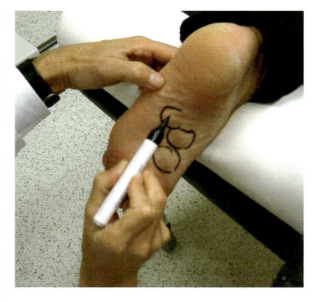

Fig. 50.3 Examination and outline of Ledderhose disease on foot sole

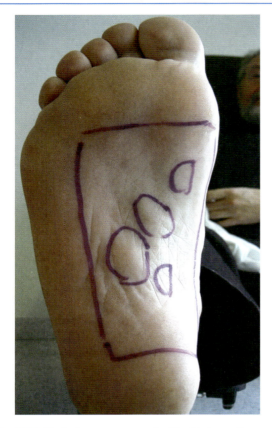

Fig. 50.4 Typical treatment portal of Ledderhose disease on foot sole

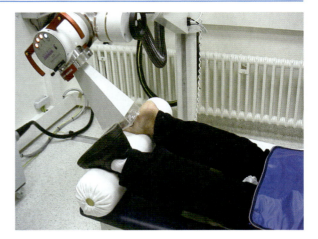

Fig. 50.5 Treatment setup of Ledderhose disease at orthovolt machine using 125-kV photons; lead apron for pelvic protection

50.2.5 Documentation

All findings were prospectively documented on specific charts and forms (see Appendix "Documentation"): visible and palpable nodules, cords, or other findings were sketched onto the skin surface with ink marker (Figs. 50.3 and 50.4), then measured with a linear ruler, and finally archived using digital photographs or acetate foils. Possible clinical symptoms were inquired, classified, and documented in a special questionnaire prior to RT onset. The same procedures and physical exams were conducted at 3 and 12 months and at last FU (FU) after completion of RT (RT group) or after first visit (control group). For the evaluation of the long-term and last FU, similar structured questionnaires were mailed and if required, some additional phone calls were conducted with all patients; in case of any substantial changes or a progression of disease, patients were scheduled for new FU visits.

50.2.6 Statistics

The statistical analysis was performed with the software program SPSS (Chicago, IL). For categorical variables numbers and percentage values, and for continuous variables, median, mean, and range values were calculated. Statistical testing for independence of categorical and continuous variables between different groups, time points, and study endpoints included the Student-t, the Cochran–Mantel–Haenszel, and the Wilcoxon test. Univariate and multivariate analyses were performed using the logistic regression analysis. A p-value of 0.05 and lower was defined as statistical significant for two-side tests.

50.3 Results

As of January 2011, all untreated ("control") and treated patients with irradiated feet were evaluated after a minimum of 24 months FU; the mean FU was 68 (median 61; range 24–160) months.

50.3.1 Primary Study Endpoints

Regarding the RT group of 91 patients and 136 irradiated feet, a total of 6 (7%) patients and 11 (8%) feet respectively showed progression between 12 and 35 months after completion of RT; of those 5 (6%) patients and 7 (5.1%) feet respectively had salvage

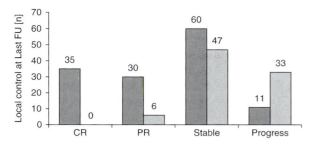

Fig. 50.6 Local control at last follow-up for RT and control group. RT group (*dark gray shaded*; n = 136) and control group (*light gray shaded*; n = 86); *CR* complete remission of LD findings and symptoms; *PR* >50% remission of LD findings and symptoms; see further details in Table 50.5

surgery (3 wide fasciectomy, 4 total aponeurectomy); one foot required a longer healing period of over 2 months. Eighty-five (93%) patients and 125 (92%) feet, respectively, had no progression of LD in long-term FU within the irradiated area and did not require any foot surgery after completion of RT (Fig. 50.6). Nine (10%) patients developed progression outside the treated RT portal or at the uninvolved foot, and two of them had additional in-field local recurrences within or at the edge of the RT portal. In long-term FU, 123 of 136 (90.4%) feet remained without progression in local control. A total of 60 (44%) feet had minor remission (change 25–50%) or remained in stable condition (change ± 25%) without increasing size and number of nodules and/or cords; 65 (48%) feet had an obvious remission (change >50%) within 1 year with regard to size and number of nodules and/or cords; of those, 30 (22.1%) had a partial remission (PR) with at least 50% remission of nodules and cords, while 35 (25.7%) feet regressed completely (CR) with freedom from all palpable nodules and/or cords (Fig. 50.6).

50.3.2 Secondary Study Endpoints: Nodules and Cords

Overall in the RT group, in 60 of 136 (44%) feet, the number and size of nodules were reduced. The mean number was reduced from 2.2 to 1.6 nodules, while the area of nodular involvement shrunk from 14 to 8 cm². Moreover, in 46/102 (45%), the number and length of cords were reduced. The mean number was reduced from 1.6 to 1.0 cords, while the mean length of the cords shrunk from 3.0 to 2.2 cm of nodules and in 61 (44.8%) feet, the number and size of cords were reduced.

50.3.3 Secondary Study Endpoints: Symptoms

Eighty-two of 91 (90%) patients of the RT group improved with regard to LD symptoms; 3 (3%) had no change and 6 (7%) patients experienced a progression of symptoms. With regard to the treated sites, a total of 121 of 136 (89%) feet experienced an improvement of any LD symptom in long-term FU. With regard to the LD site-specific symptoms, the following response rates were achieved: 71 of 86 (83%) affected feet with pain during walking and 32 of 47 (68%) affected feet with pain at rest improved; in 74 of 100 (74%) affected feet, an unpleasant pressure sensation was reduced; in 48 of 62 (77%) affected feet, an atypical and unpleasant tension sensation was reduced, and in 18 of 22 (82%), an irritating itching sensation was reduced. Prior to treatment, 118 (87%) feet were impaired by pain (P), numbness (N), and other discomforts (O); 86 (95%) patients representing 114 (83,8%) feet had functional or walking difficulties (W) due to pain and/or used orthotics in at least one affected foot. These symptoms and impairments improved in up to 90% of all sites. The patients' overall *satisfaction with the disease status* (10-point linear analogue scale) improved by 3.2 points in 81 (89%) patients; 5 patients had a stable score and in 5 patient, it increased by 1.6 points in average.

50.3.4 Treatment Side Effects

Acute side effects within the RT area developed in 36 of 136 (26.5%) irradiated feet: slight erythema and/or dry desquamation (CTC grade 1) in 29 (21.3%) and a diffuse erythema with areas of moist desquamation (CTC grade 2) in 7 (5.0%) sites; the latter situation was mostly associated with a preexisting chronic eczema or mycosis of the forefoot and foot sole. Late radiogenic changes of the skin and subcutaneous tissue (LENT grade 1) were observed in 22 (16.2%) sites, either as increased dryness of the skin or as fibrotic changes preferentially located at the vicinity of scars from previous surgical procedures. No acute or chronic radiogenic toxicity was noted beyond CTC grade 2 and/or beyond LENT grade 1.

Table 50.5 Treatment results at last follow-up with comparison of RT and control group

	All *n* (%)	RT-group	Control	Statistics
Affected feet=*N*	222	136	86	
Remission status @ last FU				
Regression	71 (32%)	65 (48%)	6 (7%)	*
– Partial remission	36 (16%)	30 (22%)	6 (7%)	*
– Complete remission	35 (16%)	35 (26%)	–	*
Minor remission or stable disease	107 (48%)	60 (44%)	47 (55%)	*
Progression	*44 (20%)*	*11 (8%)*	*33 (38%)*	*
– Inside RT field		11 (8%)	n.a.	
– Outside RT field		4 (3%) (+)	n.a.	
– Surgery	25 (11%)	7 (5%)	18 (21%)	*
– Radiotherapy	24 (11%)	4 (3%)	20 (23%)	*
Nodules				
– Remission (yes/no)	66/218 (30%)	60/136 (44%)	6/82 (7%)	*
– Mean #	2.2 (−0.1)	1.6 (−0.6)	3.8 (+1.3)	*
– Mean size (cm^2)	12 (−1)	8 (−6)	18 (+6)	*
Cords				
– Remission (yes/no)	49/162 (30%)	46/102 (45%)	3/60 (5%)	*
– Mean #	1.4 (±0)	1.0 (−0.6)	2.0 (+0.7)	*
– Mean length (cm)	2.7 (− 0.1)	2.2 (− 0.8)	3.5 (+ 1.0)	*
Symptom score (0–10)				
Status before RT/start	5.6	6.4	4.4	*
– @ 3 months FU	4.7	4.8	4.6	ns
– @ 12 months FU	3.8	3.0	5.2	*
– @ Last FU	4.2	3.2	6.2	*
Symptom change	−1.4	−3.2	+ 1.8	*
Overall satisfaction	126/222 (55%)	116/136 (85%)	10/86 (12%)	*
Symptom relief				
Any symptom	104/168 (62%)	82/104 (79%)	12/64 (19%)	*
– Pressure	79/157 (50%)	74/100 (74%)	5/57 (9%)	*
– Tension	50/ 98 (51%)	48/ 62 (77%)	2/36 (6%)	*
– Pain @ walking	73/132 (55%)	71/ 86 (83%)	2/46 (4%)	*
– Pain @ rest/stand	36/ 71 (51%)	32/ 47 (68%)	4/24 (17%)	*
Other itching, numbness	20/ 34 (59%)	18/ 22 (81%)	2/12 (17%)	*
Function improvement				
– Any improvement	50/109 (46%)	44/69 (64%)	6/40 (15%)	*
– Walking disorder	39/75 (52%)	36/49 (73%)	3/26 (12%)	*
– Obvious limp	13/33 (39%)	11/23 (48%)	2/10 (20%)	*
– Use of insoles	29/71 (41%)	26/41 (63%)	3/30 (10%)	*
– Other (sports)	20/48 (42%)	17/29 (59%)	3/19 (16%)	*

*Statistical significant values (*p* at least lower than 0.05), *ns* not statistically significant

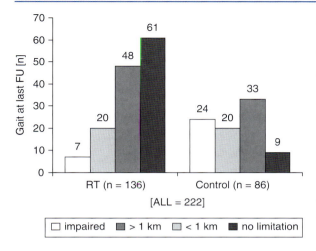

Fig. 50.7 Walking status at last follow-up for the RT group compared to control group

50.3.5 Comparison with Control Group

In comparison with the RT group, only 6 (7%) of 86 untreated sites had a "spontaneous remission"; 47 (55%) sites remained stable, but 33 (38%) feet developed progressive symptoms or measurable disease signs (nodules and cords) (Table 50.5, Treatment Results). A total of 18 of 86 (21%) sites required surgery and 20 (23%) underwent RT during FU due to progressive disease, while the RT group had a statistically significant lower rate of progression and less secondary treatments ($p<0.01$) (Table 50.5).

The mean number and size or length of nodules and cords increased in the control group compared to the RT group ($p<0.01$). The overall symptom score worsened in 41 (48%) and improved only in 10 (12%) feet; the overall symptom score in the control group increased by an average of 1.8 points compared to a decrease of 3.2 points in the RT group ($p<0.01$). In the control group, 12 sites (19%) improved with regard to any symptom and for specific symptoms such as pressure ($n=5/9\%$), tension (2/6%), and pain symptoms (4/17%) which was significantly less than in the RT group ($p<0.01$).

Functional improvement in the control group was noted in 6 (15%) sites as compared with 44 (64%) sites in the RT group ($p<0.01$). This resulted also in a significantly different long-term functional outcome in both groups, which can be seen for the difference in gait or walking function of both groups (Fig. 50.7).

50.3.6 Uni- and Multivariant Analysis

Regarding the primary endpoints "prevention of progression" and "avoidance of surgery" radiotherapy was significantly superior in long-term outcome as compared to observation alone: 11 of 136 (8%) feet in the RT and 38 of 86 (44%) feet progressed and required secondary treatment, i.e., 7 (5%) feet with surgery in the RT group and 18 (21%) in the control ($p<0.01$). For all other prognostic evaluations, only the RT group was considered: Patient-related parameters such as gender, age, family disposition, and related disorders had no significant impact on disease outcome. The only patient-related prognostic parameter was nicotine abuse. With regard to disease-related parameters, no impact was found for unilateral versus bilateral affliction, number and size of nodules and cords, and specific symptoms. Negative prognostic parameters were a progressed disease stage, a longer time from first symptoms to start of RT treatment, and a more advanced overall symptom score as well as previous surgical intervention and nicotine abuse (Table 50.6).

50.4 Discussion

50.4.1 Comparison with Other RT Studies

RT is a safe and effective treatment for management of various non-malignant disorders of the loco-motor system (El Majdoub et al. 2009; Heyd et al. 2007, 2009; Janssen et al. 2009; Rödel et al. 2002). A national pattern of care study in Germany with about 80 million inhabitants found that every year, more than 20,000 patients undergo RT for non-malignant disorders of whom almost 1,000 receive RT for symptomatic hyperproliferative disorders like hypertrophic scars, keloids, LD, and DD (Seegenschmiedt et al. 1999).

Ledderhose disease (LD) is a specific form of benign fibromatosis of the plantar fascia which is closely associated and related to Dupuytren's disease (DD) and other fibromatoses. Beatty (1938) was the first who had used RT to effectively treat DD. Thereafter, several mono-center studies assessed the potential role of RT for the management of early stages of DD (Herbst and Regler 1986; Adamietz et al. 2001; Seegenschmiedt et al. 2001; Seegenschmiedt 2007). In a current literature review, the obtained local control rates ranged from 60% to 100% after FU periods covering up to

Table 50.6 Uni- and multivariate parameters

Parameter	Univariate	Multivariate	Notes
RT versus control	$p<0.01$	$p<0.01$	Both endpoints
Gender	ns	ns	
Age	ns	ns	
Uni- versus bilateral	ns	ns	
Positive family record	ns	ns	
Comorbidity	ns	ns	
Alcohol	ns	ns	
Nicotine	$p<0.05$	ns	Progression
Time of first symptoms (months) before RT	$p<0.05$	ns	Progression
LD stage 3	$p<0.01$	$p<0.05$	Avoidance of surgery
Size/number of nodules	ns	ns	
Size/number of cords	ns	ns	
Overall symptom score	$p<0.05$		Avoidance of surgery
Prior surgical treatment	$p<0.01$	$p<0.05$	Progression

19 years (Seegenschmiedt 2007; Betz et al. 2010). Despite these favorable results for DD and the known analogy of DD and LD, the application of RT was not invented and extended to LD for a long time until the beginning of this millennium.

Our German group (Seegenschmiedtand and Atassi 2003) was the first worldwide to report on the use of RT for symptomatic primary and recurrent LD in 25 patients (with 36 feet). This pilot study assessed the treatment indication (primary versus recurrent LD), the appropriate RT technique, and the necessary clinical evaluation tools prior to and post RT to assess the treatment response. The achieved outcomes after the application of two RT series of each 15 Gy (5 × 3 Gy within 1 week) up to a total dose 30 Gy in analogy of the treatment of DD were excellent and much better than those known for RT of DD or for any surgical treatment of LD. After a median FU of more than 3 years (range 1–6.5 years FU), the further progression of LD was avoided in all patients and feet (100%); moreover, 44% sites obtained a remission of nodules and 53% sites a remission of cords, while 50% patients regained normal walking ability; overall, in 28 of 36 (78%) involved feet, a symptom regression up to total relief of symptoms was achieved. This study raised the interest in the radiotherapy community to continue the clinical research in this field.

The recently published results of a multicenter German study (Heyd et al. 2010) confirmed the findings of our first pilot study concerning remission and local control of LD, pain remission, and improvement of gait (Heyd et al. 2010). In their study, two different RT schemes (10 × 3 Gy or 8 × 4 Gy) and both mega-voltage electron beam or orthovoltage RT techniques were applied without any difference in treatment outcome. After a short median FU of almost 2 years, none of the cases showed progression of nodules/cords or an increase of symptoms occurred. Similar to our findings, complete remission was achieved in 33% (11 sites) and partial remission (reduction in number and size) was observed in 55% (18 sites); 12% (4 sites) remained unchanged, but required no surgery during FU. Pain relief was achieved in 63% and gait improved in 73%. Overall 92% of the patients were satisfied with the outcome resulting in an overall improvement of 3.5 points on the linear analogue scale (LAS) which is very similar to the findings of our own study.

The encouraging results of our updated study presented herein with long-term FU extend any reported data with regard to long-term outcome and the achievement of local control: The results are better than any reported surgical series and should promote further recruitment of patients in this RT protocol and eventually a long-term evaluation and comparison with established surgical techniques.

50.4.2 Radiobiologic Targets and Mechanisms

In this study, the proposed international staging system for LD had prognostic value for long-term outcome. The radiobiologic mechanism of RT in ML is suggested to be predominantly based on the inhibition of the fibroblast and myofibroblast proliferation which are known to be responsible for the progression of the disease. Thus, the optimal time for RT is given in patients with progressive disease. The radiosensitivity of fibroblasts is known from the treatment of other benign mesenchymal disorders (Seegenschmiedt 2007). In addition, MD specimens show an increase of growth factors produced by macrophages and platelets, including the fibroblast growth factor (FGF), transforming growth factor-beta (TGF-β), epidermal growth factor (EGF), platelet-derived growth factor (PDGF), and connective tissue growth factor (CTGF), which play a key role in the pathogenesis of ML and MD (Seegenschmiedt 2007). The impact of low RT doses on cytokine expression has been demonstrated for analgesic RT of degenerative disorders (Rödel et al. 2002, 2004, 2008), but as up to now, it remains unclear whether it plays also a role for irradiation of proliferative disorders. Hence, this should be one of the targets of future basic research.

50.4.3 Potential Side Effects of Radiotherapy

The use of ionizing radiation is associated with only mild early or late radiogenic toxicity. Minor effects, like dryness of the skin or major fibrosis, have been observed only in a minority of patients, but more often in previously operated sites than after primary RT. Usually simple skin care using moisture and greasy ointments is required to deal with these minor radiogenic sequelae. Late adverse side effects of grade 2 and more have never occurred in long-term FU. Our initial study with shorter FU and lower case numbers reported the occurrence of erythema in 14% and skin dryness in 11%, which is comparable to rates of 25.0% and 12.5% noted in the recent clinical study by Heyd et al. (2010). So far no case of radiogenic neoplasm was observed in our study. Nevertheless, the RT doses used for ML or MD are associated with a theoretical risk for induction of soft tissue sarcoma or skin cancer in the RT portals estimated to be in the range of 0.5–1% after latency periods of 8–30 years (Jansen et al. 2005; Trott and Kamprad 2006; Seegenschmiedt 2007). Usually only children and younger adults up to the age of 30 years may have an increased risk. Thus, critical indication after individual risk and benefit assessment and careful RT technique is required for this age group. However, at the present time, no single case of cancer induction has ever been reported after the use of RT for treatment of LD, DD, keloids, hypertrophic scars, or other benign hyperproliferative disorders.

50.4.4 Surgery Alone

Primary surgery is still the most recommended treatment for LD, but the available literature data indicate postoperative complications and side effects and a very high relapse rate of more than 70% depending upon the LD stage and the applied surgical techniques. The highest relapse rates of up to 100% have been observed after limited procedures including local, segmental, or wide excision procedures (LE, SE, WE) with a small safety margins of 2–3 cm around the lesion(s), while radical procedures including subtotal or total fasciectomy with much larger safety margins and with skin grafting have reduced the relapse rates to 25% (Allen et al. 1955; Alusio et al. 1996; Aviles et al. 1971; Beckmann et al. 2004; Dürr et al. 1999; Haedicke and Sturim 1989; Mirabell et al. 1990; Parnitzke et al. 1991; Pickren et al. 1951; Wapner et al. 1995; Wu 1994). The situation for recurrent LD is even worse and requires a more and more aggressive surgical approach (Landers et al. 1993). Thus, the radical total plantar fasciectomy (TPF) has been proposed as the primary surgical procedure even for early LD stages (Parnitzke et al. 1991) despite its possible long-term functional sequelae. Table 50.7 summarizes the results of the largest published studies using surgery as primary treatment. In addition, two more recent clinical studies are included which – at least in part – have implemented postsurgical RT for the most advanced LD cases (de Bree et al. 2004; van der Veer 2008).

In summary, TPF has been found to be the most successful treatment in almost all surgical studies and in particularly for advanced primary lesions and as a salvage treatment for recurrent lesions. Nevertheless, surgical treatments are also associated with a high risk for development of severe and persisting side effects including hematoma, painful scars, neuroma formation, infections, and numbness of parts of the sole (Haedicke and Sturim 1989; Wu 1994). In addition, delayed wound healing has been reported in up to 52–85% (Dürr 1999; Sammarco and Mangone 2000). Thus, less invasive and more effective treatments are still required.

50.4.5 Surgery Plus Postoperative Radiotherapy

The use of RT after surgery may improve short- and long-term outcome, but available data are limited. In one retrospective study, the relapse rate of LD after plantar fasciectomy with or without postoperative RT

Table 50.7 Results of surgical therapy for Morbus Ledderhose

Study (year)	Pts	Sites	Type of surgery	Relapse rate	Complications
Parnitzke et al. (1991)	6	7	PFE, SFE, TPF	5/7 (71%)	3 with wound healing problems 1 nerve lesion 1 chronic pain
Aluisio et al. (1996)	30	33	PFE, SFE, TPF	13/33 (39%)	4 with wound healing problems 2 nerve lesion 2 chronic pain 1 deep vein thrombosis
Dürr et al. (1999)	11	13	PFE, SFE, TPF	8/13 (62%)	4 wound healing problem
Sammarco et al. (2000)	16	21	SFE	2/16 (13%)	11 with wound healing problems 1 neuroma
de Bree (2004)	20	26	PFE, SFE, TPF + radiotherapy	Not stated; "best results" with RT	3/6 feet with RT had functional impairment
van der Veer (2008)	27	33	PFE, SFE, TPF + radiotherapy	16 (60%); 100% PFE; 25% TPF "best results" with RT	9 with wound healing problems

PFE partial fasciectomy, *SFE* subtotal fasciectomy, *TPF* total plantar fasciectomy

was evaluated over three decades (van der Veer et al. 2008): 27 patients with 33 affected feet (6 bilateral LD) underwent 40 surgical procedures and had a relapse rate of 60%; radical surgery (total plantar fasciectomy) for primary LD achieved the lowest relapse rate (25%), while limited local resection without RT resulted in the highest relapse rate (100%); the existence of multiple versus single nodule(s) was also associated with a higher relapse rate. The relapse rate for primary LD after fasciectomy was reduced with postoperative RT. Total plantar fasciectomy alone was most successful particularly for primary LD, but still compromised by a 25% relapse rate. Thus, RT may be a useful additive treatment for more complicated cases of LD treated with limited surgery. In another study from the Dutch Network and National Database for Pathology (PALGA) data from patients with LD were analyzed (de Bree et al. 2004). Twenty-six operations were performed and postoperative RT was used in six cases. Radical plantar fasciectomy was associated with the lowest relapse rate. After microscopically incomplete excisions or excision of early recurrence alone (<6 months), all lesions recurred, while the relapse rate was much lower after adjuvant RT, but RT was associated with significantly impaired functional outcome in three cases. The authors concluded that plantar fasciectomy is the operation of choice and that RT should be used very selectively because of its side effects. Nevertheless, the timing of RT was not analyzed in this study and may have provoked less favorable functional results.

Thus, a prospective randomized multicenter trial will be required to determine the type and combination of therapy which is most effective for primary and recurrent LD. In contrast to available surgical procedures, which are indicated in symptomatic or advanced ML stages or for cases refractory to conservative treatment, the more "prophylactic" implementation of RT in early LD stages may permit a highly effective prevention of symptom progression, thereby avoiding further surgery completely. Currently, any comparable data with long-term FU after surgery or RT beyond 10 years are not available, and therefore, the duration of the radiogenic prophylaxis is not known, but the published surgical series are even less conclusive with regard to long-term outcome. Although it is unclear whether RT may also reduce the recurrence rates after surgical resection in analogy to the treatment of plantar desmoid tumors (Mirabell et al. 1990), it would be of utmost interest to implement RT as a salvage option after unsuccessful surgical resection in case of signs of early relapse; however, the wound healing process should be completed at the time of RT implementation in contrast to the immediate postoperative implementation of RT for keloids.

In summary, surgical treatment of plantar fibromatosis is associated with a high recurrence rate if not conducted as a radical procedure; thus, it should be indicated only, when the LD lesions are highly symptomatic, the foot functions including gait are highly disabled and the conservative measures including RT already have failed. The role of postoperative RT needs to be further evaluated, and therefore, prospective multicenter studies will be needed to compare the different surgical procedures and to determine the type of operation that most effectively eliminates plantar fibromatosis in combination with adjuvant radiotherapy.

50.5 Conclusions

RT is the most effective treatment for primary and recurrent LD due to very low progression or relapse rates. RT permits the avoidance of primary and secondary surgical interventions due to high remission rates in various aspects of LD disease. Nevertheless, a close cooperation between foot surgery and radiation therapy is essential to improve the results for patients with recurrent LD. In addition, RT may improve long-term outcome in patients who develop an early relapse after surgery avoiding any further surgical procedures. Prospective multicenter clinical trials are needed to prove this potential new indication for radiotherapy. A national pattern of care study initiated by the German Cooperative Group of Radiotherapy for Benign diseases (GCG-BD) will investigate the current role and treatment standards of RT for LD and DD in all German RT institutions to assess the potential number of patients for this indication and the chances of a prospective multicenter study.

Appendix A

LEDDERHOSE Disease (LD) - Documentation

Date of first Assessment └ ┘└ ┘└ ┘

Name .... Surname........................ DOB └ ┘└ ┘└ ┘

General Data :   please fill in either " No " = N; " Yes " = Y

Ledderhose Disease in Family?   └ ┘ Parents .... └ ┘ Siblings ....

Related Disorders?   └ ┘ Peyronie Disease └ ┘ Dupuytren Disease

....   └ ┘ Knuckle Pads   └ ┘ Keloid

Predisposing Disorders?   └ ┘ Diabetes mellitus └ ┘ Epileptic Disorder

....   └ ┘ Liver Disease (Cirrhosis etc.) : ....

....   └ ┘ Perfusion Disorder (Hypoxia) : ....

Trauma / Injury of Feet?   └ ┘ when / which : ....

Smoking └ ┘; Alcohol └ ┘; Usual Hand work / Activity: └ ┘ rough or └ ┘ fine activity;

Which professional activities?   ....

Which sports / leisure activities? ....

When were first symptoms observed? .... (Estimation in months)

Symptoms	Right Foot		Left Foot	
Itching & Burning sensation?	└ ┘ N	└ ┘ Y	└ ┘ N	└ ┘ Y
Tension while walking?	└ ┘ N	└ ┘ Y	└ ┘ N	└ ┘ Y
Pressure while walking?	└ ┘ N	└ ┘ Y	└ ┘ N	└ ┘ Y
Pain at rest?	└ ┘ N	└ ┘ Y	└ ┘ N	└ ┘ Y
Pain while walking?	└ ┘ N	└ ┘ Y	└ ┘ N	└ ┘ Y
First skin changes?	└ ┘ N	└ ┘ Y	└ ┘ N	└ ┘ Y
First palpable "nodules"?	└ ┘ N	└ ┘ Y	└ ┘ N	└ ┘ Y
First palpable "cords"?	└ ┘ N	└ ┘ Y	└ ┘ N	└ ┘ Y
Retraction of Tows?	└ ┘ N	└ ┘ Y	└ ┘ N	└ ┘ Y
Any other complaints? (free text)	└ ┘ N	└ ┘ Y	└ ┘ N	└ ┘ Y

Any progression of symptoms or obvious signs of Ledderhose Disease?

[　] No [　] Yes, within [　] last 4 weeks: ....

[　] last 3 months: ....

[　] last 12 months: ....

[　] last [　] years: ....

Any "interuption or dormancy"? [　] no [　] yes, how long :....................................

When an which physicians or medical specialist(s) have you consulted? ....

[　] Family Doctor; [　] Orthopedist; [　] Other discipline(s): ....

Which Medication or Other Therapy has or had been applied in the past?

Therapy :	Right Foot	Left Foot
Cortison /Steroids		
Allopurinol		
Antirheumatics / Antiphlogistics		
Vitamines		
"Enzymes"		
Glucosamine		
Others:		
Local Injection (Date, Outcome?)		
Local Ointments		
Other Treatments		
Radiotherapy (Date, Outcome?)		
Surgery (Date, Outcome?)		

50 Long-Term Outcome of Radiotherapy for Primary and Recurrent Ledderhose Disease

Physical Examination / Date ⌊ ⌋ ⌊ ⌋ ⌊ ⌋ **(prior / post Tx ....)**

Physical Findings	Right Foot					Left Foot				
Toes	D 1	D 2	D 3	D 4	D 5	D 5	D 4	D 3	D 2	D 1
Symptoms (S)										
Skin Fixation (F)										
Node(s) (#) (N) [size/cm²]										
Cord(s) (#) (C) [length/cm]										
Function deficit(s) – DIP-joint										
– PIP-joint										
– MTP-joint										
Walking/Gait										
Pain Symptoms (0–10)										
Pressure (0–10)										
Tension (0–10)										
Other Symptoms (0–10)										
Overall Symptom Score (0–10)										

Symptoms at Foot Sole (plantar); = P; Symptoms at Forefoot / Toe (digital) = D; combined symptoms = PD;

Change after Tx: (Improvement / ↑) +++ (100%) / ++ (50%) / + (25%) / 0 / – (25%) /–/– (↓ / Deterioration)

Remission Stage: ⌊ ⌋ **Progression**   ⌊ ⌋ **Progression**
                   ⌊ ⌋ **Stable Disease**   ⌊ ⌋ **Stable Disease**
                   ⌊ ⌋ **Remission (%) : ....**⌊ ⌋ **Remission (%): ....**
                   ⌊ ⌋ **Overall Symptom Score. (0–10)**

Free Notes:

Signature: ....

References

Adamietz B, Keilholz L, Grünert J et al (2001) Radiotherapy in early stage Dupuytren's contracture. Strahlenther Onkol 177:604–610

Allen RA, Woolner LB, Ghormley RK (1955) Soft tissue tumors of the sole with special reference to plantar fibromatosis. J Bone Joint Surg [Am] 37A:14–26

Alusio FV, Mair SD, Hall RL (1996) Plantar fibromatosis: treatment of primary and recurrent lesions and factors associated with recurrence. Foot Ankle Int 17:672–678

Aviles E, Arlen M, Miller T (1971) Plantar fibromatosis. Surgery 69:117–120

Beatty SR (1938) Roentgen therapy of Dupuytren's contracture. Radiology 30:610–612

Beckmann KT, Baer W et al (2004) Plantarfibromatose: Therapie mit totaler Plantarfasziektomie. Zentralbl Chir 129:53–57

Betz N, Ott OJ, Adamietz B, Sauer R, Fietkau R, Keilholz L (2010) Radiotherapy in early-stage Dupuytren's contracture. Long-term results after 13 years. Strahlenther Onkol 186(2):82–90

Cavolo DJ, Sherwood GF (1982) Dupuytren's disease of the plantar fascia. J Foot Surg 21:610–612

Classen DA, Hurst LN (1992) Plantar fibromatosis and bilateral flexion contractures: a review of the literature. Ann Plast Surg 28:475–478

de Bree E, Zoetmulder FA, Keus RB, Peterse HL, van Coevorden F (2004) Incidence and treatment of recurrent plantar fibromatosis by surgery and postoperative radiotherapy. Am J Surg 187(1):33–38

Delgadillo LA, Arenson DJ (1985) Plantar fibromatosis: surgical considerations with case histories. J Foot Surg 24: 258–265

Dürr HR, Krödel A, Troullier H et al (1999) Fibromatosis of the plantar fascia: diagnosis and indications for surgical treatment. Foot Ankle Int 20:13–17

El Majdoub F, Brunn A, Berthold F et al (2009) Stereotactic interstitial radiosurgery for intracranial Rosai-Dorfman disease. A novel therapeutic approach. Strahlenther Onkol 185:109–112

Fetsch JF, Laskin WB, Miettinen M (2005) Palmar-plantar fibromatosis in children and preadolescents: a clinicopathologic study of 56 cases with newly recognized demographics and extended follow-up. Am J Surg Pathol 29: 1095–1105

Godette GA, O'Sullivan M, Menelaus MB (1997) Plantar fibromatosis of the heel in children: a report of 14 cases. J Pediatr Orthop 17:16–17

Haedicke GJ, Sturim HS (1989) Plantar fibromatosis: an isolated disease. Plast Reconstr Surg 83:296–300

Herbst M, Regler G (1986) Dupuytrensche Kontraktur. Radiotherapie der Frühstadien. Strahlenther 161:143–147

Herovici C (1961) Picropolchorme. Histoligical technic for the study of supporting tissue. Pathol Biol (Paris) 9:387–388

Heyd R, Tselis N, Ackermann H et al (2007) Radiation therapy for painful heel spurs. Results of a prospective randomized study. Strahlenther Onkol 183:1–7

Heyd R, Buhleier T, Zamboglou N (2009) Radiation therapy for prevention of heterotopic ossification about the elbow. Strahlenther Onkol 185:506–511

Heyd R, Dorn AP, Herkströter M, Rödel C, Müller-Schimpfle M, Fraunholz I (2010) Bestrahlung in frühen Stadien des Morbus Ledderhose [Radiation therapy for early stages of morbus Ledderhose]. Strahlenther Onkol 186:24–29

Jansen JT, Broerse JJ, Zoetelief J, Klein C, Seegenschmiedt HM (2005) Estimation of the carcinogenic risk of radiotherapy of benign diseases from shoulder to heel. Radiother Oncol 76(3):270–277

Janssen S, Johann H, Karstens H (2009) Endokrine Orbitopathie – Wie effektiv ist die Strahlentherapie? Strahlenther Onkol 185:61–62

Johnston RE, Collis S, Peckham NH et al (1992) Plantar fibromatosis: literature review and unique case report. J Foot Surg 31:400–406

Kashuk KB, Pasternack WA (1981) Aggressive infiltrating plantar fibromatosis. J Am Podiatry Assoc 70:491–496

Lam WL, Rawlins JM, Karoo RO, Naylor I, Sharpe DT (2010) Re-visiting Luck's classification: a histological analysis of Dupuytren's disease. J Hand Surg Eur 35:312–317

Landers PA, Yu GV, White JM et al (1993) Recurrent plantar fibromatosis. J Foot Ankle Surg 32:85–93

Ledderhose G (1897) Zur Pathologie der Aponeurose des Fußes und der Hand. Langenbecks Arch Klin Chir 55:694–712

Luck JV (1959) Dupuytren's contracture; a new concept of the pathogenesis correlated with surgical management. J Bone Joint Surg Am 41:635–664

Mirabell R, Suit HD, Mankin HJ et al (1990) Fibromatoses: from surgical surveillance to combined surgery and radiation therapy. Int J Radiat Oncol Biol Phys 18:535–540

Mornex F, Pavy JJ, Denekamp J, Bolla M (1997) Scoring system of late effects of radiations on normal tissues: the SOMA-LENT scale. Cancer Radiother 1(6):622–668, Review. French

Parnitzke B, Decker O, Neumann U (1991) Morbus Ledderhose. Die plantare Fibromatose – klinische Aspekte. Zentralbl Chir 116:531–534

Pentland AP, Anderson TF (1985) Plantar fibromatosis responds to intralesional steroids. J Am Acad Dermatol 12:212–214

Pickren JW, Smith AG, Stevenson AG et al (1951) Fibromatosis of the plantar fascia. Cancer 4:846–856

Rao GS, Luthra PK (1988) Dupuytren's disease of the foot in children: a report of 3 cases. J Plast Surg 28:475–478

Rödel F, Kamprad F, Sauer R et al (2002) Funktionelle und molekulare Aspekte der antiinflammatorischen Wirkung niedrig dosierter Strahlentherapie. Strahlenther Onkol 178:1–9

Rödel F, Schaller U, Schultze-Mosgau S et al (2004) The induction of TGF-β1 and NF-κB parallels a biphasic time course of leukocyte/endothelial cell adhesion following low-dose x-irradiation. Strahlenther Onkol 180:194–197

Rödel F, Hofmann D, Auer J et al (2008) The anti-inflammatory effect of low-dose radiation therapy involves a diminished CCL20 chemokine expression and granulocyte/endothelial cell adhesion. Strahlenther Onkol 184:41–47

Sammarco GJ, Mangone PG (2000) Classification and treatment of plantar fibromatosis. Foot Ankle Int 21:563–569

Seegenschmiedt MH (2007) Morbus Dupuytren/Morbus Ledderhose. In: Seegenschmiedt MH, Makoski HB, Trott KR, Brady LW (eds) Radiotherapy for non-malignant disorders: contemporary concepts and clinical results. Springer, Berlin/Heidelberg/New York, pp 161–191

Seegenschmiedt MH, Attassi M (2003) Strahlentherapie beim Morbus Ledderhose – Indikation, und klinische Ergebnisse. Strahlenther Onkol 179:847–853

Seegenschmiedt MH, Katalinic A, Makoski HB et al (1999) Strahlentherapie von gutartigen Erkrankungen: eine Bestandsaufnahme in Deutschland. Strahlenther Onkol 175: 541–547

Seegenschmiedt MH, Olschewski T, Guntrum F (2001) Optimierung der Radiotherapie beim Morbus Dupuytren: erste Ergebnisse einer kontrollierten Studie. Strahlenther Onkol 177:74–81

Strzelczyk A, Vogt H, Hamer HM, Krämer G (2008) Continuous phenobarbital treatment leads to recurrent plantar fibromatosis. Epilepsia 49:1965–1968

Trott KR, Kamprad F (2006) Estimation of cancer risk from radiotherapy of benign diseases. Strahlenther Onkol 182: 431–436

Trotti A, Byhardt R, Stetz J, Gwede C, Corn B, Fu K, Gunderson L, McCormick B, Morrisintegral M, Rich T, Shipley W, Curran W (2000) Common toxicity criteria: version 2.0. an improved reference for grading the acute effects of cancer treatment: impact on radiotherapy. Int J Radiat Oncol Biol Phys 47(1):13–47

van der Veer WM, Hamburg SM, de Gast A, Niessen FB (2008) Recurrence of plantar fibromatosis after plantar fasciectomy: single-center long-term results. Plast Reconstr Surg 122(2): 486–491

Wapner KL, Ververelli PA, Moore JH et al (1995) Plantar fibromatosis: a review of primary and recurrent surgery. Foot Ankle Int 16:548–551

Wu KK (1994) Plantar fibromatosis of the foot. J Foot Ankle Surg 33:98–101

Source for Statistics

McDonald JH (2009) Handbook of biological statistics, 2nd ed. Sparky House Publishing, Baltimore, pp 88–94 http://udel.edu/~mcdonald/statcmh.html

Medical Management of Peyronie's Disease

51

Ma Limin, Aaron Bernie, and Wayne J.G. Hellstrom

Contents

51.1	**Introduction**	429
51.2	**Clinical Manifestations and Evaluation**	430
51.3	**Medical Therapy**	430
51.3.1	Oral Agents	430
51.3.2	Intralesional Pharmacotherapy	433
51.3.3	Topical Therapy and Iontophoresis	433
51.3.4	Other Medical Treatments	434
51.4	**Conclusion**	435
References		435

M. Limin
Department of Urology,
Health Sciences Center, Tulane University,
New Orleans, LA, USA

Department of Urology,
Affiliated Hospital of Nantong University,
Nantong, China

A. Bernie • W.J.G. Hellstrom (✉)
Department of Urology,
Health Sciences Center, Tulane University,
New Orleans, LA, USA
e-mail: whellst@tulane.edu

51.1 Introduction

Peyronie's disease (PD), or induratio penis plastica (IPP), is a connective tissue disorder characterized by the formation of plaques or masses of fibrous tissue involving the tunica albuginea layer of the penis. These plaques usually cause palpable penile scar tissue leading to dorsal, ventral, or lateral penile angulation, intermittently painful erections, and often erectile dysfunction (ED) (Gholami et al. 2003; Bella et al. 2007; Greenfield and Levine 2005). PD was first documented in the literature in 1561 by Fallopius, and was further described and named after Francois Gigot de la Peyronie in 1743. PD may present as penile curvature, indentation, shortening, or an hourglass deformity. Epidemiological studies have shown an overall prevalence of PD ranging from 3% to 7.1% (Schwarzer et al. 2001; Smith et al. 2005; Rhoden et al. 2001; La Pera et al. 2001; Pryor et al. 2004), which is much higher than previous estimations. PD often occurs in conjunction with Dupuytren's contracture and Ledderhose Disease, fibrosis in the palm of the hand and sole of the foot, likely because of a genetic linkage between the two diseases (Bjekic et al. 2006).

The etiology and molecular pathogenesis of PD remains undefined and is likely multifactorial. A variety of hypotheses have been proposed. The traumatic hypothesis suggests that fibrosis is caused by ischemia and inflammation after penile trauma or repetitive microvascular injury during activities such as sexual intercourse (Devine et al. 1997). Another hypothesis observed that the majority (75.8%) of PD patients exhibit at least one immunological abnormality, invoking an autoimmune etiology (Schiavino et al. 1997). Other factors associated with scar or plaque formation

C. Eaton et al. (eds.), *Dupuytren's Disease and Related Hyperproliferative Disorders*,
DOI 10.1007/978-3-642-22697-7_51, © Springer-Verlag Berlin Heidelberg 2012

include the following: cytokines, vasoactive factors, serotonin, platelet-derived growth factors, transforming growth factors as well as fibrin (Vernet et al. 2005; Sasso et al. 2007), all of which may play a role in the pathogenesis of PD. In addition, genetic predisposition may serve as a contributing factor (Mulhall 2003). Oxidative stress has become a common concept as contributing to plaque growth in PD (Sikka and Hellstrom 2002). Similar to PD, Dupuytren's contracture has been linked to many of these theories, including increased fibroblast activity and damage to tissue from oxidative stress. These commonalities further strengthen the link between Dupuytren's contracture and PD.

Some invasive procedures, such as radical retropubic prostatectomy, may have an effect on the penis and lead to plaque formation (Tal et al. 2010). Recent controversy surrounds the relationship between androgens, regulators of collagen metabolism, and PD development (Karavitakis et al. 2010). Given this wide variety of hypotheses, a multifactorial concept of PD is likely.

51.2 Clinical Manifestations and Evaluation

The most common complaints of men with PD include:
1. Painful erection, mainly in the acute or early phase
2. Shortening of the penis with or without an erection
3. A palpable penile plaque or induration
4. Curvature of the penis during erection, with dorsal curvature being most frequent (followed by ventral and lateral bending of the penis)
5. Sexual dysfunction or ED

The overall risk for PD-specific ED at any age is approximately 30% (Gholami and Lue 2001). Clinically, the disease undergoes an imprecise transition between two phases: an acute inflammatory phase lasting 6–16 months and thereafter a chronic phase. The former is characterized by penile pain, sometimes even when flaccid, and there are often dynamic changes causing evolving penile malformations. Pain may be persistent, but usually does not interfere with sexual function. Rarely patients may complain of being awakened in the morning with a painful erection. The acute phase is usually self-limiting, and the associated penile pain resolves spontaneously. The chronic phase typically signals a stable penile deformity, without significant discomfort.

Comprehensive assessment of the PD patient allows the clinician to diagnose the disease correctly, and guides appropriate treatment. Unfortunately, there is still no universally accepted standard for evaluation. In general, the initial subjective report by the patient can be achieved by obtaining a comprehensive patient history and chief complaint as well as using a standardized questionnaire, such as the Peyronie's Disease Index (PDI) (Wiltink et al. 2003) Ancillary questionnaires such as International Index of Erectile Function (IIEF), Derogatis Interview for Sexual Functioning (DISF), and the Social Desirability Scale are complementary and helpful to assess patients' sexual function and quality of life. Besides routine genitourinary examination, a physical exam should include evaluation of the hands and feet for indications of systemic fibromatosis (e.g., Dupuytren's contracture or Ledderhose Disease) (Levine and Greenfield 2003). The objective evaluation includes penile length measurement, plaque characteristics (number, size, and location), erectile function, and penile curvature, all of which are helpful in deciding disease severity (Smith et al. 2005). Penile duplex Doppler ultrasonography is commonly employed to document plaque characteristics (size, calcification, etc.) and vascular status of the penile erection (arterial and venous components).

51.3 Medical Therapy

Since the first description of PD in the medical literature, many treatments have been described, although even today, no optimal treatment modality has been established. Without doubt, a more complete understanding of the cellular and molecular components involved in the development of this fibroproliferative disorder will become necessary for complete disease control, appropriate treatment, and likely cure. Despite no one optimal therapy, a wide range of nonsurgical options (Table 51.1) are currently available and may reduce or at least stabilize the penile deformity and improve sexual function in men with PD.

51.3.1 Oral Agents

51.3.1.1 Vitamin E
Vitamin E is a fat-soluble vitamin with antioxidant and DNA repair properties as well as capacity for immune

51 Medical Management of Peyronie's Disease

Table 51.1 Current medical treatment modalities used in Peyronie's disease

Oral therapy	Intralesional therapy	Topical therapy	Other medical therapies
Vitamin E: Antioxidant, DNA repair, and immune system modulation capacity. Low cost and minimal side effects	*Steroids*: Anti-inflammatory effect. Little evidence of efficacy in PD treatment	*Verapamil*: Used topically, it has been shown to decrease pain, plaque size, and curvature. May not penetrate tunica albuginea well by itself	*Penile electroshock wave therapy (ESWT)*: Causes direct damage to plaques, induces inflammatory reactions. Not first-line therapy
Colchicine: Anti-microtubular and decreased leukocyte adhesion effects. Possible decrease in pain, plaque size, and curvature	*Verapamil*: Calcium channel blocker. Used widely with minimal side effects; recent trials suggest minimal clinical benefit	*Iontophoresis*: Often added to topical therapies with verapamil and dexamethasone. Results are promising, but few studies have validated efficacy	*Radiation therapy*: Possibly positive effects on PD due to anti-inflammatory actions. Small studies show improvement in pain. Radiation may promote fibrotic plaques in some cases
Potaba: Increases activity of monoamine oxidase. Potentially stabilizers PD	*Collagenase*: Bacterial enzyme, degrades collagen. Studies have shown up to 65% of patients with reduced curvature		*Combination therapy*: Combinations such as vitamin E/colchicine, ESWT/intralesional verapamil, and L-carnitine/intralesional verapamil have been tried with varied success. More studies are needed
Tamoxifen: Antiestrogen, decreased production, and blocking of TGF-β. Mixed studies of improvement (up to 80% pain reduction) in PD	*Interferon-alpha-2b*: Inhibits fibroblast proliferation and decreases collagen production. Clinical trials have shown reduction in curvature and plaque size vs placebo		
L-arginine: Amino acid, stimulates NOS activity, acts as antifibrotic agent. Animal studies show promising results	*Orgotein*: Cu-Zn superoxide dismutase with anti-inflammatory action. 63% success rate in small trial, yet to be validated with larger studies		
L-carnitine: Amino acid, increases mitochondrial respiration. Mixed studies on successful results.			
Pentoxifylline: PDE-5 inhibitor, antifibrogenic action. Good results in randomized controlled studies (36.9% response in treatment vs 4.5% in placebo)			
Propoleum: Small studies reporting 77% success rate in treatment; lack of data			

system modulation. It was the first oral therapy to be published in a peer-reviewed journal for the treatment of PD. Though the exact effectiveness of vitamin E has not been verified, it is still widely used because of its low cost, absence of side effects, and theoretical free radical oxygen scavenging effects. Others may prescribe vitamins because it can provide some pain relief in the acute phase of PD and alleviate psychologic distress caused by this condition (Hellstrom 2009; Suzuki et al. 1999). Some urologists do not recommend vitamin E for the treatment of PD because of reports of increased risk of cardiovascular events (Lonn et al. 2005).

51.3.1.2 Colchicine

Colchicine is an oral anti-microtubular agent that decreases fibrosis and collagen deposition, leukocyte adhesion and motility, and cellular mitosis. Although a small trial demonstrated pain relief, decreased plaque size, and curvature after treatment with colchicine (Akkus et al. 1994), the efficacy of colchicine remains controversial. A recent study showed that colchicine was no better than placebo in improving pain, penile curvature, or plaque size (Kadioglu et al. 2000; Safarinejad 2004). Colchicine also carries adverse effects such as gastrointestinal disturbances, bone marrow suppression, and elevated liver enzymes.

51.3.1.3 Potassium Aminobenzoate (Potaba)

Potaba is a part of the vitamin B complex family and exerts an antifibrotic effect by increasing the activity of monoamine oxidase in tissues. Though it has been used for more than 50 years in the treatment of PD, a recent study did not show significant reduction in pain, plaque size, or penile curvature. However, it should be noted that potaba may be useful in stabilizing the disorder, which is postulated to occur by preventing progression of penile curvature during the early acute phase (Weidner et al. 2005). The most commonly reported side effect is gastrointestinal disturbance, which often leads to patients discontinuing the therapy.

51.3.1.4 Tamoxifen

Tamoxifen is a nonsteroidal antiestrogen that is postulated to act by both reducing the production of TGF-β by fibroblasts and blocking TGF-β receptors. These actions may inhibit the inflammatory response, thereby reducing fibrogenesis in PD. A short uncontrolled study established improvement in pain relief (80%), plaque size (34%), and penile curvature (35%) with tamoxifen therapy (Ralph et al. 1992). However, these successful results were questioned by a recent placebo-controlled study, which did not show statistically significant differences between tamoxifen treatment and placebo (Teloken et al. 1999). Because of this, tamoxifen is not currently recommended for first-line PD treatment. The common side effects of tamoxifen include gastrointestinal distress and alopecia.

51.3.1.5 L-Arginine

L-arginine is a nonessential amino acid that acts as a precursor for the synthesis of nitric oxide (Andrew and Mayer 1999). Inducible nitric oxide synthase (NOS) is expressed in the fibrotic plaques of PD, and long-term suppression of NOS exacerbates fibrosis of tissue. L-arginine, which stimulates NOS activity and nitric

oxide synthesis, inhibits collagen synthesis, induces fibroblast/myofibroblast apoptosis, and acts as an antifibrotic agent. There have been reports in animal models of PD that the L-arginine treatment can result in an 80–95% reduction in plaque size and the collagen/fibroblast ratio (Valente et al. 2003). Further validation with controlled clinical studies in humans with PD is needed.

51.3.1.6 L-Carnitine

L-carnitine is formed in the body from the amino acids lysine and methionine. L-carnitine increases fat usage as an energy source by transporting fatty acids into the mitochondria of cells, increasing mitochondrial respiration, and decreasing free radical formation. A study by Biagiotti et al. showed L-carnitine to be significantly more effective than tamoxifen in reducing penile pain as well as altering disease progression. In addition, L-carnitine has fewer side effects than tamoxifen (Biagiotti and Cavallini 2001). Although results of this study are encouraging, a placebo-controlled study of L-carnitine did not show improvement in pain, curvature, or plaque size (Safarinejad et al. 2007). Because of these conflicting results, more studies are needed with this prospective agent.

51.3.1.7 Pentoxifylline

Pentoxifylline is a PDE-5 inhibitor with both anti-inflammatory and antifibrogenic properties. It decreases the amount of TGFβ and increases fibrinolytic activity, which is proposed to reverse the fibrotic process observed in PD. The latest randomized placebo-controlled study in 2009 reported 36.9% of patients with a positive response, versus only 4.5% seen in the placebo group. Improvement in penile curvature, plaque size, and IIEF score were significantly greater in patients treated with pentoxifylline versus placebo (Safarinejad et al. 2010). The results of this recent study are promising, and mandate more studies to determine optimal dose and treatment duration.

51.3.1.8 Propoleum

Information regarding the composition, mechanism of action, and efficacy of propoleum is limited, as the substance is patented in Cuba and its use restricted to that country. Currently, there are only three papers regarding the composition, mechanism of action, and efficacy of propoleum, all published by the same group of authors (Lemourt et al. 1998, 2003a, b). They reported that 77% of patients accomplished improvement in penile curvature, and penile plaques were reduced by an average of 0.64 cm (with 23% of patients showing complete resolution). Unfortunately, these results cannot be confirmed for accuracy and reliability because of the limited data and lack of randomized control trial studies.

51.3.2 Intralesional Pharmacotherapy

51.3.2.1 Steroids
Steroids contribute a powerful anti-inflammatory effect through inhibition of phospholipase A2 and suppression of the immune response, making them excellent candidates for intralesional therapy in PD. However, the use of steroids is currently discouraged in the treatment of PD due to little conclusive evidence confirming their benefit. Unfortunately, adverse events such as local tissue atrophy, fibrosis, and immune suppression have been reported with steroids (Vernet et al. 2005). In addition, these side effects make later surgical intervention for PD more difficult. A recent retrospective study suggested local steroid therapy may be justified during the acute phase of PD (Demey et al. 2006), but placebo-controlled trials are still needed.

51.3.2.2 Verapamil
Verapamil, a calcium blocker, influences fibroblast metabolism by inhibiting local extracellular matrix formation and increasing collagenase activity. Clinically, verapamil is used widely with a standard injection dose of 10 mg given every 2 weeks for 12–24 weeks. Verapamil injections are safe and well tolerated, with beneficial response reported for men with mild and moderate PD (Bella et al. 2007; Greenfield and Levine 2005; Hauck et al. 2006; Hwang et al. 2003; Levine et al. 2002). However, a number of studies have shown that verapamil therapy outcomes are not so beneficial (Bennett et al. 2007; Shirazi et al. 2009). Thus, the effect of intralesional verapamil still remains controversial. Future multicenter randomized control trials are certainly needed. Adverse effects include nausea, lightheadedness, penile pain, and ecchymosis; all of these symptoms are mild in nature. Recently, intralesional injection of nicardipine, another calcium antagonist, has demonstrated good results when used during the transition period from acute to chronic phases of PD (Soh et al. 2010).

51.3.2.3 Collagenase
Collagenase is a purified bacterial enzyme that targets interstitial collagen for enzymatic degradation. It was first used intralesionally to treat PD in 1982, and 65% of the patients in this study reported a reduction in penile curvature, with the best results obtained in those with small plaques (less than 2 cm in length) and minor deformity (less than 30° curvature) (Gelbard et al. 1982, 1985, 1993). A non-placebo-controlled study showed decreases in mean deviation angle, plaque width, and length in men whose treatment was followed for 6 months. More than 50% of patients achieved a subjective improvement when surveyed during this small study (Jordan 2008). A double-blind, placebo-controlled, multicenter study is currently in the late trial phases to confirm efficacy and tolerability. Side effects of intralesional collagenase include injection-site pain, ecchymosis, and corporal rupture.

51.3.2.4 Interferon-Alpha-2b
Interferon-alpha-2b is believed to act in an immunomodulatory fashion. Duncan et al. (1991) found that interferon injection into plaques can inhibit fibroblast proliferation, decrease production of extracellular matrix collagen, and increase the production of collagenase. A recent multicenter study by Hellstrom et al. (2006) demonstrated that improvement in curvature was observed in 27% of PD patients (absolute 13.5°) and plaque size (54.6%) for treated men vs. 8.9% in control patients. Adverse effects include sinusitis, flu-like symptoms, and minor penile swelling, all of which can be effectively treated with OTC nonsteroidal anti-inflammatory agents.

51.3.2.5 Orgotein
Orgotein, a drug version of Cu-Zn superoxide dismutase, is a new anti-inflammatory agent. Its first use for intralesional injection in patients with PD was reported by Wagenknecht et al. in 1996 with an overall success rate of 63% in 117 cases. No placebo-controlled study has been published and this agent has been withdrawn from the US market due to reports of severe allergic reactions. Adverse effects include pain, swelling, stiffness, dysesthesia, and skin rashes (Trost et al. 2007).

51.3.3 Topical Therapy and Iontophoresis

Verapamil is a commonly used topical therapy in the treatment of patients with PD. Its effectiveness in a recent three arm trial over 9 months demonstrated a significant improvement in eliminating pain with erection (100%), decreasing the size of plaque (84.7%), decreasing curvature (61.1%), and improving erection quality (81.8%) compared to placebo (Fitch et al. 2007). Recently, the true efficacy of topical preparations has been questioned because effective tunica albuginea tissue concentrations of verapamil are not achievable through topical application (Martin et al. 2002).

To decrease the limitations of this type of drug penetration, iontophoresis has been recommended to increase the delivery of transdermal medications to the target tissues. Iontophoresis is an attractive treatment option since it offers a less invasive approach than injections when delivering the required drug to target tissues. There have been few studies reporting the efficacy of iontophoresis in combination with verapamil and dexamethasone in plaque reduction (43–82%), decrease in curvature (37–84%), and pain elimination (88–96%) (Di Stasi et al. 2003, 2004; Greenfield et al. 2007; Riedl et al. 2000). In fact, the treatment method itself may contribute to the improvement of symptoms, because the electrical energy delivered with iontophoresis may lead to wound healing and/or remodeling (Ojingwa and Isseroff 2003).

51.3.4 Other Medical Treatments

51.3.4.1 Penile Electroshock Wave Therapy (ESWT)

ESWT acts by causing direct damage to penile plaques, leading to an inflammatory reaction with increased macrophage activity. This intervention produces plaque lysis, improved vascularity, and plaque resorption. Some authorities suggest that the development of contralateral scarring of the penis results in "false straightening" (Taylor and Levine 2008). The first randomized control trial study by Palmieri showed that ESWT provided beneficial effects on Visual Analogue Scale (VAS), IIEF-5, and QoL scores, without significant effect on plaque size or penile curvature (Palmieri et al. 2009). Currently, ESWL is not recommended as first-line therapy for PD.

51.3.4.2 Radiation Therapy

Low-dose radiotherapy has been historically claimed as effective in improving penile pain, which may be related to anti-inflammatory effects. In one study, Incrocci noted that radiotherapy quickens symptomatic, natural, and spontaneous improvement and for that reason should be limited to patients with significant penile pain (Incrocci 2004). A retrospective study reported curvature reduction in 23% and pain elimination in 83% of patients who received radiation doses of 12–13.5 Gy (Incrocci et al. 2000). Unfortunately, radiation therapy increases the production of fibrogenic cytokines, which may worsen the fibrotic process involved in PD (Mulhall 2003). Radiation has been used to reduce penile pain associated with PD, but is not currently recommended due both to a paucity of randomized, controlled trials (Akin-Olugbade and Mulhall 2007) and to in vitro evidence that its use can actually lead to increased expression of the fibrogenic cytokines PDGF and bFGF (Mulhall et al. 2003). Additionally, recent work has shown that prostate irradiation can cause damage to smooth muscle cells in the arteries supplying the corpora cavernosa, leading to erectile dysfunction (van der Wielen et al. 2009). Therefore, further research is needed before radiation therapy can be recommended as a routine treatment modality for PD. This research should address concerns about the potential fibrogenic effects of ionizing radiation on arterial smooth muscle, explore possible side effects such as erectile dysfunction, and might also investigate the efficiency of RT in various stages of PD, because in Dupuytren's Disease, RT has been reported to be most efficient in the early, proliferating stage of disease (Seegenschmiedt et al. 2012).

51.3.4.3 Combination Therapy

A placebo-controlled study by Cakan reported that combination therapy with oral vitamin E and colchicine achieved significant improvements in curvature and plaque size in patients with early-stage PD (Cakan et al. 2006). Another non-placebo-controlled combination therapy study of ESWT with intralesional verapamil injections similarly resulted in significant improvements in pain in 91.5% and plaque reduction in 49% of men (Mirone et al. 2000). Likewise, oral L-carnitine combined with intralesional verapamil may be a useful therapy for advanced or resistant PD (Cavallini et al. 2002). Other combination studies involving oral vitamin E+L-carnitine and intralesional interferon+oral vitamin E failed to show significant differences compared to monotherapy (Safarinejad et al. 2007; Inal et al. 2006).

51.4 Conclusion

PD is a fibrotic disorder of the tunica albuginea of the penis that has a significant impact on patient's and partner's quality of life and consumption of health care resources. For patients with mild-to-moderate PD, conservative treatments are available with documented symptomatic improvement; surgical treatments are always available for PD patients with severe deformity and associated symptoms of ED, but, as with any surgical procedure, there are recognized costs and risks. Because of this, conservative treatment is still the initial method of treatment for the majority patients presenting with PD. Currently, conservative management is limited, but evolving. New oral drugs and increasing evidence for the use of intralesional injection therapy, iontophoresis, ESWT, and combination therapy will undoubtedly enter the treatment algorithm in the coming years. Currently no medical therapy is fully effective or able to relieve all symptoms in the different disease phases for the affected patients. The main problem is that the efficacy and tolerability of the majority of treatments remains uncertain because of lack of long-term randomized controlled trials with established guidelines for evaluation and treatment. Accordingly, one of our primary goals is the development of consensus guidelines for design and conduct of trials to determine efficacy and safety of the medical treatment of PD.

References

Akin-Olugbade Y, Mulhall JP (2007) The medical management of Peyronie's disease Nat Clin Pract Urol 4:95–103

Akkus E, Carrier S, Rehman J et al (1994) Is colchicine effective in Peyronie's disease? A pilot study. Urology 44:291–295

Andrew PJ, Mayer B (1999) Enzymatic function of nitric oxide synthases. Cardiovasc Res 43:521–531

Bella AJ, Perelman MA, Brant WO et al (2007) Peyronie's disease (CME). J Sex Med 4:1527–1538

Bennett NE, Guhring P, Mulhall JP (2007) Intralesional verapamil prevents the progression of Peyronie's disease. Urology 69:1181–1184

Biagiotti G, Cavallini G (2001) Acetyl-L-carnitine vs tamoxifen in the oral therapy of Peyronie's disease: a preliminary report. BJU Int 88:63–67

Bjekic MD, Vlajinac HD, Sipetic SB et al (2006) Risk factors for Peyronie's disease: a case-control study. BJU Int 97: 570–574

Cakan M, Demirel F, Aldemir M et al (2006) Does smoking change the efficacy of combination therapy with vitamin E

and colchicines in patients with early-stage Peyronie's disease? Arch Androl 52:21–27

Cavallini G, Biagiotti G, Koverech A et al (2002) Oral propionyl-l-carnitine and intraplaque verapamil in the therapy of advanced and resistant Peyronie's disease. BJU Int 89:895–900

Demey A, Chevallier D, Bondil P et al (2006) Is intracavernosal corticosteroid infiltration really useless in Peyronie's disease? Prog Urol 16:52–57

Devine CJ Jr, Somers KD, Jordan SG et al (1997) Proposal: trauma as the cause of the Peyronie's lesion. J Urol 157: 285–290

Di Stasi SM, Giannantoni A, Capelli G et al (2003) Transdermal electromotive administration of verapamil and dexamethasone for Peyronie's disease. BJU Int 91:825–829

Di Stasi SM, Giannantoni A, Stephen RL et al (2004) A prospective, randomized study using transdermal electromotive administration of verapamil and dexamethasone for Peyronie's disease. J Urol 171:1605–1608

Duncan MR, Berman B, Nseyo UO (1991) Regulation of the proliferation and biosynthetic activities of cultured human Peyronie's disease fibroblasts by interferons-alpha, -beta and -gamma. Scand J Urol Nephrol 25(2):89–94

Fitch WP 3rd, Easterling WJ, Talbert RL et al (2007) Topical verapamil HCl, topical trifluoperazine, and topical magnesium sulfate for the treatment of Peyronie's disease–a placebo-controlled pilot study. J Sex Med 4:477–484

Gelbard MK, Walsh R, Kaufman JJ (1982) Collagenase for Peyronie's disease experimental studies. Urol Res 10: 135–140

Gelbard MK, Lindner A, Kaufman JJ (1985) The use of collagenase in the treatment of Peyronie's disease. J Urol 134: 280–283

Gelbard MK, James K, Riach P et al (1993) Collagenase versus placebo in the treatment of Peyronie's disease: a double-blind study. J Urol 149:56–58

Gholami SS, Lue TF (2001) Peyronie's disease. Urol Clin North Am 28:377–390

Gholami SS, Gonzalez-Cadavid NF, Lin CS et al (2003) Peyronie's disease: a review. J Urol 169:1234–1241

Greenfield JM, Levine LA (2005) Peyronie's disease: etiology, epidemiology and medical treatment. Urol Clin North Am 32:469–478, vii

Greenfield JM, Shah SJ, Levine LA (2007) Verapamil versus saline in electromotive drug administration for Peyronie's disease: a double-blind, placebo controlled trial. J Urol 177:972–975

Hauck EW, Diemer T, Schmelz HU et al (2006) A critical analysis of nonsurgical treatment of Peyronie's disease. Eur Urol 49:987–997

Hellstrom WJ (2009) Medical management of Peyronie's disease. J Androl 30:397–405

Hellstrom WJ, Kendirci M, Matern R et al (2006) Single-blind, multicenter, placebo controlled, parallel study to assess the safety and efficacy of intralesional interferon alpha-2B for minimally invasive treatment for Peyronie's disease. J Urol 176:394–398

Hwang JJ, Uchio EM, Patel SV et al (2003) Diagnostic localization of malignant bladder pheochromocytoma using 6-18 F fluorodopamine positron emission tomography. J Urol 169: 274–275

Inal T, Tokatli Z, Akand M et al (2006) Effect of intralesional interferon-alpha 2b combined with oral vitamin E for treatment of early stage Peyronie's disease: a randomized and prospective study. Urology 67:1038–1042

Incrocci L (2004) Radiotherapeutic treatment of Peyronie s disease. Expert Rev Pharmacoecon Outcomes Res 4:235–242

Incrocci L, Wijnmaalen A, Slob AK et al (2000) Low-dose radiotherapy in 179 patients with Peyronie's disease: treatment outcome and current sexual functioning. Int J Radiat Oncol Biol Phys 47:1353–1356

Jordan GH (2008) The use of intralesional clostridial collagenase injection therapy for Peyronie's disease: a prospective, single-center, non-placebo-controlled study. J Sex Med 5:180–187

Kadioglu A, Tefekli A, Koksal T et al (2000) Treatment of Peyronie's disease with oral colchicine: long-term results and predictive parameters of successful outcome. Int J Impot Res 12:169–175

Karavitakis M, Komninos C, Simaioforidis V et al (2010) The relationship between androgens, regulators of collagen metabolism, and Peyronie's disease: a case control study. J Sex Med 7(12):4011–4017

La Pera G, Pescatori ES, Calabrese M et al (2001) Peyronie's disease: prevalence and association with cigarette smoking. A multicenter population-based study in men aged 50–69 years. Eur Urol 40:525–530

Lemourt Oliva M, Filgueiras Lopez E, Rodriguez Barroso A et al (1998) Clinical evaluation of the use of propoleum in Peyronie's disease. Arch Esp Urol 51:171–176

Lemourt Oliva M, Rodriguez Barroso A, Bordonado Ramirez R et al (2003a) Study of propoleum dosage in Peyronie's disease. Arch Esp Urol 56:814–819

Lemourt Oliva M, Rodriguez Barroso A, Puente Guillen M et al (2003b) Propoleum and Peyronie's disease. Arch Esp Urol 56:805–813

Levine LA, Greenfield JM (2003) Establishing a standardized evaluation of the man with Peyronie's disease. Int J Impot Res 15(Suppl 5):S103–S112

Levine LA, Goldman KE, Greenfield JM (2002) Experience with intraplaque injection of verapamil for Peyronie's disease. J Urol 168:621–625; discussion 625–626

Lonn E, Bosch J, Yusuf S et al (2005) Effects of long-term vitamin E supplementation on cardiovascular events and cancer: a randomized controlled trial. JAMA 293(11):1338–1347

Martin DJ, Badwan K, Parker M et al (2002) Transdermal application of verapamil gel to the penile shaft fails to infiltrate the tunica albuginea. J Urol 168:2483–2485

Mirone V, Palmieri A, Granata AM et al (2000) Ultrasound-guided ESWT in Peyronie's disease plaques. Arch Ital Urol Androl 72:384–387

Mulhall JP (2003) Expanding the paradigm for plaque development in Peyronie's disease. Int J Impot Res 15(Suppl 5):S93–S102

Mulhall JP, Branch J, Lubrano T et al (2003) Radiation increases fibrogenic cytokine expression by Peyronie's disease fibroblasts. J Urol 170:281–284

Ojingwa JC, Isseroff RR (2003) Electrical stimulation of wound healing. J Invest Dermatol 121:1–12

Palmieri A, Imbimbo C, Longo N et al (2009) A first prospective, randomized, double-blind, placebo-controlled clinical trial evaluating extracorporeal shock wave therapy for the treatment of Peyronie's disease. Eur Urol 56:363–369

Pryor J, Akkus E, Alter G et al (2004) Peyronie's disease. J Sex Med 1:110–115

Ralph DJ, Brooks MD, Bottazzo GF et al (1992) The treatment of Peyronie's disease with tamoxifen. Br J Urol 70:648–651

Rhoden EL, Teloken C, Ting HY et al (2001) Prevalence of Peyronie's disease in men over 50-y-old from Southern Brazil. Int J Impot Res 13:291–293

Riedl CR, Plas E, Engelhardt P et al (2000) Iontophoresis for treatment of Peyronie's disease. J Urol 163:95–99

Safarinejad MR (2004) Therapeutic effects of colchicine in the management of Peyronie's disease: a randomized double-blind, placebo-controlled study. Int J Impot Res 16:238–243

Safarinejad MR, Hosseini SY, Kolahi AA (2007) Comparison of vitamin E and propionyl-L-carnitine, separately or in combination, in patients with early chronic Peyronie's disease: a double-blind, placebo controlled, randomized study. J Urol 178:1398–1403; discussion 1403

Safarinejad MR, Asgari MA, Hosseini SY et al (2010) A double-blind placebo-controlled study of the efficacy and safety of pentoxifylline in early chronic Peyronie's disease. BJU Int 106:240–248

Sasso F, Gulino G, Falabella R et al (2007) Peyronie's disease: lights and shadows. Urol Int 78:1–9

Schiavino D, Sasso F, Nucera E et al (1997) Immunologic findings in Peyronie's disease: a controlled study. Urology 50: 764–768

Schwarzer U, Sommer F, Klotz T et al (2001) The prevalence of Peyronie's disease: results of a large survey. BJU Int 88:727–730

Seegenschmiedt MH, Keilholz L, Wielpütz M, Schubert Ch, Fehlauer F (2012) Long-term outcome of radiotherapy for early stage Dupuytren's disease: a phase III clinical study. In: Dupuytren's disease and related hyperproliferative disorders, pp 349–371

Shirazi M, Haghpanah AR, Badiee M et al (2009) Effect of intralesional verapamil for treatment of Peyronie's disease: a randomized single-blind, placebo-controlled study. Int Urol Nephrol 41:467–471

Sikka SC, Hellstrom WJ (2002) Role of oxidative stress and antioxidants in Peyronie's disease. Int J Impot Res 14:353–360

Smith CJ, McMahon C, Shabsigh R (2005) Peyronie's disease: the epidemiology, etiology and clinical evaluation of deformity. BJU Int 95:729–732

Soh J, Kawauchi A, Kanemitsu N et al (2010) Nicardipine vs. saline injection as treatment for Peyronie's disease: a prospective, randomized, single-blind trial. J Sex Med 7(11): 3743–3749

Suzuki H, Komiya A, Yuasa J, Suzuki N (1999) Clinical investigation of penile Peyronie's disease treated conservatively. Impotence 14:29–32

Tal R, Heck M, Teloken P et al (2010) Peyronie's disease following radical prostatectomy: incidence and predictors. J Sex Med 7:1254–1261

Taylor FL, Levine LA (2008) Non-surgical therapy of Peyronie's disease. Asian J Androl 10:79–87

Teloken C, Rhoden EL, Grazziotin TM et al (1999) Tamoxifen versus placebo in the treatment of Peyronie's disease. J Urol 162:2003–2005

Trost LW, Gur S, Hellstrom WJ (2007) Pharmacological management of Peyronie's disease. Drugs 67:527–545

Valente EG, Vernet D, Ferrini MG et al (2003) L-arginine and phosphodiesterase (PDE) inhibitors counteract fibrosis in the

Peyronie's fibrotic plaque and related fibroblast cultures. Nitric Oxide 9:229–244

van der Wielen GJ, Vermeij M, de Jong BW et al (2009) Changes in the penile arteries of the rat after fractionated irradiation of the prostate: a pilot study. J Sex Med 6:1908–1913

Vernet D, Nolazco G, Cantini L et al (2005) Evidence that osteogenic progenitor cells in the human tunica albuginea may originate from stem cells: implications for peyronie disease. Biol Reprod 73:1199–1210

Wagenknecht LV (1996) Differential therapies in various stages of penile induration. Arch Esp Urol 49:285–292

Weidner W, Hauck EW, Schnitker J (2005) Potassium paraaminobenzoate (POTABA) in the treatment of Peyronie's disease: a prospective, placebo-controlled, randomized study. Eur Urol 47:530–535; discussion 535–536

Wiltink J, Hauck EW, Phadayanon M et al (2003) Validation of the German version of the International Index of Erectile Function (IIEF) in patients with erectile dysfunction, Peyronie's disease and controls. Int J Impot Res 15: 192–197

Part VIII
Future Perspectives

Editor: Charles Eaton

The Patient's Perspective and the International Dupuytren Society

52

Wolfgang Wach

Contents

52.1	**Introduction**	441
52.2	**A Personal History**	441
52.2.1	One Problem and Two Success Stories	441
52.2.2	A Different Perspective	442
52.3	**What Do Patients Want? (Generalization)**	443
52.4	**What Can Patients Do?**	444
52.4.1	Individual Contributions	444
52.4.2	Global Cooperation	445
52.4.3	Dupuytren Symposium	445
52.4.4	International Dupuytren Award	445
52.5	**Conclusion**	445
References		446

52.1 Introduction

A patient's perspective – how useful is it? Is a personal history of any general interest? Can a generalized patient's perspective be useful data without its personal background? Is a patient's perspective different from a doctor's perspective? Has it any value for research?

Let us look at answers to these questions.

This chapter is also an attempt to build a bridge from a personal history to an internationally active organization, the International Dupuytren Society.

52.2 A Personal History

52.2.1 One Problem and Two Success Stories

At the age of 35, I noticed my first nodule. It appeared in the palm of my right hand, below the ring finger. When I noticed it, it had a diameter of 1–2 mm and a friend visiting me, a medical doctor, looked at it and diagnosed Dupuytren's. He was just coming from a conference where he had listened to a paper describing radiotherapy of Dupuytren's disease and immediately suggested that I have the nodule irradiated. Within weeks of the radiotherapy, the nodule vanished and was not palpable anymore. This was 28 years ago. The nodule never returned and my finger is still straight and fully functional. The only side effect (so far) was slightly increased dryness of my skin and today I can no longer tell whether the skin in the irradiated area is still dryer or not. So, to me that was a total success.

My mother developed her first nodule at the age of 80. My father never showed any signs of Dupuytren's disease.

W. Wach
International Dupuytren Society,
Westerbuchberg 60b, 83236 Übersee, Germany
e-mail: w.wach@dupuytren-online.info

C. Eaton et al. (eds.), *Dupuytren's Disease and Related Hyperproliferative Disorders*,
DOI 10.1007/978-3-642-22697-7_52, © Springer-Verlag Berlin Heidelberg 2012

If my mother had died earlier, like her parents did, there would be no family history of this disease. One day genetics may be able to tell the full family history.

Five years later another nodule started to grow, this time in my left palm, again below the ring finger. Being naïve and afraid of radiation (which is not naïve), I wondered whether the nodule might disappear without radiotherapy. So I did nothing. Sure enough the nodule grew, eventually developed a cord that grew into the palm and into the finger, beyond my PIP joint. When the extension deficit reached 20–25° I had surgery. I traveled quite a distance to consult a hand surgeon who was expert in Dupuytren's disease. The surgeon removed all diseased tissue and a sector of the aponeurosis to minimize the risk of recurrence. The extension deficit was completely removed. The wounds healed well with very little scarring (Fig. 52.1a, b). That was 10 years ago. Since then I experienced no recurrence, that finger is still straight and fully functional. Another success story.

Figure 52.1 makes me doubt the interpretation of Dupuytren's disease as exaggerated wound healing. My wound healing is excellent, the scarring minimal, certainly no keloids. Dupuytren's disease may have common characteristics with wound healing but it is still fundamentally different.

52.2.2 A Different Perspective

While the surgery itself was very successful, its side effects were, for a patient, somewhat frightening. I was not prepared for the size of the wound and the first undressing was a shock. More importantly my hand swelled considerably and while I regained my straight finger, I lost the ability to make a fist. It was about 2 months before I could passively make a fist and it took another 3–4 months before the swelling was completely gone. Physiotherapy helped a little but not dramatically. It could be that its effect was mostly psychological, i.e., the fact that someone cared about my hand and kept telling me that it would get better.

More frightening to me was that within a couple of months, I developed six new nodules, three in each hand, and all were quickly growing and all in areas where I had no visible disease before the surgery. I already had one diseased finger, which had not fully recovered from the surgery yet, and I now had six new affected fingers. I saw myself embarking on a series of operations, each one causing further nodules and requiring further operations. That was *really* scary. After wasting some time with useless homeopathic therapies, I remembered radiotherapy. I had major difficulties finding a clinic providing it, but eventually I succeeded and RT helped to keep my growing nodules at bay.

This experience raised several questions:

a. In the clinic's statistics, my operation showed up as successful and rightly so. But personally I perceived it as painful, with a long recovery period and massive disease extension. Whose perspective is the right one, the surgeon's or mine? In research, typically the surgeon's data are used. Is that how it should be? Shouldn't the success of a treatment be

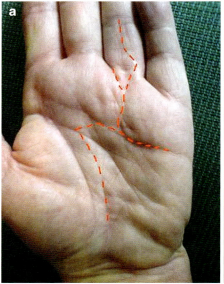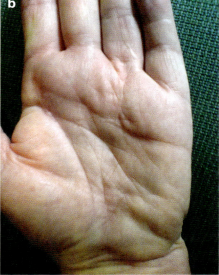

Fig. 52.1 Limited fasciectomy on the left hand. (**a**) Incision; (**b**) the well-healed cuts

judged by the patient? When going to a restaurant, I would not want the cook to judge the quality of my dinner. He may be the expert but I prefer my own judgment. However, viewing things from a research point of view, can you trust patients in what they tell about their treatment? In the last few years, the interest in patients' perspective has been growing, e.g., in conjunction with Health Technology Assessment (Facey et al. 2010). With regard to Dupuytren's contracture, surgical treatment was evaluated in the UK from a patient's perspective. Not surprisingly the results turned out more on the critical side and led to this conclusion: "Our study shows good correction can be achieved by surgery, but that treatment has a high complication rate and a significant rate of recurrent contracture" (Dias and Braybrooke 2006). So far most patient-oriented publications seem to emerge from the United Kingdom (as another Dupuytren example: Jerosch-Herold et al. 2012, and addressing more general aspects Garratt et al. 2002; NICE 2011).

b. My massive spread of Dupuytren's disease after surgery is probably not typical but it is not unique either. It is not totally surprising, as we all know that trauma can trigger Dupuytren's disease (Elliot and Ragoowansi 2005), especially when the patient is genetically predisposed. Now Dupuytren's surgery is a major trauma and a Dupuytren's patient is certainly predisposed for this disease. How frequent is spreading of the disease after surgery? More research is needed there. Where does disease extension come from and could it have been predicted? The root causes are as unclear as the root cause of Dupuytren's disease itself, but probably I had pre-stages of the disease (whatever that means), prior to surgery, in those areas where I afterward quickly developed new nodules. Could those pre-stages be detected before the surgery? Possibly not but nobody really looked for them.

c. My difficulties after surgery and my long search for a radiotherapy clinic brought me into contact with other patients and with medical doctors, all equally frustrated about the little knowledge about this disease and its treatments. Together, in October 2003, we started the Dupuytren Society (http://www. dupuytren-online.info). This was the point where I stepped beyond my own personal history and into the more general aspects of patient experience and the Dupuytren Society.

52.3 What Do Patients Want? (Generalization)

Patients want a cure, that is all. For Dupuytren's disease, unfortunately, there is no cure. So the next best option is a treatment that improves the personal disease situation. For Dupuytren's disease this might be getting fingers functional again, reducing pain, or reducing/stopping disease progression. The latter two aspects are equally valid for Ledderhose disease.

With several treatment options available, it is essential to have information about what those treatments are, what they can do, when they are best applied, and what side effects they might have. From its start the Dupuytren Society has been a nonprofit organization for physicians and patients, dedicated to informing about treatment options, supporting patients, and supporting research. One of the first steps that the Dupuytren Society undertook was installing a web site and a patients' forum. In 2003, not much information on Dupuytren's disease was available on the Internet. Today our English forum alone has 1,400 registered users and 19,000 posts. The web site has 600 visitors per day and probably reaches about 100,000 patients per year.

What we need is an understanding of what treatment is best in which situation. Fifty years ago Vernon Luck stated, "In the past, little attempt has been made to classify the stage of the disease and then employ therapeutic methods based upon the predominant stage of the process" (1959) and, unfortunately, this is still true. We need a commonly agreed-on treatment concept for Dupuytren's disease, something a bit like Table 52.1.

Although Table 52.1 illustrates what we are looking for, it has several flaws as well.

a. The relationship between the stage of the disease and the most appropriate treatment is too simplistic. For example, a very old patient having a contracted finger in stage 3 might not tolerate surgery anymore and

Table 52.1 Therapies for different stages of Dupuytren's disease

Stage	N	N/1	1	2	3	4
Radiotherapy	•	○				
Collagenase injection				•	○	
NA/PNF			○	•	○	○	○
Hand surgery				•	•	•	•

"*NA*" stands for needle aponeurotomy, also called percutaneous needle fasciotomy (*PNF*). The disease staging is extended Tubiana staging (Adamietz et al. 2001), • = very efficient, usually applied in this stage, ○ = efficient, occasionally applied in this stage

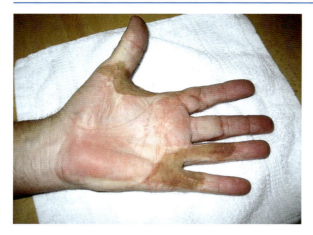

Fig. 52.2 Hand of a patient after several surgeries, including dermofasciectomy

NA or a collagenase injection might be preferable. The same might be true for patients with wound healing problems or recurrent disease. Radiotherapy is effective in the early stage of the disease but might also help after surgery. Figure 52.2 shows the hand of a patient who had 15 operations on his hand, including four dermofasciectomies for recurrent surgeries, and an aggressive disease extension shortly after his 15th surgery. He was treated with radiotherapy 4 years ago which stabilized his situation. He has been without new symptoms since that time.

We need a treatment concept that takes into account the actual situation of the patient, i.e., we need a *situation-specific treatment concept*.

b. Table 52.1 simplifies the various treatment options. For example, hand surgery offers a broad range of techniques, not only with regard to incisions but also how much to remove where (e.g., whether or not to leave the aponeurosis intact? (Rayan 2012; Meinel 2012)). Even for hand surgeons, it is probably difficult if not impossible to decide which technique is best in class. Cost, recovery time, and recurrence would be good criteria but we do not even have a common definition of how to measure recurrence. Instead of reporting x percent recurrence after y years, it would be better to measure a mean recurrence period but that would require longer observation, at least fairly beyond that mean value. Even the definition of recurrence varies widely (Dupuytren Society 2010).

c. We are using the extension deficit for defining stages of contracture but we do not yet have a standardized, repeatable way to measure an extension deficit and yield identical results, irrespective of the person performing the measurement. This may not be relevant for the consideration of which treatment to choose in a specific situation, but it is certainly relevant if we measure improvement due to treatment or the efficiency of means for rehabilitation.

In summary, patients need clear advice what treatment is best in their specific situation and they want it from the doctor who treats them. They do not want to travel from specialist to specialist and get different advice depending on what the doctor or clinic specializes in. If they need rehabilitation, they want a clear concept and someone to help them implement it. Today we are lacking most of this. The typical advice is: "Don't do anything. Wait until you have a real problem and then have surgery." Frankly, that is too simple. We need to disseminate information about available treatment options and their pros and cons.

52.4 What Can Patients Do?

52.4.1 Individual Contributions

The first thing for a patient to do is to become an informed patient. Resources will be treating doctors, the Internet, patient organizations, literature, and communication with other patients. The next step might be supporting other patients by communicating experience, by supporting forums, and, of course, by joining the Dupuytren Society. Supporting research is more difficult for patients. From other diseases we know of a few extraordinary examples, like Augusto and Michaela Odone (1994) finding with "Lorenzo's oil" a means to somewhat stabilize ALD, or more recently Tim Parks' approach to relieving pelvic pain (Parks 2010). These are admirable, exceptional contributions. For the normal patient, contributions will rather be participating in research projects by donating tissue or reporting results. Under the aspects of Evidence-Based Medicine, reporting personal observations has gained bad reputation as "anecdotal" but while such anecdotal evidence does not justify general treatment recommendations, observations from patients might still indicate new areas for research that have so far been ignored. The Dupuytren Society provides a forum for these observations and takes additional, organizational steps in supporting research.

52.4.2 Global Cooperation

The International Dupuytren Society acts globally because this is a global disease. We are cooperating with other organizations, especially with the Dupuytren Foundation in the USA with which we share the same goals and objectives. The International Dupuytren Society represents Dupuytren's patients in patients' organizations like IAPO (International Alliance of Patients' Organizations) and deals with national organizations, like NAKOS (Germany), or recently in supporting NICE (NHS UK) in the assessment of radiotherapy for early Dupuytren's Disease (NICE 2010).

52.4.3 Dupuytren Symposium

A prime effort to foster and support research was organizing, in cooperation with the Dupuytren Foundation, the conference on Dupuytren's Disease and related conditions in Miami 2010 (Dupuytren Symposium 2010). The goal of this symposium was to promote a global collaborative effort to develop better treatment options. We wanted to bring together experts from all over the world (which resulted in participants from 17 countries), encourage collaboration between specialists in their common field, increase awareness and understanding of research efforts in other fields, bring together clinical experience and research, and in general encourage research and collaboration to bring us closer to our common goal of understanding and healing Dupuytren's disease. This book shows that this certainly was worth the effort.

I believe it was Paul Zidel who at the conference raised the question, "does a Dupuytren's contracture serve a useful teleological purpose?" We all are implicitly assuming that Dupuytren's is caused by some sort of malfunction, for example overproduction of collagen, and we think about ways to correct this malfunction. The above question is probably not addressed in this book because we were not able to answer it but I cannot get it off my mind anymore. Maybe Dupuytren's contracture is a reasonable response of our body to constantly pulling on the initial nodule that fixes skin and connective tissue together. A bent finger successfully stops this pulling. This is just one of many open questions.

We are planning to organize further conferences in regular intervals, the next one to be held in 2015 in Europe. We hope that this will help in creating a global community of physicians and researchers, yielding synergy and progress toward better treatment options.

52.4.4 International Dupuytren Award

A recent and prominent effort to support and foster research is the International Dupuytren Award instituted by the Dupuytren Society (Dupuytren Award 2010). The Award recognizes exceptional scientific publications on research or clinical treatment of Morbus Dupuytren and/or Morbus Ledderhose. Research can be awarded in the areas of therapy, epidemiology, pathogenesis, genomics, or in other areas which improve the understanding and treatment of these diseases. The International Dupuytren Award will be given annually and the winner is selected by the Scientific Advisory Board of the Dupuytren Society.

The Dupuytren Award was presented for the first time in 2010 for research published in 2009. It was awarded to the PhD thesis "Therapy-resisting Dupuytren's disease - new perspectives in adjuvant treatment" by Prof. Ilse Degreef of the Katholicke Universiteit Leuven, Belgium. The Award was presented at the Annual Meeting of German Hand Surgeons (DGH 2010) in Nuremberg, Germany (Fig. 52.3a, b).

52.5 Conclusion

A patient's perspective in the first place is always a personal history: in the case of Dupuytren's disease, a history of concern, irritation, seeking for information and treatment options. The International Dupuytren Society is an example of how this frustration can lead to a productive collaboration of physicians and patients, one which is helping other patients and, might, one day help finding a cure for this disease.

Fig. 52.3 (**a**) Prof. Ilse Degreef speaking at DGH 2010 about "New perspectives of adjuvant treatment in Dupuytren's disease." (**b**) International Dupuytren Award 2010

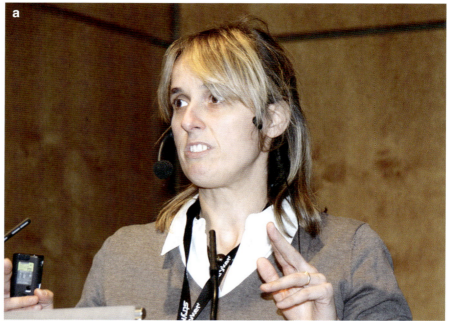

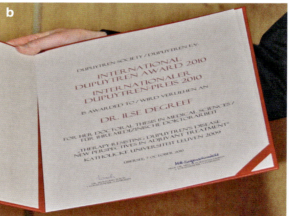

Acknowledgments This is a great place to thank all members and supporters of the International Dupuytren Society for their considerable, unpaid efforts, and their donations which provide the bulk of our funding. We are especially grateful for the support by the Society's Scientific Advisory Council and the great cooperation of the Dupuytren Foundation. Special thanks go to Judith Proctor for carefully reading and improving manuscripts and web sites. Last not least, the International Dupuytren Society gratefully acknowledges the financial support of German health insurance companies for ongoing expenses and of AOK for the Dupuytren conference in Miami 2010.

References

Adamietz B, Keilholz L, Grünert J, Sauer R (2001) Radiotherapy in early stage Dupuytren's contracture. Strahlenther Onkol 177:604–610

Dias JJ, Braybrooke J (2006) Dupuytren's contracture: an audit of the outcome of surgery. J Hand Surg [Br] 31:514–521

Dupuytren Award (2010) http://www.dupuytren-online.info/dupuytren_award.html. Accessed Oct 2010

Dupuytren Society (2010) Techniques of hand surgery. http://www.dupuytren-online.info/dupuytren_surgery_techniques.html. Accessed Oct 2010

Dupuytren Symposium (2010) http://dupuytrensymposium.com/, Accessed Oct 2010

Elliot D, Ragoowansi R (2005) Dupuytren's disease secondary to acute injury, infection or operation distal to the elbow in the ipsilateral upper limb - a historical review. J Hand Surg [Br] 30:148–156

Facey K, Boivin A, Gracia J, Hansen HP, Lo Scalzo A, Mossman J, Single A (2010) Patients' perspectives in health technology assessment: a route to robust evidence and fair deliberation. Int J Technol Assess Health Care 26:334–340

Garratt A, Schmidt L, Mackintosh A, Fitzpatrick R (2002) Quality of life measurement: bibliographic study of patient assessed health outcome measures. BMJ 324(7351): 1417

Jerosch-Herold C, Shepstone L, Chojnowski A, Larson D (2012) Severity of contracture and self-reported disability in patients with Dupuytren's contracture referred for surgery. In: Dupuytren's disease and related hyperproliferative disorders, pp 317–321

Luck JV (1959) Dupuytren's contracture: a new concept of the pathogenesis correlated with surgical management. J Bone Joint Surg Am 41:635–664

Meinel A (2012) Palmar fibromatosis or the loss of flexibility of the palmar finger tissue. A new insight into the disease process of Dupuytren contracture. In: Dupuytren's disease and related hyperproliferative disorders, pp 11–20

NICE (2010) Radiation therapy for early Dupuytren's disease. http://guidance.nice.org.uk/IPG368. Accessed Jan 2011

NICE (2011) Patient and public involvement. http://www.nice.org.uk/getinvolved/patientandpublicinvolvement/patient_and_public_involvement.jsp. Accessed Jan 2011

Odone A, Odone M (1994) More on lorenzo's oil. N Engl J Med 330:1904–1905

Parks T (2010) Teach us to sit still – a sceptic's search for health and healing. Harvill Secker/Random House, London

Rayan G (2012) Dupuytren's disease – anatomy, pathology, and presentation. In: Dupuytren's disease and related hyperproliferative disorders, pp 3–10

IDUP: Proposal for an International Research Database

53

Charles Eaton, Michael Heinrich Seegenschmiedt, and Wolfgang Wach

Contents

53.1	**Introduction**	449
53.2	**Data Collection and Data Restrictions**	450
53.3	**Contributing and Extracting Data**	450
53.3.1	Which Clinics Will Participate and Benefit?	450
53.3.2	Uploading Data	450
53.3.3	Updates, Anonymity, and Redundant Data	451
53.3.4	Extracting Data	451
53.4	**Technical Aspects**	452
53.4.1	Database Requirements	452
53.4.2	Data Structure	452
53.5	**Financial and Legal Aspects**	453
53.6	**A Prototype and Its Future**	453
References		454

C. Eaton
The Hand Center, Jupiter, FL, USA
e-mail: eaton@bellsouth.net

M.H. Seegenschmiedt
Strahlenzentrum Hamburg Nord, Hamburg, Germany
e-mail: mhs@szhh.info

W. Wach (✉)
International Dupuytren Society, Westerbuchberg 60b, 83236
Uebersee, Germany
e-mail: w.wach@dupuytren-online.info

53.1 Introduction

Although Dupuytren's disease is far from being a rare condition and each year tens of thousands, if not hundreds of thousands, of patients are treated, published data is typically based on a relatively small number of cases (recent, arbitrarily picked examples, mostly published in 2010: Lilly and Stern 2010; Rayan et al. 2010; Takase 2010; Watt et al. 2010; Jerosch-Herold et al. 2011). Data sets are typically fewer than 100 patients. Exceptions are mostly literature reviews and genomic research. The reason for these statistically small sets of data is probably that authors usually can only access data from their own clinic, and even those have rarely been collected systematically over the years. It is therefore tempting to envision an international database that consolidates data from many clinics in a standardized manner and provides them in large quantities to research projects, without giving away personal information of patients.

Another benefit of such a database could be the support for standardization of treatment. At present most treatments differ from one clinic to another. As the amount of treatment data increases in the database, this information might help to identify best practices and define standards for treatments.

The purpose of this chapter is to describe concept and prototype of an International Dupuytren database, a project abbreviated as IDUP.

C. Eaton et al. (eds.), *Dupuytren's Disease and Related Hyperproliferative Disorders*,
DOI 10.1007/978-3-642-22697-7_53, © Springer-Verlag Berlin Heidelberg 2012

53.2 Data Collection and Data Restrictions

The purpose of IDUP is supporting research. This requires a standardization of data structure and data content. To get started we decided to initially limit the data in IDUP to:
(a) Surgical data, including NA and collagenase
(b) Radiotherapy data

We considered those two types of data as similar enough to be merged into a single database and different enough to learn about problems of data consolidation. Other treatments, like injection of steroids, use of oral or topical medications, can be added after the initial phase has been completed. It is critical to begin with a data structure that is flexible and extendable enough to accommodate future requirements of documenting and researching new treatments.

We decided to focus on data from patients with Dupuytren's disease. Although it is important to document the presence of diathesis factors such as Ledderhose and Peyronie's, detailed staging and treatment information on these related conditions will not initially be collected. The database can be extended later, once enough experience with Dupuytren's disease has been accumulated and IDUP is up and running smoothly.

Finally, we decided to focus on clinical treatment data and, at least for the time being, to exclude data for basic research, e.g., for genomics or cell studies. We are aware that their need for large quantities of data is also very high but those data have quite different structures and including them from the very beginning would have considerably complicated coordination, database design, and prototyping. This is simply a matter of practicality. We would very much like to support basic research and include this data in the database, provided it makes sense. We have to start small and build upward.

53.3 Contributing and Extracting Data

53.3.1 Which Clinics Will Participate and Benefit?

The vision is that many clinics from all over the world load their data into IDUP and that clinics providing data can also retrieve data. IDUP will reside on the Internet with strictly controlled remote access for registered and approved users only. On a very high level, it could look like in Fig. 53.1.

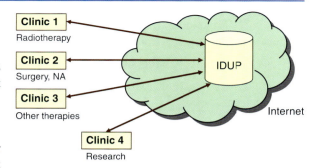

Fig. 53.1 Basic concept of the International Dupuytren database IDUP

The downloading of data will be of interest for research projects and for clinics involved in research. They will be the ones that benefit from IDUP. Therefore, at least initially, the clinics uploading data will be the only ones that are also downloading data. Participating in the project and uploading data entitles them to access the data pool.

53.3.2 Uploading Data

The uploading of data is technically probably the most demanding and critical part of IDUP. It would be tempting to define a standard electronic format in which data can be uploaded into IDUP. This would be easy and versatile to implement, but unfortunately it would likely also constitute a road block. We cannot assume that data worldwide is available in a consistent format as it is in Sweden, for example (Wilbrand 2010), which would strongly facilitate a disease register or database. Rather we have to assume that each clinic has its own more or less proprietary system to collect in-house data and only very few, if any, of the clinics will devote resources and funds to convert their internal data into another format for uploading into IDUP. Therefore, IDUP will need a flexible import module that can be easily configured by an IDUP administrator to import many different formats (Fig. 53.2).

Each clinic would get its own, specifically configured version of the interface and with this data can then be uploaded by the clinic, automatically and without further support. This sounds like pie in the sky, but it is feasible, e.g., DHL's logistic software FCI (= Flexible Customer Interface) does exactly this and includes an Admin tool for configuring the importing of data.

A manual input form could allow manual entry of data into IDUP. This manual input form will output

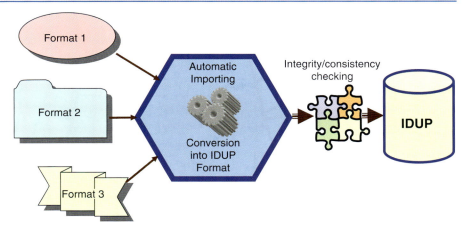

Fig. 53.2 Configurable data import module of IDUP, able to import various formats. Integrity/consistency checking analyzes the uploaded data and compares them to already stored data to avoid uploading of redundant data from the same clinic

data in the IDUP format. Those data will then not need to pass through the IDUP Import Module of Fig. 53.2 but can immediately be checked for integrity and consistency and then stored in IDUP. The manual input form (Fig. 53.3) can either be used for uploading small amounts of data or it might also be used for a local version of IDUP, within a clinic, to enter data into a local database that might create patient records, communicate with billing software or IDUP.

53.3.3 Updates, Anonymity, and Redundant Data

Initially we will probably be able to get complete data sets, i.e., data of treatments that include the patient's characteristics, disease history, the treatment details, and results. However, patients will eventually come back for review, for treatment of recurrence or for treatment of other parts of the hand. When those data are being uploaded, IDUP has to recognize that a record already exists for the specific patient and has either to append the new data or overwrite the old data. Otherwise we would end up with redundant data sets, which would eventually render the database useless.

To uniquely identify a patient within IDUP, we plan a two-stage identifier for each record: The first part will be a clinic identifier and the second part will be a patient identifier. Only the clinic itself will be able to identify a real patient with these data, within IDUP the patient will stay anonymous. But IDUP will be able to identify the patient when additional or redundant data are being uploaded and can decide how to handle them.

There is one issue that can be resolved in a patient register, like the Swedish one, but not within IDUP: If a patient is treated in one clinic and then moves on to another clinic and both clinics participate in IDUP, the patient's treatment will result in two distinct records within IDUP. They will probably have similar patient's histories but IDUP would not be able to recognize that both records refer to the same patient. At present we do not see a way to avoid this while maintaining strict anonymity, but it is not so different to today's situation where patients have no country-wide patient ID, except for a few countries that use personal identity numbers like Sweden (Wilbrand 2010). This is a shortcoming we will have to live with, but we remain open to suggestions that may help solve the problem.

53.3.4 Extracting Data

Compared to the data import, data extraction is technically easy because we control the database. What we perhaps need is a little data warehouse where the user can define selection criteria and then is able to download matching data as CSV strings or Excel or some other convenient format. It could be useful to have a data viewer displaying statistical results of the data filtering before the actual download starts. There is a chance that we can configure some standard reporting tool to do the job.

There are yet some caveats associated with download data: We must assure that specific patients cannot be identified through the downloaded data and we must make sure that specific clinics cannot be identified via downloads. We do not want someone to use IDUP for running evaluations of clinics. We believe that we can

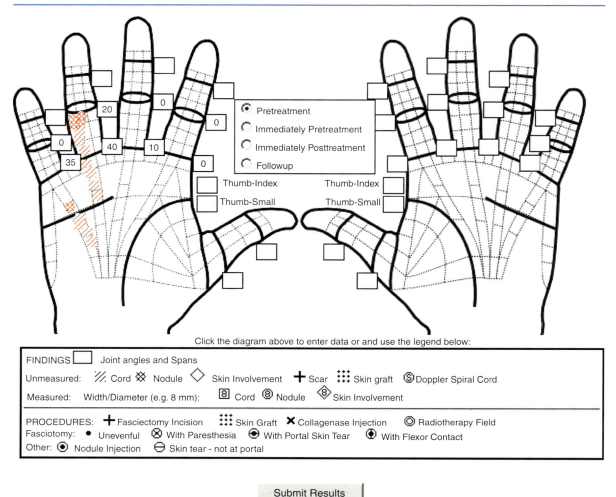

Fig. 53.3 Manual input form for IDUP (Courtesy of Charles Eaton)

meet both requirements by hiding the clinic identifier to the outside world. Each clinic would know its own identifier but not that of other clinics. Clinic identifiers would have some arbitrary structure, not just a sequential number that might be guessed.

53.4 Technical Aspects

53.4.1 Database Requirements

The database will necessarily need to reside on an Internet server and it should use a robust, easy to configure and administer database. Other requirements are more difficult to estimate. IDUP will support initially only a few clinics, growing to perhaps 50 clinics. Initially we would not be importing pictures into IDUP; thus, the required storage space will be driven by database records only. IDUP might eventually hold 100–500k records and will require around 50 GB of space. The amount of parallel users at any time will probably be low, 10 should be more than ample.

We decided to use a MySQL database and a WAMP tool set (details are interesting only for the software gurus). The database will be remotely administered.

53.4.2 Data Structure

Obviously the data structure is an important feature of this database. It has to be general enough to accommodate various types of treatments and it has to be flexible and expandable enough to adapt to future requirements of new treatments, new disease aspects, and new research. We have already developed an initial data structure but will stick here with the basics. More details are available from the International Dupuytren Society.

There can be more than one record per patient (1: N relation). Patients are identified by a patient ID that is created from the clinic ID+the clinic's patient ID. Several types of records will be used. The record type PatInfo will be available only once per patient. The other record types can appear more than once per patient.

A patient can have several record types:

System information (SysInfo): Clinic ID, country, when imported, when last edited, edited by whom – these fields will be filled by IDUP automatically

Patient information (PatInfo): patient ID, age/date of birth, gender, previous treatments in other clinics, related diseases, habits, trauma, hereditary info

Pre-status (PreStat): current symptoms, angle (for fingers), date of examination

Treatment (Treat): for example, (a) surgery (b) NA (c) radiotherapy (d) other therapy; each using its own fields

Post-status (PostStat): status, angle (for fingers), date of examination (e.g., same as treatment date), improvement? worse? recurrence? extension?

Post treatment (PostTreat): (e.g., splint, physiology), start date, duration, comment

The current plan for IDUP is to only load data from patients that have already completed their treatment. The first upload of data for a specific patient should therefore at least contain:

- SysInfo – PatInfo
- Sysinfo – PreStat
- Sysinfo – Treat
- Sysinfo – PostStat

Checking a patient's status after treatment can extend over a longer period of time, and may result in several PostStat records for this patient. These can be loaded sequentially into IDUP and can either be full records overwriting the old ones or partial records such as:

- SysInfo – PatInfo (optional ID only) – PostStat
- SysInfo – PatInfo (optional ID only) – PostTreat

New treatment of the same patient in the same clinic will require the same records as the initial treatment and will result in a second record for the same patient.

53.5 Financial and Legal Aspects

Financially we need to distinguish between the initial development of the database, its eventual extension, and the maintenance, which would include configuring and testing the importer (import interface), for additional clinics. The initial investment will probably be in the range of 20–30,000 USD, the annual running expense probably in the 5,000 USD range. This is not much for what it can achieve but is still considerable, if not too much, for a single clinic or university. Funding is obviously required. Charging for downloads would alleviate but not solve this issue. We would rather not charge for downloads.

There are a variety of legal aspects, such as who owns uploaded data. Also, the requirements for investigational board review supervision and data protection differ from country to country, so we will need to study the local legal requirements before including a new country. Another, still unclear aspect is intellectual property of the database concept.

53.6 A Prototype and Its Future

To gain experience in loading data from different clinics and therapies into a common database, we embarked on building a prototype. Currently, this prototype resides on the Internet on http://www.idup-online.de and is password protected. It uses a MySQL database. The clinics participating in this prototype were those of two authors of this paper, Charles Eaton, The Hand Center, Florida, USA, as the surgery/NA test case, and Heinrich Seegenschmiedt, then at Alfried-Krupp-Klinik, Essen, Germany, representing radiotherapy.

The prototype has a bilingual user interface (English and German) (Fig. 53.4). For the time being it has 240 data fields, organized as described above. It has a simple data viewer but neither an automatic upload nor a download capability. A few features of the user administration are available as well as a simple user guide.

What we have learned from the prototype is that the merging of data from different clinics is feasible and less difficult than one might expect, because they all refer to the same disease. Questions regarding the patient history are pretty similar in both clinics. The way that data is stored internally in each clinic is very, very different though. This will be a challenge for a future automatic importer. For the time being, data

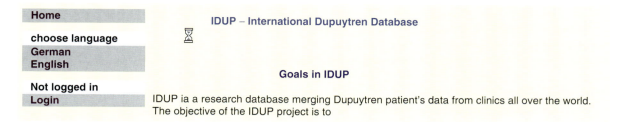

Fig. 53.4 IDUP prototype; start page

entry for the prototype is manual, which is feasible for a prototype but not when uploading data in large quantities.

The IDUP prototype is now on hold due to lack of further funding. It can be expanded into an active research database once funding of development and maintenance have been resolved. Support for projects such as this is one of the key goals of the Dupuytren Foundation and the International Dupuytren Society– to make progress in the understanding and treatment of Dupuytren's disease and related conditions.

Acknowledgments The authors would like to thank the German health insurance companies AOK, Barmer, and DAK for jointly funding development of the initial IDUP prototype, Dupuytren Society for providing resources at no charge, and CAL Computer Aided Logistics GmbH, Munich, Germany, for consulting in database design.

References

Jerosch-Herold C, Shepstone L, Chojnowski A, Larson D (2011) Severity of contracture and self-reported disability in patients with Dupuytren's contracture referred for surgery. J Hand Ther 24(1):6–10

Lilly SI, Stern PJ (2010) Simultaneous carpal tunnel release and Dupuytren's fasciectomy. J Hand Surg Am 35(5):754–759

Rayan GM, Ali M, Orozco J (2010) Dorsal pads versus nodules in normal population and Dupuytren's disease patients. J Hand Surg Am 35(10):1571–1579

Takase K (2010) Dupuytren's contracture limited to the distal interphalangeal joint: a case report. Joint Bone Spine 77(5):470–471

Watt AJ, Curtin CM, Hentz VR (2010) Collagenase injection as nonsurgical treatment of Dupuytren's disease: 8-year follow-up. J Hand Surg Am 35(4):534–539, 539.e1

Wilbrand S (2010) Registries in Dupuytren's disease. Paper presented at "Dupuytren's disease symposium" Stony Brook, New York, April 2010. Private communication, unpublished

The Future of Dupuytren's Research and Treatment

54

Charles Eaton

Contents

54.1	**Introduction**	455
54.2	**Genetics and Demographics**	455
54.2.1	Work in Progress	455
54.2.2	Demographic Research Possibilities	456
54.3	**Cell Biology**	457
54.3.1	Dysregulation	457
54.3.2	Disease Models	457
54.3.3	Pinpointing the Problem	458
54.3.4	Available Interventions	459
54.4	**Mechanical Measurements and Procedures**	459
54.4.1	Angles	459
54.4.2	Skin Involvement	461
54.4.3	Anatomic Mapping	462
54.4.4	Imaging	462
54.5	**Questions and Unsolved Problems**	464
54.6	**International Task Force**	465
54.6.1	Goals	465
54.6.2	Guidelines for Clinical Registries	467
54.6.3	Outline for Global Collaboration	468
References		468

C. Eaton
The Hand Center, Jupiter, FL, USA
e-mail: eaton@bellsouth.net

54.1 Introduction

How do we find a cure for Dupuytren's? Surgeons have held the steering wheel of the Dupuytren ship for nearly 200 years. If it were simply a matter of devising a better procedure, we would have it by now. The reason we do not is that Dupuytren's is not a local surgical disease. It is a medical condition which does not yet have a medicine. This must change, as it has in other arenas: Surgery was the traditional treatment for rheumatoid arthritis, peptic ulcer disease, prostatic hypertrophy, anal cancer, tuberculosis, and other medical conditions before effective medical treatments were developed. As with these conditions, a biologic treatment will be preferable to a mechanical one, and this requires progress in our basic understanding of the disease process. We do not need a better operation. We need a different approach. Dupuytren's is part genetic, part biological, part mechanical. Cross-collaboration across multiple specialties will provide the most powerful tools to find a cure.

54.2 Genetics and Demographics

54.2.1 Work in Progress

We have new genetic tools and very interesting research all around the world, but we are still hindered by the lack of a standard animal model, and lack of a good starting point – we have not yet clearly identified the problem chromosome, much less the specific gene. Several genes may be involved to various degrees and the majority of us might carry this genetic potential for Dupuytren's

C. Eaton et al. (eds.), *Dupuytren's Disease and Related Hyperproliferative Disorders*,
DOI 10.1007/978-3-642-22697-7_54, © Springer-Verlag Berlin Heidelberg 2012

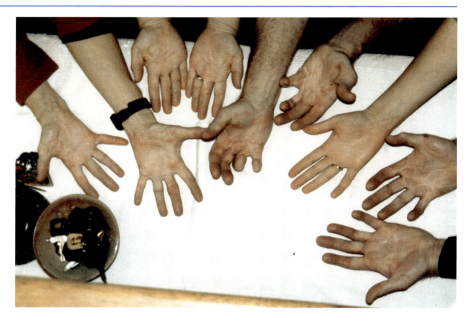

Fig. 54.1 Family with Dupuytren's (Courtesy of Dr. William Van Wyk, Ft Worth, TX)

disease. As with cancer genetics, Dupuytren's may start as a simple slight mutation of a normal gene. There is a frustrating assortment of possibilities. Could Dupuytren's start from a neonatal retroviral infection, a spontaneous mutation, a pathologic interaction of several normal genes? Dupuytren's is disproportionately common in Europe compared to Africa, so much so that it begs the question: Is it a European gene, or just the opposite – a gene from Africa which confers a special resistance to the causative factor of Dupuytren's? In addition, the results of existing genetic publications are conflicting, which may reflect more on differences in tissue processing and analysis technologies than on the true nature of Dupuytren's.

We need to augment our basic genetic research with better demographic information. As Degreef has pointed out, we do not even know whether Dupuytren's is one condition or several, like diabetes. Maybe it is not unpredictable as much as it is heterogeneous. The concept of Dupuytren' diathesis was the first step toward quantifying biologic, rather than the surgical, severity, and this has been extended from knuckle pads, Ledderhose and Peyronie's to include risk factors of bilaterality, radial hand involvement, male gender, more than 2 fingers involved, and age of onset under 50, all independently associated with higher risk of early recurrence (Abe et al. 2004; Hindocha et al. 2006; Degreef and de Smet 2011). Additional factors such as strong family penetrance (Fig. 54.1) and the pattern of involvement of ectopic disease (Fig. 54.2) may also be predictive of disease progression and responsiveness. Studies which do not take these factors into account are comparing apples and oranges – in the dark. We need to use these to document the phenotypic expression of Dupuytren's in all future studies. As the genetic risk for Dupuytren's is fairly common, it might be the most effective research strategy to focus on identifying genetic patterns associated with aggressive Dupuytren's. Are there specific genes for aggressive Dupuytren's? Also, the fastest way to get meaningful results of treatment is to study patients with aggressive Dupuytren's, because they have a high likelihood of early recurrence which reduces the sample variation, compresses the time needed for results, and magnifies the effects of treatment. We need better information to provide better treatment counseling to patients and genetic counseling to families strongly affected by Dupuytren's.

54.2.2 Demographic Research Possibilities

Further demographic studies may yield additional clues regarding risk factors. *Birth month* has been associated with a variety of conditions, including multiple sclerosis (Staples et al. 2010), tobacco addiction (Riala et al. 2009), low fertility (Kemkes 2010), type I diabetes (Kahn et al. 2009), Celiac disease (Lewy et al. 2009), myopia (Mandel et al. 2008), longevity (Vaiserman and

Fig. 54.2 Knuckle pads. Knuckle pads involving multiple digits and unusual locations, such as the thumb interphalangeal joint (**a**), distal interphalangeal joint (**b**), or metacarpophalangeal joint (**c**). These may be associated with biologically aggressive Dupuytren's

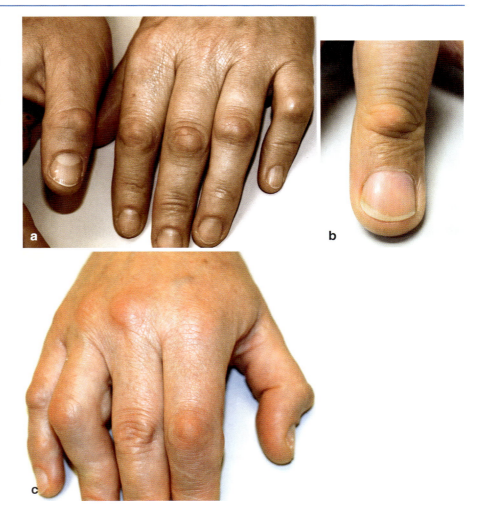

Voitenko 2003), schizophrenia (Kinney et al. 1999), autism (Zerbo et al. 2011), and others. Theories of influence include possible seasonal differences in sunlight-derived vitamin D, seasonal pesticide use, seasonal viral exposure, and others. A large analysis of birth months in Dupuytren' patients would be simple and might provide additional information regarding risk factors and etiology. *Increased parental age at birth* has also been found to influence DNA methylation (Adkins et al. 2011) and is a risk factor for a number of conditions, including schizophrenia and other common mental disorders (Naserbakht et al. 2011; Krishnaswamy et al. 2011), adult non-Hodgkin's lymphoma (Lu et al. 2010), Down's syndrome (De Souza et al. 2009), and common early childhood cancers (Johnson et al. 2009). Evaluation of parental age in Dupuytren's patients might lead to similar insights.

54.3 Cell Biology

54.3.1 Dysregulation

The commonly accepted theory is that Dupuytren's is a problem of dysregulation, loss of homeostasis, loss of normal feedback control of a normal process, a normal biologic process which is very, very slightly out of control. Developing an effective intervention requires finding and understanding the broken point in the control mechanism.

54.3.2 Disease Models

If Dupuytren's represents a slight abnormality in a normal process, what is that process? Zidel has asked:

Does a Dupuytren's contracture serve a useful teleological purpose? One theoretical framing is that Dupuytren's is a wound contracture response gone awry. Support for this includes hemosiderin deposition in Dupuytren tissues as evidence of microtrauma (Larsen et al. 1960) and association of Dupuytren's with local trauma (Connelly 1999) and heavy manual labor (Descatha 2012). However, in the majority of cases, wounding or local trauma is not a definitive part of the history. In this textbook, Meinel (2012) has described a mechanism of contracture as tissues becoming fixed in their resting position by fibrosis rather than active contracture, but this does not explain the origin of the fibrotic process. Also in this textbook, Millesi (2012) reviews evidence to suggest that Dupuytren's is a secondary consequence of abnormal viscoelastic characteristics of the palmar fascia. This leads to another theoretical framing, that Dupuytren's is a dysregulation of the normal process of connective tissue remodeling to normal mechanical stress. Repeated mechanical stress of tendons results in increased tendon stiffness, and aponeurosis structures are intrinsically stiffer than free tendons (Magnusson et al. 2008). Tendon strain results in release of tendon TGF-beta (Yang et al. 2004; Skutek et al. 2001; Kjaer et al. 2006). Strength training in the elderly produces increased tendon stiffness, which may protect active elderly patients from tendon injury (Reeves et al. 2003). Such changes – increase in stiffness – are the same as found by Millesi in the palmar fascia (Millesi 2012). This response is blunted by estrogen (Hansen et al. 2008), which would be consistent with the striking gender differences in the incidence of Dupuytren's in premenopausal women age matched with men. Similarly, gene regulation for structural and regulatory components of tendon is altered by acute resistance exercise, but with gender-related differences (Sullivan et al. 2009). Similar genetic, cytokine, and mechanical responses to strain occur in ligaments (Kim et al. 2002; Nakatani et al. 2002) and are accentuated by abnormally high glucose levels (Li et al. 2008).

It may be fruitful to rethink Dupuytren's along the lines of these normal tissue responses. Although the palmar aponeurosis is embryologically distinct from the palmaris longus tendon, it functions anatomically as an aponeurosis for this tendon, and is tightened by it. Tension from the palmaris longus, small as it is, appears to be a provoking factor: Dupuytren's is less common in hands with congenital absence of the palmaris (Powell et al. 1986); excision of the palmaris reduces early recurrence after fasciectomy for Dupuytren's (Nieminen and Lehto 1986). Beyond this, the palmar fascia is elastic, but only half as elastic as palmar skin (Yamada and Gaynor 1970), and so absorbs the majority of shear forces applied to the palmar skin via the vertical septal fibers. The different disease presentations in the hand and foot may simply reflect differences in mechanical stresses: The plantar fascia has a fixed bony origin and retains a unidirectional orientation; the palmar fascia has a tendinous origin which stretches it to a greater degree, and the palmar fascia folds in flexion. This may be why foot disease usually remains nodular only, while the palm progresses to contracture, which is consistent with Meinel's hypothesis (Meinel 2012). Further understanding of the chemical messengers which regulate normal tissue response to normal mechanical stress may profile a single step in which Dupuytren's tissues differ.

54.3.3 Pinpointing the Problem

Chemical messenger feedback controls can break down in many ways: overproduction, underproduction, lack of sensitivity, abnormal molecules acting independently, and so on. Where can we look for inspiration? There are two recent breakthroughs which may serve as role models for Dupuytren investigation: Imatinib and Anti-TNF drugs.

Imatinib (Gleevec/Glivic) was developed specifically to treat chronic myelogenous leukemia (CML). An abnormal gene found in CML produces an abnormal protein, BCR-Abl. This protein stimulates production of white cells and also blocks DNA repair, eventually causing a lethal blast crisis. Because both the gene and its product are abnormal, there is no normal feedback loop to turn off the production of BCR-Abl. Imatinib was specifically engineered to block the biologically active area of the BCR-Abl molecule, restoring normal cell production regulation. The molecular precision of this intervention results in a powerful desired effect with disproportionately low incidence of side effects.

Although the pathobiology of rheumatoid arthritis (RA) has not been as clearly defined as CML, a similar approach has worked to develop disease-modifying treatments. One of the key factors overproduced in RA and other conditions is tumor necrosis factor-alpha (TNF). The source of TNF is debated, but it is agreed that TNF is responsible for a number of pathologic changes of this disease as well as ankylosing spondylitis, Crohn's disease, psoriasis, and others. Strategies to reduce TNF activity include monoclonal anti-TNF antibodies such as adalimumab (Humira) and engineered proteins such as etanercept (Enbrel) which bind as receptors to TNF.

Imatinib and anti-TNF drugs are models to follow because they provide a precisely focused attack on a single step in underlying pathobiology, not to mask it, not to slow it down, but to stop it. The development of each of these treatment approaches required an enormous amount of work to tease apart and expose a critical component of dysregulation to target, and then develop a means to do so. The same will likely be true for Dupuytren's. We need a similar cocktail of brilliance, persistence, and serendipity. As clinical trials of anti-TGF drugs are performed for more life-threatening diseases (Gambarin et al. 2009; Bournia et al. 2009; Cordeiro 2003), it may be possible to "piggyback" observations on effects of Dupuytren's found incidentally in study participants.

54.3.4 Available Interventions

As our understanding of the biology grows, there are many options to test biologic interventions in clinical studies with available information – top down, rather than bottom up. TGF-beta-1 is clearly a key player in the pathologic biology. In vitro, *tamoxifen* blocks the effect of TGF-beta on Dupuytren myofibroblasts (Kuhn et al. 2002), and Degreef et al. (2012) have shown that perioperative oral tamoxifen improves the results of fasciectomy. Should we be injecting palms with a depot version of Tamoxifen or applying Tamoxifen as a topical hand cream? TGF-beta works by blocking *nitric oxide*–induced myofibroblast dedifferentiation (Hinz et al. 2007). Should we be studying the effect of putting nitropaste on the palms? The metabolic precursor to nitric oxide is *arginine*. Should we do trials of arginine supplementation? *Botox* is not just the botulinium toxin – it also contains C3 transferase exoenzyme, which blocks several steps in the pathway of fibrosis (Witt et al. 2008). Botox is being reported as a treatment for keloid scars and botox has been

shown to reduce contracture, adhesions, and fibrosis after experimental surgical wounds (Lee et al. 2009a; Namazi and Torabi 2007). We should be looking at this and all options to begin clinical trials with available materials.

There is also a growing body of evidence to look more seriously at diet and dietary supplements from viewpoints of both demographics and intervention. Just to scratch the surface, in vivo studies have shown therapeutic effects of TGF-beta-related fibrosis by curcumin (in turmeric) (Punithavathi et al. 2003; Gaedeke et al. 2004), ginsan (in ginseng) (Ahn et al. 2011), fish oil (Peake et al. 2011), flaxseed oil (Lee et al. 2009b), quercetin (flavonoid found in green tea and a number of fruits and vegetables) (Phan et al. 2004), and detrimental effects on TGF-beta-mediated fibrosis by excessive dietary salt (Yu et al. 1998) and dietary cholesterol (Nanji et al. 1997). Looking at this, it is not hard to imagine that some of the demographic or racial differences in the incidence of Dupuytren's might be due to cultural differences in diet, and that this should be further investigated.

54.4 Mechanical Measurements and Procedures

How do we best evaluate Dupuytren's? What is important?

54.4.1 Angles

We can measure angles with a goniometer, but this has the inherent inaccuracy of measuring individual joints in a situation for which multiple joints are affected by a single mechanism. Summarizing the contracture as a composite angle is an imperfect solution, as the mechanics of the metacarpophalangeal (MCP) and proximal interphalangeal (PIP) joints are quite different. Composite angle measurements of the MCP + PIP joints fail to include distal interphalangeal joint involvement, but more importantly do not at all represent the substantial effect of carpometacarpal joint motion, which can alter distal joint measurements by 20–40° in the ring and small fingers (Fig. 54.3). This needs better standardization. One option would be to make measurements of active extension while flattening

Fig. 54.3 Measurement inaccuracy due to carpometacarpal motion. Measurement of active extension of distal joints affected by a shared cord. Each pair shows active extension allowing (*left*) vs. blocking (*right*) CMC flexion. CMC flexion allows hyperextension of the MCP joint with secondary additional flexion of the PIP joint. Blocking the CMC joint in extension increases the measured contracture at the metacarpophalangeal joint and may decrease the proximal interphalangeal joint measurement. (**a**) MCP/PIP measurements: 20H/70 vs. 25/55; (**b**) MCP/PIP Measurements: 15H/55 vs. 75/50. This introduces a large element of error comparing passive vs. active extension, but extends beyond this: Most patients automatically flex the CMC joint with active composite extension; some, paradoxically, do just the opposite. We need a more consistent measurement system

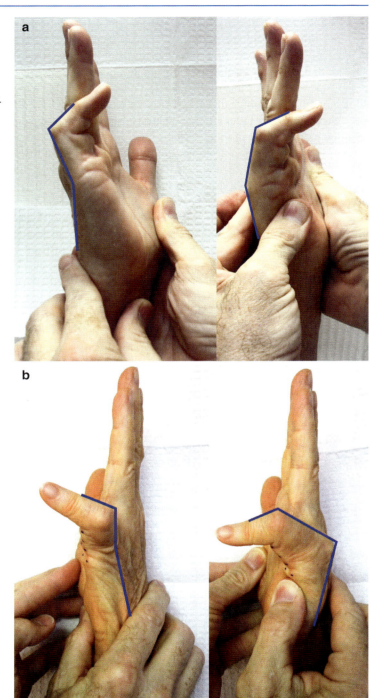

the transverse palmar arch with the patient's palm held against a flat surface extending up to the distal palmar crease. Standardization is also lacking in the choice between measurements expressed as either total extension deficit (which includes MCP hyperextension as a negative value) or composite contracture (which does not). We need better standardization of angle measurements.

Fig. 54.4 Skin involvement as an index of biologic aggressiveness. Skin involvement is an index of biologic aggressiveness which is not easily quantified. (**a**) Hypothenar skin involvement with pitting, papillary ridge prominence, erythema, and wrist crease involvement. (**b**) Close-up of highlighted area in figure a. (**c**) Thumb nodule with papillary ridge prominence and nodule erythema. These are all indicators of aggressive disease. How can this finding be quantified? How should this affect treatment recommendations?

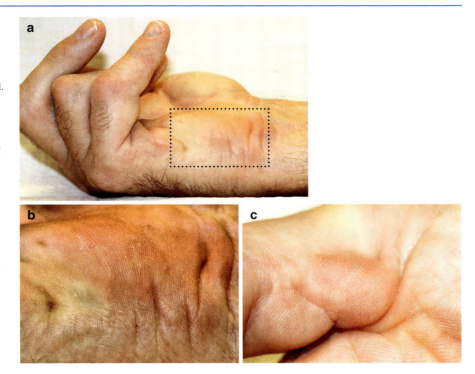

54.4.2 Skin Involvement

The skin is both a predictor and a problem in patients with aggressive Dupuytren's disease (Hueston 1985). The extent of skin involvement can be described qualitatively in terms of dermal firmness, papillary ridge prominence, pits, dimples, erythema (Fig. 54.4), and loss of transverse shear mobility.

These descriptions are difficult to quantify. Skin involvement presents a problem for fasciectomy, as the normal subdermal plane is obliterated, and also for fasciotomy, as the affected skin loses elasticity and does not unfurl. More importantly, the lack of an objective measurement is a hindrance to developing a reproducible assessment of the relationship of skin involvement to disease severity and treatment outcome. One available option to quantify hardness of nodules is an industrial durometer (Fig. 54.5) or ophthalmic surface contact tonometer (Falanga and Bucalo 1993; Thurston 1987). This objective measurement could be used for documentation of the effectiveness of biologic intervention.

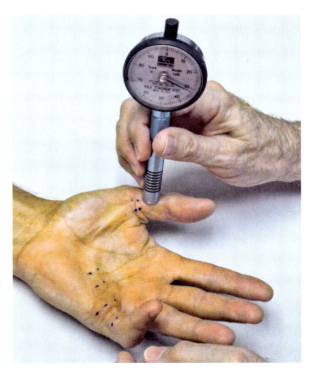

Fig. 54.5 Quantifying Dupuytren nodule firmness with a commercially available durometer

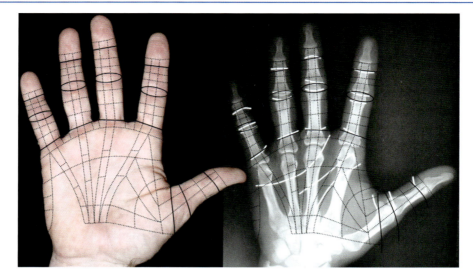

Fig. 54.6 Documentation grid for Dupuytren's based on skin crease landmarks and common areas of involvement. This also correlates with the underlying skeletal structures. This system is based on skin crease landmarks and common patterns of involvement by Dupuytren's, and is applicable to the documentation of both findings and interventions. A modified version of this, developed by Eaton and Wach, allows documentation of both soft tissue notes and range of motion measurements in the same area (Fig. 54.7). A web page version of this type of diagram could be used for quick graphical data entry of findings and procedures into a centralized online database

Fig. 54.7 Summary grid allowing documentation of palmar findings and range of motion measurements in a single diagram

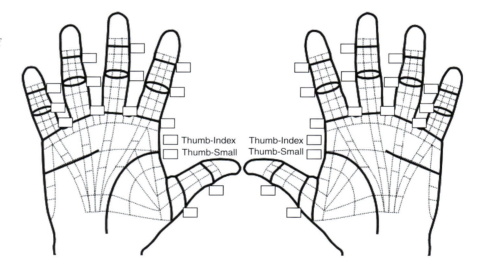

54.4.3 Anatomic Mapping

Another murky area of documentation is the exact location of the findings of cords, nodules, scars, and of the intervention of injections, incisions, or radiation. Without a standard naming system for locations, there cannot be a true investigation into the relevance of the exact location of involvement, either for staging or for evaluating the results of treatment. One attempt to address this problem is a grid system developed for documentation of needle aponeurotomy (Fig. 54.6).

54.4.4 Imaging

54.4.4.1 Doppler Tones/Doppler Imaging

Current ability to preoperatively identify normal structures and mechanically important cords is crude. The

54 The Future of Dupuytren's Research and Treatment

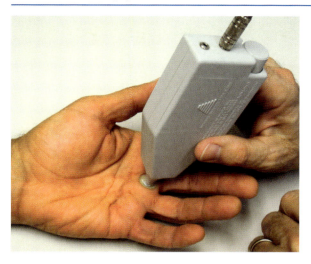

Fig. 54.8 Handheld Doppler assessment of suspected spiral cord using an 8-MHz Doppler

unpredictable anatomic changes involving neurovascular bundles remain a stumbling block for surgical approaches, and particularly for minimally invasive techniques. An 8-MHz Doppler tone assessment may be used to identify superficially displaced neurovascular bundles when Dupuytren cords lie beneath soft fleshy prominences (Fig. 54.8), but false-negatives are possible. Doppler imaging is a promising improvement (Fig. 54.9), but higher resolution imaging technology is needed.

54.4.4.2 MRI/MRA

MR assessment of Dupuytren's is hindered by the resolution of current equipment, orientation issues due to multiplanar deformities of the fingers, and lack of intraoperative availability. MRI is probably most useful in identifying additional pathology such as flexor tendon

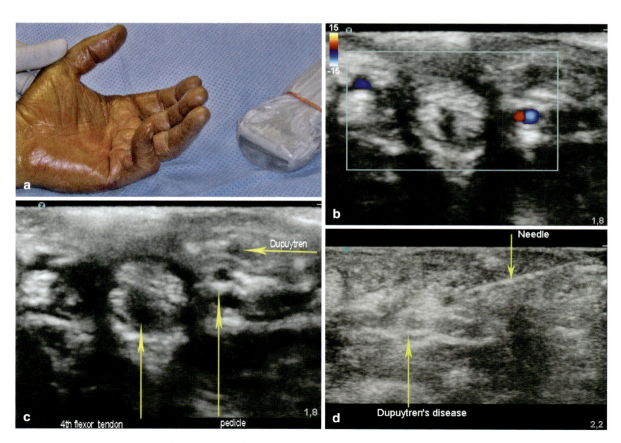

Fig. 54.9 Ultrasound imaging palmar structures during needle aponeurotomy. (**a**) Hand and Ultrasonic probe. (**b**) Doppler visualization of vascular flow in palmar digital arteries. (**c**) Visualization of tendon, pedicle, cord. (**d**) Visualization of Dupuytren cord and aponeurotomy needle within the tissues (cases of Somesh D Beeharry MD, Head of Department Hand Surgery, Hopital A Schweitzer, 68,000 Colmar, FR)

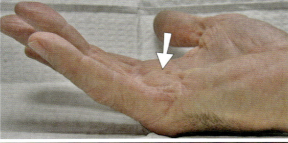
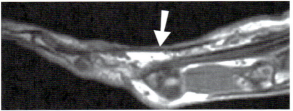

Fig. 54.10 MRI of a palmar Dupuytren's cord (*arrow*). Although clearly seen here, this is the exception rather than the rule

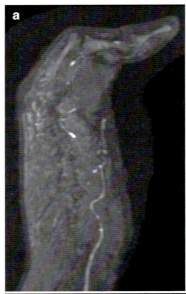
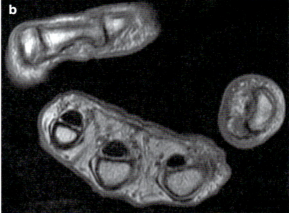

Fig. 54.11 MRA of small finger involvement. (**a**) Digital vessels are difficult to visualize in Dupuytren's, even in this 3D MRA reconstruction. (**b**) Difficulty orienting the proper imaging direction due to multiplanar contractures (case of Dr. Andrew Nelson, Hand Center of Waterbury, Waterbury, CT)

bowstringing (Figs. 54.10–54.12). MRI may be helpful in providing a quantitative noninvasive measure of cellularity of affected areas, which is an index of biologic activity (Yacoe et al. 1993), but this potential staging tool has not been investigated yet on a large scale.

54.5 Questions and Unsolved Problems

When a biologic intervention for Dupuytren's is developed, the need for mechanical treatment will be reduced, but not eliminated. Many questions remain unanswered regarding clinical management:

- What are the relative indications for any specific treatment? When is it most appropriate to perform radiotherapy, enzymatic fasciotomy, needle fasciotomy, open fasciotomy, segmental fasciectomy, wide fasciectomy, or dermofasciectomy and grafting?
- What are the relative indications for skin graft, skin flap, engineered skin substitute, and barrier technologies such as methylcellulose (Degreef and de Smet 2012) or fat graft (Khouri 2010)?
- What is the best treatment from the patient's perspective (Wach 2012)?
- What is the best definition of recurrence? Should this include combined evaluation of angle measurements and tissue firmness measurements?
- What is the best assessment of functional effects of Dupuytren's?
- What are the best options to prevent or treat secondary tendon issues (Fig. 54.13)?
- What are the best options for patients with concomitant diseases (Fig. 54.14)?
- How best to avoid postoperative stiffness (Fig. 54.15)?
- What is the best time to intervene? On which patients?
- What is the optimum management of biologically aggressive Dupuytren's (Fig. 54.16)?
- What is a sensible decision tree for the treatment of recurrent disease?
- What is the role of radiotherapy in early disease or for early recurrence after surgical intervention?

54 The Future of Dupuytren's Research and Treatment

Fig. 54.12 MRI identification of issues complicating Dupuytren's management. (**a**) Recurrent small finger contracture after two fasciectomies shows bowstringing of the flexor tendon. (**b**) Disuse atrophy and hypovascular hypothenar musculature secondary to chronic small finger flexion contracture

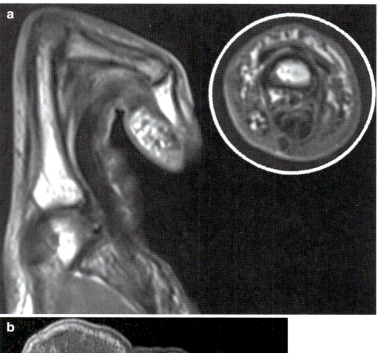
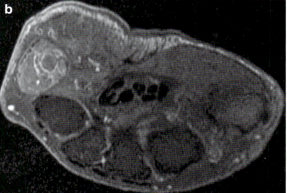

- What is the role of external fixation devices for fixed contracture?
- What is the role of splinting, with or without a procedure?
- What is the role of manual therapy?
- What is the best advice for patients with Dupuytren's regarding occupation, physical activities (handball, racquetball, tennis, golf, gardening, motorcycle, yoga, rowing, fishing, pushups, weight training), hand massage, stretching exercises?
- What determines the location of primary involvement?
- What is the best global treatment algorithm including all choices of intervention, taking into consideration local involvement, systemic factors, and response to prior treatment?
- What do we have to do to find a cure?

54.6 International Task Force

54.6.1 Goals

What do we do from here? We need to organize and carry out large-scale global collaborative studies aimed at developing better treatment options for Dupuytren's and related conditions. How do we make this happen?

It is worth repeating: Dupuytren's is not a surgical disease – it is a medical condition in need of a medicine. We need to all get on the same page. We need to input data into a global registry. The variability and unpredictability of Dupuytren's means that large numbers of patients, very large data sets will be needed to generate meaningful insights, regardless of whether the research is looking at

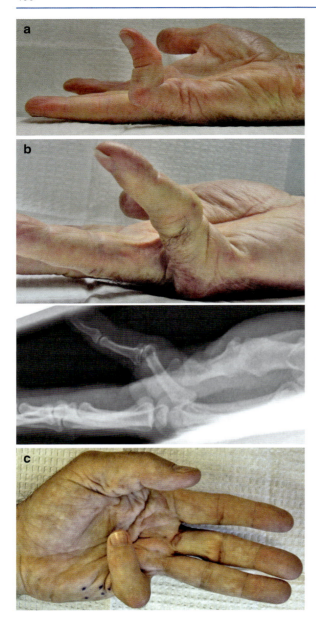

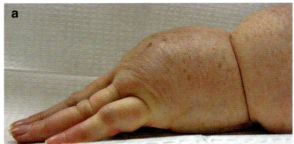

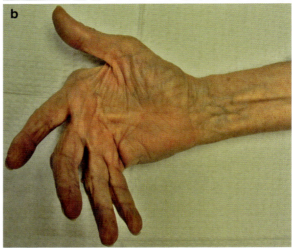

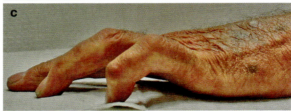

Fig. 54.13 Questions and problems: tendon issues secondary to chronic Dupuytren contractures. Once established, these become persistent forces which lead to recurrent deformity despite correction of the primary Dupuytren contracture. They require surgical reconstruction in addition to intervention for the Dupuytren's contracture. Dupuytren's with secondary (**a**) Boutonniere, (**b**) Proximal interphalangeal joint volar plate insufficiency with locking hyperextension and secondary joint changes (**c**) Radial sagittal band rupture. How can these issues be avoided, and what is the best approach when they have developed?

Fig. 54.14 Dupuytren's complicating and being complicated by additional conditions. (**a**) Dupuytren's and lymphedema. (**b**) Dupuytren's and rheumatoid arthritis. (**c**) Dupuytren's and claw posture from ulnar nerve palsy. What is the best approach for each of these situations? What is the best approach for the more common combination of Dupuytren's and trigger finger affecting the same digit (Kuehlein 2012)?

Single studies can be completely misleading, despite apparent statistical rigor (Lehrer 2010). This is a daunting task.

Fortunately, four things are in our favor:
- Dupuytren's is common. Large numbers are out there, waiting to be collected and analyzed.
- The power and availability of automated large-scale data analysis is greater than it has ever been.
- Patients with Dupuytren's are interested in giving their time to help the effort to develop better treatment options, and are increasingly organized online

genetic, demographic, cellular, or clinical data. The immensely complex nature of biologic systems strains the limits of conventional statistical analysis:

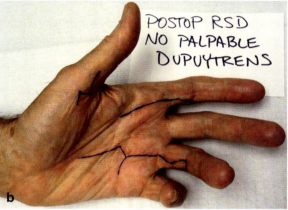

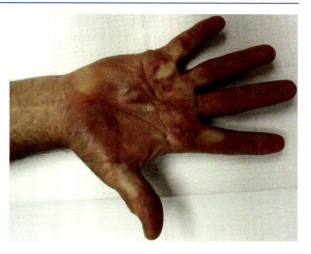

Fig. 54.15 Tissue reaction after fasciectomy for Dupuytren's contracture. (**a**) proximal interphalangeal joint contracture after fasciectomy with no residual palpable cords. (**b**) Contractures of operated and un-operated digits developing during postoperative inflammatory period after fasciectomy. Postoperative stiffness remains an occasional, unpredictable, and unsolved issue after fasciectomy. How can this change?

Fig. 54.16 Biologically high-risk Dupuytren's. This young patient has early onset bilateral disease, Ledderhose, diffuse nodular palmar involvement with tight skin, itching, tender nodules, and vasomotor instability with red, cold, sweaty palms. He has a high chance of aggressive, treatment-resistant disease and inflammatory complications after fasciectomy. He needs a disease-modifying treatment, not a procedure. What needs to be done to find a cure, an intervention at this stage to prevent the inevitable development of contractures in this patient?

(Wach 2012). Patients are a great resource to share their professional skills of marketing, programming, fund raising, and other aspects of the group effort.
- The Internet and web-enabled database technology allows the development of online data entry and analysis. This will be the key to data standardization and collection (Eaton et al. 2012).

54.6.2 Guidelines for Clinical Registries

The use, methods, and usefulness of clinical registries have grown with the availability of online collaboration. Meticulous preparatory attention to detail is the prerequisite to good quality data. Guidelines for effective clinical registries have been suggested by Alpert (2000):

1. Standardized disease definitions should be employed and stated clearly in the methods sections. All participants in the data collection should be completely familiar with these disease definitions.
2. Sampling techniques should also be standardized and followed with great care.
3. Randomized selection of hospitals or clinics is strongly encouraged. Community-wide data collection is even better.
4. All participants should have a clear understanding of the information being sought for each entry on the data sheet.
5. All collected data should be reported. Selection or exclusion of some centers or some data forms increases bias.
6. All original data sheets or electronic submissions should be centralized. Analysis should be performed by a central data collection and analysis center.
7. A professional statistician should monitor the data collection and analysis.
8. Each data sheet or electronic submission should be carefully examined by the central data center to ascertain completeness and accuracy. Individual investigators should be promptly queried concerning incomplete or confusing responses.

9. The registry protocol should be reviewed at each participating center by an institutional review board for studies involving human subjects. Appropriate consent for participation must be obtained.
10. The names of all participating investigators should appear in the published report of the registry.
11. Sponsorship for the trial should be clearly stated in all published reports so that commercial bias can be easily identified.
12. One principal investigator or a small steering committee should be designated to maintain administrative order, adjudicate disagreements, and encourage timely submission of documents and data analysis.

54.6.3 Outline for Global Collaboration

What is the next step? We need to establish a central online framework to foster communication and project development, which fits well with available web technology:

- Establish a web site to function as a central organizing location. The domain names Dupuytrens.org and DupGroup.com have been reserved for this purpose.
- The web site should have secure access to allow
  - Membership Directory
  - Patient resources and opportunities to collaborate
  - Literature Repository
  - Secure Data Collection for Clinical Registry Projects
    - Research Organization Section
    - Research project topic requests
    - Project proposals
  - Goals
  - Lead Investigators/Participant requirements/ Sign up
  - Budget/Funding requirements/Resources
  - Timeline
    - Ongoing projects: progress
    - Completed Projects
  - Discussion Forums
- Long-term funding resources for the core infrastructure (minor) and research funding (major)

Tools for creating and maintaining a project of this nature are well established and affordable. We need to develop an interdisciplinary study concept for integration of all available treatment modalities in a stepwise approach. The initial manpower and direction for this project have been through the Dupuytren Society http://www.dupuytren-online.info and the Dupuytren Foundation http://DupuytrenFoundation.org. All that is needed now is for you to join the effort.

Acknowledgments This chapter and this book would not exist without the sustained efforts of patients with Dupuytren's, looking for better options and working to get their physicians to listen to them.

References

Abe Y, Rokkaku T, Ofuchi S, Tokunaga S, Takahashi K, Moriya H (2004) An objective method to evaluate the risk of recurrence and extension of Dupuytren's disease. J Hand Surg 29B(5):427–30

Adkins RM, Thomas F, Tylavsky FA, Krushkal J (2011) Parental ages and levels of DNA methylation in the newborn are correlated. BMC Med Genet 12:47

Ahn JY, Kim MH, Lim MJ, Park S, Lee SL, Yun YS, Song JY (2011) The inhibitory effect of ginsan on TGF-ß mediated fibrotic process. J Cell Physiol 226(5):1241–1247

Alpert JS (2000) Are data from clinical registries of any value? Eur Heart J 21(17):1399–1401

Bournia VK, Vlachoyiannopoulos PG, Selmi C, Moutsopoulos HM, Gershwin ME (2009) Recent advances in the treatment of systemic sclerosis. Clin Rev Allergy Immunol 36(2–3): 176–200

Connelly TJ (1999) Development of Peyronie's and Dupuytren's diseases in an individual after single episodes of trauma: a case report and review of the literature. J Am Acad Dermatol 41:106–108

Cordeiro MF (2003) Technology evaluation: lerdelimumab, Cambridge Antibody Technology. Curr Opin Mol Ther 5(2): 199–203

De Souza E, Alberman E, Morris JK (2009) Down syndrome and paternal age, a new analysis of case-control data collected in the 1960s. Am J Med Genet A 149(6):1205–1208

Degreef I, de Smet L (2011) Risk factors in Dupuytren's diathesis: is recurrence after surgery predictable? Acta Orthop Belg 77:27–32

Degreef I, de Smet L (2012) Cellulose implants in Dupuytren's surgery. In: Dupuytren's disease and related hyperproliferative disorders, pp 207–211

Degreef I, Tejpar S, de Smet L (2012) Highly-dosed Tamoxifen in therapy resisting Dupuytren's disease. In: Dupuytren's disease and related hyperproliferative disorders, pp 379–386

Descatha A (2012) Dupuytren's disease and occupation. In: Dupuytren's disease and related hyperproliferative disorders, pp 45–49

Eaton Ch, Seegenschmiedt MH, Wach W (2012) IDUP – proposal for an International Research Database. In Dupuytren's disease and related hyperproliferative disorders, pp 449–454

Falanga V, Bucalo B (1993) Use of a durometer to assess skin hardness. J Am Acad Dermatol 29(1):47–51

Gaedeke J, Noble NA, Border WA (2004) Curcumin blocks multiple sites of the TGF-beta signaling cascade in renal cells. Kidney Int 66(1):112–120

Gambarin FI, Favalli V, Serio A, Regazzi M, Pasotti M, Klersy C, Dore R, Mannarino S, Viganò M, Odero A, Amato S, Tavazzi L, Arbustini E (2009) Rationale and design of a trial evaluating the effects of losartan vs. nebivolol vs. the association of both on the progression of aortic root dilation in Marfan syndrome with FBN1 gene mutations. J Cardiovasc Med (Hagerstown) 10(4):354–362

Hansen M, Koskinen SO, Petersen SG, Doessing S, Frystyk J, Flyvbjerg A, Westh E, Magnusson SP, Kjaer M, Langberg H (2008) Ethinyl oestradiol administration in women suppresses synthesis of collagen in tendon in response to exercise. J Physiol 586:3005–3016

Hindocha S, Stanley JK, Watson S, Bayat A (2006) Dupuytren's diathesis revisited: Evaluation of prognostic indicators for risk of disease recurrence. J Hand Surg 31A(10):1626–34

Hinz B, Phan SH, Thannickal VJ, Galli A, Bochaton-Piallat ML, Gabbiani G (2007) The myofibroblast: one function, multiple origins. Am J Pathol 170(6):1807–1816

Hueston J (1985) The role of the skin in Dupuytren's disease. Ann Royal Coll Surg Engl 67:372–375

Johnson KJ, Carozza SE, Chow EJ, Fox EE, Horel S, McLaughlin CC, Mueller BA, Puumala SE, Reynolds P, Von Behren J, Spector LG (2009) Parental age and risk of childhood cancer: a pooled analysis Epidemiology 20(4):475–483

Kahn HS, Morgan TM, Case LD, Dabelea D, Mayer-Davis EJ, Lawrence JM, Marcovina SM, Imperatore G (2009) Association of type 1 diabetes with month of birth among U.S. youth: The SEARCH for Diabetes in Youth Study. Diabetes Care 32(11) 2010–2015

Kemkes A (2010) The impact of maternal birth month on reproductive performance: controlling for socio-demographic confounders. J Biosoc Sci 42(2):177–194

Khouri R (2010) Extensive percutaneous aponeurotomy and lipografting: a new treatment alternative for Dupuytren's disease. 2010 Miami Dupuytren Symposium http://www.youtube.com/DupuytrenFoundation#p/u/0/fmWiC5V76YI. Accessed Jan 2, 2011

Kim SG, Akaike T, Sasagawa T, Atomi Y, Kurosawa H (2002) Gene expression of type I and type III collagen by mechanical stretch in anterior cruciate ligament cells. Cell Struct Funct 27:139–144

Kinney DK, Levy DL, Yurgelun-Todd DA, Lajonchere CM, Holzman PS (1999) Eye-tracking dysfunction and birth-month weather in schizophrenia. J Abnorm Psychol 108(2):359–362

Kjaer M, Magnusson P, Krogsgaard M, Boysen Møller J, Olesen J, Heinemeier K, Hansen M, Haraldsson B, Koskinen S, Esmarck B, Langberg H (2006) Extracellular matrix adaptation of tendon and skeletal muscle to exercise. J Anat 208:445–450

Krishnaswamy S, Subramaniam K, Ramachandran P, Indran T, Abdul Aziz J (2011) Delayed fathering and risk of mental disorders in adult offspring. Early Hum Dev 87(3):171–175

Kuehlein B (2012) The influence of Dupuytren's disease on trigger fingers and vice versa. In: Dupuytren's disease and related hyperproliferative disorders, pp 249–253

Kuhn MA, Wang X, Payne WG, Ko F, Robson MC (2002) Tamoxifen decreases fibroblast function and downregulates TGF(beta2) in Dupuytren's affected palmar fascia. J Surg Res 103(2):146–152

Larsen RD, Takagishi N, Posch JL (1960) The pathogenesis of Dupuytren's contracture experimental and further clinical observations. J Bone Joint Surg [Am] 42A:993–1007

Lee BJ, Jeong JH, Wang SG, Lee JC, Goh EK, Kim HW (2009a) Effect of botulinum toxin type a on a rat surgical wound model. Clin Exp Otorhinolaryngol 2(1):20–27

Lee JC, Krochak R, Blouin A, Kanterakis S, Chatterjee S, Arguiri E, Vachani A, Solomides CC, Cengel KA, Christofidou-Solomidou M (2009b) Dietary flaxseed prevents radiation-induced oxidative lung damage, inflammation and fibrosis in a mouse model of thoracic radiation injury. Cancer Biol Ther 8(1):47–53

Lehrer J (2010) The Truth Wears Off: Is there something wrong with the scientific method? New Yorker, December 13, 2010. http://www.newyorker.com/reporting/2010/12/13/101213fa_fact_lehrer#ixzz1MM1hgQ3u. Accessed Jan 2, 2011

Lewy H, Meirson H, Laron Z (2009) Seasonality of birth month of children with celiac disease differs from that in the general population and between sexes and is linked to family history and environmental factors. J Pediatr Gastroenterol Nutr 48(2):181–185

Li H, Liu D, Zhao CQ, Jiang LS, Dai LY (2008) High glucose promotes collagen synthesis by cultured cells from rat cervical posterior longitudinal ligament via transforming growth factor-beta1. Eur Spine J 17:873–881

Lu Y, Ma H, Sullivan-Halley J, Henderson KD, Chang ET, Clarke CA, Neuhausen SL, West DW, Bernstein L, Wang SS (2010) Parents' ages at birth and risk of adult-onset hematologic malignancies among female teachers in California. Am J Epidemiol 171(12):1262–1269

Magnusson SP, Narici MV, Maganaris CN, Kjaer M (2008) Human tendon behaviour and adaptation, in vivo. J Physiol 586(1):71–81

Mandel Y, Grotto I, El-Yaniv R, Belkin M, Israeli E, Polat U, Bartov E (2008) Season of birth, natural light, and myopia. Ophthalmology 115(4):686–692

Meinel A (2012) Palmar fibromatosis or the loss of flexibility of the palmar finger tissue. A new insight into the disease process of Dupuytren contracture. In: Dupuytren's disease and related hyperproliferative disorders, pp 11–20

Millesi H (2012) Basic thoughts on Dupuytren's contracture. In: Dupuytren's disease and related hyperproliferative disorders, pp 21–26

Nakatani T, Marui T, Hitora T, Doita M, Nishida K, Kurosaka M (2002) Mechanical stretching force promotes collagen synthesis by cultured cells from human ligamentum flavum via transforming growth factor-beta1. J Orthop Res 20(6):1380–1386

Namazi H, Torabi S (2007) Novel use of botulinum toxin to ameliorate arthrofibrosis: an experimental study in rabbits. Toxicol Pathol 35(5):715–718

Nanji AA, Rahemtulla A, Daly T, Khwaja S, Miao L, Zhao S, Tahan SR (1997) Cholesterol supplementation prevents necrosis and inflammation but enhances fibrosis in alcoholic liver disease in the rat. Hepatology 26(1):90–97

Naserbakht M, Ahmadkhaniha HR, Mokri B, Smith CL (2011) Advanced paternal age is a risk factor for schizophrenia in Iranians. Ann Gen Psychiatry 10(1):15

Nieminen S, Lehto M (1986) Resection of the palmaris longus tendon in surgery for Dupuytren's contracture. Ann Chir Gynaecol 75:164–167

Peake JM, Gobe GC, Fassett RG, Coombes JS (2011) The effects of dietary fish oil on inflammation, fibrosis and oxidative stress associated with obstructive renal injury in rats. Mol Nutr Food Res 55(3):400–410

Phan TT, Lim IJ, Chan SY, Tan EK, Lee ST, Longaker MT (2004) Suppression of transforming growth factor beta/smad signaling in keloid-derived fibroblasts by quercetin: implications for the treatment of excessive scars. J Trauma 57(5):1032–1037

Powell BWEM, McLean NR, Jeffs VJ (1986) The incidence of a palmaris longus tendon in patients with Dupuytren's disease. J Hand Surg [Br] 11B:382–384

Punithavathi D, Venkatesan N, Babu M (2003) Protective effects of curcumin against amiodarone-induced pulmonary fibrosis in rats. Br J Pharmacol 139(7):1342–1350

Reeves ND, Maganaris CN, Narici MV (2003) Effect of strength training on human patella tendon mechanical properties of older individuals. J Physiol 548:971–981

Riala K, Hakko H, Taanila A, Räsänen P (2009) Season of birth and smoking: findings from the Northern Finland 1966 Birth Cohort. Chronobiol Int 26(8):1660–1672

Skutek M, van Griensven M, Zeichen J, Brauer N, Bosch U (2001) Cyclic mechanical stretching modulates secretion pattern of growth factors in human tendon fibroblasts. Eur J Appl Physiol 86(1):48–52

Staples J, Ponsonby AL, Lim L (2010) Low maternal exposure to ultraviolet radiation in pregnancy, month of birth, and risk of multiple sclerosis in offspring: longitudinal analysis. BMJ 340:c1640

Sullivan BE, Carroll CC, Jemiolo B, Trappe SW, Magnusson SP, Døssing S, Kjaer M, Trappe TA (2009) Effect of acute resistance exercise and sex on human patellar tendon structural and regulatory mRNA expression. J Appl Physiol 106:468–475

Thurston AJ (1987) Conservative surgery for Dupuytren's contracture. J Hand Surg [Br] 12(B):329–334

Vaiserman AM, Voitenko VP (2003) Early programming of adult longevity: demographic and experimental studies. J Anti Aging Med 6(1):11–20

Wach W (2012) The patient's perspective and the International Dupuytren Society. In: Dupuytren's disease and related hyperproliferative disorders, pp 441–447

Witt E, Maliri A, McGrouther DA, Bayat A (2008) RAC activity in keloid disease: comparative analysis of fibroblasts from margin of keloid to its surrounding normal skin. Eplasty 8(8):e19

Yacoe ME, Bergman AG, Ladd AL, Hellman BH (1993) Dupuytren's contracture: MR imaging findings and correlation between MR signal intensity and cellularity of lesions. AJR Am J Roentgenol 160(4):813–817

Yamada H, Gaynor F (1970) Strength of biological materials. The Williams & Wilkins Company, Baltimore, pp 104–225

Yang G, Crawford RC, Wang JH (2004) Proliferation and collagen production of human patellar tendon fibroblasts in response to cyclic uniaxial stretching in serum-free conditions. J Biomech 37(10):1543–1550

Yu HC, Burrell LM, Black MJ, Wu LL, Dilley RJ, Cooper ME, Johnston CI (1998) Salt induces myocardial and renal fibrosis in normotensive and hypertensive rats. Circulation 98(23):2621–2628

Zerbo O, Iosif AM, Delwiche L, Walker C, Hertz-Picciotto I (2011) Month of conception and risk of autism. Epidemiology 22(4):469–475

Index

A

Accessory collateral ligaments (ACL), 216, 244, 246, 298–299
ACL *See* Accessory collateral ligaments
Affymetrix microarray, 110, 111, 162, 163
Anatomy, 3–10, 15–18, 22, 106–107, 169–171, 177, 190, 197, 198, 200, 202, 204, 245, 251, 252, 261–263, 268–269, 272, 292, 298, 306, 458, 462–463
Angiogenesis, 70, 395
Animal model, 62, 81, 101–107, 176–178, 188, 397, 455
Antiproliferative activity, 387–391
Apligraf®, 373–377
Aponeurotomy, 39–40, 256, 267–279, 281, 289–292, 382, 443, 462, 463
Association study, 88, 90, 94, 96, 116
Athymic rat model, 102–103, 177, 181

B

Barrier, 177, 207–210, 376, 377, 464
Benign disease, 96, 115, 121, 161, 167, 360, 364, 419, 421, 423
Bioengineered, 373–377
Bosnia, 123–127, 350
Boyer, B.A., 200–202
Burn scar, 77–82, 180, 214

C

Cadaveric, 197, 202, 261–263
Calcium, 54–55, 80, 168, 404, 431, 433
Causation, 46–48, 77, 93, 95–96, 298, 456
Cell-cell interaction, 69–74, 95, 158
Cell growth, 70, 71, 73–74, 98, 112, 180, 388–391
Cell-matrix interactions, 95, 132
Cell migration, 63, 109, 136, 144, 152–156, 158, 172, 377
Cellulose implant, 207–211
Central slip attenuation (CSA), 244, 246, 247, 299, 306
Cline, H. Sr., 39, 46, 195–204, 281, 289, 293
Collagen, 5, 22, 40, 53, 62, 69, 78, 98, 101, 131, 143, 152, 161, 168, 176, 187, 218, 300, 307, 343, 351, 373, 379, 394, 401, 411, 430, 445
Collagenase, 33, 37, 40, 80, 99, 102, 135–139, 144, 148, 155, 168, 176, 219, 300, 323, 343–346, 351, 377, 396–397, 404–405, 431, 433, 443–444, 450
Collagen fibrillogenesis, 135
Compliance, 56, 102–103, 299, 314, 335, 358

Connective tissue, 11–12, 16–19, 22–24, 32, 53, 54, 57, 109, 132, 133, 333–334, 349, 350, 360, 377, 393, 395, 401, 421, 429, 445, 458
Contraction, 11, 16–20, 53–58, 61, 69–71, 74, 78, 81, 109, 111, 138, 143–148, 161–165, 176–180, 189, 191, 199, 210, 219, 227, 228, 232, 233, 243, 289, 297, 333, 360, 373, 374, 380, 394, 411
Contracture
  release, 214, 228, 235, 269, 298–299, 301, 323, 324, 331, 333–339
  severity, 40, 77, 256, 317–321, 324, 330, 344–346, 374
Controlled clinical trial, 181, 344–346, 351, 377, 432
Cooperation, 334–335, 351, 364, 423, 445
Cooper, Sir Astley, 46, 198–199, 349–350
Cost, 27–34, 339, 431, 435, 444
Crisscrossing peritendinous fibers, 14, 15
Croat, 123–126
Cryosurgery, 80, 404–407
Cryotherapy, 401–407
CSA *See* Central slip attenuation
Cytostatic drugs, 387

D

DC *See* Dupuytren's contracture
DCP *See* Dorsal cutaneous pads
DDN *See* Dorsal Dupuytren's nodules
Dermofasciectomy, 28–30, 32, 33, 37, 39, 41, 99, 172, 190–191, 215–219, 233, 236, 239–240, 306, 309, 318, 323–331, 374, 376, 444, 464
Diabetes, 9, 32, 35, 81, 88, 90, 109, 116, 119, 123–127, 223, 229–230, 239, 249, 308, 343–344, 350, 353, 356, 404, 409, 412, 413, 456–457
Differentiation assay, 168, 171
Digital fasciectomy, 18, 19, 245, 297
Digit Widget™, 81, 297, 301–303
Disabilities of the Arm, Shoulder and Hand (DASH), correlation with flexion contracture, 318–320
Disease progression, 8–9, 27, 33, 37, 55–56, 101–102, 106, 107, 109, 151–158, 165, 219, 252, 350, 351, 354, 358–360, 364, 373, 394, 396, 411, 416, 420–421, 432, 443, 456
Distraction, 299–303
Dominance of flexed fingers, 16, 20
Dorsal cutaneous pads (DCP), 7–8
Dorsal Dupuytren's nodules (DDN), 7–9

C. Eaton et al. (eds.), *Dupuytren's Disease and Related Hyperproliferative Disorders*,
DOI 10.1007/978-3-642-22697-7, © Springer-Verlag Berlin Heidelberg 2012

Dupuytren Award, 445, 446
Dupuytren, G., 45, 77, 197, 200–201, 281, 349–350, 373
Dupuytren Foundation, 445, 454, 468
Dupuytren Society, 351, 404, 441–446, 453, 454, 468
Dupuytren surgery, 204, 207–211, 261–263, 318, 373–377, 443
Dupuytren Symposium, 81–82, 445
Dynamic external fixation, 297–303

E

ECM *See* Extracellular matrix
EMT *See* Epithelial-mesenchymal transition
Epidemiology, 7, 10, 28, 32, 33, 46, 88–90, 123–127, 429, 445
Epigenetic regulation, 65
Epithelial cells, 61–62, 65
Epithelial-mesenchymal transition (EMT), 54, 62, 63
Extension block, 11, 16, 20, 309, 334
Extracellular matrix (ECM), 54–57, 61, 70, 73, 79, 95, 98,
    101–102, 107, 111–112, 131–134, 136, 138, 140, 144,
    147, 151–154, 158, 162, 172, 187, 360, 377, 394–396, 433

F

FACS *See* Fluorescence activated cell sorting
Familial, 29, 35, 88–90, 94, 115–122, 144
Fasciotomy/Fasciectomy, 18, 27–31, 33, 36–41, 197, 199–202,
    204, 208, 227, 235, 256, 257, 267–269, 271, 276, 279,
    281–287, 289, 290, 293–295, 297, 309, 312–313, 323,
    333–339, 344, 351, 373, 443, 461, 464
FC *See* Flexion contracture
Fibroblast-populated collagen lattice (FPCL), 144–148,
    152–156, 162–164, 176–181
Fibroblasts, 56, 62, 103–106, 136, 138–140, 143–148,
    162, 176–177, 352, 396, 401–402, 404
Fibrocytes, 352, 402
Fibrosis, 71–74, 101–107, 210
Fibrosis diathesis, 207–210, 258, 259, 380
Firebreak, 208
Flaps, 178, 227–233, 235–242
Flexion contracture
    correlation with DASH, 318–320
    pre-operative, 214, 298–299, 303
Flexion contracture (FC), 6, 101, 124, 200, 214, 227, 229,
    231, 233, 243, 245, 247, 290, 294, 295, 297–303,
    307, 318–320, 330, 343, 465
Fluorescence activated cell sorting (FACS), 168–172
Foot, 9, 17, 24–26, 36, 196, 354, 374, 401, 403, 405,
    410–417, 422, 423, 429, 458
FPCL *See* Fibroblast-populated collagen lattice
FTSG *See* Full thickness skin graft
Full thickness skin graft (FTSG), 151, 190–192, 213–219,
    228, 229, 232, 233, 235, 236, 239–240, 256, 257,
    259, 260, 286, 323
Future of Dupuytren's research, 455–468

G

Garrod's pad, 36, 121, 252
Garrod's disease, 7, 353, 356, 409, 412, 413
Gene expression, 63–65, 80, 97–98, 101–104, 106, 107, 110,
    111, 134, 138, 145–148, 158, 161, 162

Genes, 21, 63–65, 87, 88, 90, 93–99, 101–107, 109–112,
    115–117, 122, 131–134, 137, 139, 140, 144, 145,
    147–148, 154, 158, 164, 165, 181, 360, 395, 402,
    455–456, 458
Genetics, 9, 21, 35, 48, 80, 81, 87–90, 93–99, 109, 115–117,
    121, 122, 131, 144, 204, 289, 380, 385, 409, 413, 429,
    430, 443, 455–458, 466
Genetic study, 95, 98–99, 115–122
Genetic susceptibility, 90, 98
Gene transcription, 63–65, 90, 96, 140, 165
Genomics, 445, 450
Glove splint, 334–337

H

Hand therapy, 33, 36, 216, 229, 282, 305–314, 318, 324–326,
    328, 331, 375
Healing, 22, 38–39, 41, 61, 69–71, 74, 78–82, 131, 133, 136,
    138, 176, 187–191, 193, 201, 204, 207, 221–225, 232,
    233, 236, 238–240, 252, 256, 299, 307, 310–311, 314,
    360, 374, 376, 377, 384, 385, 391, 395, 396, 401, 407,
    416–417, 421, 422, 434, 442, 444, 445
Heritability, 29, 94
Herzegovina, 123, 126
Heterodigital flap, 227–233
Homodigital flap, 228–230, 232, 233
Hydroxyproline, 132, 135, 145, 146, 148
Hypertrophic, 17, 18, 58, 64–65, 69–74, 78–81, 132, 175,
    179–181, 188–190, 193, 306–308, 311, 314, 353, 364,
    401, 412, 413, 419, 421

I

IDUP, 449–454
IGFBP-6 *See* Insulin-like growth factor binding protein-6
Implant, 71, 177, 189, 207–211, 395–396
Improving statistics, 283, 416
Improving surgical outcome, 211, 385
Incidence, 21, 28, 32, 33, 35, 38, 46, 89, 94, 115, 121, 144,
    207–208, 217–219, 250, 267, 291, 292, 309, 343–344,
    373, 404, 409, 411, 458, 459
Incision, 19, 23, 38, 45, 110, 188, 191, 192, 201–203, 208–210,
    214, 221–225, 227, 228, 233, 235–237, 239–241, 249,
    251, 252, 259, 261, 282, 285–286, 311, 314, 374–377,
    388, 405, 442, 444, 462
Induratio penis plastica (IPP) *See also* Peyronie's disease, 429
Injectable collagenase, 33, 99, 102, 323, 343–346, 351,
    404–405, 443–444
Insulin-like growth factor binding protein-6 (IGFBP-6), 161–165
International Dupuytren Society, 441–446, 453, 454
Intralesional injections, 433–435
In vitro, 19, 54–56, 62–64, 70, 80, 102, 144, 147, 158, 168,
    171–173, 176–181, 300, 379, 380, 385, 390–391, 395,
    396, 434, 459
Iontophoresis, 313, 431, 433–435
IPP *See* Induratio penis plastica
Isometric contraction, 19, 55

J

Jacobsen flap, 235–242

Index

K

Keloid, 22, 81, 175, 176, 179, 180, 187–190, 193, 353, 356, 361, 364, 385, 403, 412, 413, 419, 421, 422, 442, 459

L

Lateral band release, 244, 246
LD *See* Ledderhose disease
Ledderhose disease (LD), 9, 36, 81, 119, 121, 189, 209, 252, 306, 351, 353, 354, 356, 357, 361, 363–364, 401, 402, 404, 409–425, 429, 443
LF *See* Limited fasciectomy
Limited fasciectomy (LF), 37, 38, 40, 203, 204, 213, 215, 216, 218, 219, 259, 261, 281–287, 290, 323, 338, 373, 374
Linkage analysis, 88, 90, 96
Little finger, 124, 143, 192, 197, 233, 235–242, 263, 330, 335–338, 345, 379, 381
Long-term outcome, 349–368, 384, 409–425
Long-term splinting, 18, 335, 338
Loss of tissue mobility, 15–18, 333, 461

M

Matrix, 55, 61, 69–71, 73, 74, 79, 95, 101–102, 107, 111–112, 131–138, 140, 144, 148, 151, 162, 163, 172, 187–188, 300, 360, 377, 394–398, 433
Matrix metalloproteinases (MMPs), 73–74, 79, 80, 98, 99, 136, 137, 139, 144–148, 300, 394–397
Mechanotransduction, 138–140
Minimal invasive release, 351
Minimally invasive Dupuytren's surgery, 208, 210–211, 260, 334
MMPs *See* Matrix metalloproteinases
Morbus Ledderhose, 353, 361, 401, 422, 445
Muslim, 124–126
Myofibroblast differentiation, 19, 54, 56, 61–65, 152, 161–165, 309, 390, 394, 396–398
Myofibroblasts, 8, 17, 22, 53, 69, 79, 94, 101, 109, 131, 143, 151, 167, 176, 187, 207, 219, 308, 343, 350, 374, 379, 388, 394, 402, 411, 432, 459

N

NA *See* Needle aponeurotomy
NDD *See* Non-Dupuytren's disease
Necrosis, 37, 102, 221–225, 235, 238, 239, 290, 300, 307–308, 405–406, 412, 459
Needle aponeurotomy (NA), 256, 267–279, 289–292, 443–444, 450, 453, 462, 463
Needle fasciotomy, 38, 40, 41, 227, 312, 313, 337, 351, 464
Needle release, 268, 269, 274, 275, 278, 279, 312, 313
Neo-adjuvant, 381, 384, 385
Night-time splinting, 276, 279, 306, 312, 323–331
Nodules, dorsal, 7–9
Non-Dupuytren's disease (NDD), 9–10
Non-malignant disorders, 33, 409, 419
Non-surgical treatment, 27, 33, 40–41, 102, 189, 193, 255–256, 338, 344, 346, 387, 413

Notch signaling, 63, 64
No-tension, 306–310, 313, 314

O

Occupation as risk factor, 45–46, 48, 116
Open palm technique, 38–39, 204, 221, 227–228, 230, 232, 244, 246
Orthotics, 306–314, 404, 411, 413, 417

P

Palmar
    aponeurosis, 3, 9, 11, 12, 14–18, 22, 24–26, 38–39, 45, 81, 177, 197, 199–204, 216, 222, 360, 373, 458
    cutaneous branch, 261–263
    fibromatosis, 11–20
    skin incision, 202, 236, 261
    soft tissue, 12–14, 16, 269, 299
Pathogenesis, 9, 26, 54, 61, 88, 94–96, 98, 107, 115, 131, 133, 151–152, 167–173, 181, 333–334, 350, 360, 361, 421, 429, 430, 445
Pathology, 3–10, 16–17, 22, 26, 53–55, 58, 69–74, 107, 109, 115, 126, 133, 136, 167, 168, 175, 177, 178, 189, 191–193, 202, 228, 229, 240, 256, 261, 292, 305, 308, 343, 350, 360, 361, 380, 385, 394, 396, 398, 456, 459, 463–464
Patient's perspective, 441–446
Pedigrees, 88, 90, 115–122
Percutaneous fasciotomy, 267, 268
Percutaneous needle fasciotomy (PNF), 18, 20, 37, 39–40, 171–173, 256, 281–287, 293–295, 323, 333–338, 344, 443
Perinodular fat, 94, 167–173
Peyronie's disease, 36, 81, 119, 121, 209, 252, 356, 361, 404, 409, 412, 429–435
Plantar aponeurosis, 24, 25, 102, 401
Plantar fascia, 9, 353, 401, 403, 405, 410, 411, 419, 421–422, 458
Plantar fibromatosis, 401–407
Plater, F., 197, 204, 289, 293, 349
PNF *See* Percutaneous needle fasciotomy
Postoperative, 18, 19, 33, 41, 200, 201, 203, 204, 209, 217–218, 221, 223–225, 231–232, 238–241, 250, 252, 260, 269, 273, 283–285, 290, 291, 294, 295, 298, 299, 307–314, 334, 336, 337, 344, 351, 377, 380, 382–384, 387, 391, 393, 464, 467
Postoperative therapy, 36, 229, 305–307, 421–422
Prevalence, 7, 8, 10, 27–34, 89, 93, 115, 116, 123–127, 207–208, 250, 251, 255, 317, 343, 350, 402
Prodrugs, 387–391
Prognostic factors, 204, 359, 363, 364
Proliferation, 9, 10, 17, 22, 25, 26, 48, 98, 102, 107, 112, 152, 158, 161, 165, 178, 180, 203, 219, 351, 352, 360, 361, 364, 387–391, 394, 397, 401, 402, 420–421, 431, 433
Prototype, 449, 453–454
Proximal interphalangeal (PIP) joint, 7, 8, 18, 36, 168, 192, 201, 216, 236–240, 243–247, 252, 267, 297–299, 303, 306, 307, 314, 318, 336, 338, 343, 349, 376, 382, 383, 459, 460, 466, 467
Proximal interphalangeal (PIP) joint release, 232, 244–247

R

Radiation therapy, 351, 404, 413–415, 434
Radiotherapy, 33, 36, 37, 40–41, 188, 193, 349–368, 381, 409–425, 434, 441–445, 450, 452, 453, 464–465
Real-time PCR, 103, 106, 110, 145, 162, 163
Recurrence, 10, 36, 80, 102, 109, 115, 151, 168, 187, 207, 214, 232, 235, 250, 255–260, 268, 273, 276, 281, 289, 294, 317, 346, 373, 379, 387, 393, 442
Relaxin, 80, 377, 393–398
Research, 21, 32–33, 41, 46, 69, 78, 81, 88, 90, 93–94, 112, 116, 173, 188–189, 256, 289, 318, 319, 324–326, 338, 339, 377, 380, 401, 403, 404, 413, 420, 421, 434, 442–445, 449–468
Research database, 449–454
Rho kinase, 54
Risk factor, 36, 46, 48, 90, 98–99, 109, 116, 123, 127, 252, 306, 308, 350, 356, 404, 411, 413, 456, 457

S

Sandwich flap, 106, 177–179
Scar, 5, 54, 58, 65, 69–74, 77–82, 175, 176, 179–181, 187–193, 210, 214, 229, 236, 240, 256, 260, 268, 275, 295, 306–308, 311, 314, 325, 330, 334, 338, 350, 351, 355, 356, 364, 373, 375–377, 393–394, 396, 398, 401–403, 411–413, 417, 419, 421, 429–430, 442, 459, 462
Scar revision, 190–191
Screening of prodrugs, 387–391
Segmental fasciectomy, 18, 38, 208–210, 255–260, 286, 381, 384, 385, 464
Self-reported disability, 317–321
Self-reporting, 260
Serb, 123–126
Severity of contracture, 317–321
Silicone finger bed, 336–339
Skin graft, 39, 151, 190–192, 204, 214, 216, 217, 228, 229, 232, 233, 235, 236, 239–240, 244, 259, 268, 286, 299, 309, 323, 374–377, 405, 411, 421, 452, 464
  over nodule, 94, 167, 168, 172, 228, 259
  shortage, 190–192, 232, 235, 236, 244, 267
α-Smooth muscle actin (α-SMA), 53, 54, 56–58, 62–65, 101–103, 105–107, 147, 156, 208, 388–390, 397
Splint, 198, 199, 201, 209, 216, 217, 229, 240, 246, 276, 294, 308, 310, 311, 313, 324–331, 333–338, 453
Splinting, 18, 36, 41, 80, 81, 203, 204, 209, 244, 276, 279, 299, 301, 306, 307, 311, 312, 314, 318, 323–331, 333–339, 351, 381, 465
Static night splinting, 18, 324, 330, 333–339
Statistical validity, 318, 331
Stem cells, 53, 62, 80, 167, 168, 171, 172, 352
Stress adaptation, 17
Stress fiber, 57
Surgery for Dupuytren's contracture, 124, 195–204, 256, 282, 305–308

Surgical approach, 203, 421
Surgical outcome, 211, 380–381, 385

T

Tamoxifen, 80, 178–179, 181, 379–385, 432, 459
Taqman® low density arrays (TLDA), 145, 146
Technique, 18, 33, 70, 88, 190, 207, 214, 221, 227, 235, 244, 256, 267, 281, 289, 293, 298, 324, 351, 373, 374, 379, 405, 411, 444, 463
Tendon sheath, 5, 6, 11, 12, 14–16, 202, 216, 233, 244, 268, 271, 272, 276, 298, 403, 410
TGF-β *See* Transforming growth factor beta
TIMPs *See* Tissue inhibitors of metallo proteinases
Tissue engineering, 69–74, 374–376
Tissue inhibitors of metallo proteinases (TIMPs), 97, 137, 139, 144, 145, 147, 148, 397
Tissue remodeling, 53–55, 58, 62–63, 458
TLDA *See* Taqman® low density arrays
Transcriptional regulation, 64–65
Transforming growth factor beta (TGF-β), 56–58, 64, 79, 80, 90, 95–97, 101, 102, 106, 109, 138, 151, 152, 162–165, 175–181, 219, 360, 379, 394–397, 421, 459
Translational research, 398
Treatment options, 32, 33, 35–38, 40, 41, 80, 102, 193, 208, 255–256, 289, 323, 338–339, 344, 345, 351, 353, 354, 405, 411, 413, 434, 443–445, 465
Type I collagen, 103, 105–106, 133, 135, 138, 152, 162, 164

V

Vasodilation, 395, 397, 398
Volar plate, 244, 245, 276, 298, 302, 303, 466

W

Wound healing, 22, 38, 39, 41, 69, 70, 78–81, 131, 136, 138, 176, 187–191, 193, 221, 223, 232, 233, 239, 307, 310, 311, 314, 360, 377, 384, 385, 391, 395, 396, 401, 421, 422, 434, 442, 444
W-plasty, 190

X

Xiaflex, *See also* collagenase 346

Y

YV-plasty, 192

Z

Z-plasties, 190, 191, 221, 222, 227, 228, 232, 233, 235, 239, 244, 259–260, 286, 374

Printing: Ten Brink, Meppel, The Netherlands
Binding: Stürtz, Würzburg, Germany